Penguin Reference Books
Medicines: A Guide for Everybody

Professor Parish is a distinguished physician, university teacher and researcher. He
has dedicated himself to encouraging the appropriate and safe use of medicines and
his influence has been world-wide. He is a Doctor of Medicine, Member of the
Royal College of Surgeons, Fellow of the Royal College of General Practitioners
and a Member of the Faculty of Community Medicine of the Royal College of
Physicians.

Peter Parish

Medicines:
A Guide for Everybody

Sixth Edition

Penguin Books

PENGUIN BOOKS

Published by the Penguin Group
27 Wrights Lane, London W8 5TZ, England
Viking Penguin Inc., 40 West 23rd Street, New York, New York 10010, USA
Penguin Books Australia Ltd, Ringwood, Victoria, Australia
Penguin Books Canada Ltd, 2801 John Street, Markham, Ontario, Canada L3R 1B4
Penguin Books (NZ) Ltd, 182–190 Wairau Road, Auckland 10, New Zealand

Penguin Books Ltd, Registered Offices: Harmondsworth, Middlesex, England

First published 1976
Reprinted with revisions 1977
Second edition 1979
Third edition 1980
Fourth edition 1982
Fifth edition 1984
Reprinted with revisions 1987
Sixth edition 1987
Reprinted with revisions 1989

10 9 8 7 6 5 4 3 2 1

Copyright © Peter Parish, 1976, 1977, 1979, 1980, 1982, 1984, 1987, 1989
All rights reserved

Printed and bound in Great Britain by
Cox & Wyman Ltd, Reading, Berks
Photoset in Linotron 202 Times by
Rowland Phototypesetting Ltd
Bury St Edmunds, Suffolk

This book is dedicated to Pat and to our children,
Catherine, Richard and Christopher

Contents

Part Three
Pharmacopoeia

Introduction

Each year the consumption of drugs increases. Few of us would deny the immense relief from pain and suffering which some of these provide but many of us are now beginning to question the appropriateness of their seemingly indiscriminate prescribing by doctors and use by individuals. Their increasing consumption is, inevitably, associated with increasing risks from adverse drug effects, and we ought to ask ourselves whether their production, sales promotion and prescription are always in the interests of the individual who seeks relief from his symptoms.

Unfortunately, these comments apply to both prescription and over-the-counter drug preparations. The intervention of a doctor may not necessarily offer protection for the consumer. It is a sad fact that a high proportion of adverse drug effects caused by prescription drugs could have been predicted and prevented by prescribing doctors. These dangers are increased because poor communication between doctor, pharmacist and patient often leaves the consumer in almost total ignorance of the benefits and risks of any drug preparation he takes.

It is against such a background that I decided to write this book, in order to provide information about drugs to people who have no medical training or knowledge – information which might also interest and benefit doctors, pharmacists, nurses, medical students and others. However, I have written it principally for the lay person, because I see no reason why knowledge which is available to those within the medical profession should not be shared by those outside it.

Many may disagree with me – particularly some of my medical colleagues. Some may argue that by providing information about the risks of drugs I will make the reader unnecessarily anxious; that patients given such information will not comply with their doctor's instructions; that they may, in fact, reject a drug treatment altogether out of fear, and that they may lose some of the real benefits that can accrue from the appropriate use of drugs. They may also argue that such knowledge may make some patients more 'demanding' about their drug treatments; and finally they may argue that patients do not want to know – that the element of faith in the doctor and his treatment forms a 'magical' core to healing which would be lost if the patient were given knowledge about the drugs being prescribed for him.

Let me give my answers to some of these fears. With regard to patients' anxiety being increased by greater knowledge, I would argue that we cannot allow a situation where 'ignorance is bliss' to exist in drug treatment. Firstly, because the risks of inappropriate drug use can be serious and, secondly, because those risks are largely avoidable. With the information provided in this book the reader will become aware that all drug treatments involve balancing benefits with risks and that appropriate use of drugs will lessen the risks and improve the benefits. He should, therefore, be reassured about the benefits of appropriate drug treatment rather than made anxious about the risks. The pharmaceutical industry is continually striving to increase the benefits and decrease the risks of their products. But they cannot be responsible if these are not prescribed and used properly. The appropriate use of drugs, based upon knowledge of their benefits and risks, will not only benefit the consumer but should be in the best interest of doctors, pharmacists, pharmaceutical industry and governments.

As for the argument that knowledge may affect the way the patient complies – recent studies have shown that at least two out of five patients never take their prescribed drugs as directed by their doctors and collections of unused prescribed drugs from householders indicate that a large proportion are never taken. These observations and other studies of patients' use of prescribed drugs demonstrate that a patient is in any case free to take a prescribed drug if and when he thinks fit. Surely, therefore, appreciation of how to obtain maximum benefits for minimum risks from a drug should help him in his decision to take a course of treatment as directed by the doctor.

As for making the patient more demanding – if the patient is to benefit from the use of prescribed drugs, then this can be aided by his participating with the doctor in the decision to use a particular drug treatment. He can only do this if he knows something about drugs. Doctors often complain about the 'ignorance' of their patients, which hinders their understanding of treatment and the carrying out of instructions. Yet at the same time they are reluctant to 'educate' the patient by giving him more information about the drugs which are prescribed for him: I see such knowledge as being of benefit to both patient and doctor because I see it as enabling them to work together towards the most appropriate treatment.

This sharing of knowledge need not alter the patient's respect for his doctor; after all, this is often described by patients in terms which praise his manner, sympathetic approach, understanding and so on, i.e., in terms of the doctor's social attributes as well as his professional attributes. Patients with knowledge should not be seen as posing any threat to doctors. From the patient's perspective, if an individual feels that knowledge about drugs will weaken his faith in his doctor and his treatment then, of course, he does not have to read this book. Nor do those who do not wish to know, or those who think it will make them anxious.

In the area of over-the-counter drugs I hope this book will help those who wish to identify those drugs which will benefit them most. It should also help them to choose, from amongst the thousands of proprietary drug preparations available, those preparations which contain the drugs most suitable for their needs.

I would like to see an increase in self-treatments, including appropriate use of drugs; but without knowledge this is difficult. You will find that in this book I suggest that you discuss the selection of a particular drug preparation with a pharmacist, who because of his professional training has a very great knowledge of drugs.

However, self-treatment is unlikely to improve until the individual has greater knowledge about the structure and function of his body and how it responds to disease, stress and injury. This depends upon the sharing of knowledge between doctors and laymen – I hope this book is a step in that direction.

In its preparation I have been supported and encouraged by three colleagues and friends, Gail Eaton, Gerry Stimson and Barbara Webb. They have been a major influence upon my thinking and I owe them a great debt of gratitude for giving me added perspectives when studying health care. I am also grateful to Bill Williams for his support, Penny Leach for her common-sense advice, Esther Sidwell for her editing, Peter Merry and Paul Spencer for their advice, Anne Booker, Sheila Goodall, Elsie Gratrix, June McCullum and Vickie Littlejohns for their help in preparing the manuscript, and Peter Wright for being such a patient editor.

Minneapolis, 1975   Peter Parish

Introduction to the Second Edition

Each year only a few of the many drug preparations introduced on to the market represent significant pharmacological advances and only time will tell whether the benefits from the use of these drugs will outweigh the risks. The latter depend in a large part upon how appropriately they are used and yet, regretfully, we continue to see the same cycle of use repeated – exaggerated claims, widespread publicity and use, the appearance of adverse effects, and the subsequent and inevitable warnings about the dangers of inappropriate use.

The majority of new drug products represent minor changes in chemical structure, different formulations (tablets, capsules, elixirs), different doses, different durations of action (e.g., sustained release preparations) and combination preparations of different drugs in varying doses. In addition, many branded drug products are withdrawn each year and fashions in the use of certain drug treatments also change, as does the intensity of the sales promotion of different drug products and groups of drugs. Such changes may make a book of this sort appear to outdate rapidly. However, this is not the case since most of the constituent drugs in the various products remain the same and so, usually, do basic principles of drug treatment.

It is against such a background that I have tried to make this second edition as up to date as possible. In a book of this size it is not possible to include all the branded drug products which are available on prescription or over the counter. However, I have discussed most commonly used 'generic' drugs and it should not be difficult for the reader to check the generic name of a drug and to look it up in this book.

In addition to its use by patients, it has been encouraging for me to learn that this book is being used by doctors, nurses, pharmacists and dentists. I hope this sharing of knowledge will encourage the appropriate and safe use of medicines, and that the second edition makes a further contribution to this, my main objective in writing it.

Finally, I wish to thank Felicity Lee for her assistance in preparing this second edition, Alan Buckingham for his meticulous editing, Julie Routledge for preparing the subject index and Lyn Bond for her unfailing encouragement and help.

Cardiff, November 1978   Peter Parish

Introduction to the Fifth Edition

The contents of this fifth edition have been extensively revised and updated and, in particular, Part Three (which contains details of specific medicines) has been considerably expanded to include almost all currently available prescription and non-prescription medicines.

As I mention in the Introduction to the second edition, this book is written against a background of change and fashions in drug treatments, so that it is difficult to keep up to date with trends and innovations. The best advice I can give you, the readers, is that you should always purchase the most recent edition of this book and destroy previous editions. This may sound wasteful but if you consider that a new edition of the *British National Formulary* (BNF) is provided free to each prescribing doctor every six months and a new edition of the *Monthly Index of Medical Specialities* (MIMS) is also provided free every month, you will understand the importance which the Department of Health (which sponsors the BNF) and the pharmaceutical companies (who support MIMS by their advertisements) attach to keeping prescribing doctors up to date. As the consumers of all these medicines you too must keep yourselves as up to date as possible if you are to understand the benefits and risks of available drug treatments. I hope that this fifth revision and subsequent revisions will help you to do this.

The revision and expansion of Part Three has been possible because of the significant assistance given to me by Pat Colleypriest, Felicity Lee and Beth Rimmer and I wish to express my sincere thanks to them. I also wish to thank Lyn Bond, Dorothy Cotton and Lynn Goward for their valuable help in preparing the manuscript, and Jane Stevens for proofreading Part Three.

Cardiff, 1984   Peter Parish

How to Use this Book

To help you assess the benefits and risks of any drug which you may take this book is divided into three parts. Part One should give you sufficient knowledge to understand how a drug works in the body and how it may produce desired and undesired effects. In Part Two drugs used to treat commonly occurring disorders are discussed and each section ends with comments on the drugs suggested. In Part Three the drugs are listed alphabetically; the uses and adverse effects of individual drugs are given, and the precautions which should be observed.

Part One should be read by everyone; Part Two should be used for reference, for information on groups of drugs; Part Three should be used for reference, for information on individual drugs. Having read about a drug in Part Three always read in Part Two about the group of drugs to which it belongs.

There are Several Points to Remember in Using this Book

Remember, although drug treatments of particular disorders are discussed, this book is not about treatments as such but about drugs. I have included most of the commonly used drug groups. Some I have excluded because their use is highly technical, e.g., general anaesthetics and immunosuppressive drugs. Also, discussion of groups of drugs used to treat tropical diseases has been omitted.

Lists of drugs to avoid during **pregnancy** and **breastfeeding** have not been included. This is because they will always be changing as different drugs are added. Also there is a great risk in giving such lists insofar as drugs which are not included might be regarded as absolutely safe.

The general term '**blood disorder**' indicates a disorder of red or white blood cells produced by a drug's effects upon the blood-forming tissues in bone marrow or upon the blood cells themselves.

Certain drugs may enhance the effects of **alcohol**. This can be described in pharmacological terms but for simplicity is referred to as 'increasing' the effects.

Brand names are distinguished from **generic names** by their capital initial letter.

Except in general discussions about groups of drugs, **adverse effects** of individual drugs are not listed in Part Two. Always refer to Part Three to check on these.

Part One
PRINCIPLES OF DRUG USE

1 Basic Principles

Patients often say to me 'Doctor, those tablets that you prescribed for me – they're not *drugs*, are they?' I have to explain that all medicines are drugs and that coffee, tea, cola, cocoa, tobacco and alcohol are also drugs. The patient's anxiety is natural, because the word 'drugs' has become associated with the abuse of mind-active drugs by certain groups of people. This misconception has resulted in a belief that medicines are good and drugs are bad; as one headmaster said to another, 'If I were not on tranquillizers I think I would have finished up on drugs'! What then is a drug? A drug may be defined as any substance which can alter the structure or function of the living organism. Air pollutants, pesticides and vitamins, as well as virtually any chemical, may be regarded as drugs. Therefore, all medicines are drugs but not all drugs are medicines. Those drugs used as medicines have been selected because they possess or are thought to possess useful properties. They are used to relieve physical or mental symptoms, produce an altered state of mind, to treat, prevent or diagnose disease, and to prevent and end pregnancy.

The term drug does not indicate the way that it is used, whether medically or non-medically, legally or illegally, prescribed by a doctor or not. Similarly the term medicine does not refer specifically to a drug in liquid form; medicines can also be given as tablets, capsules, linctuses, inhalations, injections and so on.

Until this century most drugs used in treatment were obtained from plants. Now only a few drugs are obtained from a natural source and most of these are highly purified to remove any unwanted or harmful effects.

The action of a drug is a complex physical and chemical process which may take place locally in certain cells, organs or special tissues; or more generally upon most cells in the body. Some drugs act outside the cell, some on its surface and others within the cells. In most cases we still know very little about how drugs actually act within the body; but we know a good deal about the effects of that action.

The effect of most drugs is to stimulate or to depress certain biochemical or physiological functions within the body. Some, such as the antibiotics, have little effect on the body tissues; they have their effect instead on infecting organisms in those tissues.

The effects of drugs can be used to attack disease in several different ways. The most obvious example is the cure of disease by drugs such as antibiotics, which destroy the invading organisms that were making the patient ill. Drugs whose effects are used in this way are known as antibacterial drugs. At the other end of the spectrum are the drugs whose effects can be used to prevent disease, such as the vaccines. In between these two extremes, there are drugs whose effects can be used to alter actual body processes, in order to change the course of a disease process. They include such drugs as anticoagulants (anti-blood-clotting drugs), which are used, for example, in thrombosis, to lessen blood clotting. There are drugs which can be used to replace elements which the body cannot take in or absorb – such as vitamin B_{12} for the patient with pernicious anaemia – and there are drugs which can be used to give the body what it fails to manufacture for itself – such as thyroid hormone for the patient with an inactive thyroid gland. Finally, of course, there are all the drugs which are given because their effects relieve symptoms, and they include everything from painkillers and tranquillizers to antacids and decongestants.

Any drug produces some undesired effects along with the desired effects for which it was administered. For a drug to be a useful medicine, it must produce more beneficial than harmful effects. If it does not make you better at least it should not make you worse. Unfortunately many people do not recognize adverse drug effects (sometimes called 'toxic effects') in themselves. Drugs are described by their most important useful effect, and it does not occur to the patient that the morphine which he is considering only as a pain reliever, an analgesic, is causing his constipation or his sleepiness or his tight chest. Even doctors appear to be reluctant to consider the possibility that their treatment has made the patient worse; they may try to combat the new troubles with further drugs, thus starting up a new chain of adverse effects.

It must always be remembered that a drug's effects are like shot-gun pellets – some land on target, others do not. We must therefore try to think of a drug in terms of its full spectrum of benefits and risks. This is discussed further in Chapter 2.

Drug effects, both beneficial and harmful, are much affected by the way in which the drug is introduced into the body – the method of administration.

Methods of Administration

There are four routes by which a drug may reach the body. Topical administration means applying the drug to the skin (e.g., ointments) or to the mucous membranes (e.g., vaginal tablets) or up the nose (intranasally).

Inhalation means simply that the drug is breathed into the lungs (e.g., aerosols for asthma, or general anaesthetics). Enteral administration means that the drug is given either by mouth or via the rectum. Parenteral administration means that the drug is injected. An injection may be made directly into a nerve for local effect, as when the dentist deadens a painful tooth, or it may be made into the spinal cord fluid as in spinal anaesthesia. Otherwise, injections are either intravenous – made into a vein; intramuscular – made into a muscle; subcutaneous – made under the skin or intradermal – into the skin.

Some intramuscular injections are now given in prolonged release forms. These are called 'depot' injections; the drug is slowly absorbed from the injection site over a period of hours, days or weeks – e.g., certain insulins, steroids and tranquillizers. These 'depot' injections are not without long-term dangers and the convenience they offer to you or your doctor should not be allowed to mask these – if you are receiving one of these treatments you should carry an appropriate warning card with you.

Injections ensure that the drug reaches a high concentration in the blood very quickly. Intravenous injections may produce almost instantaneous effects, as mainlining drug abusers know. But no injection is without risk or difficulty. The drug has to be soluble; dosage must be very exact and the injection must take place under sterile conditions. Injections are therefore usually reserved for cases where a rapid effect is essential, or the drug is poorly absorbed from the gut or the patient cannot take it by mouth.

The taking of drugs by mouth is the most convenient way. Some drugs may be absorbed from the mouth itself (e.g., glyceryl trinitrate tablets are allowed to dissolve under the tongue for the treatment of angina). Most are swallowed and absorbed from the stomach and intestine. There are some disadvantages to taking drugs by mouth – some drugs may irritate the stomach and produce vomiting; others may be destroyed by the acid in the stomach or by digestive juices. These may need a special coating (called enteric coating) to protect them until they reach the intestine, or they may be administered via the rectum as a suppository.

Absorption

The rate and extent to which a drug reaches the blood-stream (absorption) determines the time between taking the drug and the onset of its action. As we have seen, parenteral routes ensure quick entry into the blood-stream, but absorption into the blood-stream from the gut is very variable. Rates of absorption can vary from person to person and from time to time in the same person. The best-known example is probably the absorption of alcohol. Hot food taken with alcohol delays its absorption. The presence of any food in the stomach also delays absorption to some extent, while alcohol taken when the stomach is empty will 'go to your head' almost immediately.

Rates of absorption are also dependent upon the solubility of the drug and of the other materials (excipients) used in making it into a tablet or capsule. Drugs given in solution are absorbed more quickly than tablets or capsules swallowed whole. Absorption from these depends upon many factors, including size and solubility of particles, chemical form, and various manufacturing processes such as the compression force used to make the tablet. These can all affect the rate at which a tablet breaks up and the particles separate in the gut before dissolving, which is the important step in absorption.

Distribution

Once a drug has been absorbed into the blood-stream, its concentration in the tissue fluids around its target area will determine its effectiveness. This depends on the concentration of the drug in the blood. As we have seen, different routes of administration can give varying initial blood levels – with intravenous routes giving the highest levels quickly; and whatever the route of administration, different formulations of drugs can give different rates of absorption into the blood, with highly soluble drugs being absorbed most quickly. But even when a drug has been put into the body and absorbed into the blood-stream, different types of drug behave differently. Some can pass throughout the whole body, entering or passing through the plasma, the fluid inside as well as outside cells, the spinal fluid and across the placenta into an unborn baby. Other drugs are much more limited in their effects being, for example, 'filtered' by the placenta, or confined to action in the fluid outside cells.

Some drugs are fairly quickly absorbed, and well distributed around the body in the blood-stream, but are quickly and easily excreted. Aspirin, for example, is normally excreted within a few hours, so that for a headache a once-only dose has time to be effective, but continuous treatment for arthritis requires regularly repeated doses.

Other drugs work quite differently, being very slowly excreted by the body because they accumulate in various tissues and form long-acting depots of the drug. At the beginning of treatment it takes several days for the depot of the drug to accumulate, so high starter doses are normally given. Once the depot has built up, only maintenance doses are needed, to keep the level of the drug in the blood-stream adequate.

A few drugs actually bind themselves to the proteins of the blood itself, so that once present in the blood-stream the drug remains there for a long period. Suramin, a drug used to treat sleeping sickness, is so tenacious of the blood proteins that a single dose will protect against the illness for three months or more.

Bones and teeth act as reservoirs for certain drugs. Lead, for example, accumulates in bones, while the antibiotic tetracycline is stored in both bones and teeth. Many unfortunate children have teeth yellowed by this drug, given to them when they were babies or young children, or to their mothers while they were in the womb.

Other specialized organs act as reservoirs for some drugs. For example the anti-malarial drug mepacrine reaches a concentration in the liver many times greater than the concentration in the blood after only a single dose. Even body fat can act as a storage depot of a fat-soluble drug, so that a fat person may store much more of such a drug than a thin person.

Drug Metabolism

Drug metabolism means the alteration of a drug from one chemical structure to another. This transformation within the body usually results in the inactivation of a drug so that it can be eliminated from the body. This may be called drug breakdown or biotransformation. Occasionally a drug is not active until it has been transformed in the body. For example, the drug pivampicillin is more readily absorbed from the gut than ampicillin and converted (hydrolysed) in the tissues and blood to the active antibiotic ampicillin. A drug such as pivampicillin is described as a *pro-drug*. Drug metabolism involves complex chemical and physical processes which usually take place in the liver. Note how your body reacts to drugs; once a drug has been administered, the body's main concern is to try to get rid of it.

Elimination

The concentration of a drug in the tissues rises when the rate of absorption exceeds the rate of elimination. Eventually these rates become equal and thereafter elimination exceeds absorption. The kidneys are the important organ involved in the elimination or excretion of a drug; less important is the bile system, the lungs, sweat and other body secretions. Drugs excreted in the faeces are usually unabsorbed drugs which have been taken by mouth (note how dark your stools are when you take iron tablets) or breakdown products excreted in the bile. Drugs may also be excreted in breast milk and affect the baby. Ninety-five per cent of alcohol is metabolized and the small amount of unchanged alcohol is eliminated in the breath, urine and sweat.

Dosage

There is a relationship between dosage of a drug and its effectiveness. Unfortunately the relationship is a very complex one. Any drug will obviously be ineffective if the dose given is too small to produce effective levels in the blood-stream, or the formulation is such that the drug cannot be absorbed, or with some drugs, the interval between doses is so great that the drug has been eliminated before the next dose starts to be absorbed. The effects of a drug can be increased by increasing the dosage. But by doing this you also increase whatever adverse effects the drug may have (see p. 30). If we enjoy the relaxing effects of a glass of whisky, we cannot make ourselves more pleasurably relaxed by taking twice the quantity. We simply become unpleasantly drunk.

The dose of a drug required to produce a specified level of effect in fifty per cent of individuals is known as the median effective dose. The dose required to produce toxic effects in fifty per cent of individuals is known as the median toxic dose. The ratio of these two is called the therapeutic index and it gives an indication of a drug's safety and the relationship between benefits and risks.

Some drugs do not have one single therapeutic index, but many. The antihistamines are an example: they are useful in allergic disorders, but often cause drowsiness. One therapeutic index for antihistamines might therefore refer to the ratio between their beneficial action in relieving allergic symptoms and their adverse effect of making the patient sleepy. But that same adverse effect of sleepiness becomes the desired effect of the antihistamine when a manufacturer includes it in a preparation marketed to promote sleep. So another therapeutic index is constructed, this time looking at the ratio between the drug's sleep-inducing properties and other adverse effects.

Drug Testing and the Placebo Effect

Therapeutic indices are initially worked out on animals but in the end they have to be applied to the effect of actual drugs given to real patients. As we have already seen, innumerable factors to do with the patient, such as the state of his digestion, his weight, his age and so forth, may alter a drug's effects. To complicate drug testing further the placebo effect operates in all sorts of unpredictable ways in different individuals. The word 'placebo' means 'I shall please'. It is used to describe any effect of a 'treatment' which is not due to the action or effects of the drug, but which occurs as a result of the patient's expectations of that treatment. Usually the effect of such a 'treatment' is good; if you think something will make you feel better it often will. But the placebo effect can operate the other way too: people given dummy tablets in drug trials may complain of side-effects such as headaches, nausea or giddiness.

Most of the medical practice of past centuries was based on placebos; there were very few effective drugs known, and treatment therefore rested on the faith the patient had in his doctor and his 'medicines'. Now many highly effective drugs have been discovered, and their very effectiveness has strengthened the faith which both patients and doctors have in drugs, so that the placebo effect is still as general as ever. It shows itself most clearly in the testing of pain-killers and sedatives. When such drugs are tried against dummy tablets, around four out of ten patients report improvement after taking the inactive tablets. And the effect does not only operate when you are given dummy tablets, it works when real medicine is given too. The more sure you are that the drug (or operation or other procedure) will do you good, the more likely it is to work well for you. *Your faith in the doctor who prescribes for you or the neighbour who suggests a pill or the advertisement which persuades you to buy one over the counter will all have some effect on how effective the drug will be for you.*

Scientific drug testing has to allow for these faith-healing elements as well as all the other factors that influence a drug's effectiveness. In order to allow for them, it is necessary to know as much about them as possible. It is also essential to know as much as possible about the disorder which the drug is intended to cure or ameliorate. Perhaps the first essential is to understand the disorder's 'natural history'. For example, a cold (coryza) lasts for about three to four days if no treatment is given; an effective cold cure would have to shorten this duration of illness.

The selection of a proper sample of patients for the drug trial is important too. They must be representative of the population who are to be offered the new treatment, i.e., their age, sex, social group and many other factors should be considered as well as the disease being treated. The size of the sample of patients must be statistically representative, and the drug dosage must be carefully and realistically chosen.

Once a sample of patients and a drug regimen have been chosen, the drug-testers have to find a way of preventing placebo effects from distorting their results. This is usually done by using what is called a double-blind technique. Identical tablets (or linctuses or injection ampoules) are made up, half containing the drug to be tested and the other half containing either an established drug (against which the new one is to show its worth) or some inert 'dummy' substance. Half the patients are given the true drug, half are given the dummy, and their responses are compared. Or half the patients may start with the real drug and then change to the dummy tablet after a suitable period, the other half of the sample starting with the dummy tablets and changing to the drug. The point, of course, is that neither the patient nor the prescribing doctor knows at any given time whether the 'drug' is real or fake, new or old. In this way the patient's expectations about treatment, and the extent to which he is influenced by his doctor, are kept out of the picture.

The results of the trials are subjected to highly complex statistical analyses. They may take several years from start to finish, and cost the drug companies a great deal of money, with no guarantee that at the end they will find that they have an effective, safe, marketable drug. So it is not surprising that many of the drugs in common use have never been subjected to such trials. Many of them would fail under scientific scrutiny, yet people swear by them. *Because of the placebo effect many of us feel better just because we have consulted a doctor, even before we swallow the first pill. Clearly our own opinions on effective 'cures' are often quite unreliable.*

Unfortunately there are many disorders for which there is no cure. In the absence of a real cure and in the presence of patients many of whom react favourably to *anything* which is done to help them, 'treatments' tend to proliferate. *It is a good rule of thumb that if many treatments are in use for the same disease it is because there is no real treatment known for that disease.* If one treatment had ever been scientifically shown to be effective, it would have displaced all other treatments for that disorder. But people find it very difficult to accept lack of treatment. Even the most unorthodox and expensive treatments will always be glowingly recommended by some patient who preferred any action to none. Hair clinics and skin clinics, for example, perpetuate a range of expensive treatments largely on a basis of 'personal recommendation' from one patient to the next. Similarly non-prescribed drugs, herbs and 'health' foods can be widely and profitably sold even where scientific testing would show them to be totally useless.

It should be obvious, then, from what I have said so far, that testimonials from people about a preparation are not worth the paper they are written on. Even less attention should be paid to preparations sponsored by actors and footballers and so on – they are paid to do it. Similarly, be careful about being taken in by television commercials and newspapers articles dealing with various preparations – the products advertised are nearly always expensive and gimmicky versions of drugs which are available much more cheaply.

2 The Use of Drugs

Drug Regimen

Some drugs are taken occasionally as a single dose – for example, two aspirins for a headache. Others are taken daily as a single dose, such as a sleeping tablet taken each bedtime. A few drugs are prescribed to be taken when necessary such as glyceryl trinitrate taken to relieve the pain of angina, or an antacid taken when indigestion is troublesome. But the majority of prescribed drugs are taken at intervals throughout the day for several days, or even for weeks or years at a time.

Decisions about drug regimen, dosage and the interval between doses, are largely based on two considerations, both of which were discussed in detail in Chapter 1. Firstly the doctor must consider the length of time which this particular drug in this particular dosage takes to reach effective levels in the blood, and how quickly it starts to be eliminated from the body. Secondly he must consider the therapeutic index for the drug. If the index is small, so that the effective level in the blood is rather close to the toxic level, then the dose will have to be very carefully controlled if adverse effects are to be prevented. If the index is large, then there is more leeway and more than adequate doses can be given without much risk of adverse effects which may reduce the number of doses to be taken daily.

Some drugs, for example antibiotics, can only do their work properly if the blood level is kept steady throughout the twenty-four hours. If the patient leaves a ten-hour gap between doses during the night, bacteria have a chance to re-assert themselves so that the drug faces a two steps forward and one back situation. In such cases the doctor will probably prescribe the drug to be taken six hourly rather than four times daily.

Drugs which gradually build up and accumulate in the body are much more difficult to control than drugs which act rapidly and are readily excreted. Sometimes patients who are put on antidepressant drugs do not fully understand that the unpleasant side-effects will appear almost at once but the beneficial ones will be delayed for as much as two weeks. They decide that the drug is making them worse rather than better, and either abandon treatment or fail to stick to the regimen laid down by the doctor. Similarly patients given phenobarbitone for sedation may not realize that even while their regular dosage is producing the desired effect, the drug is accumulating in their bodies, being put in faster than it can be excreted. When such a patient stops taking the pills he will still have phenobarbitone in his body for several days. The breakdown products of a major tranquillizer called chlorpromazine have been detected in the urine of patients many months after their last dose.

Obviously you should follow your doctor's instructions about taking any drug very carefully, and check with him before you alter either the dosage or the interval between doses. The way in which drugs are taken can be important too. Most drugs, as we have seen, are absorbed better if they are taken when the stomach is empty. It makes sense therefore to take them before meals. But some drugs, for example aspirin and anti-rheumatic drugs, may irritate the stomach if it is empty. They are better taken after meals. Most drugs are better absorbed if they are taken in solution, so that soluble aspirin tablets taken in water will be more quickly effective than ordinary aspirin tablets which do not dissolve in water, but many pills and capsules are not soluble and must be swallowed whole with a good drink of water. A few drugs, such as tetracycline, are ineffective if taken with milk.

Many drugs are available in a wide variety of forms. For example, children can be given syrups and sweetened suspensions of drugs.* People who suffer gastric irritation from drugs can often take the same medicine in the form of suppositories or of specially coated tablets which protect the stomach from the drug until it reaches the intestines. Whatever the form of drug you are taking it is important to remember what it actually is. A suppository has just as much effect on the body as does a pill. Some drugs should never be taken together, so that any doctor who is prescribing for you must be told of anything you are already taking – including alcohol – and so must the pharmacist from whom you buy medicines over the counter.

Often a drug will appear to have made you better before you have taken the full course prescribed by the doctor. To stop taking it without consulting him may be harmful. The most usual example is probably antibiotics given to children. The child has tonsillitis and a high temperature; the doctor prescribes an antibiotic to be given for five days, but in two days the temperature is down and the child feels better. The mother stops giving the drug and very probably puts it away in the medicine cupboard for use without consulting the doctor, next time someone has a sore throat. The original patient may have got better because the disorder cured itself, but equally he may have got better because the antibiotic had started its work. In that case the bacteria have been decimated but not destroyed and the

* Many medicines for children have a syrup base and therefore are very harmful to teeth.

illness will reappear in a few days, but this time with the added complication that the bacteria may have become resistant to that antibiotic. At the same time, the bottle of medicine which the mother stored away may have a short shelf-life, such that it becomes useless after ten days; it should not be stored or used on another occasion without the doctor's advice.

Anyone who is prescribed or buys over the counter a drug he does not intend to use immediately should tell the pharmacist. The form in which the drug is dispensed may well affect its shelf-life, and many formulations will only remain effective for a short period of time. An ancient bottle of antibiotic eye drops dredged from the back of a cupboard may well do more harm than good. Active drug ingredients are often mixed with others (called 'excipients' or 'vehicles') to mask their bitter taste, for example, or to give an ointment easy spreading properties or to make it smell nice; these excipients may themselves cause adverse effects.

Interactions between Drugs

A drug interaction is the modification of the effects of one drug by another. Some drug interactions are used intentionally for therapeutic purposes, but most arise from unplanned combinations of drugs. Obviously the more drugs you take the more likely it is that some of them will react adversely with each other. The patient who takes over-the-counter drugs at the same time as prescribed ones, without telling the prescribing doctor what he buys from the pharmacist, may be at risk.

Most doctors are against the use of medicines containing several active drugs because it is impossible to vary the dosage or time schedule of each drug separately and because if adverse effects arise it is difficult to know which drug is responsible for them. For example phenacetin has been widely used for many years as one constituent in minor pain-killers. A few patients who consumed such mixtures daily over a long period developed fatal kidney damage. Phenacetin is now considered to be the culprit, but it would have been indicated sooner had its consumption not been confused with the use of aspirin and caffeine and other ingredients in such combined pain relievers. Do not be impressed by advertisements which stress that products contain more than one active ingredient, and that they are approved by doctors. Several drugs are not necessarily more effective than one, and it would be surprising if such mixtures were not approved by doctors since the drug companies employ doctors to advise them!

If the combined effect of two drugs is greater than the effect of each alone they are said to act synergistically. If the combined effect is less than the sum of the two they are said to be antagonistic. The combined effects of drugs with similar actions are usually referred to as additive. The 'normal' dose of a drug may become an overdose if it is given with another drug with which it interacts. Overdosage may also arise from additive effects. Most of the mind-active drugs, for example, have additive effects with alcohol. The patient who drinks moderately when taking tranquillizers may unexpectedly become very drunk indeed.

Drug interactions may cause adverse effects or simply make a drug ineffective. For example, the antibiotic tetracycline may interact with calcium salts (for instance, in milk) or magnesium salts (as in many indigestion remedies) to form an unabsorbable complex in the stomach. This interferes with the absorption of the antibiotic to a point where it cannot reach effective levels in the blood-stream.

Before embarking on the regular use of several drugs, people should consider the possibility that their need for the second or third drug may in fact be dictated by their consumption of the first. *All too often adverse drug effects arise because patients and doctors try to deal with the ill effects of one drug by taking another.*

Adverse Effects to Drugs

Some experts consider that drugs are now prescribed out of all proportion to the need for them. Collections of unused drugs from patients' houses indicate a tremendous waste of drugs; but they also suggest that multiple drug use is now very common. Furthermore, increasing numbers of drugs are bought over the counter every year, and so the risk of adverse effects from drugs acting with or against each other is increased.

Any unintended reaction from a 'normal' dose of a drug for a particular person with a particular disorder is an adverse effect. Most adverse effects of a drug have usually been observed and recorded; for example, it is known that when a patient starts to take tricyclic antidepressants he may experience blurring of vision, dry mouth, constipation and so forth. These are recognized adverse effects which wear off after one or two weeks.

If any of the processes involved in the body's use of a drug (absorption, distribution, metabolism or elimination) are altered, then a drug may have an excessive effect even when given in a 'normal' dose.

Some people may become allergic to certain drugs, and some suffer hypersensitivity reactions which are idiosyncratic (i.e. peculiar to them). These become additional recognized adverse effects of that drug over time. The commonest allergic effects are skin rashes; there may also be fever, painful joints or a swollen face, or wheezing; occasionally sensitivity of the skin to sunlight may be produced by a drug. Very rarely a patient may drop dead from anaphylactic shock following the injection of a drug to which he has become allergic during previous treatment (death from a second bee sting is an example of this). Other idiosyncratic reactions may cause jaundice (e.g., the drug chlorpromazine).

Some rare adverse effects to drugs can be due to underlying genetic disorders which are not recognized until a drug touches them off. For example, barbiturates can trigger off a first attack of a genetic disease called porphyria, which causes abdominal colic, polyneuritis (nerve damage), mental disturbances and sometimes death. Genetic factors may also influence the effect of a particular drug in a particular patient. The drug isoniazid, which is used in tuberculosis, is used up quickly in most patients. But in a few it is broken down and excreted very slowly, so that such patients run the risk of harmful effects from it. Many people believe that once they have been on a drug for some time without obvious ill effects, the appearance of adverse effects becomes unlikely. Unfortunately this is not true. The ill effects of a drug taken for a long time may be cumulative – as they are in the long-term consumption of phenacetin, which has been shown to lead to kidney damage. Or ill effects may arise spontaneously even when the patient has been on a drug for years. Furthermore certain drugs (e.g., prednisolone) can produce serious adverse effects long after the patient has stopped taking them (see pp. 218–19).

While all drugs are liable to produce some adverse effects, whether these are recognized or idiosyncratic, short-lived or long-term, the effects of single drugs or of drug interactions, some groups of people are especially vulnerable to these effects.

The Use of Drugs in Elderly Patients

'Ageing' may be restricted to certain organs or tissues or may affect the whole body. Such changes may produce ageing before the person is old in years. Whenever its onset, the ageing process can alter the delicate physiochemical processes which are involved in drug action. Ageing does not mean disease, though the older you get the more chance you have of developing a disorder, particularly of the degenerative type (e.g., arthritis). In fact, older people are often found to have multiple disorders such as anaemia, arthritis and diseases of the arteries.

With advancing age, the body burns up energy more slowly, digestion may become affected, the acid in the stomach decreases, the gut wall may lose its muscular power and the emptying of the stomach and movement of the bowels may become less efficient. The circulation may be affected and the function of the liver, kidneys and brain may all be impaired.

Whether or not these actual deteriorations have taken place, the diet of an old person may lack the basic elements which are essential for normal body functioning and for the normal use of drugs by the body. So the elderly patient is at risk whenever he or she is given drugs. Aspirin may cause bleeding from the stomach in anyone; in an elderly person such bleeding may be serious because dietary deficiencies have already led to anaemia. Constipation caused by poor diet and weakened bowel action may become serious if the patient is given codeine. Sleeping pills, sedatives or tranquillizers in 'average' doses may make the elderly person confused and unsteady; a benzodiazepine sleeping drug which would be excreted by most patients within eight hours may 'hang over' the whole of the next day.

Clearly then, fixed 'average' doses and dosage schedules should not be applied to elderly patients. They, even more than the rest of us, need careful tailoring of drug dosages to their particular needs, current health and social circumstances. Sometimes failure to provide this highly personal prescribing leads to tragic results. A patient who has become confused on tranquillizers may be considered senile and admitted to a psycho-geriatric unit, where more drugs are given to control the confusion – a vicious circle which may lead to the patient finishing his days on a hospital bed. The same kind of outcome may follow the prescribing of drugs to lower the blood pressure of elderly patients. The drugs reduce the volume of blood reaching the heart and brain, thus putting the patient at risk and mimicking symptoms of senility in someone who already has an insufficient blood supply to their organs. Another group of drugs called diuretics make the kidneys pass out more water and salt in the urine. This makes the patient empty his bladder more frequently, and, in the elderly patient, this often leads to incontinence. A drug-induced problem may be the final straw to a harassed family.

In order to avoid such tragedies, *the fewest possible drugs should be given to elderly patients, and in the minimum dosage which is effective for them, even if this is far less than the 'average'*.

The Use of Drugs by Pregnant Women

In the early weeks of pregnancy the placenta (or afterbirth) is developing. Until it is fully formed, any drug circulating through the mother's body may enter the embryo. In later months the placenta acts as a barrier, protecting the developing baby from moderate doses of non-fat-soluble drugs. Fat-soluble drugs, and drugs given in high dosage, will continue to cross the barrier throughout pregnancy. Yet the baby's liver is not sufficiently developed to deal with the breakdown of drugs and its kidneys are not sufficiently developed to excrete them – but of course they return to the mother through the umbilical vein for her to break them down and excrete them from her body.

From the moment the female egg is fertilized, complex processes are set in motion. The egg embeds itself in the wall of the uterus (womb); the cells of the fertilized egg start to divide and re-divide; under chemical control they start grouping and organizing themselves. Cells destined to be part of the brain, the liver, the eyes, the kidneys and so on position themselves, and the various organs start to develop. So the whole embryo baby is a group of cells, all dividing and being chemically organized.

In the first chapter of this book we stated that, while we know a good deal about the effects of drugs within the body, we know very little about how those effects are produced; how the drugs actually act on the cells. So we do not know much about how drugs act upon the cells that make up a developing baby either. We really know little more than that some drugs may produce abnormalities (teratogenesis) and that these are more likely when the drug is taken within the twelve weeks after conception. You will not need to be reminded that thalidomide produced abnormalities in some five or six thousand babies. It is particularly sad when it is realized that thalidomide was just another sedative with no particular advantage over other established drugs, and that it was taken for minor symptoms. However, this tragedy led, though at terrible cost to the children involved, to widespread publicity and recognition of the danger by the medical profession and by governments.

Governments and pharmaceutical companies have increased and improved the testing of *new* drugs for possible dangers during pregnancy. But there are thousands of prescribed drugs and over-the-counter drugs on the market which have never been tested. Pregnant women take so many drugs, including tea, coffee, alcohol, cigarettes, aspirin and antacids, that it is very difficult to discover the relationship between any abnormality in the baby and drugs used by the mother in pregnancy. There is some evidence that mothers of abnormal babies tend to have taken more drugs than other mothers, but we do not know whether the abnormality is a direct result of the drug-taking, nor, if it is, whether it is the combinations of drugs or one specific one which causes the trouble. We do not even know whether prolonged drug use in both men and women may lead to some mutant change in the genes and thus cause abnormalities in their children either at birth or later in life.

Only a few drugs are actually known to produce abnormalities. Smoking, for example, puts the unborn baby's life at risk and also leads to smaller babies; tetracycline can affect bone growth and stain teeth; anti-convulsant drugs have been associated with the risk of club foot and of cleft palate. Then there are a few drugs which can damage the baby by affecting its blood supply, such as excessive vitamin A, which affects the placenta. Yet others may damage the baby after it is fully developed; hormones for example may affect sexual development; iodine and anti-thyroid drugs may lead to the baby being born with a thyroid goitre. Finally, of course, the baby may develop an overall reaction and even be born already addicted to narcotics.

What conclusions should we draw from this state of affairs? Without being alarmist *it is probably best to try and avoid taking any non-essential drugs in pregnancy or if you are trying to become pregnant*. If your doctor must prescribe drugs for you, he will choose among those which have been tested and shown to be safe.

Drug Use During Breast Feeding

The taking of some drugs whilst breast feeding may lead to toxic effects in the baby. Some drugs pass through the milk and work directly in the baby's body. Therefore, any drug should be taken with caution by breast-feeding mothers. Some drugs can become concentrated in the mother's milk, e.g., iodine, which can then produce goitre in the baby; some tranquillizers (e.g., diazepam; Valium) can produce lethargy and weight loss in the baby, oral anticoagulants can produce bleeding and there are many other examples. *For many drugs there is insufficient information available, therefore any drug should be taken with caution by breast-feeding mothers. It is always best to consult your doctor or pharmacist.*

The Use of Drugs in Babies and Children

If you have read Chapter 1 of this book you will realize that the way the body deals with drugs is very complex and relies on healthy, mature and functioning organs. You will remember that the liver has to bring about the breakdown (biotransformation) of drugs, so that the kidneys can excrete them. In babies, the liver and kidneys are still immature. Some of the enzyme and other systems involved in drug breakdown and excretion are not fully developed. Ineffectively broken down or incompletely excreted, almost any drug may cause adverse effects.

Babies are also much more sensitive than older people to changes in the salt and water balance in their bodies. Drugs which alter this balance – such as drugs with a diuretic effect, or drugs which cause diarrhoea – may cause serious adverse effects. Equally any drug whose effect is made worse by a change in salt and water balance may have adverse effects in babies.

Infants are growing and developing. Drugs which have few adverse effects in an adult may interfere with growth or development in a baby, or may have adverse effects on the infant's mechanisms for controlling his body temperature or on his new developing muscle control or coordination.

All these factors apply also to toddlers and, to a lesser extent, to children too. Dosage is therefore absolutely critical. Any liquid medicine should be administered via a 5 ml spoon given to you by the pharmacist. If the instructions say '1 teaspoonful' they mean 5 ml. A domestic teaspoon may hold 4 or 7 ml and such inaccuracy could be dangerous. Similarly if any dilution of the medicine is required, this should be carried out by the pharmacist when the drug is dispensed; it should never be left to the mother to estimate the right quantity of a drug with a label saying 'dilute in 5 parts of water'.

On the whole too many drugs are given to babies and children. Mothers have been led to expect a prescription every time they take their child to the doctors and many doctors seem unable to resist prescribing anti-diarrhoeal remedies, cough medicines and antibiotics. Antibiotics in particular are often used inappropriately. The mother says 'Doctor always gives him an antibiotic when he gets these nasty colds.' The very statement is a command. Many of those 'nasty colds' are caused by viruses against which antibiotics are totally ineffective. In such a situation their only possible value is in protecting the child against the possibility that the cold may be followed by a bacterial invasion of the chest, throat or ears. With common colds and other virus infections of the nose and throat secondary infections are the exception rather than the rule. Doctors ought to stop thinking that patients expect drugs at every consultation and try giving reassurance, explanation and sound advice instead. Equally, mothers should not expect a prescription to relieve their child's every symptom.

Drug Use in Kidney Disease

Most drugs are excreted by the kidneys so that any impairment can lead to toxic levels of a drug or one of its breakdown products in the blood-stream. Drugs must therefore be used with *caution* in patients with impaired kidney function, particularly those that are excreted entirely by the kidneys. The dose of the drug must be decreased and/or the interval of time between doses should be increased. (*Note warning on drug use in the elderly.*) Drugs that are known to damage the kidneys should be avoided. For specific drugs refer to Part Two, but *always check with your doctor or pharmacist*.

Drug Use in Liver Disease

Many drugs are broken down in the liver so that severe liver disease may affect the metabolism of a drug and lead to toxic levels of the drug in the blood-stream. The liver is also involved in the manufacture of certain proteins in the blood to which drugs attach themselves. A serious liver disease will reduce the amounts of these proteins in the blood-stream (hypo-albuminaemia), thus allowing less protein for the drugs to attach themselves to and causing a toxic level of 'free' drugs in the blood-stream.

The clotting of blood depends on clotting factors made in the liver – any reduction in these by liver disease will lead to a greater sensitivity to oral anticoagulant drugs such as phenindione and warfarin.

All drugs should be given with caution to patients with liver disease, particularly drugs which depress brain function and drugs which affect fluid and salt balance in the body (e.g., carbenoxolone, corticosteroids).

Some drugs can actually damage the liver. These may be predictable effects and related to the dosage or they may be completely unpredictable and particular to the individual patient, i.e., they are idiosyncratic. You must be aware of the warnings with individual drugs – see Part Two and *always consult your doctor or pharmacist if you suffer from liver disease*.

The Use of Drugs by Drivers

To achieve the high degree of mental and physical skill, coordination and judgement required to drive any motor vehicle safely, a driver must be fully awake, alert, calm and concentrating. Yet every day thousands of motorists drive while under the influence of drugs which are bound to affect their skills to some extent.

The drug most usually indicted after a motor accident is of course alcohol. The mechanisms by which alcohol affects the body are discussed in detail in Chapter 3. Moderate amounts of alcohol impair driving ability to some extent. Often this impairment is not noticed by the driver himself. Because the alcohol has relaxed him and made him less inhibited than usual he may even feel that he is driving particularly well. In high doses alcohol produces disorientation and confusion, blurred vision and poor muscle control. Such a driver is extremely lucky to get home without hurting himself or somebody else. Alcohol is not a suitable drug for drivers under any circumstances.

Unfortunately many of the other drugs which impair driving ability do this to an even greater extent if they are combined with even a very little alcohol. For example, many cough remedies and cold 'cures' contain drugs which affect the nervous system. Because they have been bought over the counter, the patient gives no thought to their possible effects on his driving. On their own they might not impair it seriously, but when he has also had a drink with his friends before driving home from work he may be quite unfit to drive.

Even more dangerous are the many drugs which are prescribed by doctors without any warning to the patient about their possible effects on driving ability. These include many of the most commonly prescribed groups of drugs such as antihistamines, stimulants, sleeping drugs, sedatives, tranquillizers, antidepressants, slimming drugs, drugs used to treat blood pressure, anti-spasmodics, drugs used to treat nausea or vomiting in pregnancy, or motion sickness, and insulin, used to treat diabetes. Obviously it would be impossible to forbid any person taking any of these groups of drugs to drive a car. The effects depend on the person, the situation, the dose. What one can and must do is to point out the possible effects of these drugs on driving skill, and above all the danger of combining them with alcohol and then driving.

The rule is that any drug with an effect (whether intended or not) on the brain or the nervous system is likely to have some effect on driving ability. If a drug prescribed for you makes you feel drowsy, nervous, tense, dizzy, faint, trembly, makes it difficult for you to concentrate or blurs your vision, then you can be sure that your driving skills are impaired. (Of course other skills may also be impaired, particularly those calling for a combination of manual skills, experience and alertness; this may affect those in charge of complex machinery, airline pilots, train drivers, etc.)

The Use of Drugs in Patients with Stoma

Enteric coated and **sustained-release** preparations of drugs should not be used, particularly by patients with ileostomies – they will not have time to release their active drug.

Laxatives, enemas and **bowel wash outs** should not be used by ileostomy patients – they may produce severe dehydration. Bulk-forming laxatives (e.g., bran) are best. Codeine phosphate, loperamide and diphenoxylate may be used to treat diarrhoea.

Antacids containing magnesium salts may produce diarrhoea and those containing aluminium salts produce constipation.

Diuretics should be used with caution because they may easily produce dehydration and loss of potassium. If necessary, a potassium-sparing diuretic should be used (p. 184).

Patients on **digoxin** should be given liquid preparations of potassium because of the dangers of low blood potassium levels in patients receiving digoxin (pp. 157–8).

Morphine and related pain relievers (e.g., codeine, dextropropoxyphene, in **Distalgesic**) may produce troublesome constipation in colectomy patients.

Iron preparations may produce loose motions and may need to be given by intramuscular injections.

Warnings to Patients on Long-term Drug Treatment

Several groups of drugs, discussed in detail in Part Two, may give rise to very serious adverse effects when other drugs are given to the patient, or when he undergoes dental treatment, or requires emergency treatment even for a minor injury at an outpatient department. *The first rule for anyone undergoing long-term drug treatment should be to tell any medical personnel about his drugs*. In most cases warning cards are issued to such patients. If issued they should always be carried. In that way the patient can be sure that the hospital will have the information it needs should he be admitted unconscious after an accident.

1.   Corticosteroids

These drugs, especially prednisolone, are frequently used to treat rheumatoid arthritis, allergic diseases, skin diseases, eye diseases and asthma.

During periods of anxiety, stress or injury, the body requires and produces more corticosteroids. This natural response by the adrenal glands is prevented by treatment with corticosteroids. The patient's body is already living with large amounts of corticosteroids in the blood-stream, so the adrenal glands do not respond by producing extra in times of stress. Patients having such treatment are therefore liable to develop a state of acute adrenal insufficiency if they have an accident, a surgical operation or even an acute infection. Even the stress of an ordinary dental procedure can be enough, in such a patient, to produce faintness, weakness, nausea, vomiting and finally collapse.

If you are on these drugs or have had treatment with them even for only one month in the preceding two years, you should always carry your warning card with you.

2.   Anticoagulants

These drugs lessen the blood's ability to clot. They are most often used to prevent the extension or recurrence of a thrombosis (clot) in a vein or in the chambers of the heart. Patients taking these drugs tend to bleed easily, and bleeding, even from a minor injury, can be difficult to stop. *You should always carry your warning card with you.*

3.   Anti-diabetic Drugs

Any patient on anti-diabetic treatment may experience a drastic fall in blood sugar (hypoglycaemia) with weakness, faintness or even collapse, if he misses out a meal in order to have an anaesthetic. Patients on anti-diabetic tablets must discuss any proposed dental anaesthetic with their dentist and with their doctor. Those who are taking insulin, especially if the total dose is high, should be admitted to hospital if they require dental anaesthesia.

4. Antidepressants

Those antidepressant drugs which belong to the group of monoamine oxidase inhibitors may produce adverse effects when taken with certain other drugs and with certain foods. *Patients on these drugs should be issued with warning cards, and should carry them.* Stimulant drugs, such as the amphetamines, and pain relievers, such as pethidine and morphine, can be highly dangerous to patients on these drugs.

Another group of antidepressants, the cyclic compounds, makes some patients sensitive to adrenaline and similar substances. A local anaesthetic given for dental treatment or for the stitching of a minor injury may make the heart race and send the blood pressure up. Dentists and casualty department doctors should be told if you are on cyclic antidepressants, so that they can give local anaesthesia without adrenaline.

5. Drugs Used to Treat Raised Blood Pressure

Many drugs used to treat raised blood pressure may react with a general anaesthetic to produce a severe drop in blood pressure which can be very dangerous. *If you are taking a drug of this type make sure you have a note on you.*

6. Sedatives and Tranquillizers

These may increase the depressant effects of general anaesthetics upon the brain, particularly the breathing centre. *Make sure you carry a warning card or note with you.*

3 Dependence on Drugs

Everybody has their own picture of what they think a 'drug addict' is like. Yet many people would be hard put to it to define drug addiction in a way which covered all the possible types of person who might be addicted and all the possible types of drug they might be addicted to. Because of these problems of definition and because of the extent to which the term addiction has been misused in popular parlance, most authorities are now in favour of substituting the general term 'drug dependence' and then following it with a description of the type of dependence they mean.

In general, drug dependence can be defined as a psychological and/or physical state which results from the taking of a drug. It is associated with a compulsion to go on taking the drug either because of the 'desired' effects it produces, or because of the ill effects if it is not taken, or both.

Defined in this general way it is clear that most of us are at least psychologically dependent on a great many substances we do not usually talk about as 'drugs'. Many of us feel we cannot start the day without coffee, cannot enjoy a rest without a cup of tea or are deprived if we do not have a much-more-than-adequate meal. And we are psychologically dependent on all kinds of other things in our daily lives too, from sex and sport to television and the newspapers. So psychological dependence is not *necessarily* a bad thing. What we have to decide is whether this dependence is producing problems – mentally, physically or socially – bearing in mind that different people will see different things as problems.

The person who is dependent on drugs may have such a craving for his drug, such a compulsion to go on taking it, that he goes on even when he knows full well that he is causing harm to himself (e.g., smoking).

Physical dependence is a condition in which repeated use of a drug leads to certain symptoms when the drug is stopped. Not all drugs that cause psychological dependence cause physical dependence, but all those that produce physical dependence produce psychological dependence also. The 'withdrawal symptoms' that arise when a drug is taken away from someone physically dependent on it can be extremely severe. Among the most usual are vomiting, convulsions, trembling and confusion. Without the drug, the body goes to pieces. If no help is offered the patient may die. Physical withdrawal symptoms can always be instantly relieved by the administration of a dose of the drug which caused the dependence. In some cases one drug can replace another in this respect. Tranquillizers, for example, can relieve the symptoms of alcohol withdrawal. In instances like these, there is said to be cross-dependence between the two drugs.

Many of the drugs which can cause dependence also cause tolerance in the user. This simply means that the person's body becomes accustomed to a certain intake of the drug so that in order to derive a similar effect from it he has to increase the dose. The double scotch which makes a novice drinker feel pleasantly intoxicated will barely affect the seasoned drinker. Some drugs are capable of producing tremendous tolerance. Constant users of opium and morphine for example can take and tolerate doses which would be fatal to ordinary people.

Just as there can be cross-dependence between drugs so too there can be cross-tolerance. A heavy drinker may need much more sleeping drug to 'knock him out' than a teetotaller.

A wide range of drugs which alter mood can cause drug dependence. But we are still very ignorant about who will become dependent on which drugs under what circumstances. Some drugs are highly likely to cause dependence and some individuals are highly likely to become dependent. On the whole dependence seems most likely to arise when three factors come together; a potential drug of dependence, a 'vulnerable' personality and some adverse aspect of the environment. Whether the risk becomes reality depends on many other complex, socio-psychological factors which affect that individual.

Alcohol

Alcohol is one of the most widely used and misunderstood of drugs. In Western societies it is conventionally taken in social situations, where it is regarded as a stimulant. In fact it is not a stimulant at all but a sedative whose effect, as with so many other drugs, depends on the mood and the social circumstances of the taker. Its apparent stimulant effect arises from its ability to free us from some of the restraints which normally govern our behaviour, relieving anxieties and releasing tensions. At a party such effects tend to give us a feeling of well-being and friendliness. Other people's anecdotes seem funnier and one's own flow freely. Yet the same quantity of alcohol taken alone by an unhappy depressed individual will not lift his mood; it is more likely to remove his controls so that he weeps helplessly. Taken at bedtime such a dose will simply make you sleepy. Taken during a jealous quarrel it may make the drinker extremely aggressive. And even though the party-goer *feels* confident and therefore efficient he is actually much less so than before. His increased sexual desire will not lead to a better sexual performance; his easy flow of conversation will be less perceptive than it is when he is sober and if he goes home and tries to read or to study he will find that his ability to concentrate is impaired.

The effects of alcohol on mood are not the only effects which are misleading. A drink of alcohol opens up the small blood vessels in the skin, so that the skin becomes warm and flushed (vasodilatation) and may cause sweating. The person who has taken alcohol therefore *feels* warmer than before but is, in fact, being cooled as more blood reaches the surface of the skin and therefore the outside air. To drink alcohol to make yourself feel warmer when you come in from the snow may be perfectly sensible, but to drink it in preparation for going out into the cold, or to 'keep you warm' while out, can be dangerous.

Alcohol may give you a warm comfortable feeling inside, and temporarily banish uneasy feelings arising from indigestion or other stomach troubles. But in fact alcohol increases the secretion of gastric acid and may cause irritation and inflammation. It is therefore quite the wrong drug to put into a stomach that is already disturbed. Heavy drinkers often have chronic gastritis; people with peptic ulcers should abstain; and, above all, alcohol should never be taken with aspirin, which is also irritant to the stomach.

The effects of alcohol on the brain and nervous system are proportionate to the *blood alcohol level*. The effects are more marked when the level in the blood is rising than when it is on the way down again. They are also very marked when the level in the blood rises very rapidly because a large amount of alcohol is taken quickly and rapidly absorbed. The drug is absorbed from the stomach, small intestine and colon. Absorption from the stomach is slowed by the presence of food or of milk; it is also slower when the alcohol is taken in large volumes, e.g., as beer, the latter also contains a lot of carbohydrate which slows absorption. Once the alcohol has left the stomach and reached the intestine it is unaffected by the presence or absence of food. This is why patients who have had part of their stomachs removed absorb alcohol very rapidly and may become easily drunk.

Once absorbed into the blood, alcohol is distributed to all the body tissues, including fat; a thin person may experience greater effects from a drink of alcohol than does a fat person. The alcohol is then burned up at the rate of about 10 ml per hour. About 95 per cent of it is broken down in the body, the rest being excreted in the sweat, tears, bile, gastric juice, saliva and the breath. The alcohol excreted in the breath has a fixed relationship to that which is present in the blood. It is therefore possible to estimate the blood alcohol level from the alcohol in expired air, and this is the principle used in breathalyser tests.

Since the body can use and excrete only about 10 ml of pure alcohol per hour (about two teaspoonfuls), you can see that during an evening's continuous drinking the drug is bound to accumulate in the body. Thus much longer than the usual time between refills is needed for the body to get rid of each drink.

In high doses alcohol produces drunkenness, disorientation and confusion, blurred vision, slurred speech, poor muscle control and often nausea and vomiting. As the dose increases breathing becomes depressed; coma follows, and if some of the overdose is not got rid of in vomit, it may be followed by death. Intoxication with alcohol is followed by a 'hangover' which makes you feel sick, weak and dizzy, and gives you aches and pains all over. Even moderate amounts of alcohol, and even a slight hangover, impair driving ability. Alcohol is a factor contributing to a large percentage of road traffic accidents. *Nobody should drive when he has been drinking*.

A great many of us are psychologically dependent on alcohol. We may associate a nightly drink with the end of the working day and the beginning of the evening's relaxation; or we may feel unable to face social occasions without it; or use it to calm us down whenever we must face unusual stress. We use alcohol as a social prop and as a coping mechanism. The use of alcohol so frequently that it impairs health or adversely affects family, employment or other interpersonal relationships on a continuing basis can be termed 'alcoholism'.

Those who do become physically dependent on alcohol have usually passed through a period of many years of extreme psychological dependence and therefore regular daily drinking of increasing quantities. Alcoholism is thus a term used to describe the very wide range of disorders which may result from drinking alcohol. The end results of high alcohol intake and poor diet include alcoholic cirrhosis of the liver* and disorders of the brain. Others are the indirect results of alcoholism, caused by the neglect of personal care, which is common among alcoholics. Malnutrition, and other disorders resulting from it, lead to a high risk of infections and other illnesses. The alcoholic is also liable to mental illness, fits, loss of memory and sexual impotence.

Tolerance to frequent use of alcohol is often interpreted as a sign of *masculinity*. This is exploited by the multi-million-pound promotional machine of the brewing industry, which plays on the conviction that being able to consume large quantities of alcohol without falling down is a sign of 'manliness'. An illogical conviction to say the least. While tolerance to alcohol may include learning to function apparently normally after heavy doses, it does *not* include being able to tolerate a lethal dose of the drug.

---

* In recent years there has been observed an increase of alcoholic cirrhosis of the liver among women and it is being suggested that women develop this disorder more readily than men.

Alcoholics often die of acute alcohol poisoning, although as stated earlier vomiting and coma may prevent the taking of a fatal dose.

The withdrawal of alcohol from a chronic heavy drinker who is physically dependent on the drug may produce nausea, agitation, anxiety, confusion, tremors, sweating, cramps, vomiting, rise in temperature and hallucinations. These withdrawal effects are referred to as *delirium tremens* ('the DTs').

If no help is offered, such as tailing off the use of alcohol gradually, or obviating the worst effects with tranquillizers, the patient may move on into convulsions, coma and death.

In most alcoholics it takes years to produce the degree of physical dependence necessary for these extreme withdrawal effects. But this is at least partly dose-dependent. Physical dependence can take place within a few weeks if the daily dosage is very high.

Alcoholism is often said to 'run in families'. In fact alcoholism itself cannot be inherited. What can be passed on from one generation to the next is whatever psychological genetic factors made the first victim turn to alcohol as a coping mechanism in the first place, together with the stress of living with an alcoholic and the influence of his example.

Cross-tolerance and cross-dependence occur between alcohol, sleeping drugs, sedatives and tranquillizers. A man who tolerates a great deal of alcohol will need a larger dose of a sleeping drug than his teetotal brother. Unfortunately this cross-tolerance does not affect the lethal dose of any of these drugs, it merely narrows the gap between the dose that is effective and the dose that is dangerous. Many deaths from overdosage arise from mixing alcohol with these drugs, and from taking more and more in an attempt to make them effective.

Warning: Whatever drugs you are prescribed or purchase, always check with your pharmacist whether it is advisable or not to drink alcohol whilst taking them.

Tobacco

The main drug in tobacco is nicotine. In addition to nicotine, tobacco smoke contains hundreds of other chemicals as well as appreciable amounts of tar (which many consider to be causative agents in producing cancer) and carbon monoxide gas (which many consider to be a cause of heart disease). Smoking may give pleasure, relieve tension or stimulate according to the personality of the user and the situation in which smoking occurs. Psychological dependence is common, tolerance occurs and physical dependence is possible. In addition, there is an association between cigarette smoking and cancer of the lungs, chronic bronchitis, coronary artery disease, arterial diseases, peptic ulcers, raised blood pressure and adverse effects on the unborn baby (pp. 32–3). One of the greatest advances in this decade in the field of preventive medicine (and surely all health-care services should aim at prevention) has been the discovery of the relationship between cigarette smoking and these diseases. To stop smoking is one of the most important steps you can take to ensure health. Yet, even knowing the risks, people carry on smoking – which shows how severe is the psychological dependence produced by tobacco.

The inhaled smoke from one cigarette may yield as much as 6 to 8 mg of nicotine (cigar smoke, 15 to 40 mg) and from 4 to 38 mg of tar. About 90 per cent of nicotine in inhaled smoke is absorbed into the body compared with about 25 to 50 per cent if it is not inhaled. Because marked tolerance to nicotine develops rapidly once an individual begins to smoke regularly, few people realize that it is one of the most toxic of all drugs. The lethal dose is only 60 mg. There is more than this quantity in one packet of ten cigarettes, even though this amount is not absorbed if the tobacco is smoked. (A toddler who eats a cigarette should be treated as if he had taken tablets from the medicine cabinet.) Non-smokers who regularly sit in smoky environments may run similar but reduced risks to smokers and there is some evidence of increased risk of cancer of the lung among 'non-smoking' relatives of smokers.

In small doses, or in the tolerant individual, nicotine first stimulates and then depresses the functions and endings of certain nerves supplying the gut, heart and circulation. It causes vasoconstriction (closing down) in the tiny blood vessels of the skin; speeds up the pulse and causes a rise in blood pressure and increased bowel activity. It is absorbed from the lungs, the gut and the skin. It breaks down in the liver and is excreted by the kidneys. Traces are also excreted in breast milk (0·5 mg/l in a heavy smoker).

Nicotine poisoning leads to acute nausea, salivation, abdominal pain, vomiting, diarrhoea, sweating, headaches, dizziness, confusion, weakness and disturbances of hearing and vision. Untreated these are followed by a dramatic rise in blood pressure, very rapid pulse, difficulty in breathing and finally death.

Barbiturates, Sedatives and Anti-anxiety Drugs (Benzodiazepines)

Anti-anxiety drugs, sleeping drugs and sedatives (e.g., barbiturates and benzodiazepines) all depress brain function. They are all capable of producing drug dependence although some are much more dangerous than others in this respect.

As with alcohol, there are many patients who are psychologically dependent on such drugs, and some who are physically dependent. Thousands of individuals take two sleeping pills every night and are sure that they would not sleep without them. Deprived of the pills they might feel psychologically disturbed, and would take up to six weeks to sleep properly. At the other extreme there is the true addict who is physically dependent on barbiturates, and takes them by intravenous injection to maximize their effect.

All these drugs produce some degree of tolerance in the individual who takes them regularly. Indeed the way to be sure that a sleeping pill will work for you when you really need it, is to make sure that you do not get into the habit of taking it when you do not really need it. Reliance on such drugs either means that they are not useful when they are needed, or that larger doses must be taken.

Tolerance to the barbiturates is dangerous because while the individual becomes tolerant to the sedative or intoxicant effects he does not become tolerant to the lethal ones. He may need a larger and larger dose to make him sleep, but it does not take a larger and larger dose to kill him.

Cross-tolerance occurs between all these drugs and between any one of them and alcohol. As we saw in the previous section, many fatal overdoses arise from a combination of alcohol drinking and some of these drugs.

The symptoms of intoxication with any of these drugs show themselves most clearly in barbiturate intoxication. There is difficulty in thinking coherently, slurred speech, little concentration. The individual becomes emotional, irritable, suspicious (paranoid); he may also become depressed and suicidal. His gait may be unsteady and his vision blurred. In long-standing dependence there may also be a poor state of general health and nutrition associated with the dependence.

If an individual does become physically dependent on any of these drugs he may suffer from withdrawal symptoms if they are suddenly stopped. These vary markedly in degree, depending upon which drug is responsible, how long the individual has been taking it and in what dosage. But they may include anxiety, restlessness, trembling, weakness, abdominal cramps, vomiting, hallucinations, delirium, fits and even death.

Amphetamines

The amphetamines are discussed on pp. 83–4, dealing with stimulant drugs.

While different doses may produce different effects in different people, many individuals after a moderate dose taken by mouth feel alert, happy, full of energy. In the Second World War these drugs were widely used among the armed forces to combat fatigue. After the war their use spread.

Students, nightshift workers and long-distance drivers found that they could stay awake and alert more easily with their help; athletes used them to increase their performance while doctors prescribed them both to lift the mood of depressed patients and to help would-be-slimmers.

Towards the end of the sixties many young multi-drug-users took to amphetamines and then discovered that their effects could be enormously increased (and distorted) if they were taken intravenously instead of orally. Such amphetamine use was known as a 'speed trip'.

But patients who took amphetamines in this way for 'kicks' sometimes experienced truly disastrous adverse effects. They became paranoid and extremely aggressive; they developed the symptoms of full-blown schizophrenia, together with physical ill effects such as chest and abdominal pains, and fainting. Chronic users developed sores and ulcers, infections, liver damage, high blood pressure and sometimes bleeding into the brain. Users who developed bad effects (bad trips) became known in their own drug-taking subculture as 'speed freaks', and the drug underworld itself turned against amphetamine use with such slogans as 'speed kills'. Not unnaturally public and medical opinion turned against the amphetamines also, and over a period of a very few years there was a drastic reduction both in the non-medical and medical use of these drugs.

Tolerance develops to the amphetamines, to the adverse effects as well as the mood effects. Addicts may use hundreds of milligrams in a day – far above the dose that would kill an ordinary patient.

The type of physical dependence caused by these drugs is not fully understood. Withholding the drug from a chronic user does not produce the florid withdrawal symptoms of, say, alcohol or the barbiturates. Indeed it was claimed for years that the amphetamines produced no physical dependence and were therefore 'non-addictive'. But withdrawal does produce a marked 'let-down' effect, showing itself in extreme fatigue, lengthy sleep, increased appetite, depression and changes in electrical brain traces (electroencephalograph).

Cocaine

Cocaine is obtained from the leaves of the coca plant. It is a stimulant with high potential for abuse. Its effects are similar to those produced by amphetamines. It is known as 'coke', 'snow', 'gold dust', 'bernice', 'lady', 'she', 'Dama Blanca' etc.

The taking of cocaine is surrounded by ritual and socio-recreational influences. Description of its subjective effects is therefore difficult because any drug experience is a complicated interaction between social and cultural influences, individual expectations, the psychological make up of the individual and his responses and idiosyncrasies to the drug. The dose taken can vary significantly between takers and so can the adverse effects which are dependent upon the dose, frequency of dosage and the way it is taken. Also, individual sensitivity to unwanted effects may vary widely – these can include depression, psychological dependence, anxiety and psychoses, all qualitatively similar to the unwanted effects produced by amphetamines.

Cocaine may be taken by mouth (Andean Indians chew coca leaves as a social ritual and as a mild stimulant). It may be *snorted* up the nose where it is rapidly absorbed through the nasal lining to produce stimulation (the individual becomes talkative and full of energy and self-confidence). Snorting produces effects which last for about 20–40 minutes. Repeated snorting (every 20–30 minutes) leads to agitation, suspiciousness and paranoia. Regular use causes the lining membrane of the nose to shrink (cocaine rhinitis or cocaine sniffles). The nose can shrink and occasionally the septum which separates the nostrils can perforate.

Other ways of taking cocaine include smoking and injection into a vein (which produces an immediate amphetamine-like effect, p. 83). Repeated and regular injections of cocaine can led to intense anxiety, severe paranoia and hallucinations – again very similar to amphetamine psychosis.

Psychological dependence to cocaine occurs but whether it produces physical dependence is open to debate. Withdrawal symptoms do not occur if the drug is suddenly stopped but severe depression does occur which is viewed by some as a withdrawal state. The depression is dose related. Death can occur from overdose, causing fits and arrest of breathing. Marked tolerance to cocaine develops, so that users can tolerate high doses. There is no cross-tolerance or cross-dependence with the amphetamines.

The taking of cocaine with alcohol or other depressant drugs (e.g. benzodiazepines) can produce alarming behaviour since cocaine produces excitement and increases the energy whilst alcohol and related drugs produce poor judgement.

Cocaine damps down the appetite, produces disturbed sleep and although initially it may produce sexual arousal and delayed orgasm, its continued use may lead to sexual disinterest. The appeal of cocaine as an aphrodisiac owes more to its socio-cultural status than to its pharmacological effects.

Narcotic Pain Relievers (Opium, Morphine, Heroin etc.)

Morphine and narcotic pain relievers are discussed on pp. 189–91. The term narcotic in this book refers to drugs which are obtained from, or are pharmacologically related to drugs obtained from the opium poppy plant, *Papaver somniferum.*

The use of opium and opiate drugs goes back over thousands and thousands of years. The subjective effects produced by them vary considerably amongst individuals and under different situations. What may produce a warm feeling of peace in one person may produce nausea, drowsiness, lethargy, dizziness and changes in mood in another. They reduce the desire for sex and food and reduce aggression. Some regular users may lead 'normal' lives, for example, doctors or other professionals with comparatively easy access to drugs; others may become social outcasts or steal to get the money to buy drugs on the black market.

Tolerance to the various effects of narcotics develops when the drugs are used frequently so that the addict who seeks a 'kick' or 'high' has continuously to increase the dose in order to achieve the same effects. In this way addicts may tolerate doses far in excess of those which would be tolerated by non-addicts. However, tolerance is not the same for the different effects produced by these drugs; for example, an addict who may tolerate very high doses of morphine may still show the small pupils and constipation which a non-addict would show with a 'normal' dose.

The development of physical dependence on narcotics is related to the size and frequency of dose taken, the length of time over which it is used, the particular drug and the personality of the user. In some individuals, regular use of small doses over even a few days (perhaps following a painful accident) can cause some degree of physical dependence. Others in similar circumstances would not notice when the drug was withdrawn provided that the pain it was given for had eased.

The severity of withdrawal symptoms is therefore closely related to all these factors. A patient who has been taking large doses of codeine for years is unlikely to have physical withdrawal symptoms if he stops. A baby born of a narcotic-dependent mother will be physically dependent himself and may die if his acute withdrawal symptoms are not recognized. The truly physically dependent person whose drugs are withdrawn will experience an overwhelming desire to obtain more. If he is unsuccessful his first withdrawal symptoms will include watery eyes, a running nose, yawning, sweating, restlessness and sleep. Later he will become irritable, develop tremors, sneeze and yawn continuously while nose and eyes run copiously. Later still there will be weakness, depression, nausea, vomiting, diarrhoea, chilliness, sweating, abdominal cramps, pain in the back and legs and kicking movements. At this stage the skin is cold and covered with gooseflesh, giving rise to the name 'cold turkey'. Without treatment these symptoms burn themselves out in seven to ten days. But at any point they can be dramatically reversed by giving a dose of any narcotic, since cross-dependence occurs between them all.

This cross-dependence is the basis for the commonly used and often criticized methadone treatment of heroin and other opiate dependences. There are two elements to the dependence on opiates – the taking of them for the pleasurable 'high' they produce (a craving) and the taking of them to avoid unpleasant withdrawal symptoms, which in itself produces relief and pleasure without a 'high'.

Cannabis

Cannabis is obtained from *Cannabis sativa* (Indian hemp), a herbaceous annual plant which readily grows in a variety of temperate climates. Under the single heading 'cannabis' are a large variety of drug preparations made in different ways from different parts of the plant, and known by different names in various parts of the world.

The crushed leaves, flowers and twigs of the plant are called marihuana, often known as grass, pot, weed, tea, boo or Mary Jane in various parts of the West, or as *bhang* or *ganja* in India, *kif* in Morocco or *dagga* in Africa. Hemp is made only from the flowering tops of the plant. Hashish, known as hash in the West and as *charas* in India, is made from the relatively pure resin of the plants; it is at least five times more potent than the highest quality marihuana.

The use of cannabis in the East for its mood-altering effects goes back over many thousands of years. It spread to the West mainly after the First World War, but was restricted to certain groups of users. It was only in the sixties that its use spread throughout the Western world.

Marihuana is usually smoked in hand-rolled cigarettes (joints, Js, sticks, reefers), but both marihuana and hashish may be smoked by placing small pieces on the tip of a burning cigarette, or through ordinary pipes or water pipes (hookahs). Cannabis smoke is inhaled deeply into the lungs and held there for a while. Effects upon mood start almost immediately, reach a peak in about three quarters of an hour and last for several hours. Cannabis resin may be taken by mouth in tea or other beverages, on pieces of biscuit or on other foods. It is less effective by mouth than when smoked, and the effects produced by smoking may be more carefully controlled. Very little is known about the distribution, breakdown and excretion of cannabis by the body.

Our scientific knowledge of the effects and adverse effects of cannabis is extremely scanty. It is not improved by the highly emotional and biased approach which many writers take to the subject. The difficulties in making objective studies of the effects of cannabis are numerous. The strength of different preparations of the drug may vary widely, and varying quantities of inert 'filler' may be added. The effects on mood obviously vary with the strength, but they also vary with the speed and method of administration, the personality, expectations and previous drug experiences of the user, his mood and the mood and expectations of those around him. A controlled dose, smoked by a particular person at a specified rate in a laboratory, may therefore affect him quite differently from cannabis smoked at home or with friends.

The most frequently described subjective effects of the drug include a dreamy state or one of giggling happiness, feelings of timelessness and of increased awareness, feelings of great insight, free-flowing ideas and feelings of deep inward joy usually known as a 'high'. Frequently described adverse effects include anxiety, impairment of concentration and memory, and unpleasant fantasies.

On the whole desired subjective effects seem to arise most often when the drug is taken in pleasant supportive company by an experienced marihuana smoker. Markedly unpleasant effects have been described by inexperienced smokers who have taken large doses when alone. These include panic, fear of death, peculiar sensations in the limbs, suspiciousness, headaches, nausea, dizziness, confusion, depression, delusions and loss of control. Such extreme reactions are known as 'freak-outs' and are apparently rare.

Cannabis is claimed by some to produce an 'a-motivational syndrome' which is characterized by loss of interest and apathy. It has also been claimed that it produces a loss of brain tissue as seen in the elderly and in chronic alcoholics, that it produces deformity of the unborn baby and increased tendency to miscarriage, and that its L.S.D.-like effects may encourage experimentation with L.S.D. Furthermore some people claim that the drug interferes with the white blood cells and their protective role in virus infections. None of these claims are proven. They all require careful examination and further research.

Cannabis accumulates in the body. Tolerance to its effects is thought to develop and withdrawal in heavy users may produce depression and anxiety, tremor and insomnia. The long-term effects of cannabis on the individual are still undefined, its effects on driving ability have not been clearly stated, and its long-term social effects are still unrecognized.

Cannabis has proved of some use in relieving symptoms of nausea and vomiting in patients receiving treatment with anti-cancer drugs.

L.S.D.

L.S.D. (d-lysergic acid diethylamide) or simply 'acid' produces incredible effects upon the mind with minor effects on the body. It is active in minute doses. It is a semi-synthetic derivative of lysergic acid, an ergot alkaloid produced by a parasitic fungus sometimes found on rye and other grain.

It was in the mid-1940s that interest in its effects upon the mind gained publicity in scientific and medical circles. Because some of its effects seemed to resemble schizophrenia it was called a psychotomimetic (mimicking psychosis) drug and was used by psychiatrists in the vain hope that it would enable them to understand this type of disorder more clearly. However, it was eventually realized that the mind-effects of L.S.D. are different from schizophrenia and it became known as a hallucinogenic or illusinogenic drug – i.e., a hallucination- or illusion-producing drug. Subsequently in the 1950s it was used in psychotherapy and became known by the general term 'psychedelic' – mind-manifesting – a term which rapidly caught on and became applied to music, art and fashion during the early 1960s.

Psychedelic drugs have been used for thousands of years by various cultures in religious ceremonies. In the West, by the 1950s, a few academics and artists started experimenting with them. In the early 1960s the fashion quickly caught on. By the late 1960s governments had introduced legislation which made it a criminal offence to be in possession of L.S.D. It is, however, almost impossible to detect this substance because it is tasteless, odourless, colourless in solution, and can be taken in a minute dose. It can be taken by mouth, sniffed in powdered form or injected in solution. It is quickly absorbed from the gut and distributed around the body; in pregnant women it enters the unborn baby. The physical effects can include dilatation of the pupils, increase in blood pressure, rapid beating of the heart, tremor, nausea, muscle weakness, a rise in body temperature, sweating, headache, flushing of the face, goose pimples, chills, alertness, insomnia, decreased appetite, increased reflexes, and very rarely convulsions.

Like cannabis, the effects of L.S.D. on the mind are unpredictable and depend on many factors such as the personality of the individual, what he expects and has been led to expect from the drug, the place where he takes the drug and whether he is with friends who have had experience of it. The social setting in which the drug is taken may affect the response even more than the size of the dose. Larger doses prolong the duration of a 'trip' but do not seem to alter its nature or intensity.

The experiences felt under L.S.D. are very personal to the taker and may vary from one trip to another. However, there are recognized adverse effects, for example, those known as a 'freak-out', during which the individual experiences panic, fear, hallucinations and depression – symptoms just like an acute mental breakdown. 'Freak-outs' are usually of short duration but may occasionally be prolonged. Other individuals under the influence of the drug may experience fear, illusions, depression, and they may indulge in antisocial behaviour. These are called 'bad trips'. Others may re-live past experiences and undergo severe emotional feelings as past conflicts are brought to the surface. Some may experience periods of 'mad' thoughts. Others may experience increased sensory perception with a 'cross-over' of sensations (synaesthesia), so that sounds may be seen and colours and shapes appear more beautiful. Some may feel joy and peace and a feeling of transcendence of time and space, or feelings of holiness, insight and awareness.

L.S.D. occasionally triggers off a prolonged mental breakdown (psychotic episode) which may last for many months. It is impossible to predict which individual will respond to 'acid' in this way, although some claim that the drug merely triggers off an underlying psychotic predisposition which would have developed anyway. Suicide is rare but accidental deaths whilst on a 'trip' are not. These accidental deaths are thought to occur because of delusions about being able to fly or because the user feels himself to be indestructible. 'Flash-backs' or 'echoes' of experiences under L.S.D. may occur for many months. They are transient but may be disturbing if the original trip was a bad one. Tolerance to the psychedelic effects of L.S.D. develops with repeated use, although this is more related to the interval of time between dosage than to the actual dose. Paradoxically, experienced users may need a smaller dose to produce the same effects. Physical dependence does not occur and psychological dependence is unlikely when use of L.S.D. is very intermittent.

Phencyclidine (Angel Dust)

Phencyclidine hydrochloride (P.C.P. or 'angel dust'), first developed as an anaesthetic, dulls the central nervous system. It produces a schizophrenic psychosis in a person awakening from the anaesthesia or when given in doses insufficient to cause anaesthesia.

P.C.P., usually taken by smoking, inhalation or swallowing, can cause violent behaviour, thought disorders, hallucinations, a feeling of disassociation with the surroundings and temporary paralysis, as well as respiratory and kidney failure, convulsions, raised blood pressure and memory loss. Effects of a single dose can last several hours, a portion of the drug being constantly recycled as it passes through the digestive organs. Chronic users may thus constantly feel some of its effects.

Magic Mushrooms

These comprise several species of psilocybe mushrooms which grow in temperate climates. They contain chemicals related to mescaline and psilocybin which are known hallucinogenic drugs. However, these are present in only small amounts but nonetheless, taken in quantity, they can produce severe hallucinations and deaths have been reported.

Volatile Substances

Inhalation of volatile substances and gases for 'kicks' has been known for many years. They include glues, cements, dry-cleaning fluids, paints, lacquers, sprays, petrol (gasoline), kerosene, various petroleum products, lighter fuel, nail-polish remover, aerosols, nitrous oxide, ether and chloroform used in anaesthetics, and many other products. The general effects produced by these are stimulation, followed by sedation accompanied by floating, distant feelings, timelessness and illusions. Frequently they are also associated with confusion, drunkenness, slurred speech, headache, nausea and vomiting. Finally, the user goes into a stupor and then unconsciousness. Some may develop panic, fear, acute mental breakdown, antisocial behaviour and aggression.

The use of these solvents for 'kicks' may produce ulcers on the nose and mouth, liver damage, kidney damage, blood disorders, gastro-enteritis, loss of appetite, self-neglect and death due to overdosage, inhalation of vomit, damage to lung tissue or heart failure due to a disordered rhythm.

Part Two
DRUGS USED TO TREAT SPECIFIC DISORDERS*

* Products marked with an asterisk have now been taken off the market.

1 Sleeping Drugs and Sedatives

Sleep

Sleep requirements vary from person to person and so 'normal' sleep is what suits you under ordinary everyday circumstances. The amount of sleep you need is as much a part of you as your appetite or your conscience. If your sleep is disturbed for only a night or two, this is usually of no consequence; but if the disturbance persists for two or more weeks then you have a sleep problem and need to take action.

Insomnia really means sleeplessness but nowadays it is used to describe most sleeping difficulties. These include difficulty in getting off to sleep, inability to stay asleep, frequent wakenings, restless sleep – often with nightmares, early morning wakening, and sleep which is not refreshing (you wake up and continue to feel as exhausted as you did when you went to bed).

There are many causes of sleep disturbance – these may be social, physical or mental. Amongst social causes are changes in your environment such as a strange bed or bedroom, changes in temperature, noise, motion, and changes of routine like going on night work. Pain from any cause, irritation of the skin, discomfort from indigestion and muscle cramps are some of the physical causes of disturbed sleep. Emotional disorders are a common cause of persistent insomnia. However, remember that social, physical and mental factors are all interrelated. Problems at work may produce anxiety which may produce insomnia. Persistent noise at night may interfere with sleep which may cause you to worry about lack of sleep, which may then produce tension and irritability resulting in further difficulty in sleeping. The death of a close friend or relative, the loss of a job, failure at work or in an examination may trigger off psychological symptoms, a prominent one of which may be disturbed sleep.

Insomnia must always be regarded as a symptom of some underlying disorder. This is of particular importance in psychological disorders, especially in those patients who feel anxious, tense and/or miserable. In such patients insomnia may be only one of a group of mental or physical symptoms which they may experience. It is, therefore, wrong for doctors to prescribe sleeping drugs as the only form of treatment in these patients.

Drugs may even cause insomnia. For example, caffeine in tea, coffee and cocoa may keep you awake, particularly as you get older. Regular alcohol drinkers may find themselves waking early and people who take heroin or morphine may find their sleep impaired. Amphetamines, most slimming drugs, and some antidepressant drugs may keep you awake. So may some drugs used to treat nasal catarrh, colds and asthma.

We really know very little about sleep and its function. It may be related to various anatomical structures in the brain and to certain chemical changes. It produces electrical changes in the brain, eyes and muscles. These can be measured by electrical tracings of muscles (electromyograph, E.M.G.), eye movements (electro-oculograph, E.O.G.) and brain waves (electroencephalograph, E.E.G.). From these tests two main kinds of 'normal' sleep activity have been defined: a stage of non-rapid eye movements (N.R.E.M. sleep) which is followed by a stage of rapid eye movements (R.E.M. sleep). N.R.E.M. sleep is called orthodox sleep and is the stage when we 'think'; R.E.M. sleep is called paradoxical sleep and is the stage when we 'dream'. It seems that both stages of sleep are essential for health.

Breaking the Sleeping Drug Habit

Tests have shown us that sleeping drugs disrupt normal sleeping patterns. All sleeping drugs suppress paradoxical sleep but when these drugs are stopped paradoxical sleep increases. As paradoxical sleep is associated with dreaming withdrawal of sleeping drugs (even after a few nights) may result in restless sleep with dreaming and nightmares. These withdrawal effects make the individual think that he is unable to sleep without sleeping drugs, not realizing that the drug's effects have produced the disturbed sleep.

If you have been taking sleeping drugs nightly for weeks, months or years and wish to stop them you must reduce the dose very slowly over several weeks and therefore it is better to consult your doctor, who will be able to give you a small-dose preparation to help you do this. A gradual reduction in dosage over several weeks may enable you to break a long-lasting sleeping-drug habit. Even so you are bound to have restless nights until your brain gets used to sleep without drugs – this may take from one to two months.

Sleeping Drugs and Sedatives (Hypnosedatives)

Drugs in this group depress brain function; in small doses they are used as sedatives (to calm you down) and in larger doses as hypnotics (to send you to sleep).

All are habit forming so that you can quickly become psychologically dependent upon them. The restless sleep which results when you stop these drugs also strengthens your psychological dependence. This is further complicated by the observation that four in ten patients sleep well on dummy sleeping tablets so that in addition to the drug's chemical effects upon the body there appears to be something in the nightly ritual of taking sleeping tablets.

Like alcohol, they cause intoxication if taken regularly in a dosage above that normally recommended. Further, elderly and debilitated patients and patients with impaired heart, kidney or liver function may develop intoxication at 'normal' dosage. Signs of intoxication are similar to those of alcohol – confusion, difficulty in speaking, unsteadiness on the feet, poor memory, faulty judgement, irritability, over-emotion, hostility, suspiciousness and suicidal tendencies.

Physical dependence (see p. 40) may occur with resultant withdrawal symptoms when the drug is suddenly stopped. These include anxiety, trembling, weakness, dizziness, nausea, vomiting, convulsions, delirium and sometimes death. Psychological dependence is common. Tolerance may develop to these drugs. This means that you will get less effect from the same dose over time and therefore there is always the danger that you may increase the dose in order to obtain the same effects. With the barbiturates there may also be an increased breakdown in the liver, producing a decreased sleeping time and an increase in the average dose required to maintain sleep so that you start to wake earlier. Nevertheless, it is surprising how many patients stay on these drugs for years and years without increasing the dose. Even so, tolerance is a danger and if you find yourself having to increase the dose of your sedative or hypnotic to get the same effect then consult your doctor – you are in danger of becoming addicted.

If you drink alcohol regularly you ought not to take these drugs regularly. This is because alcohol is also a depressant of the brain and tolerance may develop to alcohol. It is quite easy to take an overdose of either and the combination may be fatal. Do not forget, therefore, that although you may be able to tolerate an increased dose of alcohol or hypnosedative the lethal dose of these drugs remains unaltered so that their combination can rapidly prove fatal. Another important point to remember is that hypnosedative drugs can actually make you anxious, irritable and depressed. Since your doctor probably put you on these drugs in the first place in order to control such symptoms you or he may be tempted to increase the dose in order to control these symptoms further. Yet the increased dose will actually make you worse. This also applies to alcohol, so remember if you are getting anxious and miserable despite taking more alcohol and/or sleeping drugs or sedatives it is the drugs that are having this effect. Not a few people have become trapped on this downward course which may end in suicide.

The deliberate taking of an overdose with suicidal intent accounts for most cases of overdose, but accidentally self-administered overdose is not uncommon as a result of what is called 'drug automatism'. If you take a dose of sleeping drug and fail to fall asleep you may reach out and take another dose. The effects of this increased dose may make you confused and you may take further doses without knowing (or remembering subsequently). Therefore, never keep sleeping drugs by your bedside, keep them locked in a drug cupboard in the bathroom or kitchen. Only take the recommended dose and leave the bottle in the locked cupboard. If you are responsible for, or live with, someone who is elderly, debilitated or depressed, and on sleeping drugs, then supervise their administration.

Do not forget that if you are tense or miserable, alcohol and hypnosedative drugs, although calming you at first, may eventually make you feel worse. You may sleep all right and awake feeling less tense, only to become tired, irritable and bad-tempered later in the day. One more important point to remember about these drugs (especially alcohol) is that they may reduce the effects of antidepressant drugs.

Hypnosedatives impair learned behaviour and interfere with your power to concentrate, therefore watch your driving. They may increase pain perception and if given along with pain relievers they are useful but if taken alone they may cause restlessness and confusion in the presence of pain. These drugs depress a wide range of functions in many vital organs, particularly nerves, muscles, respiration, and the heart and circulation. They may produce any state from mild sedation to confusion and unconsciousness. Like alcohol they may produce different effects according to the situation in which they are taken. At a discotheque they may produce excitement, whilst if taken on retiring to bed they may produce sleep. The combination of a strange environment (e.g., admission to a hospital ward) and a dose of hypnosedative may make elderly patients very confused and disorientated. This is a warning against the habit of giving patients sleeping drugs as a routine just because they are in hospital; although very convenient for the night staff it is often not necessary and may lead to the development of the sleeping-drug habit when the patient returns home. Also, there is some evidence that drug-induced sleep may interfere with the normal restorative functions of sleep. Hypnosedatives must be used with special caution in patients with chest and heart disorders.

Do not forget that sleep produced by drugs is *not* natural. Remember also that most sleep studies have been concerned only with brief periods of drug administration in 'normal' subjects. The effects of long-term use of drugs in patients with impaired sleep rhythm are not known.

It may be appropriate to take sleeping drugs for a night or two during periods of stress (e.g., after a bereavement) or after periods of intense work when you just cannot relax, or intermittently through long periods of stress or when travelling overnight or working shifts. In such circumstances they should only be taken for a few nights in a row, because it is accepted that the sleeping-drug habit is a real risk after several weeks of drug-induced sleep. If you have a persistent sleep problem then you ought to consult your doctor. But, of course, he does little good if he gives a quick consultation and a prescription for sleeping drugs with instructions to get more from his receptionist when you need them. Do not forget that emotional problems are a common cause of sleep disturbance and these may produce many symptoms in addition to insomnia; for example, frequent headaches, feeling anxious or tense, sad, depressed or tearful, backaches, pains in the chest, indigestion, dizziness, no energy, feeling fed up, feeling irritable, fears about your health or about going out by yourself, loss of appetite, loss of interest in sex, loss of weight, palpitations, feelings of guilt, feeling not wanted or feeling that other people are talking about you. These are only some of the group of symptoms which should help your doctor diagnose a psychological disorder and organize appropriate treatment.

If you have a psychological disorder, the use of hypnosedatives may aggravate your condition, especially if you are feeling sad or miserable. It is important to recognize what are labelled as 'depressive symptoms'. These include characteristic sleep disturbances, and anti-depressant drugs may be effective in relieving them (see p. 73). This again highlights the importance of the initial treatment of insomnia. You and your doctor need to consider together as many as possible of the factors which may be causing your insomnia.

What about those patients who have developed the habit of taking sleeping drugs every night? They are often elderly and many of them are widows. There may be no harm in letting them continue, provided they are not depressed, anxious or tense, and do not drink alcohol regularly; and provided they do not increase the dose, show signs of intoxication or have impaired kidney, heart or liver function. They may come to little harm even if they are psychologically dependent. I think it would be wrong to give them guilt feelings about being on drugs but it may be advisable to change them slowly on to a drug such as **temazepam** and then gradually try to wean them off it. Perhaps in the future, with more careful understanding of insomnia, the long-term use of sleeping drugs may decrease.

In the treatment of insomnia there are many alternatives to sleeping drugs, such as a hot bath before retiring, reading a book, taking a walk, not having too large an evening meal, cutting down on coffee, tea or cocoa in the evening, reducing smoking, reducing alcohol intake, trying to get some regular exercise and fresh air during the day and probably most important of all – being taught how to relax. The ritual just before going to bed may condition you to go to sleep – undressing, washing, etc. A milk-cereal drink may help you sleep more peacefully. A warm drink and a biscuit often helps the older patient to get off to sleep and, of course, patients with pain, discomfort and irritation of the skin need more specific treatment, as do those with other physical or psychological symptoms.

Sleeping Drugs and Sedatives (Hypnosedatives)

Benzodiazepines

chlormezanone (Trancopal)
flunitrazepam (Rohypnol)
flurazepam (Dalmane, Paxane)
loprazolam (Dormonoct)
lormetazepam
nitrazepam (Mogadon, Nitrados, Noctesed, Remnos, Somnite, Surem, Unisomnia)
temazepam (Normison)
triazolam (Halcion)

Other hypnosedatives

chloral hydrate (Noctec)
chlormethiazole (Heminevrin)
dichloralphenazone (Welldorm)
methyprylone (Noludar)
triclofos sodium

Antihistamines

promethazine (Phenergan)

Barbiturates

amylobarbitone (Amytal)
amylobarbitone sodium (Sodium Amytal) with quinalbarbitone (Tuinal)
butobarbitone (Soneryl)
cyclobarbitone calcium (Phanodorm)
heptabarbitone (Medomin)
phenobarbitone
quinalbarbitone sodium (Seconal Sodium)

Benzodiazepines

Benzodiazepines used as sleeping drugs should have a short duration of action (e.g., **triazolam**, **temazepam** and **lormetazepam**) and be given in *reduced* doses to elderly patients. This is because the long acting ones may give rise to hangover effects and because they accumulate in the body. The benzodiazepines are discussed on pp. 65–6.

Other hypnosedatives

Bromide was widely prescribed as potassium bromide during the last half of the nineteenth century and many patients developed bromide intoxication. Psychiatric wards often contained patients suffering from impaired memory, drowsiness, delirium, trembling and slurred speech, and from hallucinations and skin rashes caused by bromide intoxication. Bromide, if taken daily, accumulates to reach a toxic level over several weeks – it should not be used.

Paraldehyde was used as a hypnotic injection. It makes the breath smell because a proportion of it is excreted unchanged in the breath.

Chloral hydrate is the oldest sleeping drug. It tastes horrible and irritates the stomach. It has less effect on paradoxical sleep than the barbiturates but may cause excitement and delirium if given to a patient in pain. Acute poisoning may occur from a mixture of alcohol and chloral hydrate – known as a Mickey Finn.

Trichlorethanol is the active breakdown product of chloral hydrate and a stable form of this is available as **triclofos**. Another preparation with effects similar to chloral hydrate is **dichloralphenazone (Welldorm)** – a complex of chloral hydrate and phenazone. **Methyprylone (Noludar)** has no particular advantage over the others. **Chlormethiazole (Heminevrin)** may bring on depression in patients with manic-depressive illness. It has a short half-life and may be useful in elderly patients who easily suffer from hangover effects with longer acting drugs.

Remember: All sleeping drugs and sedatives depress brain function and they may produce tolerance and addiction, increase the effects of alcohol, interfere with ability to drive motor vehicles and operate moving machinery, and produce intoxication like alcohol.

Antihistamine Drugs

Antihistamine drugs, e.g., **promethazine (Phenergan)** produce drowsiness as a side-effect and this is sometimes used to promote sleep. Antihistamines which produce sedation are useful for promoting sleep in patients with skin irritations and in patients who may be kept awake by allergic symptoms.

There are dangers in using antihistamines to promote sleep because sleep cannot be improved just by increasing the dose. Rather, the reverse happens and after a large dose, excitation occurs which may result in restlessness and agitation. Note that the use of an antihistamine in children, in normally recommended doses, may actually produce excitement, and it would be dangerous to increase the dose.

Some anticholinergic drugs (e.g., **scopolamine**) which act on the brain (see p. 94) are also promoted as sedatives, and so are some major tranquillizers.

Barbiturates

Barbiturates produce tolerance, psychological dependence, physical dependence and withdrawal symptoms (see p. 40), they increase the action of alcohol and they were a common agent in accidental or intentional overdose. The signs of intoxication are similar to those produced by alcohol. They are involved in complex chemical processes in the liver which may affect the effectiveness of other drugs. In patients suffering from a disease called porphyria (a rare congenital metabolic disease) they can trigger off an acute attack resulting in abdominal colic, paralysis, confusion and even death.

Barbiturates and their salts should not be used as daytime sedatives or to relieve anxiety; nor should they be used to produce sleep. Their use in combination preparations with other drugs is not recommended, e.g. in combination with an antacid, pain reliever, anti-asthma drug or with an anti-angina drug.

Warning: Any drug which depresses brain function may produce addiction and problems when the drug is stopped. Benzodiazepines are no exception.

2 Drugs Used to Treat Anxiety

Diazepam (Valium) and related drugs are the drugs principally used to treat anxiety. They belong to a group of drugs known as the benzodiazepines. They were discovered in 1933 but it was not until 1960 that **chlordiazepoxide** was shown to produce 'taming' in wild animals. This taming effect was then shown to work on monkeys and, because of this, clinical trials were carried out in man which demonstrated its anti-anxiety effects. They are referred to as anti-anxiety drugs, anxiolytics, anxiolytic-sedatives, minor tranquillizers, tranquillizers or 'tranks'.

The benzodiazepines have four main properties – sedative, anti-anxiety, muscle relaxant and anti-convulsant.

Benzodiazepines Used to Treat Anxiety

alprazolam (Xanax)
bromazepam (Lexotan)
chlordiazepoxide (Librium, Tropium)
chlormezanone (Trancopal)
clobazam (Frisium)
clorazepate dipotassium (Tranxene)
diazepam (Alupram, Atensine, Diazemuls, Evacalm, Solis, Stesolid,
    Tensium, Valium)
ketazolam (Anxon)
lorazepam (Almazine, Ativan)
medazepam (Nobrium)
oxazepam (Oxanid)
prazepam

Depending on the dose benzodiazepines will calm you down but they *impair* brain function and in larger doses they send you to sleep – they are 'downers'. Common adverse effects produced by benzodiazepines include drowsiness, light-headedness, sedation, lack of coordination and difficulty in walking (ataxia). These effects may occur after a single dose as well as after repeated doses and they may persist into the following day. They may particularly affect the elderly, who may also become confused and their memory may be affected. Elderly patients may also develop incontinence or they may develop difficulties in passing urine. Other adverse effects are rare and include vertigo, headaches, stomach upsets, skin rashes, blurred vision and double vision, changes of libido, slurred speech, blood disorders and jaundice.

Warnings

Benzodiazepines should not be used in *pregnancy* because there is no convincing evidence of their safety in pregnancy. The use of high doses or prolonged use of low doses in the last three months of pregnancy or during labour has been reported to produce irregularities of the foetal heart and low temperature (hypothermia), floppy limbs (hypotonia) and poor sucking in newborn babies.

They should not be taken by breast-feeding mothers because drugs such as Valium have been shown to enter the breast milk.

The dose of benzodiazepines should be reduced in patients with long-standing kidney or liver disease and in patients with severe, long-standing chest diseases such as chronic bronchitis and emphysema.

They can reduce ability to carry out skilled tasks so that they can affect ability to drive motor vehicles and operate moving machinery. They can increase the effects of alcohol.

Benzodiazepines should be used with great caution in elderly patients because of the risks, particularly of confusion, lack of coordination and difficulty in walking and incontinence of urine. Elderly patients should be given no more than half the normal recommended daily dose for adults.

These drugs can produce opposite effects (paradoxical effects) in some people. Instead of acting as 'downers', they act as 'uppers' and the patients become excited, aggressive and confused. Underlying depression may be triggered off and the patient might become suicidal.

They can increase the effects of other drugs which depress brain function (e.g., sleeping drugs, antidepressants, pain relievers and anaesthetics). These effects when given with other drugs can be dangerous in elderly patients. They can increase the risks of using some anti-convulsant drugs, e.g., hydantoins and barbiturates (see p. 118).

Addiction to Benzodiazepines

The benzodiazepines are 'downers', they calm you down (sedation) and send you to sleep (hypnosis). Because of their effects on the brain they produce addiction in some people if taken regularly every day for four to six weeks. Addiction means that you cannot manage without them because if you stop them you get *withdrawal symptoms*.

Withdrawal Symptoms

If you stop taking benzodiazepines suddenly you develop severe anxiety, tension and panic attacks, poor concentration, difficulty in sleeping, nausea, trembling, palpitations, sweating, and pains and stiffness in your face, head and neck. You become very aware of sensations in your body, very aware of light and you can experience strange feelings of movement. You can feel depersonalized (outside of yourself) and unreal (as if you are in a dream). In severe cases you can have fits, become confused and have a mental breakdown with delusions and hallucinations. You can even get the d.t.'s (delirium tremens) – see alcohol p. 41.

These withdrawal symptoms occur two to three days after stopping short-acting benzodiazepines, e.g., **oxazepam (Oxanid)** and **lorazepam (Almazine, Ativan)**. With the others, which are longer acting, withdrawal symptoms occur in about seven days after stopping them. Withdrawal symptoms usually last from one to three weeks but can go on for months.

In mild cases, symptoms of withdrawal can be like the original anxiety symptoms and lead the doctor to continue the treatment or even increase the dose! However, do not forget that your anxiety symptoms can return, which means you need help but certainly not by regular daily use of 'downers' over months and years.

Note: You can become addicted to benzodiazepines if you take them regularly every day for as short a period of time as four to six weeks.

Long-term Harmful Effects of the Benzodiazepines on the Brain

These drugs can affect your ability to perform skilled tasks (psychomotor function) and can affect your memory. There is a possibility that their long-term use may produce effects on your brain like chronic alcoholism (p. 41).

Benzodiazepines should be taken in as low a dose as possible, as infrequently as possible and for the shortest duration of time possible. Intermittent use (e.g., for one or two weeks during a severe attack of anxiety and then several weeks without them) is better than continued use and may prevent you becoming addicted. But do not forget you should try to do *without* them as soon as is possible.

Miscellaneous Drugs Used to Treat Anxiety

Barbiturates

Before the introduction of the benzodiazepines millions of tablets and capsules of barbiturates were prescribed by doctors. Unfortunately, these drugs are much more dangerous than benzodiazepines and produced many cases of intoxication and addiction. They are very dangerous in overdosage and have produced many deaths particularly when taken with alcohol. (Note that benzodiazepines are much safer when an overdose is taken.) *Barbiturates should not be used to treat anxiety*.

Meprobamate (Equanil, Meprate, Tenavoid)

This drug is less effective than the benzodiazepines. It carries a higher risk of drug addiction and is more dangerous in overdose. It produces more adverse effects and has no benefit over the benzodiazepines.

Major Tranquillizers

Low doses of drugs used to treat serious mental illness are sometimes used to treat anxiety. These drugs, usually referred to as anti-psychotic drugs, neuroleptics or major tranquillizers are discussed on pp. 69–71.

(Note that patients with serious mental illness can develop severe anxiety which is also treated with these drugs, see p. 72).

Betareceptor Blocking Drugs (e.g., oxprenolol: Trasicor; Slow-Trasicor; propranolol: Berkolol; Inderal LA; Half-Inderal LA)

These drugs, which are discussed in detail on p. 152, are useful for relieving symptoms such as palpitations, sweating, nervous stomach symptoms and tremor which may be associated with anxiety.

Buspirone

Buspirone (Buspar) is a new anti-anxiety drug not related to the benzodiazepines but we need much more information about its benefit and risks over time.

Flumazenil

Flumazenil (Anexate) is a benzodiazepine antagonist (see part III).

3 Drugs Used to Treat Psychoses and Related Disorders

These drugs are used to treat serious psychological disorders such as schizophrenia and mania (often labelled psychoses). They are also used to treat acute confusional states, dementia, behaviour disorders and personality disorders. They are often called **anti-psychotic drugs** or **major tranquillizers**. They may also produce a state of emotional quietness and indifference called neurolepsy and they may therefore be called **neuroleptics**. In addition they may be prescribed (in small doses) for the treatment of anxiety, tension and agitation and some of them are used to treat dizziness, nausea and vomiting.

Drugs Used to Treat Psychoses and Related Disorders

Phenothiazines

chlorpromazine (Chloractil, Largactil)
fluphenazine (Moditen)
methotrimeprazine (Nozinan, Veractil)
pericyazine (Neulactil)
perphenazine (Fentazin)
prochlorperazine (Buccastem, Stemetil, Vertigon)
promazine (Sparine)
sulpiride (Dolmatil)
thioridazine (Melleril)
trifluoperazine (Stelazine)

Butrophenones

benperidol (Anquil)
droperidol (Droleptan)
haloperidol (Dozic, Fortunan, Haldol, Serenace)
trifluperidol (Triperidol)

Diphenybutylpiperidines

fluspirilene (Redeptin)
pimozide (Orap)

Thioxanthenes

chlorprothixene (Taractan)
flupenthixol (Depixol)
zuclopenthixol (Clopixol)

Others

oxypertine (Integrin)

Depot injections

flupenthixol decanoate (Depixol and Depixol-Conc.)
fluphenazine decanoate (Modecate and Modecate Concentrate)
fluphenazine enanthate (Moditen Enanthate)
fluspirilene (Redeptin)
haloperidol decanoate (Haldol Decanoate)
pipothiazine palmitate (Piportil Depot)
zuclopenthixol decanoate (Clopixol and Clopixol-Conc.)

The **phenothiazines** are the most widely used. There are between twenty and thirty products available – about half of them are used to treat psychological disorders and to treat nausea, vomiting and dizziness. Others have antihistamine properties, some relieve itching and some are used to treat disorders of movement (e.g., chorea, tics, hiccups).

These compounds are very similar in their effects and uses and therefore the first to be discovered (and still one of the most useful) will be discussed. **Chlorpromazine** was developed in 1951 following the accidental discovery of 'tranquillizing' properties in certain antihistamines to which chlorpromazine is chemically related. It produces considerable sedation, but this differs from that produced by the barbiturates because the patient on chlorpromazine may be easily roused. It impairs the ability of animals to make a conditioned response (e.g., a response to a learned signal such as an electric buzzer) but not an unconditioned response (e.g., escape). Sustained attention is impaired by chlorpromazine and it diminishes spontaneous aggressive activity so that wild animals may be tamed. It produces changes in all parts of the nervous system. It may cause involuntary movements such as tremor, dystonias and Parkinsonism with long-term use. By causing dilatation of the blood vessels in the skin and by acting on control centres in the brain it may cause the body to cool (hypothermia), affect the heart and lower the blood pressure. These effects can be dangerous in old people. It may increase the effects of all depressant drugs – alcohol, hypnotics, sedatives and anaesthetics.

Chlorpromazine controls over-active and manic patients without impairing consciousness. It relieves many symptoms of schizophrenia and modifies behaviour (makes the patient more socially compliant). It calms agitation and is useful in the treatment of drug- or disease-induced vomiting but is of no value in treating motion sickness. It has also many severe adverse effects (see Part Three).

Other drugs used to treat psychoses differ in the amount of sedation they produce; in their effects upon the blood pressure; and in the production of adverse effects such as Parkinsonism and movement disorders.* **Thioridazine** produces strong atropine-like effects (see p. 94) and in high doses may cause pigmentation of the retina and impaired vision. **Fluphenazine** has some stimulant effects and is especially likely to cause movement disorders which may be crippling and permanent. The use of these drugs depends upon balancing the benefits with the risks. The choice of drug depends upon the degree of sedation required and consideration of the wide variation in response which may be expected between patients, particularly to adverse effects. The anti-psychotic drugs therefore differ in the predominance of the effects they produce and in their adverse effects. Parkinsonism adverse effects may be suppressed by atropine-like drugs (p. 94), but they make tardive dyskinesia worse.

These drugs, which consist of several chemically related compounds, are valuable in the treatment of serious psychological disorders and have enabled patients to be treated in the community rather than being locked away in psychiatric hospitals. They are not curative but they do relieve distressing symptoms such as thought disturbances, paranoid symptoms, hallucinations, delusions, loss of self-care, social withdrawal, anxiety and agitation. Patients may need to take a daily maintenance dose for many years because it has been observed that failure to take a regular dose may lead to relapse, necessitating referral to hospital.

A high proportion of those patients who have been labelled schizophrenic can stop using the drugs after a year or two without relapse. It is therefore important that they are seen regularly by a psychiatrist; particularly when it is realized that relapse may take from two to eight weeks after stopping the drugs.

---

* These include dystonias (abnormal face and body movements), akathisia (restlessness), tardive dyskinesia (involuntary movements of jaws, tongue, face, lips and limbs).

The Treatment of Non-psychotic Disorders

Some phenothiazines and related drugs, are marketed in small-dose preparations for the relief of anxiety. Many regard this as taking a sledgehammer to crack a nut. Most anxieties do not respond well to these drugs since they reduce drive and energy. They may be useful to relieve anxiety and agitation in the early stages of treating depression; in relieving free-floating anxiety (anxiety coming on without apparent cause) in some patients; and to relieve confusion and agitation in elderly patients.

Some of them are also used to relieve nausea and vomiting and millions of tablets are prescribed every year to treat dizziness and vertigo. They have been used in the treatment of alcohol and drug dependence, but it must be remembered that most of them increase the tendency to convulsions and so their use in the treatment of withdrawal symptoms (which often include convulsions) is not recommended. Toxic confusional states resulting from infections or metabolic disorders are sometimes helped by phenothiazines, as are certain dementias. They may also be of use in disturbed mentally subnormal patients and in patients with involuntary movements. Their use to increase the effects of pain relievers in patients dying of cancer is being re-examined, although they are useful in preventing nausea and vomiting associated with the use of some morphine-like drugs. Their use in restraining over-active children and captive groups of individuals (e.g., prisoners, inmates in psychiatric or geriatric hospitals) requires investigation.

4 Antidepressant Drugs

Depression

Antidepressant drugs are prescribed to patients who are 'labelled' by their doctors as suffering from 'depression' But what is depression? We can all feel sad or happy and some of us at times may feel very happy or very sad. These feelings are part of everyday life so why do doctors talk about depression and why do some patients need drugs? Why can't they 'just pull themselves together'? The fact is that many patients who go to their doctors for help have got sick of trying to pull themselves together. They may complain of various mental and/or physical symptoms and not feel or recognize they are suffering from a psychological disorder. Unfortunately some doctors may not recognize a psychological disorder, and patients may be subjected to all kinds of investigations and physical treatments, particularly if they get referred to a hospital outpatients' department.

Of course it is impossible to separate social, physical and mental factors, but it is possible to recognize a group of symptoms which, for want of a better label, the pharmaceutical industry and doctors now call 'depression'. Admittedly there is a continuum from feeling blue to feeling severely depressed and suicidal, and from feeling tired and fed up to possessing symptoms which totally interfere with your capacity to cope with your everyday life. If you feel sad and miserable for long periods then this is not just 'feeling blue'. Doctors would call it 'depression'. There can be many reasons for depression: social factors – for example, unemployment or bereavement; physical factors – after virus infections such as influenza, because of continuous pain, irritation or discomfort, after surgery or a heart attack; and following certain kinds of drug treatment – for instance, reserpine given for raised blood pressure, and certain sulphonamide drugs. You may feel severely depressed after childbirth, during the menopause, just before a period or if you have vitamin deficiencies. But you may also be severely depressed for no obvious reason.

Some depressive episodes are labelled endogenous, i.e., doctors think it comes from inside so that the patient gets depressed for no obvious reason.

Other depressive episodes may be labelled reactive: this means there appears to be an obvious cause, such as a bereavement of a friend or relative or loss of a job. However, let me state quite clearly that these are labels. Let me repeat that you cannot separate the social from the mental from the physical, but, as we shall see later, because of antidepressant drugs doctors are now able to relieve painful physical and mental symptoms and enable patients to cope with their everyday problems of living. But this is not without its hazards – it is all too easy to tell the patient he is depressed and give him a prescription for an antidepressant drug.

Along with feelings of depression (sad, miserable, weepy, suicidal) patients may develop changes in behaviour. They may stop wanting to mix socially and start staying at home in the evenings. They may develop physiological changes such as alterations in sleep rhythm (particularly difficulty in getting off to sleep or early morning wakening), alteration in appetite, weight or sex drive, and loss of energy. They may develop physical symptoms; for example, headaches, dizziness, chest pains, palpitations, dyspepsia, diarrhoea and backache. These symptoms may make them worry about physical disease so that they become hypochondriacal and think they have a cancer, or heart disease or tuberculosis. They may develop mental symptoms and feel unreal, divorced from themselves, as if they are looking from outside at themselves; they may have difficulty in concentrating; in thinking; their memory may be affected and they may keep thinking morbid thoughts about death, dying and suicide. They may become very tense and anxious (as if something dreadful is going to happen all the time). Some develop fears (e.g., fear of seeing people; fear of going out). They may become very agitated and irritable or very withdrawn and quiet. Some become obsessive, having to do things over and over again, and some feel guilty. They may recall all sorts of things from their past lives.

This has been a very sketchy description of what doctors label as depression. Patients may experience a few or many of these symptoms. Some symptoms may be mild and some intense, and according to all sorts of factors in his upbringing, his culture, his personality and his environment, the patient will react in different ways. Certainly in Western society the puritan ethic of 'being firm and standing on one's own two feet' may produce awful feelings of guilt and unworthiness in which suicide appears to be the only way out. The whole problem is far too complex to be simply labelled 'depression'. Some patients may need individual or group psychotherapy, others may respond to counselling or to drugs, some just want a new house and a cheque for £50,000, others want a new husband or wife, all need to be taught how to relax.

The Use of Drugs to Treat Depression

The antidepressant drugs introduced since 1958 have greatly improved the treatment of some psychological disorders in some patients. This has resulted in an impressive relief from suffering in these patients and their relatives, a reduction in hospitalization and in electroconvulsive treatments, and an increasing involvement of family doctors in the treatment of disorders of this kind. We must remember that they do not 'cure', but they provide relief from distressing symptoms until such time as the underlying 'disorder' resolves itself – which happens in the vast majority of patients. Doctors prescribe these drugs because within a few weeks of treatment crippling symptoms may be relieved and the patient is able to cope – he may start to sleep better, his energy and appetite return, his interests return, his mood lifts and he may begin to see how dreadful he has felt for months or years. He may then begin to sort himself out. Here is the crunch for the doctor; having relieved the patient's symptoms he must not forget to treat the patient. The duration of treatment may be short or long and may need the help of a clinical psychologist or psychotherapist or psychiatrist; however, because the patient's symptoms are relieved he may respond that much better to such therapy. This does not mean that all depressed patients need drugs – the decision to use antidepressants should only be taken after careful consideration of all the facts by the doctor. They are used far too frequently without adequate reason.

Some of us can tolerate physical pain better than others and some of us can tolerate mental pain better than others – but at some stage we all may need help. Some of us may respond better to one drug and not to another or to one doctor and not another. Some will respond to individual therapy and others to group therapy. We all vary and it is, therefore, wrong to say that all depressed patients should receive drug therapy and it is equally wrong to say they should all have psychotherapy. What is certain, however, is that doctors within the limits of their present knowledge must aim at giving maximum benefit with minimum risks to the maximum number of patients. At present, the responsible and rational use of drugs appears to offer the most hope in this direction.

Antidepressant Drugs

There are two main groups of antidepressant drugs:
 (1) **monoamine oxidase inhibitors** (M.A.O. inhibitors);
 (2) the **tricyclic** and **other cyclic** compounds.
Before the introduction of these two drug groups, amphetamines were the principal and most popular drug treatment for depression. But because

they produce an initial lift in mood followed by a drop (let-down) and because they became widely abused drugs of dependence, they should not be used.

1. The Monoamine Oxidase Inhibitors

These are a mixed group of drugs that share the ability to block the breakdown (by the enzyme monoamine oxidase) of naturally occurring chemicals (amines) in the body. These amines (e.g., adrenaline, noradrenaline, 5 hydroxytryptamine and dopamine) are chemicals produced in response to emotion, fear and exercise and they have an effect upon mood – if they are high we may feel 'high'; if they are low we may feel 'low'.

The M.A.O. inhibitors block many other enzymes in addition to monoamine oxidase and produce numerous other effects apparently unrelated to their enzyme activity. They raise mood and lower blood pressure (some have been used to treat blood pressure). Their action also affects the way the body deals with a whole range of drugs – such as barbiturates, alcohol, analgesics (e.g., pethidine), anticholinergic drugs, particularly those used to treat Parkinsonism, and antidepressant drugs, especially imipramine and clomipramine – and chemicals in foods. The breakdown of these products is blocked and their concentration in the body increases. The M.A.O. inhibitors are probably present in the body for only a short time; but they produce long-lasting effects by irreversibly inactivating enzymes and it may take several weeks before these enzymes regenerate.

The adverse effects of M.A.O. inhibitors are greater and more serious than those of any other drug used in the treatment of psychological disorders. The risk of liver damage with currently used M.A.O. inhibitors, **iproniazid, isocarboxazid (Marplan), phenelzine (Nardil)** and **tranylcypromine (Parnate)**, is low. But these drugs may cause excessive stimulation of the brain, causing trembling, insomnia, sweating, agitation, hallucinations, confusion and convulsions. A fall in blood pressure is usual and dizziness, headaches, delayed or inhibited ejaculation, difficulty in passing urine, weakness, fatigue, dry mouth, water retention (oedema) and skin rashes may occur.

Interaction with other drugs may produce serious effects. What is called a hypertensive crisis may occur when certain drugs or foods are taken with M.A.O. inhibitors. This is caused by a sudden increase in blood pressure which may cause severe headache, bleeding into the brain, heart failure and death. The foods which may produce this interaction all contain amines such as tyramine which may affect the blood pressure. The M.A.O. inhibitors prevent the breakdown of tyramine in the liver and allow it to work at the nerve endings, releasing a chemical (noradrenaline) which sends up the blood pressure. Tyramine is present in cheese and various other foods. Patients taking M.A.O. inhibitors should always carry a warning card with them which lists the prohibited foods and drugs – see under **phenelzine**.

2. Tricyclic and Other Cyclic Compounds

These antidepressants share a basic chemical structure which consists of two, three or four benzene rings. They include:

amitriptyline (Domical, Elavil, Lentizol, Tryptizol)
butriptyline (Evadyne)
clomipramine (Anafranil, Anafranil S R)
desipramine (Pertofran)
dothiepin (Prothiaden)
doxepin (Sinequan)
imipramine (Praminil, Tofranil)
iprindole (Prondol)
lofepramine (Gamanil)
maprotiline (Ludiomil)
mianserin (Bolvidon, Norval)
nortriptyline (Allegron, Aventyl)
protriptyline (Concordin)
trazodone (Molipaxin)
trimipramine (Surmontil)
viloxazine (Vivalan)

The antidepressant properties of the parent drug (**imipramine: Praminil, Tofranil**) of the tricyclic group were discovered in 1958. **Mianserin (Bolvidon, Norval)** and **maprotiline (Ludiomil)** are examples of **tetracyclic** (four rings) antidepressant drugs. They produce effects similar to those produced by imipramine.

These drugs, although they lift mood, do not produce the same kind of lift as pep pills. In fact imipramine, one of the more stimulating tricyclics, produces fatigue, dry mouth, blurred vision, palpitations and retention of urine in 'normal' people. Continued use leads to an increase of these symptoms along with difficulty in concentrating and thinking. Some of them, such as amitriptyline and trimipramine produce a marked drowsiness. The tricyclics and cyclics are extremely useful drugs for treating depressive symptoms and lack the abuse potential of the amphetamines.

The manner in which they relieve the symptoms of depression is not understood but it is thought that they may produce an increased quantity of stimulating chemicals (amines produced by the body) at nerve endings by blocking the re-uptake of these stimulants. They do not produce a 'high' even though there are reports of imipramine producing manic excitement in some patients. They produce atropine-like adverse effects such as dryness of the mouth, constipation and difficulty in passing urine. Because these drugs may affect the eyes they should be given with utmost caution to patients with glaucoma. Similarly, their effect upon the bladder makes caution necessary when using them in patients who have an enlarged prostate gland, since the patient may develop retention of urine. Some of the drugs may affect sexual function. They may produce rapid beating of the heart, palpitations and a fall in blood pressure. Furthermore, they may produce changes on the electrocardiograph (heart tracings) and therefore they should be used with caution in patients with heart disorders.

Tolerance develops to some of the adverse effects (dry mouth, blurred vision, etc.) and within one or two weeks patients notice these symptoms less and less. At the same time their mental and physical symptoms start to disappear and they begin to feel better as each day goes by. This knowledge is important to anyone prescribing or taking antidepressant drugs because with some of them their beneficial effects are slow to develop (up to two or five weeks from starting) whereas adverse effects come on straight away. It is during these first few weeks of treatment, when adverse effects dominate the desired effects, that patients need much reassurance from the doctor and from those around them.

The tricyclics are useful because they offer a choice of drug to treat different depressive symptoms. For example, imipramine, which is re-latively non-sedating, stimulates and is therefore used to treat depressed patients who are slow and withdrawn (melancholic). Amitriptyline and trimipramine have a more pronounced sedative effect and are therefore useful for treating depressed patients who are tense, anxious or irritable. Amitriptyline and trimipramine are particularly useful for patients with sleep disorders, since the whole daily dose may be given at night and help to improve sleep. The other cyclic antidepressant drugs come somewhere between imipramine and trimipramine in their sedative properties; some sedate and some stimulate, some have reduced adverse effects but also reduced desired effects. For example, some newer ones appear to have sedative properties, to work more quickly and to produce few adverse effects, but often at the expense of reduced antidepressant effects. Some of them are safer in overdose.

Precautions When Using Antidepressant Drugs

Monoamine oxidase inhibitors should not be given to children under twelve years of age, to patients with a history of liver disease, to patients with heart failure, or to patients who have had a thrombosis or haemorrhage in the brain. They should not be given to patients with epilepsy or with a disorder of the adrenal glands which may cause episodes of high blood pressure (phaeochromocytoma). Patients should always be warned about diet and issued with a warning card. During treatment and for two weeks after stopping an M.A.O. inhibitor patients should not be given pethidine, amphetamines, ephedrine or tricyclic drugs like imipramine. The M.A.O. inhibitors increase the effects of antihistamines, barbiturates and drugs taken by mouth to treat diabetes. They may also interact with alcohol, opiates, cocaine and procaine, anaesthetics, reserpine, antihistamines, diuretics, levodopa, caffeine, various drugs in over-the-counter cough medicines and cold remedies and slimming drugs.

Tricyclic and other cyclic antidepressant drugs should be used with caution in patients with heart disease, glaucoma, in patients with overworking of their thyroid glands, or who are on thyroid drug treatment, in patients with epilepsy, or in patients with enlargement of their prostate gland. They should preferably not be given within two weeks of stopping M.A.O. inhibitor drugs. Alcohol and barbiturates may decrease their effectiveness. Patients should preferably not take barbiturates when being treated with antidepressant drugs and patients who drink regularly should be encouraged to reduce their daily intake of alcohol. Local anaesthetic solutions containing adrenaline should be given with care. Tricyclic drugs may reduce the effectiveness of some anti-blood-pressure drugs such as **guanethidine (Ismelin)**, and **clonidine (Catapres)**.

The **cyclic antidepressants** are the drugs of first choice for any depressive disorder. The selection of a particular drug depends upon the degree of sedation required. If you drive a motor vehicle or operate moving machinery then the dose of sedative tricyclic needs watching and you may need a few days off work. Instead of taking the drug in divided doses throughout the day a larger dose may be taken about one hour before going to bed. Desired sedative effects, stimulant effects and adverse effects must be balanced to obtain maximum benefit. The M.A.O. inhibitors are now used by a minority of psychiatrists and very rarely by family doctors.

Some antidepressant drugs may be stopped after six weeks to six months of treatment or a daily maintenance dose may be needed for much longer. Some patients may need to take a course of drugs intermittently (e.g., for cyclical depression).

There appears to be little dependence to antidepressant drugs in common use and rather than a desire to increase dosage, patients on antidepressants seem to do the opposite and themselves want to bring down the daily dose to its minimal effective level.

Other Antidepressant Drugs

Flupenthixol (Fluanxol) is useful in patients who are withdrawn and apathetic. **Fluvoxamine (Faverin)** is not related to the cyclic antidepressants. It depresses appetite and may be of use in treating depressed patients who overeat.

Tryptophan (Optimax, Pacitron) is an essential amino acid in the diet. On its own, combined with pyridoxine (vitamin B_6) or with another antidepressant, it has been shown to improve depression in some people.

Combined Antidepressant Preparations

Anti-psychotic drugs such as a phenothiazine or an anti-anxiety drug (e.g., a benzodiazepine) combined with an antidepressant drug in the same preparation are not recommended. This is because the dose of each constituent drug cannot be adjusted separately to the individual patient's needs and furthermore most patients require additional anti-anxiety treatment only in the first few weeks of their antidepressant treatment or intermittently in small doses during the course of their treatment.

Lithium Salts

Lithium salts (Camcolit, Liskonum, Litarex, Phasal, Priadel) are used to prevent and treat manic-depressive episodes. Lithium competes with sodium salts in the body and changes the composition of the body fluids. It is accumulative and adverse effects are related to dosage. When these appear the drug must be *stopped* immediately. Lithium should only be given under hospital supervision and weekly blood tests to estimate the plasma level should be carried out. When the dosage is stabilized these can be reduced to once every two to four weeks. Read the entry on lithium in Part Three.

5 Stimulant Drugs – Tea, Coffee, Cocoa and Cola

Coffee contains the drug **caffeine**, plus certain oils; tea contains caffeine, theobromine and tannin; cola contains caffeine, and cocoa contains caffeine, theobromine and tannin. Caffeine is also present in numerous over-the-counter tonics, 'pick-me-ups', and pain relievers. The drugs caffeine, theophylline and theobromine are usually referred to as xanthines because of their chemical structure. They produce stimulation of the nervous system, make the kidneys produce more urine, stimulate heart muscle, relax the muscles of the bronchial tubes and affect the blood pressure and circulation. Caffeine is used as a stimulant and theophylline in the treatment of bronchial spasm (e.g., asthma).

The xanthines also possess other properties which affect the heart and circulation; they increase the blood supply to the heart, dilate blood vessels in the skin, and constrict blood vessels which supply the brain. Theobromine produces less of these effects than caffeine or theophylline.

Caffeine

The use of caffeine (e.g., a strong cup of tea or coffee) to wake you up or to help you after a hangover is well founded. Caffeine stimulates the brain and all parts of the central nervous system. It stops you feeling tired and makes you think clearly. It lessens fatigue and increases muscular power to do physical work. After a dose of caffeine typists are said to type faster and with fewer mistakes. The dose of caffeine to produce stimulation varies from 100–300 mg. The final caffeine content of a cup of tea or coffee varies according to how strong a person likes his drink. The average caffeine content in a cup of tea is 50–100 mg, in coffee 100–200 mg and in cocoa 50–200 mg per cup. An average-sized bottle of a cola drink contains 35–55 mg of caffeine.

The effects of caffeine vary from person to person but a dose of 1,000 mg or over will produce adverse effects such as difficulty in sleeping, restlessness, excitement, trembling, rapid beating of the heart with extra beats, increased breathing, desire to pass water, ringing in the ears and flashes of light in front of the eyes. Caffeine increases the production of acid in the stomach and therefore patients with indigestion or stomach ulcers should restrict the amount of tea, coffee, cola or cocoa that they drink. They should preferably drink their tea or coffee with meals and add milk to the drinks. The oils in coffee may cause irritation of the gut and the tannin in tea may produce constipation.

Psychological dependence and tolerance to caffeine obviously develop and it must be accepted that the majority of us are dependent upon our daily supply of tea and/or coffee, cocoa or cola.

Warning: Coffee is a complex compound which contains many organic chemicals including not only caffeine, but tars, acids and other compounds produced during roasting and processing. Too much coffee (e.g., more than ten cups of coffee per day) can produce symptoms like anxiety neurosis – recurrent headaches, irritability, palpitations and stomach upsets. Both regular and decaffeinated coffee stimulates gastric acid secretion more than caffeine alone, therefore anyone with a peptic ulcer should avoid coffee whether decaffeinated or not. Abrupt withdrawal of coffee may be associated with headaches and other nervous symptoms which are relieved by taking coffee. The association between coffee drinking and coronary artery disease remains unproven, as does the association between coffee drinking and certain types of cancer. High coffee intake during pregnancy should be avoided and also in patients with raised blood pressure or heart disease.

6 Stimulant Drugs – Amphetamines

The term stimulant generally refers to a drug which stimulates the brain, producing increased activity and alertness. **Amphetamines** form the principal group of drugs used. Other drugs which are used by doctors to produce mental stimulation include **pemoline (Ronyl*, Volital)** and **prolintane (Villescon)**.

Amphetamines

The **amphetamines** are synthetic compounds. In many ways they produce actions and effects similar to the body's own stimulant, adrenaline. This is produced, for example, by fear, emotion or physical exertion. It lifts you up ready for what has been called fight or flight. It makes you 'high'. The amphetamines include amphetamine (previously marketed as Benzedrine), dexamphetamine (dextroamphetamine, **Dexedrine**), and methylamphetamine (previously marketed as Methedrine and Metamsustac).

Amphetamines were previously used to treat depression, as tonics, to treat over-active children and bed-wetters, and to treat patients who kept falling asleep (narcolepsy); they were also used to treat alcoholism and drug dependence. Psychiatrists even used them to get patients to talk. In addition doctors issued millions of prescriptions each year to people in order to help them lose weight.

The effects produced by amphetamines vary with dose and the rate of administration. Children respond differently from adults; in fact, as stated earlier, amphetamines have been used to calm over-active children. In moderate dosage they increase heart rate, blood pressure and blood sugar. The pupils dilate, respiration increases and the appetite decreases.

The effects on mood vary tremendously between individuals and are influenced by many factors in the environment and in the personality. In some individuals there is increased wakefulness and alertness. They become more active physically and mentally, and fatigue is delayed; thinking gets clearer and they become more responsive and aware of their surroundings – in effect more sociable. Other individuals, however, may become restless, irritable and anxious.

Amphetamines may cause nausea, headache, dry mouth, trembling, difficulty in passing water, rapid beating of the heart and chest pains, diarrhoea, constipation and inability to concentrate. Higher doses may produce panic, confusion, aggression, hallucinations, mental breakdown and heart irregularities.

On stopping the use of moderate doses patients become fatigued, drowsy and depressed. They feel 'let down' and have a strong desire to take another dose to lift themselves again. Dependence on amphetamines is discussed on pp. 46–7.

The medical use of amphetamines should be restricted to treating narcolepsy, a rare disorder. Their use in treating hyperactive children has been challenged. So too has their use in treating bed-wetting. You should not use them as slimming drugs and if you are depressed they will do you more harm than good.

Other Stimulants

Methylphenidate is a mental stimulant; it increases activity, delays fatigue, lifts mood and has little effect upon appetite or blood pressure. Its widespread use in some countries to treat over-active children should be investigated.

Claims for the benefits of other stimulants such as **pemoline (Ronyl*, Volital)** and **prolintane** (in **Villescon**) have to be treated with caution.

7 Tonics

Millions of pounds are spent every year on tonics and yet most doctors accept that there is no single substance which may be called a tonic. Pharmacologists are highly critical of the whole concept of tonics and their criticism has influenced prescribing doctors. However, although medical fashions can change quickly, patients' expectations often do not. Doctors' prescribing habits influence patients' demands so that patients often expect what they have been led to expect. For decades doctors prescribed tonics for everybody and everything, yet they are now critical of patients who ask for a tonic, even though they accept the use of a placebo.

Some doctors who cannot come to terms with prescribing an inert substance or a tonic, prescribe vitamins, iron and other remedies just to reassure themselves that their treatment may be pharmacologically active. They thus strengthen the belief in the value of vitamins and iron for non-specific symptoms.

For obvious reasons the drug companies have not rejected tonics; they spend millions of pounds each year in persuading us that we need this or that product. But instead of being purely placebo some of these tonics contain substances which may be harmful if taken over a prolonged period of time.

If you think something will do you good then it most probably will – the least it should do is cause you no harm. A tonic is something that we hope will help us to feel better. However, drug tonics are usually taken because the individual is feeling persistently run-down, physically or mentally. They are often, and quite wrongly, taken for a multiplicity of mental and/or physical symptoms, the cause of which may be fairly straightforward – such as convalescence from an attack of influenza – or quite complex and due to a serious underlying physical or psychological disorder. The reasons which make people feel that they need a tonic are complex and include social, physical and mental factors. Therefore, there is no such thing as a universal tonic – someone who is anaemic will require a blood test and specific treatment; someone who is depressed needs specific treatment, as does someone with an underlying physical disease. The idea that a tonic can help anybody just is not true. When you see a footballer or actor recommending a remedy in the press or on television remember that he is doing it for the money.

If you feel persistently run-down and/or fed-up then see your doctor. He should check your medical history, your physical, mental and social state, and advise and treat you accordingly.

Many over-the-counter tonics are based on the principle that if you belch and have your bowels opened then you are living life to the full. Some tonics are very expensive foods containing malt, wheat germ or bone marrow. A popular 'tonic' these days contains 23·5 per cent liquid glucose which is no substitute for a well-balanced nutritious diet.

Iron salts are often included in tonics because many individuals believe and have been led to believe that anaemia is a common cause of feeling run-down. You may develop iron-deficiency anaemia because your diet is low in iron and/or because you are losing blood regularly through, for example, heavy periods or a bleeding peptic ulcer. However, iron deficiency is only one cause of anaemia and doctors cannot recognize the type of anaemia from which you may be suffering without carrying out blood tests. Incredible variations have been reported when groups of doctors have been asked to estimate the degree of anaemia in a particular patient. Yet patients still believe that a doctor has some magical power to diagnose anaemia without blood tests; this is because doctors in the past have used anaemia and iron treatment in a placebo situation. As a consequence many patients will say to their doctor 'I think I am anaemic, can I have some iron, please!' Of course, drug companies and health stores cash in on this belief. The same applies to vitamins; there is an optimum daily intake to prevent vitamin-deficiency disorders and there is a recommended dose for treating these disorders. The principle that if one hundred units will make you feel good then one thousand units will make you feel even better just is not true. We are seeing too many disorders – some of them serious – produced by taking too many vitamins.

Many decades ago it was found that nerve cells contain glycerophosphates; because of this the manufacture and sale of nerve tonics containing glycerophosphates and hypophosphates has proved an extremely lucrative business. This has happened despite the fact that the use of these drugs has never been shown to produce any benefit over and above that which would be produced by an inert substance. However, they are harmless and therefore useful as a placebo. Unfortunately they are mixed with all sorts of bitters (appetite stimulants), laxatives and stimulants. Some of these may produce adverse effects if taken regularly over time. Tonic wines contain hypophosphates and vitamins but people who take them must realize that it is probably the wine that makes them feel better.

Bitters, which appear in many tonics, stimulate salivation and the production of gastric juice by taste and smell. Certain alcoholic drinks are used for this purpose (aperitifs); but persistent loss of appetite is not the sort of symptom you should treat yourself.

Yeast is the basis of many tonics; again it can do you no harm on its own and it supplies you with a few vitamins. However, it is often combined with other drugs such as caffeine (you would get the same degree of stimulation from the caffeine in a cup of tea), with obsolete drugs and with rarely used pain relievers.

Over-the-counter remedies containing digestive enzymes such as pepsin and pancreatin, liver salts and bile salts are valueless. Some contain small quantities of obsolete laxatives. Health salts have nothing to do with health, and honey may make you feel beautiful if you believe that it will. There is also no evidence that if you stuff yourself full of vitamin E, you will look younger and feel more sexy.

Finally, there is no substitute for a good healthy diet and reasonable exercise and sleep. If you feel you really need a tonic then you ought to see your doctor. Otherwise take the least harmful and least expensive tonic (but only for a short period of time). Remember, the only part of a tonic that is really guaranteed to make you feel better is your belief that it is going to work.

8 Slimming Drugs

Obesity or fatness may be divided into two main types: that due to glandular disturbances, which is very rare, and simple obesity which is very common. Actually there is nothing very simple about obesity and most of us prefer to talk about being fat or overweight. This, however, implies that there is a range of normal weights to which we should conform. Because of these and the relationship between weight and diet, being overweight is said to be the commonest nutritional disorder in the Western world. In order to persuade us that this is true and in order to help us conform to these 'normal weights' a multi-million pound slimming industry has developed since the Second World War.

Being overweight may be due to having a big frame but it is usually due to fat. Stand naked in front of a mirror – if you have got rolls which shake when you jump up and down then you are fat! Being fat is mainly due to eating more food, particularly foods containing a larger number of calories, than we require for our everyday needs. This results in the storage of fat in some of us, but others appear to be able to use up the extra calories. Lack of physical exercise also predisposes to the laying down of fat. Women have more fat cells than men and there is a relationship between the number of fat cells, their size and being overweight. Hereditary factors may influence the number of fat cells we have (fat parents may have fat children – but children may also 'inherit' their parents' eating habits). The number of our fat cells may also increase up to about the age of twenty and they may increase as a result of overeating in childhood so that fat children may become fat adults. We may also become fat if our fat cells store a lot of fat and increase in size. This is due to the way we use up fats and sugars, and is related to diet and exercise. There are also glandular influences which make us put on weight and which must be regarded as normal; for example, women may put on weight in their early teens, after pregnancy and during the menopause. These may be short-term increases in weight but we must not forget that we all put on weight as we get older; women more than men. Women tend to put fat on round their bottoms and breasts and men around their abdomens.

Our appetites and the foods that we eat often have little to do with our requirements and are more determined by the eating habits we have acquired from childhood. These are related to family and environmental factors, our economic status, various customs and social requirements. Further, overeating may be as much a problem of habit as alcoholism, drug taking or smoking, and as such is as much related to our personality as it is to social and hereditary factors.

The Use of Slimming Drugs

Doctors consider that obesity requires treatment when fat deposits have raised the body weight by 10 per cent or more above the standards for people of the same age, sex and race. They point out what they think are the hazards of being fat. These include flat feet, varicose veins, osteoarthritis, gall-bladder disorders, high blood pressure, bronchitis, diabetes, complications after surgical operations, degenerative changes in heart muscle and a shortening of our lives. Doctors have certainly been successful in giving some of us the motivation to lose weight, although much of their evidence may not stand up to very close scrutiny.

Since the commonest cause of being fat is the eating of more food than is or was required, the only sensible way to reduce weight is to reduce the amount of food you eat or to alter your eating habits so that you eat a balanced diet and take in fewer calories. You should also take more physical exercise.

The Five Groups of Drugs Used to Aid Slimming

1. Drugs Which Cause Loss of Fluids

(*a*) Some patent slimming medicines contain laxatives such as **cascara**, **rhubarb** or **phenolphthalein**. These cause a loss of water from the bowel and therefore from the tissues, resulting in weight reduction. The body immediately puts to rights this water loss the next time you drink and so such medicines are useless. They could be harmful if taken regularly.

(*b*) Some doctors prescribe **diuretics** – these are drugs which interfere with the body's storage of salt and water. They act on the kidneys to make them excrete more salt and this takes water with it. The loss of water and salt results in a fall in body fluids and a subsequent temporary reduction in body weight. These diuretics also alter the body's excretion of other salts. They may be harmful and should only be taken under medical supervision for the treatment of an excess of body fluids caused by certain kidney, liver or heart diseases and in the treatment of raised blood pressure (see pp. 180–86).

2. Drugs Which Increase the Bulk of Food

Many patent slimming remedies contain **methylcellulose** or a similar substance in tablet form or as biscuits or granules **(Celevac, Cellucon, Cologel, Nilstim)** or **sterculia (Normacol, Prefil)**. These are substances which absorb water from the stomach, swell and are supposed to make you feel less hungry if taken before meals. They are not absorbed and increase the bulk of the motions taking some water with them. As slimming aids these preparations have not been proved to be of value.

3. Thyroid Extracts

Thyroid extracts are ineffective in small doses and dangerous in high doses.

4. Drugs Which Suppress the Appetite

Amphetamines. Most slimming drugs prescribed by doctors are amphetamines or related compounds. They have been widely used in the past because they stop you feeling hungry but they lose this effect after a few weeks. They do, however, stimulate, give you more energy and make you feel happy, but only for a short period of time. These effects cause some people to increase the dosage which may eventually lead to drug dependence and mental breakdown. Any possible benefit is outweighed by the dangers.

Diethylpropion (Tenuate Dospan, in Apisate), phentermine (Duromine, Ionamin). These are other drugs used to suppress appetite. Their toxic effects are similar to those of the amphetamines but they have less effect upon the heart and circulation. Their power to suppress appetite soon wears off and they may produce drug dependence of the amphetamine type. There is thus a risk of drug abuse.

Fenfluramine (Ponderax) has some chemical resemblance to the amphetamines but does not produce stimulation. It suppresses the appetite and may have an effect upon the way the body utilizes certain fats and glucose. It may rarely produce drug dependence.

Mazindol (Teronac) produces amphetamine-like effects. It is related chemically to the tricyclic antidepressant drugs and produces an antidepressant effect.

Overall, the value of drugs which stop you feeling hungry must be regarded as completely trivial when compared with diet control.

5. Starch Blockers

These comprise a protein component (**phaseolansin**) from red kidney beans which is claimed to prevent the digestion of dietary starch – the protein is said to 'lock' into amylase (an enzyme in the gut which converts starch to sugar) without changing it chemically or being absorbed. In recent years many preparations on the market in the U.S.A. just contained ground-up kidney beans and there were many reported adverse effects which led to the drugs being withdrawn from the market. Preparations available in the United Kingdom include **Calorex** and **Starchex**. Their effectiveness has never been demonstrated and they are expensive.

Occasionally, being overweight may be due to a psychological disorder. If you are a compulsive eater, excessive nibbler or a night eater then you ought to consult your doctor and be given more specific treatment for your problems, which may be psychological. However, if your doctor uses certain tranquillizers or antidepressant drugs these may, in fact, increase your appetite and make you put on more weight so he has to be careful about drug therapy if he thinks your weight problem warrants such treatment. Certainly slimming pills are not indicated because they will only make you feel more nervy or depressed. The oral contraceptive pill may also make some women put on weight and if diet fails to control this increase then it may be worth trying a lower-dose pill.

In conclusion, slimming drugs are no long-term substitute for will power and motivation. Being fat is a life-long problem and although these drugs will help you lose weight initially they have no effect upon your motivation or willpower, so that you will soon regain your weight when treatment is stopped. There is no evidence that they recondition you to a low calorie diet. The hard fact is that you must re-educate yourself to accept a change in eating and exercise habits for life. Crash diets, slimming pills, artificial powders containing a balanced mixture of carbohydrates, proteins, fats and minerals, and all the other paraphernalia of the slimming industry have only a transient effect and yet if you have a weight problem, it is usually for life. The slimming industry has, like all consumer industries, created a demand for its own products by making you feel out of fashion if you are not thin enough to conform to what they have decided is normal. If you do not overeat and if you take reasonable exercise then accept yourself as you are. But if you find yourself worrying about your weight and have tried hard for three months to lose weight then you are probably the sort of person who needs support and encouragement. Group therapy (e.g., a slimmers' club) may well be the answer in this case.

9 Drugs which Act upon the Autonomic Nervous System

The autonomic nervous system, as the name implies, is not under voluntary control. It supplies internal organs, e.g., the stomach, intestine, bronchi, heart, blood vessels, sweat glands, bladder and the eyes. It therefore controls all sorts of functions – from breathing to sexual activity and from sweating to digestion. It consists of two divisions – **sympathetic** and **parasympathetic**. These divisions oppose each other but a careful balance is maintained by special centres in the brain.

Impulses from the brain and spinal cord join the autonomic network of nerves along nerve fibres which run into ganglia (rather like electrical switchboxes). The impulses are transmitted at these junctions by chemical transmitters. The nerve fibres running to the junctions are called *pre*-ganglionic nerve fibres and they all use the same chemical transmitter – **acetylcholine**. This only works for a very short time because once it is liberated at nerve junctions to act as a chemical transmitter another chemical starts to break it down. The latter chemical is an enzyme called **cholinesterase**. Nerve fibres running *from* the nerve junctions (ganglia) are called *post*-ganglionic nerves.

Parasympathetic post-ganglionic nerves also use **acetylcholine** as a chemical transmitter – they are therefore known as cholinergic nerves, but the sympathetic post-ganglionic nerve fibres use **adrenaline** and **noradrenaline** as chemical transmitters and therefore these are known as adrenergic nerves. The central part (medulla) of the adrenal glands also produces adrenaline and noradrenaline.

Drugs which Act on the Parasympathetic Nervous System

Drugs which act like acetylcholine are called **cholinergic drugs** – they may also be called **parasympathomimetic** because they mimic the actions of the parasympathetic nervous system.

Stimulation of the parasympathetic division produces stimulation of secretory glands – salivary, tear, bronchial and sweat. It slows the heart rate, constricts the bronchi, produces increased movement of the gut, contracts the bladder and constricts the pupil. Cholinergic drugs also stimulate nerve endings in voluntary muscles, stimulate and then depress the brain, and dilate blood vessels.

Cholinergic Drugs

Cholinergic drugs mimic the actions of **acetylcholine**. There are three groups:

(1) Choline esters (**carbachol, bethanechol**) – these act at all sites like acetylcholine;

(2) Alkaloids (**pilocarpine, muscarine**) – these act selectively on those nerve endings which respond to acetylcholine;

(3) Cholinesterase inhibitors or anticholinesterase drugs (**physostigmine, neostigmine**) – these inactivate the enzyme (cholinesterase) which is responsible for breaking down acetylcholine. This allows acetylcholine to go on working.

Cholinergic drugs produce similar effects to stimulating the parasympathetic division. But not all effects occur with each drug and also the intensity of effects varies. Acetylcholine is not used in drug treatments. **Carbachol** may be used to stimulate bowel and bladder function after surgical operations. It may be given by injection under the skin or by mouth. **Bethanechol (Myotonine Chloride)** is related and may be given by mouth. **Pilocarpine** is used to constrict the pupil and decrease the pressure inside the eye in patients with glaucoma. The anticholinesterase drug **neostigmine** may be used to stimulate the bowel and bladder after surgery. **Endrophonium (Tensilon)** is used to diagnose and **neostigmine (Prostigmin)** and **pyridostigmine** are used in the treatment of myaesthenia gravis (a disease caused by defective transmission of impulses by acetylcholine and characterized by severe muscle weakness and fatigue). They are used as antidotes to neuromuscular blocking drugs (p. 94). **Ambenonium** is slightly longer acting than pyridostigmine and **distigmine (Ubretid)** is very long acting. Many related drugs are also 'used' as nerve gases and some are pesticides.

Drugs which Oppose Acetylcholine Activity

These may be called **acetylcholine antagonists** or **parasympatholytics**. They prevent acetylcholine from acting as a transmitter. There are three groups:

(1) **Anticholinergic drugs** which act principally at parasympathetic nerve endings;

(2) **Ganglion blocking drugs** which act on ganglia (and don't forget that

acetylcholine is the chemical transmitter in all ganglia – both in the parasympathetic and sympathetic divisions);

(3) **Neuromuscular blocking drugs** – these act on nerve endings in voluntary muscles.

(1) *Anticholinergic drugs*. The effects of these drugs are characterized by **atropine** and therefore they are often referred to as **atropine-like drugs**. Atropine is an alkaloid from the plant *Atropa belladonna* (deadly nightshade): it competes for the same chemical receptors as acetylcholine, thus blocking its effects. It produces the opposite effects to stimulation of the parasympathetic division – it produces dry mouth and reduces all secretions (except milk). In the stomach this reduces the amount of acid produced. It reduces sweating and bronchial secretions. It causes relaxation of muscles in the bowel, bronchi and bladder and is used to relieve muscle spasm in these organs, e.g., intestinal colic, bronchospasm. It dilates the pupils and increases the pressure inside the eyes. It increases heart rate, stimulates the brain, reduces motion sickness, and decreases the tremor and rigidity of Parkinsonism. High doses of atropine produce a rapid heart beat, dry mouth, blurred vision, dilated pupils, and restlessness. In overdose atropine produces excitement, hallucinations, delirium, mania and coma. (Note deadly nightshade poisoning.)

Other atropine-like drugs are **hyoscine (scopolamine)**, which depresses the brain and is used pre-operatively and in motion sickness; **atropine methonitrate**, which was used to treat infantile pyloric stenosis; **homatropine**, which is used to dilate the pupils; **hyoscine butylbromide**, which relaxes involuntary muscles and is used to relieve colic; **tropicamide** and **cyclopentolate**, which are used as eye-drops to dilate the pupils; and **propantheline (Pro-banthine)** which is one of several anticholinergic drugs used on their own or in combination with alkalis or sedatives in the treatment of peptic ulcers and irritable bowels. Many anticholinergic drugs have been used to treat Parkinsonism.

The principal uses of anticholinergic drugs therefore include the treatment of Parkinsonism and motion sickness, as sedatives, to dilate the pupils, to dilate the bronchi and reduce bronchial secretions, to reduce acid production by the stomach in the treatment of peptic ulcers and to relieve spasm of the gut, to treat colic, to reduce sweating and occasionally to treat heart block and slow pulse rates.

(2) *Ganglion blocking drugs*. These have been used in the past to treat raised blood pressure. They lower blood pressure by producing dilatation of blood vessels and therefore a fall in peripheral resistance. They include **mecamylamine, pempidine** and **hexamethonium**. Because they are not selective and block ganglia in both parasympathetic

and sympathetic divisions, they produce numerous adverse effects – particularly constipation.

(3) *Neuromuscular blocking drugs*. When an impulse passes down a nerve to a voluntary muscle it causes the release of acetylcholine at the nerve ending which acts as a chemical transmitter stimulating the muscle to contract. Neuromuscular blocking drugs interfere with this chemical transmission. **Curare**, used on poisoned arrows by the natives of South America, is the most famous example of this group of drugs. There are two main ways in which neuromuscular blocking drugs work. **Tubocurarine**, **gallamine** and **pancuronium** compete with acetylcholine and block the impulse being transmitted to the receptor organ in the muscles. They cause a flaccid paralysis of voluntary muscles. Drugs such as **suxamethonium (succinylcholine)** mimic the action of acetylcholine – at first they cause the muscles to contract but this effect wears off quickly and they leave the muscle no longer receptive to stimulation by acetylcholine. They are said to work by depolarization because they block the complex physicochemical process called polarization. Thus neuromuscular blocking drugs work in two ways – by competition and by depolarization. They are used in surgery to provide muscular relaxation and also in electroconvulsive therapy (ECT) to prevent injury during the induced fit.

Drugs which Act on the Sympathetic Nervous System

Those drugs that imitate the effects of stimulation of the sympathetic division may be called **sympathomimetic** drugs. Those that oppose its effects may be called **sympatholytic**.

Sympathomimetic Drugs

This group of drugs includes **adrenaline**, which is the main hormone produced by the medulla of the adrenal glands, and **noradrenaline** which is the main chemical transmitter at post-ganglionic sympathetic nerve endings. These nerves are therefore called adrenergic nerves and drugs which stimulate them are called **adrenergic drugs** – those that oppose their action are called **adrenolytic**.

Noradrenaline is produced and stored at adrenergic nerve endings and can be liberated from these stores by stimulating the nerve, or by drugs such as amphetamines, ephedrine, reserpine and guanethidine. Sympathomimetic drugs (or adrenergic drugs) may act directly on the receptors at the nerve endings of the sympathetic nervous system (e.g., **adrenaline, noradrenaline, isoprenaline**); indirectly by stimulating the liberation of noradrenaline from the stores at the nerve endings (e.g., **amphetamines**); or by both indirect and direct actions (e.g., **ephedrine, metaraminol**).

Sympathomimetic drugs act on adrenergic receptor sites which are found widely distributed throughout the body. These receptors are classified simply into alpha (α) and beta (β_1 and β_2) receptors. Stimulation of alpha receptors produces what are called alpha effects – constriction of the blood vessels in the skin and gut, a rise in blood pressure and dilatation of the pupils. β_1 receptors are principally located in the heart; stimulation produces an increase of heart rate and increased output of blood from the heart. Stimulation of β_2 receptors produces relaxation of bronchial muscles, relaxation of the uterus and dilatation of blood vessels, chiefly in muscles. Stimulation of both alpha and beta receptors in the gut produces relaxation. Alpha and beta stimulation also produces a raised blood sugar and a raised level of blood fatty acids. The mobilization of sugar from the liver is an alpha effect and from the voluntary muscles a beta effect.

Adrenaline produces both alpha and beta effects, **noradrenaline** produces chiefly alpha effects and **isoprenaline** produces beta effects.

Sympathomimetic drugs are principally used:

as nasal decongestants: read the section on drugs used to treat the common cold, p. 99;

to treat bronchospasm: read the section on drugs used to treat bronchial asthma, p. 111.

to treat low blood pressure: because they constrict blood vessels in the skin they increase resistance and raise the blood pressure (e.g., **metaraminol: Aramine**). They may be used in severe states of low blood pressure caused by coronary thrombosis, anaesthetics or drug overdose. They are not as popular as they once were.

to stimulate the heart: **dopamine (Intropin)** and **dobutamine (Dobutrex)** stimulate heart muscle and increase contractability. They are used in heart (cardiogenic) shock.

Drugs which Oppose Sympathetic Activity

These drugs oppose sympathetic activity:

(1) *Adrenergic neurone blocking drugs.* These block transmission of nerve impulses along post-ganglionic sympathetic nerves (adrenergic nerves) or their nerve endings. They include **guanethidine**. These drugs are discussed under the section on drugs used to treat raised blood pressure, p. 163.

(2) *Alpha-receptor blocking drugs.* These include **phentolamine, phenoxybenzamine** and **tolazoline**. The principal effect of these drugs is to produce dilatation of the blood vessels in the skin. They are discussed under

the section on drugs used to treat disorders of the circulation, p. 170.

(3) *Beta-receptor blocking drugs*. These are used to treat angina, disorders of heart rhythm and raised blood pressure. They are discussed on p. 152.

Summary: Drugs which Act on the Autonomic Nervous System

Parasympathetic Division

Parasympathomimetic drugs

	choline esters (e.g., **carbachol**)
Cholinergic drugs	alkaloids (e.g., **pilocarpine**)
	cholinersterase inhibitors (e.g., **neostigmine**)

Parasympatholytic drugs

Anticholinergic drugs, e.g., **atropine**

Ganglion blocking drugs (block ganglia in both parasympathetic and sympathetic divisions), e.g., **mecamylamine**

Sympathetic Division

Sympathomimetic drugs

	alpha-receptor stimulants (e.g., **noradrenaline**)
Adrenergic drugs	alpha- and beta-receptor stimulants (e.g., **adrenaline**)
	beta-receptor stimulants (e.g., **isoprenaline**)

Sympatholytic drugs

Adrenergic neurone blocking drugs, e.g., **guanethidine**

alpha-receptor blocking drugs, e.g., **phentolamine**

Beta-receptor blocking drugs, e.g., **propranolol**

Drugs which Enhance Neuromuscular Transmission

In conditions such as myasthenia gravis anticholinesterase drugs are used. They prolong the action of acetylcholine by inhibiting the action of the enzyme acetylcholinesterase which breaks down acetylcholine. They may produce adverse effects such as increased sweating, salivation, and gastric secretion, increased contractions in the gut and uterus, and slowing of the heart rate. These drugs include **ambenonium, distigmine (Ubretid), edrophonium (Tensilon), neostigmine (Prostigmin)** and **pyridostigmine**

(Mestinon). They vary according to their duration of action. Their effects can be stopped by giving atropine (an anticholinergic drug).

Muscle Relaxants

Drugs which block the transmission of nervous impulses at neuromuscular junctions are used in anaesthesia. They are usually referred to as *neuro-muscular blocking drugs* or *myoneural blocking drugs*. They make muscles relax during surgery (e.g., abdominal muscles) and they make the vocal cords relax so that a tube can be passed down into the lungs in order to give anaesthetic gases. As stated earlier, there are two groups of neuromuscular blocking drugs – those that compete with acetylcholine and block its effects (*non-depolarizing muscle relaxants*). They include **alcuronium (Alloferin), atracurium (Tracrium), gallamine (Flaxedil), pancuronium (Pavulon), tubocurarine (Jexin, Tubarine Miscible), vecuronium (Norcuron)**. The second group are *depolarizing muscle relaxants* which mimic the action of acetylcholine and cause blockage of impulses at neuromuscular junctions. **Suxamethonium (Anectine, Brevidil M, Scoline)** is the most commonly used. **Suxethonium (Brevidil E)** is used occasionally.

Muscle relaxants used to relieve pain and spasm in skeletal muscles act principally on the brain and spinal cord. Drugs used include benzodiaze-pines (e.g., **diazepam**) and **baclofen (Lioresal)**. **Dantrolene (Dantrium)** acts directly on skeletal muscles to produce relaxation but produces adverse effects on the brain. **Quinine** is useful for relieving leg cramps in bed at night.

10 Drugs Used to Treat the Common Cold

There is no such drug as a cold cure. Apart from a possibility that high doses of vitamin C may shorten the duration of a common cold, or decrease the intensity of symptoms in *some* individuals, there is no drug on the market which prevents colds or reduces their duration. But, because there is no cure, there are numerous remedies.

The common cold produces swelling and inflammation of the lining membrane of the nose which produces blockage and a runny nose. This may be accompanied by a sore throat, cough, headache, aching back or limbs and a mild fever. In an attempt to relieve these symptoms drug companies produce nose drops, inhalants, sprays, aerosols, ointments, tablets, powders, capsules, linctuses and mixtures, in all shapes, colours and sizes. Treatment is aimed at two target groups of symptoms – aches, pains and fever; blocked and runny nose.

Relief of Aches, Pains and Fever

Pain relievers such as **aspirin*** or **paracetamol** will relieve your aches and pains and will bring down your temperature. They must be taken according to the instructions on the package and with plenty of fluids. (Read about the adverse effects of aspirin and paracetamol, particularly in babies and infants, see p. 194). They will have no effect upon the duration or outcome of the cold and they may be harmful if they enable someone to do physical work when they should be resting or taking it easy. There are hundreds of pain-relieving preparations on the market and yet the choice boils down to two drugs – soluble aspirin or paracetamol.

Aspirin is the drug of choice but if you have a peptic ulcer or history of a peptic ulcer, if you get indigestion or have any stomach upset then do not take aspirin. **Paracetamol** is an alternative. *There is no point in spending money on any preparations because they fizz or taste fruity*. Furthermore, many proprietary remedies contain several drugs and so expose you to the risk of several adverse effects – these remedies are often expensive and best avoided.

---

* Aspirin should not be used for children under twelve.

Nasal Sprays

The majority of decongestant drugs belong to a group of drugs known as sympathomimetic drugs (see p. 95).

When applied locally to the surface of the nose or throat from a nasal spray these produce blanching and constriction of small blood vessels. They are used to relieve runny nose and nasal congestion. They all share the disadvantage that their use may be followed by an increase of nasal congestion ('rebound' or 'after congestion'). Some irritate the lining of the nose and sting when applied. Their effectiveness decreases with repeated use and some experts consider that they actually prolong a cold. Their repeated use may damage the lining membrane of the nose.

The use of these drugs in nasal drops or sprays should be avoided in infants and young children. Two of them, **naphazoline** and **tetra-hydrozoline**, may cause unconsciousness and a fall in body temperature in children, especially in infants. See below.

Topical nasal sympathomimetic decongestants include **ephedrine hydrochloride** nasal drops, **oxymetazoline** nasal drops and sprays (**Afrazine** nasal drops, paediatric nasal drops, **Afrazine** nasal spray, **xylometazoline hydrochloride** nasal drops and sprays (**Otrivine** nasal drops, **Otrivine** paediatric nasal drops, **Otrivine** nasal spray), **phenylephrine hydrochloride** (**Neophryn** nasal drops and sprays). Nasal applications that contain a combination of drugs include **Otrivine-Antistin** nasal drops and sprays which contain **antazoline sulphate** and **xylometazoline hydrochloride**. **Hayphryn** contains **phenylephrine** and **thenyldiamine**.

Nasal Decongestants by Mouth

Nasal decongestants are usually applied locally in the nose by nasal spray or drops, but there is increasing pressure from advertising to take such drugs by mouth. The blood vessels supplying the lining membranes of the nose have not been shown to be more sensitive to these drugs than any other vessels in the body. Nasal decongestants taken by mouth will therefore produce constriction of other blood vessels in the body and increase the blood pressure. This may be dangerous in patients who suffer from angina, coronary thrombosis, high blood pressure, diabetes or overworking of their thyroid glands, and in patients who are receiving monoamine oxidase inhibitor antidepressant drugs. Their adverse effects include giddiness, headache, nausea, vomiting, sweating, thirst, palpitations, difficulty in passing urine, weakness, trembling, anxiety, restlessness and insomnia.

Some individuals may be very sensitive to them whilst others may be able to tolerate high doses. They are best avoided.

Other drugs used to decrease nasal congestion include **belladonna alkaloids** and **antihistamines**.

The **belladonna alkaloids** (see **atropine** p. 94) reduce secretions in the upper and lower respiratory tract. They are a common constituent of proprietary cold remedies, usually in such small doses as to be totally ineffective. But, of course, if they were given in effective doses by mouth they would produce very unpleasant adverse effects.

Antihistamines are present in numerous common cold remedies and yet there is no evidence that they are of the slightest value. They are not the sort of drugs which should be taken casually – for example, they influence brain function, making you drowsy, and they may interfere with your ability to drive a motor vehicle. Their effects are increased by alcohol. They do tend to 'dry up' the respiratory tract. However, this reduces natural barriers to bacteria, and in the presence of infection this effect is considered to be harmful by some experts.

Treating the Common Cold

Drink plenty of fluids and take some rest in the early stages. Alcohol has no beneficial effect on the cold but may help you to rest. Antiseptic gargles, mouth washes and throat lozenges have no effect upon the cold virus.

Aspirin or **paracetamol** in appropriate dosage and taken with appropriate precautions are the only drugs worth taking by mouth, and even these drugs serve only to relieve pain and fever. For social emergencies (e.g., a party which you cannot get out of) a nasal spray may be used, but not repeatedly.

This may seem hard advice but to take a proprietary cold remedy which contains a decongestant, pain reliever, stimulant (e.g., caffeine) and an antihistamine is like taking a sledge-hammer to crack a nut – a nut that is in any case virtually uncrackable. No drug has a single effect and to take several drugs with many diverse effects and adverse effects in order to dry up a few square centimetres of the lining membrane of the nose is quite irrational. One last warning – individuals taking a decongestant drug by mouth could very easily take a toxic dose if they were to use a decongestant nose spray or drops as well. If you have to use a local application for a social emergency use a nose spray that is mixed with water, not oil, since the latter may be inhaled into the lungs and cause inflammation or even pneumonia.

Anti-infective Nasal Preparations

Nasal preparations containing **mild silver protein** should not be used because of the risk of argyria (a dusky-grey or blue discoloration of the skin and mucous membranes). Preparations containing **antibiotics** may be useful for eradicating local infections in the nose (see antibiotics used in skin applications, p. 272).

Catarrh

The term catarrh is not found in medical textbooks but is generally accepted to mean an inflammation of the lining of the nose and throat with the production of a discharge, e.g, nasal discharge, phlegm in the throat, snuffles in babies. Many factors are involved relating to air pollution and the spread of droplet infections in the home. Steam inhalation is the best form of treatment along with stopping smoking and/or avoiding smoky atmospheres.

11 Drugs Used to Treat Coughs

Coughs frequently serve a useful purpose, for example, to get rid of an inhaled foreign body or to cough up sputum. These coughs are said to be productive. A cough which is just dry and irritating is said to be unproductive and serves no purpose. As with cold remedies the marketing of cough medicines is a lucrative business and so the market is flooded with preparations. Many of these are mixtures containing such small doses of individual drugs as to render them pharmacologically ineffective. But, of course, a large proportion of us respond to inert mixtures – some of us responding better to one colour or taste than to others.

The aim of using cough medicines is to give comfort to those people with a productive cough and to help them cough up their sputum. For those people with a dry, irritating, unproductive cough, the aim is to suppress it. We therefore have two main groups of drugs which are used to treat coughs – expectorants and cough suppressants. Expectorants are given with the aim of liquefying the sputum, so that it is easier to cough up. Cough suppressants either work locally at the site of the irritation in the throat or they act on the cough centre in the brain, reducing the desire to cough. Some cough mixtures contain drugs which act on the conscious part of the brain producing sedation and therefore making you less aware of the irritation in your throat.

Expectorants

These act by irritating the lining of the stomach which by reflex stimulates the nerves supplying the glands in the bronchi. This is said to result in an increased production of secretions thus making the sputum more watery and easier to cough up. However, the dose required to do this would, with most of these drugs, produce stomach pains and vomiting. They include **ammonium chloride, acetates, acetic acid, bicarbonates, potassium iodide, sodium citrate, ipecacuanha, squill, creosote, eucalyptus, menthol, peppermint, sodium benzoate, tolu, benzoin compounds** and **guaiacols** (e.g., **guaiphenesin**). They are present in many cough medicines, and from the point of view of effectiveness you may as well choose them by taste or colour. There is no evidence that any drug whether given by mouth, injection, or inhalation can specifically produce expectoration either directly or indirectly via the cough reflex. Expectorant cough medicines are an expensive myth.

The stickiness of sputum depends on its degree of water content, which in turn depends upon the general degree of hydration of the body. Patients with chronic bronchitis and other chest disorders which produce dry sticky sputum may well benefit from increasing their fluid intake. **Inhalation of water or steam** may also be very useful and it does not really matter whether these are made to smell pleasant by the addition of **menthol**, **eucalyptus** or **benzoin**. The addition of a weak detergent (e.g., **tyloxapol**; **Alevaire**) may help.

Mucolytic Drugs

Some drugs have been shown to 'digest' sputum in the laboratory, but their effect upon sputum in the bronchial tubes has been variable. Cysteine compounds, e.g. **carbocisteine (Mucodyne)**, **methylcysteine (Visclair)** and **acetylcysteine (Fabrol)** by mouth may liquefy sputum and help you to cough up phlegm, but few patients appear to benefit. **Tyloxapol (Alevaire)** by inhalation is probably no more beneficial than water or steam inhalations, nor is **bromhexine** by mouth.

Cough Suppressants (Antitussives)

The most important cough suppressant in people who smoke is to stop smoking. For coughs which are caused by irritation or inflammation in the throat above the larynx (voice-box) there are hundreds of different makes of throat sweets, pastilles, lozenges, cough drops and linctuses available. Many contain **antiseptics** (such as **creosote, thymol, benzoin, cetylpyridinium, chloroxylenol, domiphen**) in doses which are totally useless but which, if given in effective antiseptic doses, could be harmful.

Most cough sweets contain **demulcents**, which are soothing substances which act on the surface of the throat, e.g., **honey, liquorice, glycerin**. Such preparations also contain pleasant smelling and tasting substances like **peppermint, eucalyptus, cinnamon, lemon, clove, aniseed**. Others contain **menthol, camphor, chloroform**. The main effect of these preparations is that their smell or taste may help you feel better. They may increase the production of saliva, which is soothing and helps to wash the inflamed surfaces of the throat. Many preparations contain a topical anaesthetic (e.g., **benzocaine**), which may reduce the pain of inflammation. Cough medicines which contain the same ingredients in liquid form are even more irrational since they are swallowed directly into the stomach and only have a fraction of a second to work locally on the throat. There is no evidence that any of these cough preparations are any more effective than sucking ordinary sweets or chewing gum.

For non-productive irritating coughs caused by inflammation below the larynx, **steam inhalations** may be very useful and can be made to smell nice by adding such substances as **menthol**. The main drugs used to suppress coughs may be divided into two groups – narcotic and non-narcotic.

Narcotic cough suppressants include **diamorphine (heroin)** and **methadone (Physeptone)**. These are discussed under the section on narcotic pain relievers, p. 189. As well as suppressing the cough reflex they also tend to dry up and thicken bronchial secretions. They are drugs of dependence and should not be used routinely.

Codeine is present in many cough medicines, usually in non-effective doses. In appropriate dosage it is an effective cough suppressant. It may cause constipation and may, very rarely, produce drug dependence of the morphine type in some patients.

Other cough suppressants include **pholcodine**, **dextromethorphan** (present in many cough mixtures), **isoaminile**, **noscapine** and **pipazethate**. They all cause constipation.

Cough Mixtures

There are numerous mixtures on the market, some containing up to ten drugs. Some are useless, some are harmful, many are expensive, some are addictive, and it is difficult to find out what some of them contain. Some mixtures sold over the counter or prescribed by doctors contain mixtures of an expectorant and a suppressant, which seems contradictory: the suppressant dries and thickens the bronchial secretions, and blocks the reflex which clears them from the bronchial tubes, whereas the expectorant liquefies the secretions.

In addition to expectorants, demulcents and suppressants many cough medicines contain **antihistamines**. Yet there is little support for the popular belief that antihistamines are of any use in treating coughs. They may produce sedation which may help at night and they have an anticholinergic effect (p. 94) which may dry the surface of the upper respiratory tract, but otherwise it is difficult to understand their popularity.

Selecting a Cough Medicine

For a dry throaty cough (i.e., caused by inflammation or irritation above the larynx) anything that may be sucked or chewed will help and there is little point in taking cough lozenges or mixtures. If the cough is very irritating it is better to take a dose of a cough suppressant along with something to suck or chew.

For a cough which is on the chest (below the larynx), which is irritating and non-productive, a straight cough suppressant is best, e.g., **codeine**, **pholcodine**, **dextromethorphan**, **isoaminile**, **noscapine**, or **pipazethate**. The choice is not critical and for the ordinary dry cough associated with a common cold only three or four doses at appropriate intervals will be required. If you find yourself having to take a cough suppressant for more than a few days then see your doctor. Also see your doctor if the cough does not clear up after one or two weeks, if your sputum turns yellow or green (you may need an **antibiotic**), if there is blood in your sputum, if your cough is associated with chest pain and/or fever or if it is associated with breathlessness. Steam inhalations are of benefit to both dry throaty coughs and to non-productive chesty coughs.

A productive cough (i.e., when you cough up sputum) may be helped by a **warm drink** and/or **steam inhalations**. A simple expectorant mixture may help (e.g., sodium chloride compound mixture), but these mixtures may produce stomach pains and upsets if taken over prolonged periods. If you have the habit of taking cough medicines every day and suffer from indigestion – then it might be the cough medicine that is causing it. *All patients with a cough should stop smoking.*

Patients with kidney or heart disorders, or with raised blood pressure, or any patients on a reduced sodium intake, should check the sodium content of any cough medicine that they purchase with their pharmacist.

Diamorphine (heroin) and **methadone** are effective cough suppressants used to control coughs in patients suffering from lung cancer or other severe lung disorders.

12 Drugs Used to Treat Disorders of the Mouth and Throat

Drugs used to Treat Disorders of the Mouth

Thrush (*candida albicans*) of the mouth is treated with **nystatin** suspension **(Nystan, Nystatin-Dome)** or with **amphotericin** lozenges **(Fungilin)**. **Polynoxylin** lozenges **(Anaflex)**, **dequalinium (Dequadin** lozenges, **Labosept** pastilles) and **natamycin** oral suspension **(Pimafucin)** are less effective. **Miconazole** oral gel **(Daktarin)** should be reserved for severe fungal infections.

Herpes infection of the mouth is very difficult to treat. Drugs worth trying include **idoxuridine** and **tetracycline** mouth bath.

Recurrent mouth ulcers (aphthous ulcers) can be very painful and treatment very disappointing. Local treatment aimed at soothing the pain and helping healing is not usually very effective. Preparations available include mechanical protectives (e.g., **carmellose paste** in **Orabase gel** (carmellose sodium, pectin and gelatin) and **Orahesive powder** (carmellose sodium, pectin and gelatin); **corticosteroids** in lozenges or pastes (e.g., **Adcortyl (triamcinolone** in **Orabase paste)**; **Corlan** pellets **(hydrocortisone)**, local anaesthetic gels and lozenges (e.g., **benzocaine** lozenges, benzocaine **compound** lozenges (contain **menthol** as well)), **Medilave gel (benzocaine** and **cetylpyridinium)** and **Oral-B** gel **(lignocaine** and **cetylpyridinium)**; **salicylate** pastes and gels (e.g., **choline salicylate** paste: **Bonjela**, **Teejel** and **Pyralvex (anthraquinone** and **salicylic acid))**; and **antibiotic** mouth washes (e.g., **tetracycline** mouth wash). **Carbenoxolone sodium gel (Bioral)** and granules **(Bioplex)** and **benzydamine (Difflam** oral rinse) may relieve pain. **Alum** or **silver nitrate** sticks applied to the ulcer may relieve pain for a short time but cause tissue damage and therefore they may actually delay healing of the ulcer.

Drugs Used to Treat Sore Throat

The commonest cause of a sore throat is a virus infection which does not respond to anti-infective treatment. Streptococcal sore throats require **penicillin** treatment and acute ulcerative disorders (Vincent's) require a drug such as **metronidazole (Flagyl)**.

Antiseptic Throat Lozenges

There is no convincing evidence that antiseptic lozenges and sprays have any benefit at all; most are combined with a local anaesthetic which relieves pain but may produce irritation. They include **benzalkonium** lozenges, **A A A spray** (**benzocaine** and **cetalkonium**), **Bradosol** lozenges (**domiphen**), **Eludril** aerosol spray (**amethocaine** and **chlorhexidine**), **Hibitane** lozenges (**benzocaine** and **chlorhexidine**). **Locabiotal** aerosol spray (**fusafungine**), **Merocaine** lozenges (**benzocaine** and **cetylpyridinium**), **Merocet lozenges** (**cetylpyridinium**) **Oralcer** lozenges (**ascorbic acid** and **clioquinol**), **Strepsils** lozenges (**amylmetacresol** and **dichlorobenzyl alcohol**) and **Tyrozets** (**benzocaine** and **tyrothricin**).

Mouth Washes and Gargles

The use of mouth washes and gargles should be restricted to the care of the mouth in debilitated patients. They include **compound sodium chloride** (salt) mouth wash, **compound thymol glycerin** mouth wash and **hydrogen peroxide** mouth wash. Brand preparations include **cetylpyridinium** (**Merocet**), **chlorhexidine** (**Corsodyl, Eludril**) which is useful for preventing plaque formation on teeth which may lead to the development of caries, **hexetidine** (**Oraldene**), **phenol** (**Chloraseptic**), **povidone-iodine** (**Betadine**), **sodium perborate** (**Bocasan**), **thymol** (**thymol** and **sodium benzoate**) and **thymol glycerin compound** (**glycerol** and **thymol**).

13 Drugs Used to Treat Disorders of the Ears

Inflammation of the external ear (*otitis externa*) may be primarily due to infection by bacteria or fungi or due to eczema secondarily to infection. It is usually treated with ear drops or ointments. Preparations usually aim at drying the ear (astringents), relieving inflammation and treating infection. The most useful astringent is **aluminium acetate** ear drops (8 or 13 per cent). Anti-inflammatory preparations include the two corticosteroid drugs **betamethasone (Betnesol, Vista-Methasone)** and **prednisolone (Predsol)**.

Anti-infective ear preparations include **chloramphenicol drops (Chloromycetin)**, **clioquinol** combined with **flumethasone** (in **Locorten-Vioform**), **framycetin (Framygen)** and **framycetin with hydrocortisone** (in **Framycort**) **Gentamicin (Cidomycin, Garamycin*, Genticin** and **Gentisone H C (gentamicin** and **Hydrocortisone))**, **neomycin** with **betamethasone (Betnesol N, Vista-methasone N)** with **hydrocortisone (Neo-Cortef)** and with **prednisolone (Predsol N)**; and **tetracycline (Achromycin)**.

Compound anti-infective ear preparations include:

Audicort (neomycin, undecenoic acid; triamcinolone and **benzocaine)**
Otosporin (hydrocortisone, neomycin and **polymyxin B)**
Ototrips (bacitracin, polymyxin B, trypsin, gelatin and **sodium chloride)**
Sofradex (dexamethasone, framycetin, gramicidin)
Soframycin (framycetin, gramicidin)
Terra-Cortril (hydrocortisone, oxytetracycline and **polymyxin B)**
Tri-Adcortyl Otic (gramicidin, neomycin, triamcinolone and **nystatin).**

Other preparations include:

Audax (choline salicylate and **ethylene oxide-polyoxypropylene glycol)**
Auralgicin (benzocaine, chlorbutol, ephedrine, hydroxyquinoline and **phenazone** in **glycerol)**
Auraltone (benzocaine, phenazone and **glycerol)**

Removal of Wax in the Ear

The cheapest and most effective drugs to use are **warm olive oil, glycerol** or **sodium bicarbonate ear drops. Dioctyl sodium sulphosuccinate (docusate sodium: Audinorm, Dioctyl, Molcer, Soliwax** and **Waxsol)** and **urea hydrogen peroxide complex (Exterol)** are of use. Organic solvents are best avoided since they cause irritation (e.g., **Cerumol (chlorbutol, paradichlorobenzene,** and **turpentine oil)**).

14 Drugs Used to Treat Bronchial Asthma

Bronchodilators

Drugs which open up the airways are called bronchodilators because they act by dilating (opening up) the bronchial tubes. They are used to reverse or decrease obstruction to the flow of air to the lungs caused by narrowing of these tubes. This occurs in bronchial asthma when narrowing of the airways is produced by spasm of the muscles in the bronchial tubes. This spasm (bronchospasm) is often associated with swelling of the lining surfaces and an increased production of secretions. Narrowing of the airways may also occur in chronic chest disorders such as emphysema and bronchitis. In these disorders the small bronchial tubes are scarred, distorted and narrowed by repeated infections (e.g. bronchitis). In addition repeated infections affect the secretory glands in the walls of the bronchial tubes and in the lining membranes. These increase in size and produce more secretions (sputum or phlegm) resulting in a productive cough. Also in such disorders as emphysema the lung tissues lose their normal 'elastic' action and this causes many small bronchial tubes to close up on breathing out. Thus the two types of obstruction to the airways produced by asthma and chronic bronchitis differ; the extent to which they can be treated by drugs also differs. Much more benefit from bronchodilator drugs may obviously be obtained when the airways are obstructed due to spasm, as in asthma, than when it is due to scarring as in chronic bronchitis. Machines (spirometers) which measure the volume of air breathed out by an individual in a given time show that these drugs may be highly effective in improving the airways in patients suffering from bronchial asthma but not very effective in patients with chronic obstructive bronchial disease (e.g., chronic bronchitis and emphysema).

There are two main groups of bronchodilator drugs – sympathomimetic compounds (adrenaline-like drugs) and theophylline derivatives.

Sympathomimetic Drugs

These drugs, as their name implies, mimic the effects of stimulating the sympathetic division of the autonomic nervous system (see p. 95). They include chemicals which are produced in the body, e.g., **adrenaline** and

noradrenaline (which is the main chemical messenger at nerve endings of the sympathetic nervous system). Numerous synthetic chemicals also mimic stimulation of the sympathetic nervous system, e.g., **isoprenaline**, **ephedrine** and **amphetamines**. Drugs which have sympathomimetic effects may act directly on the site of nerve endings (e.g., **adrenaline, noradrenaline, isoprenaline**); indirectly by causing a release of the chemical messenger **(noradrenaline)** at the nerve endings (e.g., **amphetamine**); or by both direct and indirect actions (e.g., **ephedrine**). This is a very simple description of what is really a most complex physiochemical process, which is made more complicated by factors which influence stores of noradrenaline in the body, so that sympathomimetic drugs will act differently if given for a short or prolonged period of time.

The site of action of the nerve endings are called receptor sites and these are widely distributed throughout various tissues of the body. Three types of receptors have been recognized – alpha (α) receptors and beta (β_1 and β_2) receptors (see pp. 95–6).

Drugs which stimulate beta receptors are used in treating obstruction to the airways because they relax bronchial muscles. Original sympathomimetic bronchodilator drugs act on both β_1 and β_2 receptors so that in addition to relieving bronchospasm they also produce unwanted effects upon the heart and circulation and may produce serious disorders of heart rate and rhythm. They are called **non-selective**. Drugs which dilate bronchial muscles but produce less effect upon the heart are called **selective β_2-receptor stimulants**.

The sympathomimetic drugs used to treat asthma include:

Selective Stimulants	*Non-Selective Stimulants*
fenoterol (Berotec)	**adrenaline (Medihaler-Epi; Min-i-Jet Adrenaline)**
pirbuterol (Exirel)	**ephedrine (in numerous preparations)**
reproterol (Bronchodil)	**isoetharine (Numotac)**
rimiterol (Pulmadil)	**isoprenaline (Iso-Autohaler, Medihaler-Iso,**
salbutamol (Aerolin,	**Medihaler-Iso Forte)**
Asmaven, Cobutolin,	**methoxyphenamine**
Ventodisks, Ventolin,	**orciprenaline (Alupent)**
Volmax)	
terbutaline (Bricanyl,	
Monovent)	

Selective β_2-receptor stimulants are the drugs of choice to control recurrent attacks of asthma. There is little to choose between them; **fenoterol** and **terbutaline** are longer acting than **salbutamol** and **rimiterol**.

To stop an acute attack which has developed, an aerosol containing a **salbutamol-like** drug is possibly the safest preparation to use. In emergencies **adrenaline** or **aminophylline** by injection may be used, alone or in combination with salbutamol.

Remember that it is not rational to take bronchodilator drugs every day unless there is evidence from breathing tests that they reverse airway obstruction.

The **pressurized aerosol inhaler** is the most effective and convenient method of administration for mild to moderate airways obstruction. They provide relief for 3 to 5 hours, act rapidly, produce fewer adverse effects than tablets (e.g., tremors and tension) and they deliver the drug directly to the site of action and therefore very small doses can be used. (Note that only a small proportion reaches the bronchi; the rest is swallowed.) Other special devices such as the **Bricanyl Spacer Inhaler** and the application of aqueous aerosols using a **nebulizer** may be very useful in some patients.

Theophylline Derivatives

Theophylline and its derivatives relax bronchial muscles, stimulate the respiratory centres in the brain and increase the output from the heart. They may be given by injection, by mouth and as suppositories. Their effectiveness depends upon the amount of theophylline which enters the blood-stream. **Aminophylline** is a mixture of theophylline and ethylinediamine which makes a more soluble preparation.

Ordinary tablets of theophylline and its derivatives can produce adverse effects which include tachycardia, palpitations, nausea, gastro-intestinal upsets, insomnia and convulsions. Intravenous injections may produce a rapid onset of these effects. Suppositories may produce them and also cause irritation of the ano-rectal area (proctitis). Therefore it is now more common practice to use long-acting (slow-release) preparations which need to be given no more frequently than every 12 hours. Long-acting preparations by mouth (sustained-release) of **aminophylline** or **theophylline** are very useful in patients suffering from less severe and more chronic asthma. They are useful when given at night for controlling night attacks of asthma and for preventing early morning attacks of wheezing. The sustained-release preparations produce fewer adverse effects than ordinary oral preparations but they can still irritate the stomach, produce headaches and cause caffeine-like stimulation (see p. 81). Treatment should start with s.nall doses and be gradually built up.

Theophylline-like Bronchodilators

aminophylline (Phyllocontin Continus, Theodrox)

choline theophyllinate (Choledyl, Sabidal)
diprophylline (Silbephylline)
etamiphylline (Millophylline)
proxyphylline (Thean)
theophylline (Biophylline, Labophylline, Lasma, Nuelin, Nuelin S A,
    Pro-Vent, Slo-Phyllin, Theo-Dur, Uniphyllin continus)

Note the duration of action of **theophylline** is reduced in regular smokers. It is increased by cimetidine and in patients suffering from liver damage, heart failure and severe lung disease. This may result in high blood levels producing nausea and vomiting in these patients on what appears to be a 'normal' dose. Blood level monitoring should be carried out on patients receiving a theophylline preparation.

A drug called **sodium cromoglycate (Intal)** acts on the lining surfaces of the airways to interfere with the allergic reaction in patients who develop allergic asthma. The allergic effects (spasm of the bronchial muscles and swelling of the lining membrane) are stopped or reduced if the drug is present on the airway surfaces at the time when the allergic-reaction begins – it is not effective if taken after the reaction has started. It is of use in preventing asthma in children and rhinitis (inflammation of the nasal passages) due to allergy. It is taken by inhalation and may cause bronchospasm and slight irritation of the throat especially if used during or after a respiratory infection. It may produce contact dermatitis in people who handle it. The drug is available as a dry powder in a gelatin capsule with isoprenaline **(Intal compound)** or without **(Intal)**. A special inhaler punctures the capsule, which then spins in the inspired air stream to deliver the powder into the lungs. The small dose of isoprenaline is added to cut down bronchospasm which may occur in some patients on inhalation of a dry powder. It is also available for allergic rhinitis (hay-fever) as **Rynacrom** which may be of value in some patients with seasonal hay-fever. The powder from each capsule is puffed up each nostril several times a day. It is also available as a nasal spray.

Ketotifen (Zaditen) produces similar effects to sodium cromoglycate and is taken by mouth. It has some properties of the antihistamine drugs (p. 125) and may produce drowsiness. **Nedocromil sodium (Tilade aerosol)** produces similar effects to sodium cromoglycate but also relieves inflammation.

Corticosteroids

These are discussed on p. 216. They are used in the treatment of a number of chest diseases. Their most important use is in treating patients suffering from asthma.

Corticosteroids may be used to treat asthma of varying degrees of severity. The most serious form of acute asthma attack is called status asthmaticus. In such an emergency as this, the use of corticosteroids by injection into a vein can be life-saving, although their maximum effects are not immediate and take six hours or more to work. For this reason additional treatment, such as the intravenous injection of **salbutamol** or **aminophylline**, is also required to obtain some immediate relief for the patient.

Severe attacks of asthma may be helped by the use of oral corticosteroids (e.g., **prednisolone**) starting with a high dose and slowly reducing the daily dose over a six-day period. Some patients will benefit by intermittent courses when necessary, but a few will need a maintenance daily dose of prednisolone with increased dosage during an acute attack. However, a maintenance daily dose of above 7·5 mg of prednisolone (or equivalent dosage for other oral corticosteroids) may produce serious adverse effects. In particular, the body's own production of corticosteroids is suppressed, with all the added dangers from injury, infections and surgery (read adverse effects of corticosteroids, p. 217). In order to minimize these adverse effects corticosteroids should, whenever possible, be given in the mornings in the smallest effective dose.

An alternative to oral corticosteroids may be injections of **adrenocorti-cotrophin hormone (ACTH)** which stimulates the body's adrenal glands to produce corticosteroids, but this is not without danger (see adverse effects of ACTH, p. 220). Nor do long-lasting depot injections of a corticosteroid appear to be that much safer.

One of the most effective ways of administering corticosteroids is via an aerosol. Hoarseness and thrush infections of the throat may occur with their use.

The availability of **aerosol inhalations of corticosteroids** has increased their use in the treatment of chronic asthma. The dose can be significantly reduced in aerosols and yet can be very effective; this reduces the risk of adverse effects. Corticosteroid aerosols must be used regularly to obtain maximum benefit. Preparations of corticosteroids for inhalation include **betamethasone (Bextasol), beclomethasone (Becloforte, Becodisks, Becotide**, in **Ventide**) and **budesonide (Pulmicort))**. *Note that only a small proportion reaches the lungs, the rest is swallowed and absorbed into the bloodstream. This may produce corticosteroid adverse effects (see p. 217).*

If you are on steroids ask for a warning card if you have not got one; also read the section on corticosteroids. The dose of these drugs needs careful adjustment according to the individual's age, sex and weight, and the severity of his disorder.

Corticosteroids are also used to treat certain rare chest diseases such as sarcoidosis and fibrosing alveolitis. Their use in pulmonary tuberculosis is now restricted to those patients with fluid in their pleural cavity (pleural effusion). Corticosteroids may cause old tuberculosis to flare up, and therefore patients with a previous history of tuberculosis should have their chest X-rayed at intervals and be under the care of a chest physician.

Atropine-like drugs (see p. 94) by mouth are not recommended for the relief of bronchospasm. By inhalation they may produce some relief, e.g., **ipratropium (Atrovent)**, particularly in patients suffering from chronic bronchitis. Proprietary preparations for the treatment of asthma often contain an atropine-like drug.

Antihistamine drugs (see p. 125) are of no use in treating bronchial asthma.

Combined Bronchodilator Preparations

There are numerous preparations on the market which combine a bronchodilator with other drugs, for example, with a cough expectorant, with atropine-like drugs and with sedatives. All these preparations are best avoided.

Note: young children needing long-term treatment with a bronchodilator are often given liquid preparations which are sweetened with sucrose and can produce severe dental caries. Always ask for a preparation which does not contain sugar (e.g., **terbutaline (Bricanyl Syrup)**, **reproterol (Bronchodil Elixir)**).

Drugs Used to Treat Nasal Allergy

Hay-fever and nasal allergy (allergic rhinitis) produce unpleasant symptoms which include a runny nose, sneezing and nasal obstruction. These symptoms may be relieved by **nasal decongestants** which are discussed in the section on drugs used to treat the common cold, p. 99. **Oral antihistamine drugs** are also used (p. 125). **Corticosteroids** may be of use to some individuals. These may be administered locally in the nose, e.g., **beclomethasone diproprionate (Beconase)**; **betamethasone sodium phosphate (Betnesol, Vista-Methasone)**, **budesonide (Rhinocort)**, **flunisolide (Syntaris)** and **hydrocortisone acetate** or by depot intramuscular injection (e.g., **methylprednisolone; Depo-Medrone**). **Sodium cromoglycate (Rynacrom)** may help some individuals.

15 Drugs Used to Treat Epilepsy

Epilepsy is characterized by an abnormal and excessive stimulation of the nerve cells in the brain. This results in a fit which may also be called a convulsion or seizure. The excessive stimulation taking place in the brain may be measured on an electroencephalograph (EEG). Epileptic attacks may be caused if the brain is 'irritated' by an infection (e.g., meningitis, encephalitis), by a head injury, by a tumour or by a stroke (a thrombosis or haemorrhage into the brain). The most common type of epilepsy occurs without any recognized abnormality and is therefore called idiopathic epilepsy. This produces a characteristic fit and also a characteristic EEG.

Idiopathic epilepsy includes two main types of epilepsy – grand mal (major epilepsy) and petit mal (minor epilepsy).* Grand mal epilepsy is sometimes preceded by a warning sensation or aura (e.g., flashing lights, a smell, taste or noise), which is followed by a sudden loss of consciousness, then an attack of rigidity and breath-holding, followed by twitching that may last for a minute or two. The person may empty his bladder and foam at the mouth. The attacks may be followed by coma, sleep, confusion or headache. Petit mal attacks are transient attacks of impaired consciousness which may only last a fraction of a second. There are, of course, many degrees of severity of grand mal and petit mal epilepsy. Automatism may follow both types – this is a state in which the patient carries out his normal routine without knowing that he has done so.

There are other types of epilepsy which may be localized to certain parts of the brain – focal or local epilepsy. These may start with contractions of the muscles or abnormal sensations in one area of the body and then spread (e.g., from the fingers to the arm) without the patient losing consciousness. Other local epilepsy attacks may produce sudden changes in mood, e.g., psychomotor epilepsy, which is confined to the temporal lobes of the brain.

In general, the idiopathic epilepsies – grand mal and petit mal – are controlled more easily by drugs than epilepsy secondary to brain irritation caused by injury or disease. Any general depressant of the nervous system will decrease or abolish an epileptic fit but the ones used to treat epilepsy

---

* Grand mal is now referred to as tonic-clonic seizures, petit mal as absence seizures and local epilepsy as partial (focal) seizures.

have been selected because they reduce excessive stimulation in the brain without depressing vital centres (e.g., the respiratory centre) or without sending the patient to sleep. **Bromide** was the first effective anti-epileptic drug (or anti-convulsant) but it is now obsolete. **Phenobarbitone** has been used since the 1910s and **phenytoin** was discovered in the 1930s. Since then numerous anti-convulsant drugs have been introduced.

Like the treatment of any disorder, drug treatment of epilepsy should come after such obvious principles as seeking for and treating causative factors (e.g., infection, tumour), the identification and subsequent avoidance of precipitating factors (e.g., flashing lights, stress), and an awareness of when and where the attacks may come on (e.g., in bed). The selection of the most appropriate drug and dosage regimen is critical to the individual being treated. This takes knowledge, patience and time – it may take several months to get a patient controlled on a particular drug regimen. The dose needs increasing slowly (not more frequently than every week) and if you suffer from epilepsy it needs your cooperation – you must take the drugs strictly as directed and you must record all adverse effects which you experience. You must get involved with the specialist in your treatment – ask him about the drugs and their adverse effects, also ask him about alcohol and driving and having a family and so on. You will learn that there are many false myths about epilepsy.

Anti-convulsant Drugs

These include:

1. Barbiturates	**phenobarbitone (Gardenal sodium, Luminal)**
	methylphenobarbitone (Prominal)
2. Barbiturate-related drugs	**primidone (Mysoline)**
3. Hydantoins	**phenytoin (Epanutin)**
4. Succimides	**ethosuximide (Emeside, Zarontin)**
5. Benzodiazepines	**clobazam (Frisium)**
	clonazepam (Rivotril)
	diazepam (Diazemuls, Stesolid, Valium)
	lorazepam (Ativan)
6. Other drugs	**beclamide (Nydrane)**
	carbamazepine (Tegretol)
	sodium valproate (Epilim)

The objective of treatment is to prevent fits by maintaining an effective concentration of drug in the blood and hence in the brain at all times. The aim is to achieve maximum benefit for the minimum use of drugs. No drug should be stopped abruptly and a changeover of drugs should take several weeks.

Driving

Patients suffering from epilepsy may drive a motor vehicle (but not a heavy goods vehicle or public service vehicle) provided they have been free from fits for a period of two years and if they have only had fits in their sleep over a three-year period. If you develop drowsiness from your drugs then you should not drive or operate moving machinery.

Pregnancy

The risk of anti-epileptic drugs producing abnormalities in the baby are slight and this must be balanced against the risk of stopping the drugs during pregnancy. Phenytoin can reduce the effectiveness of oral contraceptives.

The Use of Anti-Convulsants

Grand mal epilepsy and focal epilepsy. The most frequently used drugs include **carbamazepine**, **clonazepam**, **phenobarbitone**, **phenytoin**, **primidone** and **sodium valproate**.

Petit mal. The most frequently used drugs include **ethosuximide** and **sodium valproate**.

Myoclonus. Drugs used to treat this disorder include **clonazepam** and **sodium valproate**.

At the start of treatment, frequent blood-level monitoring should be carried out until the patient is stabilized. Regular monitoring of the patient should then follow in order to ensure effective blood levels, suppression of fits and minimal adverse effects. Dosage regimens should be as simple as possible and multiple drug therapy should be avoided. Children break down anti-convulsant drugs more quickly than adults and will require more regular and higher dosing throughout the 24 hours. Treatment should aim at keeping the individual free from fits for two to three years and then the drug should be slowly tapered off and stopped. Sudden withdrawal may cause status epilepticus.

Drugs Used in Status Epilepticus

Diazepam or **clonazepam** should be given intravenously. They must be given with caution because of the risk of respiratory depression and they may produce thrombophlebitis at the site of infection. If the attacks do not subside or if they return an intravenous infusion of **chlormethiazole** should be used. Intravenous **paraldehyde** is an alternative and sometimes intravenous **phenytoin sodium** may help if other drugs fail.

Parkinsonism is a disorder of the nervous system in which voluntary movement is disturbed, involuntary movements occur and the tone of muscles is altered. Voluntary movements become slow and shaky (tremor) and muscles become stiff (rigidity). The group of signs and symptoms produced are usually referred to as the 'Parkinson's syndrome' or simply as 'Parkinsonism'. There are several causes and the severity of the disorders varies between patients. A not infrequent cause these days is the long-term use of the major tranquillizer group of drugs.

To function properly, two centres in the brain responsible for controlling movement must maintain a correct balance between the chemical transmitter systems, **acetylcholine** and **dopamine**. They are thought to work like the two opposing chemical transmitters in the peripheral autonomic nervous system – acetylcholine and adrenaline. These two processes in the brain are often referred to as the cholinergic system and the dopaminergic system respectively. In Parkinsonism the dopaminergic system appears to be defective so that the control mechanisms of movement become unbalanced and the cholinergic system dominates the control. Chemical suppression of this dominance may, therefore, be applied by the use of drugs which block or interfere with the action of acetylcholine (e.g., by the use of anticholinergic drugs). Alternatively, drugs which increase the effect of the dopaminergic system will have beneficial effects (e.g., the use of levodopa or amantadine).

The main aim of treatment in Parkinsonism is to try to improve both the difficulty in starting movements and the slowness of movement (bradykinesia), and to reduce tremor and muscle rigidity.

For over a century Parkinsonism has been treated with anticholinergic drugs. Atropine was the first to be used and since then many atropine-like drugs have been used. Antihistamines have also been used (such as promethazine and diphenhydramine) but these may have helped because they produce mild atropine-like effects (read the section on antihistamine drugs). Many other drugs have been claimed to be of benefit in treating patients suffering from Parkinsonism but the real advance in recent years has been the discovery of the effects of levodopa.

Anticholinergic Drugs

There is a wide choice of anticholinergic drugs available for the treatment of Parkinsonism. These include **benzhexol (Artane, Bentex, Broflex), benztropine (Cogentin), methixene (Tremonil), orphenadrine (Biorphen, Disipal)** and **procyclidine (Arpicolin, Kemadrin)**.

The anticholinergic drugs are discussed on pp. 93–4. Their beneficial effects in Parkinsonism are very limited. Muscle rigidity and tremors may be helped but bradykinesia (slowness of movement), one of the most disturbing effects of Parkinsonism, is unaffected by them.

The adverse effects produced by these drugs are like those of atropine and are the result of their actions upon the parasympathetic division of the autonomic nervous system. These atropine-like effects include blurred vision, constipation, dryness of the mouth, retention of urine, thirst, dry skin, rapid beating of the heart, flushing, dizziness and vomiting. Toxic doses may produce high temperature, rash, hallucinations and delirium (particularly in the elderly). The different drugs available may produce some or all of these effects in varying intensities according to dosage. They should be used with caution in patients with enlarged prostate glands and in those patients with heart disorders. They should not be used in patients with closed-angle glaucoma or in patients who are receiving monoamine oxidase inhibitor antidepressants or in patients who have received these drugs in the previous fourteen days. Their effects may be increased by other drugs, e.g., major tranquillizers and antihistamines. The dosage of these drugs should be slowly reduced before stopping them since sudden withdrawal may produce severe rigidity and tremor.

Anticholinergic drugs exert an increased effect (synergistic effect) when used with levodopa and they are useful in reducing sialorrhoea (excess salivation). They are useful for reducing drug induced Parkinsonism in patients receiving anti-psychotic drugs. Tardive dyskinesia is not improved by anticholinergic drugs and may be made worse. The choice of drug is not critical and they may be taken before food if dry mouth is a problem or after food if they produce stomach upsets.

Levodopa

Levodopa (Brocadopa, Larodopa) is the chemical forerunner (precursor) of **dopamine** (which does not cross from the blood into the brain). Although levodopa is quickly converted to dopamine in the body, sufficient enters the brain to be effective if it is given in high dosage. The worst features of Parkinsonism – difficulty in starting movement and slowness of movement – improve during treatment with levodopa. This is often impressive, resulting in improvement in walking, eating and talking. The rigidity is also helped and other effects of Parkinsonism such as difficulty in balancing, drooling of saliva from the mouth and involuntary eye movements may also improve slowly. Shaking is less frequently improved.

Levodopa may produce many adverse effects which are related to dosage. These include nausea, loss of appetite, fall in blood pressure, disorders of heart rhythm, insomnia, vivid dreams, restlessness, agitation, aggression, delusions, paranoia, mania and mental depression. In particular abnormal involuntary movements (dyskinesia) of the tongue, lips, face and limbs may occur as well as jerking (tremors with muscle spasms). Levodopa should be given with caution to patients with impaired function of the heart or circulation and also to patients with psychological disorders. Its effects may be decreased by phenothiazine major tranquillizers, methyldopa and reserpine and increased by anticholinergic drugs such as atropine. It should never be given to patients receiving or who have received M.A.O. inhibitors in the previous two weeks. It should also be given with caution to patients receiving sympathomimetic drugs, e.g., isoprenaline, amphetamines, or sympatholytic drugs such as guanethidine (used to treat raised blood pressure) because of the risk of drug interactions. **Pyridoxine** (vitamin B_6) in small doses blocks the effects of levodopa and since this vitamin is often present in tonics patients taking levodopa should check with their pharmacist or doctor whether such preparations may be taken. This does not occur if levodopa is given with a decarboxylase inhibitor (see below).

A major problem with levodopa is that it is rapidly metabolized in the body into dopamine which cannot cross the blood–brain barrier whereas levodopa can. When given in high dosage sufficient levodopa enters the brain, where it is converted into dopamine. However, adverse effects of levodopa are dose related. **Carbidopa** and **benserazide** block levodopa metabolism in the body by inhibiting the enzyme dopa-decarboxylase but do not enter the brain. They cannot therefore interfere with the conversion of levodopa to dopamine in the brain. When these are given along with levodopa, the metabolism of levodopa outside the brain is blocked and the blood level of levodopa increases. An effective treatment, therefore, is to give a dose of levodopa and carbidopa or benserazide together. The addition markedly reduces the dose of levodopa necessary. When giving carbidopa or benserazide and levodopa separately there is a risk that too high a dose of levodopa may be given. Therefore a fixed-dose preparation is used, e.g., **carbidopa** and **levodopa (Sinemet)** or **benserazide** and **levodopa (Madopar)**. This also ensures the appropriate dose of each.

Amantadine

Amantadine (Symmetrel) is thought to work by acting on nerve endings to produce the release of dopamine. In some patients it may be beneficial to all three main factors of Parkinsonism – bradykinesia, rigidity and tremor – but less so than with levodopa. It may produce indigestion, excitement, difficulty in concentrating, dizziness, slurred speech, mental depression, insomnia, lethargy, nausea, loss of appetite, vomiting, discoloration of the skin, dry mouth, ankle swelling and rarely a reduction in white blood cells (leucopenia). Overdose may produce convulsions. It should be given with caution to patients with peptic ulcers, to the elderly, and to patients taking amphetamines and other stimulants. It should not be given to patients with epilepsy. It may increase the effects of anticholinergic drugs. It is sometimes used in combination with levodopa, particularly in patients who are unable to tolerate full therapeutic doses of levodopa. More study is needed to evaluate its use in the treatment of Parkinsonism.

Bromocriptine (Parlodel) stimulates dopamine receptors and is worth trying when other drugs fail. It may produce confusion and abnormal involuntary movements.

Selegiline (Eldepryl) is a monoamine oxidase (B) inhibitor which increases the effects of levodopa. It is generally used when the effects of levodopa begin to wear off.

In order to improve benefits and reduce the risks a combination of the above drugs is generally used.

17   Antihistamine Drugs

Allergy

In defence against infecting organisms, the body produces antibodies which combine with protein in the organisms to neutralize any effects which they may have upon the body. By means of this defence mechanism the body develops resistance or immunity. This often gives protection against reinfection by the same organism (e.g., you never get chicken pox twice). An antibody is a protein (globulin) which reacts only with the protein of the infecting organism (usually called an antigen) responsible for its formation. There is no cross antibody formation to other organisms (cross immunity), for example, between measles and polio. Sometimes renewed exposure to an infection produces a different or altered response – this is called allergy which is the result of the body having been sensitized to that organism. Allergy to 'organisms' is rare and most allergy is to a foreign protein (i.e., a protein not made by your body and not known to your own defence systems).

Foreign proteins (allergens) include drugs, house dust, pollens, certain foods and all sorts of things. These are usually grouped under the general term allergens. The reason why some people become sensitized and not others is not understood – we are all, for example, exposed to pollen grains and yet some of us will develop hay-fever and others will not. Nor is the nature of allergic reactions fully understood; it may be a fault in the immunity mechanisms resulting in faulty antibody protection or it may be due to an inherited defect in the tissues concerned.

The features of the allergic reaction are largely due to the release locally or into the blood-stream of a chemical called histamine and several other chemicals. A single allergen may cause reactions at several sites; thus a patient sensitive to a certain food may develop stomach symptoms, a rash and wheezing. Allergens may affect the body through the skin (e.g., contact dermatitis due to cosmetics), in the food (e.g., allergy to strawberries), by inhalation (e.g., hay-fever and asthma due to grass pollens), and by injections (e.g., insect bites and allergy to anti-tetanus serum). The resulting reactions may appear as skin rashes; swelling of the eyelids, face, lips and throat; as abdominal symptoms (vomiting, diarrhoea and colic); or commonly as hay-fever (itching eyes, running nose and sore throat) or as wheezing (asthma). Allergic reactions may be sudden and transient, e.g., sneezing, or last for years, e.g., eczema. They may be trivial, or so serious as to cause sudden death from what is called anaphylactic shock – collapse of the circulation, fall in blood pressure and acute asthma. This usually occurs in patients given an injection which contains a protein to which they have already been made sensitive by a previous injection (e.g., anti-tetanus serum; bee stings). It is rare.

One of the chemicals mainly responsible for allergic reactions is histamine; it is present in most tissues of the body and is released when cells are injured. It causes the small vessels of the body (capillaries) to open up, particularly those in the skin, making it hot and red. It also makes the vessels more permeable so that plasma flows from inside the blood vessels out into the surrounding tissues to produce swelling (oedema). When histamine is injected into the human skin it produces what is called a triple response: (i) a localized red spot which extends within a few seconds, reaches a maximum in about a minute and then becomes bluish; (ii) a bright red 'flame' spreads out from this spot and (iii) local swelling occurs forming a weal. (This reaction is often associated with itching and pain.) Histamine also causes the blood vessels in the brain to dilate, which produces a headache. It causes a fall in blood pressure and may increase the heart rate. Large doses may produce shock (collapse). It stimulates the muscles of the small bronchial tubes to produce constriction resulting in asthma and it stimulates the production of acid in the stomach. It is released in anaphylactic shock, allergy and injury. Its concentration is particularly high in the skin, stomach lining and in the lungs.

The release of histamine does not account for all allergic reactions and it is obvious that what was thought to be a straightforward antigen antibody reaction is not so. There is a whole spectrum of allergic responses both direct and indirect which accounts for the lack of effect of antihistamine drugs in some cases: in fact the drugs themselves may sometimes produce an allergic response.

Any chemical that causes tissue damage will cause the release of histamine but some drugs may do this with little sign of tissue damage. The allergic effects produced by drugs may vary from an itchy skin rash to death from anaphylactic shock. The release of histamine may be caused by a physical process – e.g., sunburn, cold, light and friction – as well as by drugs. Pressure on the skin may release histamine and some people can write their name on their skin (dermatographia). The juice of the stinging nettle contains histamine which produces a skin rash called urticaria (nettle-rash). This sort of rash may also appear in patients with psychological disorders. In fact most allergic disorders may be aggravated by emotional disturbances.

Antihistamines

H₁ Antihistamines Used to Treat Allergy

astemizole (Hismanal)
azatadine (Optimine)
brompheniramine (Dimotane)
chlorpheniramine (Alunex, Piriton)
clemastine (Tavegil)
cyproheptadine (Periactin)
dimethindene (Fenostil)
diphenylpyraline (Histryl, Lergoban)
mebhydrolin (Fabahistin)
mepyramine maleate (Anthisan)
mequitazine (Primalan)
oxatomide (Tinset)
phenindamine (Thephorin)
pheniramine (Daneral SA)
promethazine (Phenergan)
terfenadine (Triludan)
trimeprazine (Vallergan)
triprolidine (Actidil, Pro-Actidil)

For antihistamines used to treat nausea, vomiting and motion sickness see p. 132.

The conventional antihistamines block the action of histamine at peripheral (H₁) receptor sites but have no effect on its gastric acid secretory action (H₂) receptor sites. They antagonize in varying degrees most, but not all, of the effects produced by histamine. They may also reduce the intensity of allergic and anaphylactic reactions. They act, not by preventing the release of histamine, but by occupying its sites of action. They block its action on the muscles of the gut and bronchial tubes, they reduce the weal produced by histamine and they reduce hay-fever symptoms, itching skin rashes and swelling. They have no effect upon stomach secretions.

In addition to their actions in blocking the effects of histamine the antihistamines also produce other effects, particularly upon the brain. In some patients they may cause stimulation. But their usual effect is to depress the brain, leading to drowsiness and sleep; in overdose this may lead to excitation and convulsions. Their depressing effect upon the brain means that they can also be used to reduce motion sickness. Some, but not all, antihistamines have this property, and those that do may also be used to prevent nausea, vomiting and dizziness.

In effective dosage all antihistamines produce adverse effects but these vary from individual to individual and from drug to drug. The commonest is drowsiness; others include dizziness, noises in the ears, lack of coordination, fatigue, blurred vision, double vision, changes of mood, nervousness, delusions, hallucinations, insomnia and tremors, loss of appetite, nausea, vomiting, diarrhoea or constipation, dryness of the mouth, cough, frequency and difficulty in passing urine, palpitations, headache, tightness in the chest, tingling, heaviness and weakness of the hands. You may even become allergic to an antihistamine, particularly if it is applied to the skin. Very rarely, antihistamines may cause serious blood disorders.

Terfenadine (Triludan) and **astemizole (Hismanal)** produce less drowsiness than other antihistamines.

Those antihistamines that block H_2 receptors are called H_2 receptor blockers (or **H_2 antihistamines**) and are used to treat patients suffering from peptic ulcers (see p. 139). Examples of H_2 receptor blockers include **cimetidine (Tagamet)** and **ranitidine (Zantac)**.

Use of H_1 Antihistamines

There are numerous antihistamines to choose from and, bearing in mind individual variations in response, it is often a matter of trial and error before you find one that will relieve your particular allergic symptoms and produce a minimum of adverse effects.

1. Antihistamines are useful in relieving the symptoms of seasonal hay-fever (pollinosis) but they have no effect upon the cause.

2. They are virtually useless in treating asthma, including allergic asthma.

3. They may relieve allergic swelling of the face but are of little value if the swelling affects the throat and threatens life. Furthermore they are of little value in anaphylactic reactions.

4. Only about half the patients who suffer from perennial nasal congestion, running nose and sneezing (hay-fever) respond to antihistamines. Similarly they are of very doubtful and unproven value in cough medicines; in fact they may have undesirable effects because they dry the lining of the nose and respiratory tract, impairing natural defence systems. Apart from providing some relief from a running nose, they are of no benefit in treating the common cold.

5. Some skin rashes such as allergic nettle-rash (urticaria) respond well to antihistamines by mouth. Long-standing rashes are little affected.

Antihistamines by mouth may be used to relieve itching. When applied to the skin, there is a danger of producing allergic dermatitis. Given by mouth or injection they relieve the itching and swelling produced by insect bites.

6. They are of use in relieving the rash in serum sickness (an allergic reaction following the injection of a serum), but they do not help tne fever and joint pains very much.

7. They are of benefit in treating blood transfusion reactions.

8. They are of no value in treating allergic reactions affecting the stomach or gut – nausea, vomiting, diarrhoea.

9. Many drug reactions respond well to antihistamines – but do not forget to stop the drug that caused the reaction.

10. Some antihistamines are effective in preventing motion sickness.

11. Some are useful sedatives.

Warnings: You must by now realize that antihistamine drugs are complex chemicals which have many actions in the body and produce numerous effects including adverse effects ranging from loss of appetite to serious blood disorders. They increase the effects produced by alcohol and sedative drugs and interfere with your mental function. If they make you drowsy you should not drive a motor vehicle or operate moving machinery. Overdose with these drugs is serious and difficult to treat.

Antihistamines may produce alarming reactions in some children (stimulation, fever and convulsions) and reports have associated high dosages of **cyclizine**, and **meclozine** with abnormalities in new-born babies, although these reports have not been fully confirmed.

Because of the variations in response between individuals taking antihistamines it is often necessary to try different ones. If a drug does not relieve your symptoms within about three days it is unlikely to do so at all. If it produces drowsiness take it at bed-time. Always take antihistamines with food because they irritate the stomach. If you are just starting a course, try taking the first dose on a Friday and then you have the week-end to overcome or become accustomed to the adverse effects. Avoid prolonged-release preparations until you know the nature and intensity of the adverse effects caused by the antihistamine drug in question. Prolonged-release preparations are most useful taken at bed-time in order to reduce early-morning symptoms.

Desensitization (hyposensitization)

Hay-fever, urticaria, allergic asthma, contact dermatitis and other allergic disorders are often due to over-sensitivity to certain agents, e.g., foods, pollens, fur, feathers, dust, hair, mites and cosmetics. Contact dermatitis of the skin may occur to drugs (e.g., streptomycin), metals (e.g., nickel buttons on blue jeans), plants (e.g., primula), paint, resins and cosmetics. Most people get to know what they are sensitive to and can avoid that substance in future. In some cases it is not possible to identify or to avoid a particular substance, e.g., hay-fever. Therefore, skin tests to certain allergens may be carried out, although the results of these tests are often difficult to assess. If you are found to be sensitive to an inhaled allergen, e.g., grass pollen, then you may be desensitized by having a series of injections of the allergen under the skin at intervals using gradually increasing strengths. These courses are usually given in winter and may have to be repeated for several years. There are several preparations of allergens on the market, some contain a mixture of commonly occurring allergens (e.g., grass pollens) and others are prepared individually for each person's requirements after skin tests with a wide range of allergens. Desensitization is of little use in skin allergies and drug reactions. They do not cure although they may reduce the severity of the symptoms.

The value of desensitization* is very limited. It may be of benefit to patients with specific allergy to grass pollens or house dust mite. Diagnostic skin testing is unreliable. Wasp and bee venom desensitization may be of benefit. Multiple desensitization is not recommended since it may precipitate an acute allergic reaction, particularly in children.

Allergic Emergencies

An allergic emergency (anaphylactic shock) requires prompt action:

1. **Adrenaline** – intramuscularly in a dose of 0·5–1·0 mg (0·5–1 ml of 1 in 1,000 adrenaline solution) repeated every 15 minutes until improvement occurs.

2. **Chlorpheniramine** – by subcutaneous or intramuscular injection or slow by intravenous infusion: 10–20 mg when necessary to a maximum dose of 40 mg in 24 hours.

3. **Hydrocortisone** (sodium succinate or sodium phosphate) by intravenous injection in a dose of 100–300 mg.

N.B. For the use of **sodium cromoglycate** in the treatment of bronchial asthma and nasal allergy see pp. 114, 116 and read about the drug in Part Three.

The Reduction of Acid in the Stomach

H₂ antihistamines used to treat peptic ulcers are discussed on p. 139.

---

* Deaths occur every year from densitization. It should only be given where full resuscitation facilities are available.

18 Drugs Used to Treat Nausea, Vomiting and Motion Sickness

Nausea and vomiting are symptoms. These symptoms may occur with all kinds of physical disorders, some of which are quite simple and short-lived such as food poisoning, and some very serious and long-lasting, such as cancer of the stomach or a brain tumour. Drugs often cause nausea and vomiting (e.g., morphine, digitalis, oestrogens) and so may motion, pregnancy and emotion (e.g., the sight of a severely injured road-accident victim). Nausea and vomiting may serve a useful purpose – as in food poisoning – but usually they are distressing symptoms which need relieving.

There is a vomiting centre in the brain which responds to stimulations from the stomach and gut and also from the brain. Another part of the brain seems to respond to chemical stimulation. It is thought that this area is stimulated by certain drugs (e.g., morphine) and also by chemicals produced in the body (e.g., in diabetes or kidney failure). Two groups of drugs help to prevent vomiting and are thought to work on the vomiting centre. These are the anticholinergic drugs (see p. 94) and antihistamines (see p. 127). A third group, the phenothiazines (see major tranquillizers, p. 68), are useful in preventing vomiting when it is due to drugs or toxic reactions in the body. However, there is an overlap between the effects produced by these drugs. Antihistamines resemble anticholinergic drugs in some respects.

Motion Sickness

Movement can affect the organ of balance, which has associations with the vomiting centre. For example, motion produced by travelling in a car, on a boat or on a roundabout stimulates the organ of balance. This stimulates the vomiting centre, resulting in the feeling of nausea (sweating, salivation, rapid beating of the heart and the feeling you are going to vomit) and vomiting. Motion sickness is more common in children. Certain movements, e.g., swinging, will make some people sick, whilst others who are not made sick by swinging may become sick at sea. There are numerous physical, social and psychological factors involved in motion sickness: fortunately tolerance to motion develops over a period of several days.

Drugs Used to Treat Motion Sickness

The aim of drug use should be to try to prevent an attack of motion sickness developing. A short-acting drug should be taken for a short journey and a long-acting one for a long journey. Many drugs are effective, provided the right dose is taken at the right time. Unwanted adverse effects are drowsiness, blurred vision and dry mouth.

Anticholinergic drugs. These drugs may produce blurred vision, dry mouth and rapid beating of the heart (see adverse effects of atropine, p. 94). They should not be used in patients with glaucoma or in those patients who may develop retention of urine (e.g., men with enlarged prostate glands). They are short acting and are therefore useful for relieving motion sickness on short journeys (up to half a day). Their prolonged use for this purpose is not satisfactory because of troublesome adverse effects. They usually contain **atropine** or **hyoscine (scopolamine; Kwells, Sereen)**. *Alcohol should be avoided. The drugs may interfere with your ability to drive a motor vehicle.*

Antihistamine drugs. There is a marked variation between individuals in their response to antihistamines (see adverse effects of antihistamines, p. 127). *The most common adverse effect is drowsiness, but in infants and young children antihistamines may produce stimulation, making them nervous and unable to sleep. Do not drink alcohol on the same day that you have taken an antihistamine drug. They may interfere with your ability to drive a motor vehicle and they may increase the effects of other depressant drugs such as sedatives, tranquillizers and sleeping drugs.*

The antihistamines most often used to treat motion sickness are: **cinnarizine (Stugeron); cinnarizine (Marzine), cyclizine (Valoid); dimenhydrinate (Dramamine); meclozine (Sea-Legs); promethazine (Avomine)**.

Vomiting in Pregnancy

Vomiting in pregnancy is probably due to hormonal changes which occur in the early months of pregnancy. In addition there are numerous psychological, social and dietary factors. Excessive vomiting may lead to an alteration in blood chemistry, which then causes further vomiting. Although it is preferable that all 'unnecessary' drugs should be avoided during early pregnancy, some doctors continue to prescribe a great variety of drugs to control vomiting in pregnancy. These include anticholinergic drugs, antihistamines and phenothiazine tranquillizers.

The main considerations should be: how much distress is being caused by the vomiting and what effects may these drugs have upon the unborn child?

A decision in the light of these considerations is not easy. Vomiting in pregnancy is extremely distressing, the patient needs sound advice, understanding and careful support.

You and your doctor are going to see each other many times during your ante-natal care and so the initial visit, when you complain of feeling sick, is as good a time as any for your doctor to really get to know you and for you to begin to learn about what forms good ante-natal care.

Drugs Used to Treat Vomiting in Pregnancy

Anticholinergic drugs (for adverse effects, see p. 94). **Dicyclomine (Merbentyl)**.

Antihistamine drugs (for adverse effects, see p. 127). **Cyclizine*; meclozine*; promethazine (Avomine)**.

Phenothiazine drugs (for adverse effects, see p. 70, under chlorpromazine). **Chlorpromazine (Largactil); prochlorperazine (Buccastem, Stemetil, Vertigon); thiethylperazine (Torecan); trifluoperazine (Stelazine)**.

Because deficiency of vitamin B_6 **(pyridoxine)** can occur in severe continuous vomiting it is widely used to treat vomiting in pregnancy, although there has been no proof that a deficiency of pyridoxine occurs in this disorder. It is usually taken in combination with an anti-vomiting drug.

Other Vomiting Disorders

Drug-induced vomiting, post-anaesthetic vomiting, vomiting due to disease, and radiation sickness are best treated with phenothiazine drugs such as **chlorpromazine (Largactil)** or an antihistamine such as **cyclizine (Marzine)** or **promazine (Sparine)**. Anticholinergic drugs are of little use. **Metoclopramide (Gastrobid, Gastromax, Maxolon, Metox, Metramid, Parmid, Primperan)** and **domperidone (Evoxin, Motilium)** are dopamine receptor antagonists. They are very useful in relieving nausea and vomiting due to anti-cancer drugs and post-operative vomiting. Domperidone produces fewer effects on the brain (e.g., drowsiness and dystonias, particularly in children) than does metoclopramide. They both have a peripheral effect and may be better than the phenothiazines in treating sickness due to gastro-intestinal, liver or gall-bladder disease. Metoclopramide has not been found to be very helpful for motion sickness or pregnancy sickness. **Nabilone (Cesamet)** is a synthetic cannabis drug which may help to relieve nausea and vomiting caused by anti-cancer drugs.

---

* NOTE There is still a suspicion that cyclizine and meclozine may produce abnormalities in the unborn baby if given in high doses.

Dizziness (vertigo)

The term vertigo is used to describe sensations of movements within the head or in the environment. It is always accompanied by a disturbance of balance and if severe can be associated with sweating, pallor, nausea, vomiting and occasionally diarrhoea and fainting. It may be caused by disorders of the eyes, brain, organ of balance, and ears. The organ of balance may be disturbed by infections (labyrinthitis) and by drugs such as streptomycin, quinine or aspirin. Dizziness and giddiness are much more vague. They are highly subjective feelings and may be associated with all manner of disorders.

An incredible mixture of drugs are used to treat vertigo. These include the anti-vomiting drugs (anticholinergic drugs, antihistamines and phenothiazines), drugs which dilate blood vessels, sedatives, tranquillizers, antidepressants and vitamins. As often stated in this book, where there is no specific treatment for a disorder there are numerous remedies.

Ménière's Disease

This is a most unpleasant disorder which is characterized by recurrent attacks of vertigo associated with noises in the ears (tinnitus) and progressive nerve deafness. Men get it more than women and most attacks develop between the ages of forty and sixty years of age. It is self-limiting and spontaneous recovery occurs at any stage. Patients with Ménière's disease get very anxious and depressed and therefore need a lot of sympathy and understanding.

The drug treatment of Ménière's disease is as confused as the drug treatment of vertigo and dizziness. In an acute phase the patient is unwilling to move his head because he may vomit. In between attacks any of the drugs mentioned under the treatment of dizziness may be tried.

Hyoscine, an **antihistamine** or a **phenothiazine** are useful for preventing attacks. **Betahistine (Serc)** and **cinnarizine (Stugeron)** are promoted for the treatment of Ménière's disease. In an acute attack an injection or a suppository of **chlorpromazine (Largactil), cyclizine (Valoid), prochlorperazine (Stemetil, Vertigon)** or **thiethylperazine (Torecan)** is useful.

19 Drugs Used to Treat Indigestion and Peptic Ulcers

The middle and upper parts of the stomach act as a reservoir for food; the part near its outlet into the duodenum contracts and relaxes to churn and mix the food. The rate of emptying of the stomach varies with the volume of contents: the greater the volume the faster the rate of emptying. A fatty meal delays emptying; so does an increase in stomach acidity. Some drugs increase and some decrease the rate of emptying of the stomach. Another important function of the stomach is to make digestive juice. This contains hydrochloric acid (about one and a half litres are produced every day), mucus which protects the surface of the stomach and an enzyme called pepsin which helps to digest protein in food.

The stomach can get 'upset' if its lining is irritated (e.g., by aspirin or alcohol), by eating too much, by eating some unusual food or by virus or bacterial infections. The lining of the stomach can also become 'inflamed' (gastritis). This may be caused or aggravated by many things; for example, certain foods (pickles, fried food), alcohol and smoking. This irritation or inflammation may produce symptoms such as discomfort, nausea, pain, loss of appetite and heartburn. These symptoms are usually referred to as indigestion or dyspepsia. Sometimes the surface of the stomach may ulcerate to produce a peptic ulcer. A peptic ulcer may occur in the oesophagus (gullet), stomach (where it may be called a gastric ulcer) and in the duodenum (duodenal ulcer).

Relatively little is known about the factors which cause peptic ulcers but there is evidence that acid and pepsin are partly responsible. However, 'normal' stomachs do not develop ulcers. Therefore, the 'normal' lining of the stomach must be protective, and it may be something affecting this protection that causes ulcers. This may be related to the mucus that covers the surface, the ability of the mucous cells to renew themselves every few days, the nutrition of the stomach itself, its blood supply, and various chemical factors. There are other factors such as heredity (there is often a family history), seasonal factors, diet, smoking, alcohol, and particularly worry and stress.

The symptoms of peptic ulcer usually start with 'indigestion' but may start with acute pain, or bleeding or perforation. Indigestion going on for more than several days may be due to a peptic ulcer, particularly if the episodes keep recurring and if accompanied by pain rather than 'discomfort'. Pain from a duodenal ulcer often comes on when you are hungry and it wakes you in the night; whereas a gastric ulcer pain may come on fairly soon after food. Food, antacids or vomiting may relieve peptic ulcer pains.

You should always consult your doctor if you have indigestion lasting more than a few weeks or recurring at intervals – you may have a peptic ulcer. The treatment of a peptic ulcer includes advice on diet – which means taking a well-balanced diet and frequent, regular small meals. You should avoid alcohol and any foods which you know give you pain. You should stop taking coffee and avoid any drugs known to irritate the stomach; for example, aspirin, corticosteroids (e.g., prednisolone) and most drugs used to treat rheumatism and arthritis. You should also stop smoking. There is no point in filling yourself full of indigestion mixture whilst continuing to smoke and drink alcohol. If you are worried, anxious or tense then you need help and advice on sorting out the stresses which are affecting you.

The main drugs used to treat peptic ulcers fall into three groups – drugs which neutralize the acid in the stomach (antacids), drugs which reduce the production of acid by the stomach cells and drugs which help to protect the stomach lining.

1 Drugs which Neutralize the Acid in the Stomach

Antacids neutralize the acid in the stomach contents and this process relieves pain. This is a specific action and yet antacid preparations are swallowed in huge amounts by millions of people for the relief of numerous minor symptoms of indigestion totally unrelated to acid production. Unfortunately, the presence of antacids in the stomach may actually increase the amount of acid produced, so an antacid like calcium carbonate may leave the patient with more acid in his stomach than before he took the antacid – this is often called an acid rebound. You will get initial relief followed by a flare-up of pain.

Antacids relieve the pain of a peptic ulcer and if taken appropriately may help to heal ulcers.

The benefits of antacid consumption are difficult to evaluate because according to advertisements we are all suffering from 'acid indigestion'. Of course, this is not true but this carefree use of antacids distorts their real value in the treatment of disorders such as peptic ulcers, where, if taken in appropriate dosages, they can help ulcer healing.

Antacids usually consist of mixtures of various **base salts of sodium, magnesium, calcium, aluminium** and **bismuth**. The amount needed to neutralize stomach acid depends upon the rate of acid production by the stomach, the presence or absence of food, and upon the rate of emptying of the stomach. Antacids may be classified according to whether they produce an effect upon the rest of the body (systemic effect) or produce just a local effect in the stomach (non-systemic). A **systemic antacid** is absorbed into the blood-stream and produces changes in the chemistry of the blood. This effect is often of no consequence because the kidneys quickly restore the chemical balance. However, in patients with impaired kidney function this may be dangerous. **Non-systemic antacids** form insoluble compounds in the stomach which are not absorbed.

Sodium bicarbonate relieves pain rapidly, but its effects quickly wear off and it may cause changes in the blood chemistry. It releases carbon dioxide gas into the stomach which causes belching (this makes some people think it is working effect' /ely) but it may also cause distension of the stomach, which is unpleasant. It is useful for quick relief but there is nothing to recommend its continued use. Patients with impaired heart or kidney function should not use it. Also, it should not be used by patients with fluid retention (oedema) because it increases the blood salt level and may cause further retention of water by the kidneys.

Magnesium hydroxide is slow to act but its effects are fairly long lasting. **Magnesium oxide** is converted to magnesium hydroxide in water but it may not react completely with water or acid before it is emptied from the stomach. **Magnesium carbonate** is fairly slow to act. **Magnesium trisilicate** is slow to act and has a prolonged action.

Magnesium salts may cause diarrhoea and some magnesium may be absorbed into the blood-stream – they should not be used in patients with impaired kidney function.

Calcium carbonate acts quickly and effectively. Some calcium is absorbed into the blood-stream. Many patients with peptic ulcers are put on milk diets (which are high in calcium) and therefore patients who take milk and calcium carbonate regularly for long periods of time may develop a high level of blood calcium, which may cause a group of symptoms – loss of appetite, nausea, vomiting, headache, weakness, abdominal pains, constipation and thirst. This is often called the milk-alkali syndrome ('syndrome' being the term used to indicate a group of signs and symptoms). Temporary or permanent kidney damage may occur. **Calcium salts** tend to constipate; they are, therefore, often given mixed with magnesium salts.

Aluminium hydroxide is slow to act but quicker than magnesium trisilicate. It does not alter the blood chemistry because it forms insoluble complexes in the stomach. It forms these complexes with certain antibiotic drugs (tetracyclines). It may also interfere with the absorption of iron. Aluminium hydroxide is not superior to other insoluble alkalis and differences in antacid effects may vary tremendously between different commercial preparations of aluminium antacids. **Aluminium compounds** constipate; for example, aluminium silicate (kaolin) is used to treat diarrhoea. **Dihydroxyaluminium sodium carbonate** and **dihydroxy-aluminium aminoacetate** are alternatives but have not been shown to be more effective.

Bismuth salts are not very effective as antacids and may produce toxic effects when absorbed.

The Use of Antacids

Antacids relieve the pain of uncomplicated peptic ulcer. They are also useful in relieving the pain of hiatus hernia and inflammation of the gullet (oesophagitis). They are less effective in gastritis, in which acid production is often reduced. None of the available antacids is ideal. They vary in their rate and duration of action and in the amounts required to neutralize the acid contents of the stomach. Liquid preparations and powders mixed with water are more effective than tablets. Tablets should be sucked slowly between meals; their routine use after meals to prevent symptoms is of no use. Because no specific antacid can be recommended, mixtures are generally used. Mixtures also help to avoid bowel complications such as diarrhoea from magnesium salts and constipation from calcium or aluminium salts.

Antacids interfere with the absorption of many drugs and should not be taken with other medicines. Some have a high sodium content (salt) and should not be used by patients having treatment for raised blood pressure, heart failure, liver failure or in pregnancy – *always check with your pharmacist or doctor*.

Some antacid mixtures contain drugs which disperse wind (e.g., **activated dimethicone**) and drugs which spread the antacid over the surface of the stomach and act as anti-foaming agents. These latter include **co-dried gels** and **complexes of silicates and alginic acid**. They are useful in the treatment of gastro-oesophageal reflux and hiatus hernia.

For repeated use, preparations containing systemic (absorbable) antacids such as sodium bicarbonate should be avoided. Comparable antacid preparations are not necessarily equivalent in their ability to neutralize the acid. Do not forget that the speed of action of antacids depends upon their ability to neutralize the acid in the stomach. This depends principally upon the speed with which they dissolve and the rate of emptying of the stomach. The choice is really what suits you and the right dose is what relieves *your* symptoms. The most expensive are not necessarily the best.

2. Drugs which Reduce Acid Production by the Stomach

Anticholinergics

These drugs are called anticholinergic because they block cholinergic nerves (see p. 93). They are used to treat peptic ulcers because cholinergic nerves supply the stomach and their stimulation leads to an increased production of gastric juices (which includes acid). These nerves also increase muscle movement in the stomach and gut. Anticholinergic drugs, therefore, reduce acid production and reduce spasm of the stomach wall, which reduces pain.

There are many anticholinergic drugs on the market and some of them such as the **belladonna alkaloids** have been very popular for the treatment of peptic ulcer symptoms. However, these preparations tend to produce adverse effects such as blurred vision, dry mouth, rapid beating of the heart, retention of urine and constipation. These are called **atropine-like** effects because they are classically produced by atropine and are not very pleasant. Other anticholinergic drugs are available which do not produce so many of these adverse effects; for example, **propantheline (Pro-Banthine), poldine (Nacton)** and **dicyclomine (Merbentyl)**.

Anticholinergic drugs may be of use in treating peptic ulcers if given in a high dose at night – this helps to reduce the acid production which occurs during sleep. However, despite the fact that they are widely prescribed and appear in all kinds of mixtures, authoritative medical opinion remains divided about their value. Because of their anticholinergic side-effects they should not be given to patients with glaucoma. They should be given with caution to patients with enlarged prostate glands, the elderly, and to those with heart disease. In patients with coronary heart disease, the rapid beating of the heart which these drugs produce may cause angina. They should not be given to patients taking monoamine oxidase inhibitor antidepressant drugs. Antihistamines, phenothiazine, major tranquillizers and tricyclic antidepressants may increase the atropine-like effects of these drugs.

Anticholinergic drugs are seldom used these days.

Pirenzepine (Gastrozepin) is a selective muscarinic anticholinergic drug. It inhibits gastric acid and pepsin secretion. It produces fewer adverse effects than the other anticholinergic drugs since it does not enter the brain. It may produce dry mouth and visual disturbances.

H_2-receptor Blockers

Acid production can be reduced by using an H_2 antihistamine drug which blocks the histamine receptors in the stomach.

The H_2 antihistamines **cimetidine (Dyspamet, Tagamet), famotidine**

(Pepsid PM), **nizatidine (Axid)** and **ranitidine (Zantac)** heal peptic ulcers, particularly duodenal ulcers. They are also of use in reflux oesophagitis. *Note:* It is important to establish whether a gastric ulcer is malignant or not because these drugs will mask the symptoms of a gastric cancer and cause a delay in diagnosis.

The reduction in gastric acid may be associated with the growth of bacteria which produce nitrosamines from nitrates in the food. This could produce cancer although this has not been reported in patients. Initial treatment should preferably last for four to six weeks. A daily maintenance dose of cimetidine or ranitidine will prevent relapse but do not forget that they do not cure; after stopping them, ulcers may recur. Nonetheless, their use has reduced complications from peptic ulcer disease and also reduced the need for surgery.

Adverse effects produced by **cimetidine** include diarrhoea, dizziness, skin rashes, photosensitivity (sensitivity to sunlight) and joint and muscle pains. It has an anti-male hormone effect (anti-androgenic) and produces reversible impotence and enlargement of the breasts in men (gynaecomastia). In elderly patients and in patients with impaired kidney function it may produce mental confusion. It should be used with caution therefore in the elderly and in patients with impaired kidney function. It should also be used with caution in patients with impaired liver function. Cimetidine stops certain enzyme activities in the liver and it therefore slows the breakdown and increases the effects of drugs such as oral anticoagulants, phenytoin, benzodiazepines and beta-blocking drugs. **Ranitidine** does not produce these effects in the liver nor does it appear to produce anti-androgenic effects or mental confusion. It may produce diarrhoea, headache, dizziness and skin rashes.

3. Drugs which Protect the Stomach Lining

Liquorice wood has been used in various herbal indigestion mixtures for centuries. But when in 1948, crude powdered liquorice extract was tried in patients suffering from peptic ulcers it was found that one in five developed serious adverse effects which included high blood pressure, irregular heart beats and muscle weakness. However, research on it continued and in the early 1960s it was shown that liquorice extracts are of use in the treatment of gastric ulcers. Two derivatives of liquorice are available – **carbenoxolone** (**Biogastrone**, **Duogastrone**, in **Pyrogastrone**) and **deglycyrrhizinised liquorice** (**Caved-S, Rabro**).

Carbenoxolone has been shown to increase the rate of healing of ulcers. It protects the stomach lining from attack by pepsin and acid and it increases mucosal mucus production.

It may cause salt and water retention, and a reduction in blood potassium level. This may result in weight gain and swollen ankles, a rise in blood pressure, and heart failure. The low blood potassium may cause muscle weakness. It should be given with caution to elderly patients and to those with impaired heart or kidney function or raised blood pressure. It should not be continued for more than four or six weeks and it may be necessary to give additional potassium salts and/or a diuretic drug (see p. 180).

Deglycyrrhizinised liquorice (Caved-S, Rabro) is prepared from liquorice residue after the remaining glycyrrhinic acid has been removed (it is from this acid that carbenoxolone is obtained). It contains less than three per cent of the acid and produces no salt or water retention, or reduction in blood potassium. It is also less effective.

De-Nol (tri-potassium di-citrato bismuthate). This is a complex bismuth preparation (not a salt) which forms a protective layer over the ulcer lining. It is active only when the stomach contents are acid. See directions on use in Part Three.

Sucralfate (Antepsin) protects the ulcer lining from acid and pepsin attack. It is a complex of aluminium hydroxide and sulphated sucrose, see Part Three.

Ulcer Treatment

In addition to antacids there have been numerous fashions consisting of bland diets, milk diets, bed rest and sedatives. Some rigid 'ulcer diets' have made patients much worse and there is no real evidence that in the end they do the patient any good.

Try the combined effects of the following: stop smoking, stop drinking alcohol and coffee; if you have symptoms suggestive of a psychological disorder (tension, irritability, depression, insomnia, etc.) get expert help; try to reduce external pressures; take regular, frequent small meals; avoid foods that upset you; do not take any preparation containing aspirin, corticosteroids, anti-rheumatic drugs or any other drug that irritates the stomach; try to get sufficient rest, exercise, fresh air and sleep and eat a nutritious diet. Consult your doctor about appropriate drug treatment.

Drugs Acting on the Gall-bladder

Chenodeoxycholic acid (Chendol, Chenofalk) and **ursodeoxycholic acid (Destolit, Ursofalk)** are used to treat patients with mild symptoms and small or medium sized cholesterol gallstones which are radiolucent to X-rays. Patients need to be in hospital and monitored by X-ray and therefore require hospital supervision. Gallstones recur in one in four patients within one year of stopping treatment. Read about each drug in Part Three. Ursodeoxycholic acid produces diarrhoea less frequently than chenodeoxycholic acid and liver disfunction has been reported with chenodeoxycholic acid. **Dehydrocholic acid** is used to improve drainage from the gall duct after surgery.

20 Drugs Used to Treat Diarrhoea

An acute attack of diarrhoea is unpleasant and can be exhausting. If associated with vomiting in babies and infants it may be very dangerous because of the risk of dehydration. This requires immediate treatment and, therefore, any baby or infant who develops vomiting and diarrhoea should be seen by a doctor. Similar precautions apply to very elderly and debilitated patients. In most of us, apart from typhoid fever and certain bacillary and amoebic dysenteries, an attack of diarrhoea is usually self-limiting and of no consequence. It may be regarded as the body's way of getting rid of a noxious substance; and so some regard its treatment as unnecessary and possibly harmful. Others regard diarrhoea as an unpleasant symptom warranting drug treatment. Certainly, if it goes on for more than a day then it can be quite exhausting. It may also ruin a holiday. In addition to plenty of fluids and a bland diet it is therefore worth taking one of the popular remedies. The treatment of chronic diarrhoea (e.g., ulcerative colitis, Crohn's disease) is quite different.

Drug Treatment of Diarrhoea

Drug treatments of diarrhoea include drugs which reduce the number of bowel movements by acting on the contents of the gut or upon the wall of the gut, and anti-infective drugs which are used to treat bacterial or amoebic infections. These are often given in various combinations.

Drugs which Alter the Bowel Contents

Inert powders are used to form bulk and carry away irritant substances. These include **activated charcoal; aluminium salts** (e.g., **kaolin**); **pectin** (a purified carbohydrate product obtained from citrus fruits); **activated attapulgite** (a hydrated magnesium aluminium silicate) and **calcium carbonate (chalk)**. Bulk-forming laxatives (see p. 149) made from **starches** or **cellulose** are sometimes used in chronic diarrhoea. These bulk-forming substances (e.g., **methylcellulose, ceratonia, ispaghula, sterculia, psyllium**) modify the frequency of the motions because they absorb water *but* they do not reduce the loss of water and salts.

Drugs which Act on the Bowel Wall

Opium drugs (see p. 189). Opium drugs slow down movement of the bowel wall. They are still the most effective agents for treating diarrhoea. They are often mixed with kaolin or chalk. **Codeine phosphate** is very useful on its own. Fortunately, with these drugs, the dose to stop diarrhoea is much less than the dose which produces adverse effects.

A frequently prescribed proprietary preparation for the treatment of diarrhoea (**Lomotil**) contains **diphenoxylate** and a small dose of **atropine**. Diphenoxylate is related to pethidine and is used to treat diarrhoea because of its constipating effects. It should not be used in patients with impaired liver function. *It should not be given to children*.

Anticholinergic drugs. **Belladonna** and **related drugs** reduce the movements of bowel muscles and reduce spasm (which causes colic). They may produce atropine-like effects such as dry mouth, dizziness and blurring of vision. In mild diarrhoea they may relieve pain and reduce the number of bowel movements. They are not much use in severe diarrhoea nor in the chronic diarrhoea of ulcerative colitis and similar disorders.

Loperamide (Imodium) acts on the muscles of the gut and slows down movements.

Anti-infective Drugs

Numerous anti-diarrhoea remedies contain **antibiotics** mixed with powders (e.g., kaolin) or with mixtures which contain anticholinergic drugs. But after decades of excessive use of antibiotics in patients suffering from diarrhoea most authoritative opinion is now against their widespread use except in specific infections such as typhoid fever and certain dysenteries.

Antibacterial drugs may alter the normal bacterial content of the gut which may result in a super-added fungal infection (moniliasis). With some bacterial infections antibiotics may also prolong the period when the patient can pass on the disease as a carrier. They may also increase the risk of relapse, interfere with subsequent bacterial diagnosis, promote the development of resistant organisms and cause rashes. They should not be used routinely.

Treatment of an Acute Attack of Diarrhoea

The greatest risk from diarrhoea is the loss of large volumes of water containing salts of sodium and potassium. The loss of these salts and water is dangerous in babies and infants and requires urgent treatment. Patients require **rehydration**, i.e., the priority is the urgent replacement of lost water and salt.

It has been found that the addition of glucose to an oral salt solution greatly improves the absorption of salts and water through the gut wall into the blood-stream. Because of this finding it is important that any rehydration fluid contains both salts and glucose.

There are several preparations of these **salt/sugar solutions** (e.g., **Dioralyte, Electrolade, Electrosol, Paedialyte, Rehidrat).** These are mixtures of sodium chloride, glucose and other salts, usually available as powders for making up into solution. In emergency you can make a solution up at home but you must be careful. Dissolving the sugar and the salt in the *correct* volume of water is very important since too concentrated a solution can, in infants, produce the risk of too much salt absorption leading to convulsions.

A **simple sugar/salt solution** contains one level teaspoonful of household salt (5 ml) and eight level teaspoonfuls of sugar in *one* litre of water. To correct dehydration you will need 50–100 ml/kg of body-weight (kg = 2·2 lb) given over a 3–4 hour period. To replace fluids lost in ongoing diarrhoea you will need to give 50 ml per stool for small infants, 100 ml per stool for older infants, 200 ml per stool for older children and 400 ml per stool for adults. In addition the following amounts of fluids should be taken as water, fruit juices, tea or diluted cow's milk – small infant: 150 ml/kg over 24 hours; older infants: 120 ml; young child: 100 ml; and adults 80 ml/kg of body-weight over 24 hours.

It is best not to eat for 24 hours and most patients with acute diarrhoea should **avoid milk and milk products.** This is because the diarrhoea may produce a deficiency of the enzyme in the gut which breaks down lactose in the milk and the lactose may make the diarrhoea worse.

The drug treatment of diarrhoea takes second place to rehydration. Drugs commonly used to treat diarrhoea include **codeine phosphate, kaolin** mixed with an opium drug (**kaolin and morphine mixture**), **a chalk and opium mixture, diphenoxylate with atropine (Lomotil)** and **loperamide (Arret; Imodium).**

To avoid an attack of diarrhoea on your continental holiday, preventive methods, such as not eating salads, sea food, ice cream and cold meats, and not drinking the tap water, are best.

Drugs used to treat chronic diarrhoea (e.g., ulcerative colitis, Crohn's disease) include **corticosteroids** (p. 215), **sulphasalazine (Salazopyrin), azathioprine (Azamune, Imuran)** and **sodium cromoglycate (Nalcrom).** Read about each drug in Part Three.

21 Drugs Used to Treat Constipation

Drugs used to treat constipation are called laxatives. They are extensively misused – the result of the mistaken belief that there is some relationship between regular daily emptying of the bowels and health. It does not matter if you have your bowels opened two to three times a day or two to three times a week. It only matters if you develop a change in bowel habit; if you only go a day or two over the normal for you, this again does not matter.

We usually talk about **laxatives** when we wish to produce a soft, formed, easy-to-pass motion and a cathartic or **purgative** when we wish to produce fairly quick and fluid emptying of the bowel. Laxatives are harmless when taken infrequently but their continued use over long periods of time may lead to complications such as fluid and salt loss. This may make you feel tired, weak and thirsty. Calcium loss may occur and lead to bone softening and the bowel wall may become permanently damaged and inflamed.

The taking of laxatives is only occasionally necessary; for example, after childbirth, after an operation for piles or some other condition around the anus, after some abdominal operations, after a coronary thrombosis and in elderly or debilitated bedridden patients. Apart from these cases the use of a laxative is seldom indicated and you certainly will be no healthier if you drink a glass of health salts every morning.

The most natural treatment for simple constipation is a **high fibre diet**. You should increase the amount of indigestible waste products in your diet which is easily achieved by eating more fruit, leafy vegetables and by adding bran to your diet in the form of a processed cereal or as bread or scones. If you have a long-standing problem then in addition to diet make sure that you drink plenty of fluids, take regular exercise and develop a habit of trying to empty your bowels just after a meal when food entering the stomach stimulates the large bowel to empty its contents into the rectum, which produces the urge to go. Never neglect a feeling that you want to empty your bowels. The same advice applies if you have developed a laxative habit, but, in addition, slowly try and reduce the dose over a period of time.

Laxatives should never be taken regularly and they should never be taken to relieve abdominal pains, cramps, colic, nausea or any other symptom whether associated with constipation or not. You may have, for instance, an acute appendicitis and the taking of laxatives could cause the appendix to rupture and give rise to peritonitis. If in doubt you should always consult your doctor, particularly if you pass blood in the motions, if you are developing the laxative habit, or if you develop a change in bowel habits.

The occasional use of laxatives is not harmful but the danger is that you will develop the laxative habit – when you have taken one dose of laxative your colon will be empty and it may take several days for it to fill and give you the urge to go again. Unfortunately, some patients cannot wait that long before taking another dose. A regular routine develops and the bowel action becomes so abnormal that it is then unable to function properly and the person will be totally reliant upon the use of these drugs. These warnings refer to all laxatives which include the much-advertised taking of health salts before breakfast and numerous patent health remedies. In fact many of these contain irritant purgatives now regarded as obsolescent.

There are four main groups of drugs used to treat constipation: stimulant, saline, lubricant and bulk-forming.

1. Stimulant Laxatives

These include **bisacodyl (Dulcolax), cascara, castor oil, danthron (Dorbanex,** * in **Co-Danthrasate, Normax), fig, senna** (in **Agiolax, Senokot, X-Prep), sodium picosulphate (Laxoberal, Picolax)**. There are so many preparations on the market which contain stimulant laxatives that it would be impracticable to list them all. Stimulant laxatives increase large bowel movements by irritating the lining and/or stimulating the bowel muscles to contract. They may cause cramps, increased mucus secretion and excessive fluid loss. Response to dosage varies tremendously and what may produce stomach cramps and diarrhoea in one person may have no effect in another.

Senna, cascara and **danthron** may colour the urine red, cause excessive loss of fluids and if taken for a long time may cause patchy pigmentation of part of the bowel (colon). This is not serious and is reversible on stopping the drug. **Phenolphthalein** may cause allergic skin rashes and colour the urine pink. **Bisacodyl** is related to phenolphthalein. It may be used as a suppository as well as taken by mouth. Another popular suppository contains **glycerin,** gelatin and water (**Glycerol suppositories**). **Castor oil** differs from the other stimulant laxatives because it works on the small

---

* The manufacturers of Dorbanex, which contains danthron, stopped manufacturing in February 1987 because studies suggested that long-term high-dose administration of danthron is associated with the development of cancer in the intestine and livers of rodents. There is no evidence that danthron produces cancer in humans.

bowel and therefore produces an effect in about three hours. The others act on the large bowel and work in six to twelve hours. Bisacodyl suppositories work in half to one hour.

2. Saline Laxatives (Osmotic Laxatives)

These are **salts of magnesium, sodium** or **potassium** in various mixtures. They are incompletely absorbed and increase the bulk of the bowel contents by causing it to retain **water** (a process called osmosis). Some of them are made fizzy by adding sodium bicarbonate and fruity by adding weak acids such as citric and tartaric. These salts may take fluids from the body and cause dehydration, and should therefore be taken with large drinks of water. They include **magnesium sulphate (Epsom salts, Andrews liver salts), magnesium hydroxide (Milk of Magnesia), sodium sulphate (Glauber's salts), sodium potassium tartrate (Rochelle salts) and potassium bitartrate (cream of tartar).** Eno 'Fruit Salt' contains **sodium bicarbonate** plus **citric** and **tartaric acid**. They are commonly called health salts, which is reasonable enough if health is defined as bowel movements and belching. Health salts containing sodium salts should never be given to patients with congestive heart disease because they cause salt and water retention. Likewise they should never be taken by patients on diuretic drugs since these drugs are given to get rid of salt from the body. Also magnesium health salts should never be given to patients with impaired kidney function since about twenty per cent of magnesium may be absorbed from the gut and as it is excreted by the kidneys any impairment may lead to an accumulation of magnesium in the blood resulting in magnesium intoxication (sharp drop in blood pressure and respiratory paralysis).

Lactulose (Duphalac) is a non-absorbable synthetic disaccharide sugar. It increases the fluid bulk of the motions and leads to stimulation of bowel movements. It also increases the bacterial content of the bowel. It may cause nausea, diarrhoea and wind.

3. Lubricant Laxatives (Faecal Softeners)

There are three types of lubricant laxatives: **mineral oils (liquid paraffin), dioctyl sodium sulphosuccinate (docusate sodium: Dioctyl,** in **Normax,** and mixed with **bisacodyl** in **Dulcodos**) and **poloxamer** (in **Dorbanex***). **Liquid paraffin** softens and lubricates the motions. Its use should be avoided since it interferes with absorption of carotene (pre-formed vitamin A), vitamin A and vitamin D. In pregnancy it may reduce the absorption of vitamin K and produce a disorder of blood clotting. Young, elderly and debilitated patients may inhale a few drops into their lungs when they swallow liquid paraffin and this may cause a type of pneumonia. It may also be absorbed from the gut and cause swelling of lymph glands in the gut wall, the liver and spleen. It may also leak from the anus in the night and cause irritation (pruritus ani). **Dioctyl sodium sulphosuccinate** and **dioctyl calcium sulpho-succinate** lower surface tension and are used in the pharmaceutical industry as emulsifying or wetting agents. They soften the motions in twenty-four to forty-eight hours and are present in numerous laxative preparations. They are also used to soften wax in the ears. **Poloxalkol** is another surface active agent which acts as a lubricant laxative.

4. Bulk-forming Laxatives

These are substances which increase the bulk of the bowel content which stimulates the bowel muscles to become active. In addition they dissolve or swell in water to form a soft mass which helps to lubricate the passage of the motions. They usually take twelve to twenty-four hours to work. Some bulk-forming laxatives are naturally occurring substances such as **gums, e.g., agar, tragacanth; ispaghula husks (Fybogel, Isogel, Metamucil, Reg-ulan** and **sterculia (Normacol)** – these are present in numerous proprietary laxatives. Others are semi-synthetic like **methylcellulose (Celevac, Cellu-con, Cologel)**. They must be taken with plenty of fluids because of the risk of bowel obstruction in elderly or debilitated patients. Gums may cause hypersensitivity resulting in skin rashes and hay-fever/asthma-like symp-toms. **Bran (Fybranta, Lejfibre)** is a by-product of the milling of wheat and contains about 20 per cent of indigestible cellulose. It is an effective bulk laxative and may also help to prevent certain bowel disorders such as diverticulitis.

Which Laxative to Take

For the occasional attack of constipation which you feel needs treating and where diet has failed, use a stimulant laxative (e.g., senna, cascara or bisacodyl) or a saline laxative (e.g., magnesium sulphate). In bedridden, elderly or debilitated patients a simple bulk laxative, such as bran, may be effective. If this does not work try a semi-synthetic compound like methyl-cellulose but make sure that the patient, provided his bladder control is normal, drinks plenty of fluids. Lactulose is an alternative. After oper-ations on the anus, after childbirth or where you do not want to have to strain, a lubricant laxative, such as dioctyl sodium sulphosuccinate (docu-sate sodium) is probably the best. Always take the smallest effective dose as infrequently as possible.

Bran

Bran comes from the outer layers of wheat grain and its fibre content varies from 30 to 50 per cent depending on the milling process and on the variety of wheat. It is present in such foods as wholemeal bread and certain breakfast cereals. It is very useful for treating constipation, and for treating diverticulosis and it may help patients suffering from irritable bowel syndrome. It is also of use in treating constipation associated with haemorrhoids, anal fissure and ulcerative colitis affecting the lower end of the colon. There are numerous products available to which bran has been added (e.g., special breads, biscuits and cereals) or you can buy 'pure' bran to add to cereals, etc. The choice is not critical but everyone should switch from white bread to wholemeal bread and high fibre cereals and reduce or try to stop eating sugary foods and foods made from refined flour. You must take an adequate amount of fluids to avoid obstruction from bran.

Rectally Administered Laxatives

When the faeces are impacted, laxatives administered rectally may be useful. (Remember in the elderly, impacted faeces due to constipation may present as diarrhoea, a watery leakage of faeces around the impaction.) Preparations available include **bisacodyl suppositories (Dulcolax), phosphate enemas (Fletchers'), phosphate suppositories (Beogex), dioctyl sodium sulphosuccinate (Dioctyl syrup used as an enema, Klyx enema, Fletchers' Enemotte), arachis oil (Fletchers'), magnesium sulphate (Fletchers'), osmotic enemas (Micolette Micro-enema, Micralax Micro-enema, Relaxit Micro-enema), oxyphenisatin (Veripaque)** and **glycerol suppositories.**

22 Drugs Used to Treat Angina

Angina pectoris is the term used to describe attacks of pain from the heart of short duration and without evidence of lasting damage to the heart muscle. It is caused by a disorder of the coronary arteries which supply the heart. This results in a deficient supply of blood to part of the working heart muscle causing a lack of oxygen and pain. *Coronary thrombosis* implies an attack of pain from the heart due to a thrombosis in a coronary artery; it may or may not be accompanied by evidence of damage to heart muscle. This damage or scarring results from the cutting off of the blood supply to part of the muscle and is called *myocardial infarction*. Narrowing and closure (coronary occlusion) and spasm may produce a similar effect.

In most patients angina occurs only on effort and goes off on resting – this is because on effort the heart has to do more work and the heart muscle requires more oxygen. If the coronary arteries are not healthy enough to supply the extra oxygen, the muscle starts to ache. As soon as the patient rests, the heart has to do less work, oxygen demand falls and the pain goes off. Many factors can trigger off an attack of angina and people vary tremendously in their response to treatment. For these reasons the assessment of drugs in relieving angina is very difficult. Most of these drugs are aimed at improving the blood supply and therefore the oxygen supply to the heart muscle.

Drugs used to treat angina include those used to treat an acute attack or to prevent an attack over the short term and those used to prevent attacks over the long term. They belong to three major groups – organic nitrates and nitrites and inorganic nitrites, beta-receptor blocking drugs and calcium antagonists.

Nitrites and Nitrates

Amyl nitrite and **glyceryl trinitrate (nitroglycerin, trinitrin)** have been used for over one hundred years. Organic nitrites and nitrates and inorganic nitrites have similar actions and effects. Their basic action is to relax involuntary muscles, particularly those in the walls of blood vessels. This results in dilatation of blood vessels and various other effects. High doses of these drugs reduce the return and output of blood to and from the heart – so much so that a 'normal' individual may faint if kept standing up after a high dose of one of these quick-acting drugs. The general effects lead to a reduction of work-load for the heart and therefore less oxygen is needed. In addition these drugs improve the coronary artery blood flow. Anginal pain is relieved and can also be prevented. These drugs increase the amount of exercise a patient can do before getting an attack of angina, and they relieve or prevent the attack of pain.

Proprietary preparations available include:

Glyceryl trinitrate – **G T N 300 mcg** tablets, **Nitrocontin Continus** sustained-release tablets, **Coro-Nitro** Spray and **Nitrolingual** aerosol sprays, **Percutol** ointment for application to the skin, **Suscard Buccal** for dissolving in the mouth, **Sustac** sustained-release tablets, **Deponit** and **Transiderm-Nitro** self-adhesive dressings to apply to the skin, and **Tridil**, **Nitrocine** and **Nitronal** injections.

Application of **glyceryl trinitrate to the skin** is a new way of maintaining blood levels of the drug and so providing a prolonged prevention against attacks of angina.

Longer-acting nitrates by mouth are used to prevent attacks coming on. They include: **isosorbide dinitrate** – **Cedocard, Isoket, Isordil, Soni-Slo, Sorbichew** (chewable tablets), **Sorbid, Sorbitrate** and **Vascardin**. **Isosorbide mononitrate (Elantan, Imdur, Ismo, Monit, Mono-Cedocard), pentaerythritol tetranitrate (Cardiacap, Mycardol)**.

Adverse effects of the nitrites and nitrates are related to their vasodilation, they include throbbing headache, flushing, a fall in blood pressure on standing, and rapid beating of the heart. The headache may be troublesome initially but usually goes over time. Glyceryl trinitrate tablets can easily lose their effectiveness and you can tell this if they lose the burning sensation when you suck them. Ask your pharmacist how to store them.

Read about specific preparations in Part Three.

Beta Adreno-receptor Blocking Drugs (Beta-Blockers)

These include **acebutolol (Sectral), atenolol (Tenormin), betaxolol (Kerlone), bisoprolol (Emcor, Monocor), labetalol (Labrocol, Trandate), metroprolol (Betaloc, Lopresor), nadolol (Corgard), oxprenolol (Apsolox, Slow-Pren, Slow-Trasicor, Trasicor), penbutolol (in Lasipressin) pindolol (Betadren, Visken), propranolol (Angilol, Apsolol, Bedranol, Berkolol, Inderal, Sloprolol), sotalol (Beta-Cardone, Sotacor), timolol (Betim, Blocadren)**.

Many patients develop angina in response to an emotional upset. This is because the heart beats faster in response to fear, panic, tension, anxiety, excitation or aggression. This increases its work-load and in the presence of a deficient coronary artery blood supply, anginal pain will develop. The rapid beating of the heart is caused by stimulation through nerve endings called beta-receptors. Drugs can prevent this stimulation by blocking these receptors. This blocking will also prevent stimulation which occurs during exercise.

Beta-receptor blocking drugs have a marked effect when the heart is being stimulated by exercise, emotion or adrenaline-like drugs. They reduce the effects of such stimulation to produce slowing of the rate and a reduction in the force of contraction of the heart. Some of them reduce the rate of conduction of impulses through the conducting system of the heart. The overall result from beta-receptor blockers is a reduction in the volume of blood pumped out by the heart during each contraction and a decreased oxygen consumption because the heart has to do less work.

They reduce the response of the heart to stress and exercise and are used to treat angina, to lower blood pressure and to correct abnormal rhythms. These drugs may also be used to treat patients who develop heart symptoms in response to stress or tension.

Beta-receptor blocking drugs can trigger off heart failure in patients who are near to such a state. They may make heart block worse and they should be used with caution in pregnancy. In patients with asthma, bronchospasm and bronchitis they may cause constriction of the bronchial tubes. They should be used with caution in patients undergoing an anaesthetic for surgery. They should also be given with caution to patients taking oral anti-diabetic drugs. Note that discontinuance of beta-receptor blocking drugs after long-term therapy in a patient with angina must be done *gradually* and under the careful supervision of a doctor. Sudden stopping in these circumstances has caused heart attacks (myocardial infarction).

In addition to being used to treat angina and to prevent a second and/or subsequent myocardial infarction they are now frequently used to treat patients suffering from raised blood pressure (see p. 161). They are also used to treat migraine, anxiety, tremor, thyrotoxicosis and glaucoma (used topically). They are all equally effective but there are differences between them which may affect choice in treating individual disorders and patients.

Oxprenolol, pindolol and **acebutolol** retain some stimulating effects in addition to their blocking effects – this is called intrinsic sympathomimetic activity (ISA). They tend to produce less slowing of the heart. They also produce less coldness of the hands and feet which is a problem with some other beta-blockers.

Atenolol, nadolol and **sotalol** are soluble in water and are therefore less likely to enter the brain to produce adverse effects such as poor sleep and nightmares. Fat-soluble beta-blockers can produce these effects because they enter the brain. Some beta-blockers have a short duration of effect and have to be given two to three times daily; however, these are usually available as slow-release preparations which means they need only to be taken once daily. As stated earlier, in patients with asthma, beta-blockers may also block the nerve endings supplying the bronchi and trigger off an asthmatic attack. In these patients it is important to use beta-blockers that have less effect on beta receptors in the bronchi and a more selective effect on beta-receptors in the heart, e.g., **metoprolol, atenolol, acebutolol**. Nonetheless, *it is better to avoid beta-blockers in patients with asthma whenever possible*.

Beta-blockers can make disorders of the circulation worse, affect glucose levels in diabetic patients, and they can mask some of the symptoms of low blood sugar (hypoglycaemia) in patients taking anti-diabetic drugs, including insulin. They should therefore be used with utmost caution in diabetic patients.

Practolol (Eraldin) was withdrawn from general use because it caused the oculo-mucocutaneous syndrome – dryness and scarring of the conjunctivae of the eyes, a skin rash like psoriasis and fibrosis of the peritoneum in the abdomen. It is still used in hospitals by intravenous injection to slow very fast heart rates.

Calcium Antagonists (Calcium-Channel Blockers)

Calcium-Channel blocking drugs or antagonists reduce the work of the heart by blocking the entry of calcium ions into the heart muscle cells and thus reducing the strength of contraction and slowing electrical conduction of impulses through the heart. They also decrease muscle contractions in veins and arteries producing vasodilatation. Many calcium antagonists are now available – **diltiazem (Britiazim, Calcicard, Tildiem), lidoflazine (Clinium), nicardipine (Cardene), nifedipine (Adalat), nimodipine (Nimotop), prenylamine (Synadrin), verapamil (Barkatens, Cordilox, Securon, Univer)**. They differ according to the three main effects of calcium antagonism which they produce – i.e., vasodilator effects, reduced heart muscle contractility and reduced conduction of impulses.

Calcium antagonists lower the oxygen requirement of heart muscle but unlike beta-blockers they do not greatly reduce the heart rate. They may be used in combination with beta-blockers or when beta-blockers are not indicated. They should be used with caution in elderly patients. Caution is also needed when using calcium antagonists along with a beta-blocker, an antihypertensive drug, or digoxin, since there is a risk of a fall in the blood pressure, excessive slowing of the heart, or heart failure.

Other Drugs Used to Treat Angina

Patients with angina who suffer from anxiety or tension may benefit from intermittent use of an anti-anxiety drug; patients should stop smoking, take regular moderate exercise, eat a balanced diet and watch their weight.

Coronary artery disease may be related to blood fat levels in certain patients. The use of drugs to lower blood fat levels is discussed on p. 101.

The Drug Treatment of Angina

Glyceryl trinitrate is the drug of choice in the treatment or prevention of individual attacks of angina. You should learn your own dosage regimen. Relief of pain takes about two minutes. Many patients take their tablet just before the onset of exertion which they know will produce pain, for example, going upstairs or before sexual intercourse. This gives protection from pain for about 20–30 minutes.

The use of **isosorbide dinitrate**, if taken under the tongue, may produce longer relief from angina, but in general long-acting preparations such as pentaerythritol tetranitrate have been of less value than the short-acting ones.

The aim of long-term treatments of angina is to try to get a more steady drug effect without having to anticipate or experience an attack. The **beta-receptor blockers** delay the onset of pain and the long-term use of these drugs has been shown to reduce the number of anginal attacks and the consumption of glyceryl trinitrate. If beta-receptor blockers fail, then it is worth trying a **calcium antagonist**.

23 Drugs Used to Treat Heart Failure

In the failing heart the volume of blood in the heart chambers during relaxation of the muscles increases. This causes them to stretch which interferes with their pumping capacity when they contract. More blood accumulates in the chambers causing a back-pressure to build up in the blood vessels returning blood to the heart. This back-pressure may cause congestion of the lungs and produce breathlessness and disorders of respiration. If the back-pressure affects the right side of the heart where blood from all over the body is returned then the pressure builds up in the veins and back to the tissues. This produces an increase of fluids in the tissues called oedema (dropsy). Oedema may also be due to other causes such as impaired kidney or liver function and so one usually talks about cardiac (heart) oedema or congestive heart failure.

Drugs used to treat heart failure fall into three main groups: **digoxin** and related drugs to improve the contraction of the heart, **diuretics** to get rid of excess fluid and **vasodilators** to reduce the load on the heart.

Digoxin and Related Drugs

They include **digoxin (Lanoxin)**, **digitoxin**, **lanatoside C (Cedilanid)**, **medigoxin** and **ouabain**.

These drugs have been used for centuries to treat heart failure. They are called cardiac glycosides, and are found in a number of plants. **Digitoxin** is prepared from the leaves of *Digitalis purpurea* (purple foxglove) and **digoxin** is prepared from the leaves of *Digitalis lanata* (white foxglove). **Prepared digitalis** is a crude mixture obtained from powdered leaves of both types of foxglove plant. **Strophanthus** is extracted from the seeds of the plants *Strophanthus kombé* and *S. gratus*. Also from *S. gratus* is extracted **ouabain (strophanthin-G)**. Yet another cardiac glycoside is obtained from the fleshy bulb of the 'sea onion' *Urginea (Scilla) maritima*. Digitoxin is slower acting than digoxin; ouabain is the most rapidly acting.

Digoxin and **digitoxin** are the most commonly used of this group of drugs. They have similar actions and effects but they differ in the rate at which they start to act and in the duration of their effects. They act mainly on the heart. They increase both the force of contraction of the heart muscle and the work done by the heart without increasing its oxygen consumption.

In heart failure they cause the heart muscles to work more efficiently; this causes increased output from the heart, reduction of back-pressure, decrease in the size of the heart and a reduction in blood volume. The latter is produced by the effects of a more efficient circulation of blood to the kidneys resulting in more urine being produced. They are therefore used principally to treat heart failure. Secondary to the circulatory improvement mentioned above, they reduce heart rate by reducing sympathetic drive to the heart (i.e. they reduce adrenaline-like actions). They also make the heart sensitive to impulses from the vagus nerve, which slows the heart rate. In addition they slow down the rate at which electrical impulses pass from the heart's pacemaker (the part of the heart where electrical impulses start) to the rest of the heart. They are equally effective in treating oedema and/or respiratory complications caused by heart disease. They are also used to regulate disorders of heart rate.

When taken by mouth digoxin and digitoxin are adequately absorbed, although significant variation in absorption between different brands of digoxin has been demonstrated. Digoxin is almost completely excreted unchanged in the urine, whereas digitoxin is mainly broken down in the liver to inactive products; the latter is therefore safer to use in patients with impaired kidney function. They are slowly excreted and are accumulative. Digitoxin is the most slowly excreted.

Intoxication

Digoxin and related drugs cause signs and symptoms of intoxication when taken in high doses, and can produce dangerous adverse effects which may prove fatal. Yet despite our knowledge about the effects and uses of these drugs and despite the fact that every medical student is taught about them, a high proportion of adverse drug effects which take place in hospitals are due to intoxication with them.

Every prescribing doctor should be aware of the effects and adverse effects of these drugs. They are extremely valuable if used appropriately and yet serious adverse effects occur because some doses are not adjusted carefully, according to the needs of the individual. Too much at once or too much for too long can be dangerous. Cumulative effects may develop. Furthermore, the dangers of their use when combined with diuretics are well documented.

Loss of appetite, nausea and vomiting are the earliest indications of overdose. Nausea is an important warning and vomiting can be most distressing to a patient with heart failure. They may also cause diarrhoea and abdominal discomfort or pain. These symptoms disappear in a few days but they are generally avoidable. They must be distinguished from similar symptoms which occasionally develop in heart failure. Headache, fatigue and drowsiness may also occur and elderly patients may become confused.

The most frequent and well-recognized adverse effect on the heart is the appearance of extra heart beats. If these extra heart beats occur after each regular beat then you get what is called coupling – a good clue that the patient has been overdosed. Toxic amounts interfere with the passage of electrical impulses from the pacemaker down the main transmission paths between the upper and the lower chambers of the heart. This leads to missed or dropped heart beats and sometimes to partial or complete heart block, which means that the pacemaker has lost control and the upper and lower chambers of the heart are beating independently. This is a dangerous adverse effect and should be suspected if the heart rate drops below 50 beats per minute. However, an increase in rate is sometimes the first evidence of poisoning because of excitatory effects upon the heart muscle. This is a particular hazard in patients who are also receiving diuretics (these may reduce the blood potassium, which sensitizes heart muscle to the effects of digoxin-like drugs). The rapid beating of the heart may become quite irregular, which if it affects the lower chambers (ventricles) may cause sudden death.

Dosage with these drugs involves two problems: the amount required to produce the desired effects as quickly as possible in someone not previously on the drug (initial digitalization) and the amount required to maintain the good effects with minimal adverse effects (maintenance dosage). There is a wide variation in individual response and therefore these two problems need skill and care. The 'right' dose for an individual patient is that which proves right for him. Regular blood-level measurements should be carried out and the doses adjusted accordingly.

Diuretics

These reverse the salt and water retention which occurs in heart failure as the body attempts to keep the blood volume raised in order to *compensate* for the failing heart. This causes an increased *pre-load* on the heart. Reduction in circulating volume with diuretics reduces the congestion in the lungs and elsewhere, reduces oedema, reduces breathlessness and reduces the workload on the heart. Initially a potent short-acting diuretic is needed (e.g., a loop diuretic such as **frusemide**, **bumetanide** or **ethacrynic acid**). These are then usually replaced by a **thiazide** diuretic for maintenance therapy. Since digoxin-induced disorders of rhythm are more common with a low blood potassium and since diuretics produce a fall in blood potassium it is important to take **potassium supplements** (see p. 186). Alternatively, a diuretic which spares potassium such as **amiloride** or **triamterene** may be given along with a thiazide diuretic (see p. 181). In addition, moderate salt restriction in the diet is recommended. The diuretics are discussed in greater detail on pp. 180–86.

Vasodilator Drugs

In the failing heart, as output drops the peripheral blood vessels begin to close down in order to maintain blood pressure. This closing down is called vasoconstriction and as it increases, the heart finds it more and more difficult to pump blood against the increased pressure. In order to reduce this after-load pressure on the heart, drugs which open up the blood vessels are used: these are called vasodilators.

There are three main groups of vasodilators available for use in heart failure: those which principally affect the venous system and reduce *pre-load* pressure on the heart by reducing the volume of blood returning to the heart (e.g., **nitrates**), those which principally affect the arterial system and reduce the *after-load* by reducing the resistance to the flow of blood from the heart (e.g. **hydralazine**), and those which act on both the venous and arterial systems and reduce both *pre-load* and *after-load* (e.g., **prazosin**).

Nitrates produce dilatation of veins, and increase in the pooling of venous blood and reduce the return of blood to the heart. This reduces the pressure on the heart and helps it to pump more efficiently. Since they are rapidly absorbed from the gut and broken down in the liver it is best if they can be chewed or sucked and the drug absorbed through the mouth into the blood-stream, thus by-passing the liver. The rapid breakdown of these drugs as they pass through the liver after absorption from the gut may mean that very little drug actually reaches the circulation to produce an effect, thus there are several preparations available which are designed to try to get round this problem. Nitrates cause a small fall in blood pressure, a small increase in heart rate and very little change in output.

Hydralazine works on the arterial system; it causes a fall in peripheral resistance, increased cardiac output and improves the blood flow through the kidneys. **Prazosin** has an effect on both the arterial and venous systems, as does **nitroprusside**.

Captopril (Acepril, Capoten) and **enalapil (Innovace)** are ACE inhibitors (see p. 165). They block the formation of angiotensin II (see p. 162) and reverse the constriction of arteries. This produces a fall in resistance to the flow of blood, a fall in blood pressure and a reduced workload on the heart (after-load). They also reduce the blood volume because they improve the blood supply to the kidneys and increase the excretion of salt and water in the urine. In addition, they stop the production of aldosterone (p. 163) and therefore reverse the retention of salt and water caused by aldosterone.

24 Drugs Used to Treat Disorders of Heart Rhythm

Drugs used to treat disorders of heart rhythm show a wide variation in their chemical structure, their site of action in the body and their clinical use. In addition some drugs have more than one action. They are often grouped into four classes:

Class I contains those drugs which possess local anaesthetic properties and which affect the surfaces of the cells (membrane stabilizing properties) in the conducting system causing a reduction in the triggering-off of spontaneous beats. Drugs in this group include **quinidine (Kiditard, Kinidin Durules, procainamide (Pronestyl), disopyramide (Dirythmin, Rythmodan), phenytoin (Epanutin), tocainide (Tonocard), mexiletine (Mexetil), flecainide (Tambocor)** and **lignocaine (Xylocard)**.

Class II drugs reduce the potential for disordered rhythm which occurs in response to stimulation of the heart of adrenaline-like chemicals. These include the **beta adreno-receptor blockers** (p. 152) which block the effect of these chemicals and **bretylium (Bretylate)** which blocks the release of adrenaline-like substances.

Class III drugs prolong the resting phase of the heart. These include **amiodarone (Cordarone X)**.

Class IV drugs are calcium channel blockers (see p. 154). They depress the passage of impulses through the conducting system.

Digoxin is the drug of choice for treating a disorder of heart rhythm called atrial fibrillation. **Atropine** may be used to treat slow heart rate (bradycardia) after a myocardial infarction and bradycardia caused by beta-blocking drugs (p. 152). The latter may be used to treat certain types of tachycardia (rapid heart rate).

The treatment of a disorder of heart rhythm (arrhythmia) requires a precise diagnosis using an electrocardiograph. According to the disorder of rhythm one or more of the drugs listed will be used. Read the entry on each drug in Part Three.

25 Drugs Used to Treat Raised Blood Pressure

The blood is forced around the body under pressure from the contractions of the heart. The blood pressure depends principally upon the amount of blood being pumped out by the heart and the resistance it meets as it enters smaller and smaller blood vessels.

The range of 'normal' blood pressure varies considerably between individuals, and at different times in the same individual. It is influenced by many factors, for example – age, sex, physical exercise, food, smoking, drugs and changes in posture. Emotion particularly may send your blood pressure up whereas sleep sends it down. Repeated blood pressure recordings when you are up and about often give lower levels overall than just a single casual recording.

An individual is only considered to have a raised blood pressure (**hypertension**) if the pressure is consistently raised, in the absence of any factors which may cause a temporary increase during the recording. There are two groups of hypertension – one is very common and because we do not know what causes it we call it **essential or idiopathic hypertension.** The other group is called **secondary hypertension** because it is caused by a known disorder such as kidney disease, toxaemia of pregnancy, narrowing of the main artery from the heart or of an artery supplying a kidney or a tumour (phaeochromocytoma) of the sympathetic nervous system found most often in the adrenal glands.

The blood pressure recording consists of two readings – the upper reading is the pressure at the point when the contractions (systole) of the heart forces the pulse wave of blood through the artery from which the pressure is being recorded (this is usually the artery at the front of the elbow). This is called the systolic blood pressure. The second reading is the pressure recorded between the pulse waves when the heart is relaxed, and filling with blood (diastole) ready for the next pumping action – this is called the diastolic blood pressure. The readings are recorded as the systolic over the diastolic pressures – e.g., 120/80.

The systolic blood pressure may be raised on its own by emotion, fever, pregnancy and old age, when the arteries harden and narrow. A raised diastolic blood pressure appears to be more related to resistance to the flow of blood caused by constriction of the peripheral arteries.

We are interested in high blood pressure because there is an increased predisposition to illness and death amongst people with a blood pressure raised above the 'normal'. High blood pressure has been found to be more common among patients with coronary artery disease and there appears also to be a connection between high blood pressure and disease of the blood vessels; for example, disease of the blood vessels supplying the brain may produce an increased risk of a stroke. Sustained high blood pressure may also be associated with heart failure and kidney damage (which in turn causes an increase in pressure since damaged kidneys may produce a chemical which increases the blood pressure). High blood pressure may also damage blood vessels in the eye.

We know very little about what causes essential hypertension. Blood pressure increases with age; in early life the pressure is higher in men than in women but from middle age (around about 45 years) the pressure becomes higher in women than in men. Men are much more likely than women to develop complications such as coronary artery disease and in men the higher the pressure the higher is the risk of premature death. Hereditary, dietary, environmental, psychological and racial factors have all been considered to try to account for the development of essential hypertension. Raised blood pressure is also considered (by some) to be related to obesity so that reduction in weight may help although differences in thickness of the arm (at the point where the cuff is applied when measuring the blood pressure) may also alter the recordings.

Factors Causing a Raised Blood Pressure

The arterial blood pressure is determined by the output from the heart (cardiac output) and the resistance to the flow of blood as it is pumped into smaller and smaller blood vessels at the periphery (peripheral resistance). This peripheral resistance varies according to the calibre (or narrowing) of the blood vessels and the thickness (or viscosity) of the blood. These are in turn controlled by the following mechanisms.

Special blood pressure receptors in the main arteries in the neck (baroreceptors) detect changes in blood pressure – a fall in blood pressure causes the baroreceptors to send messages to the vasomotor centre in the brain which triggers off an increase in sympathetic stimulation to the heart, causing an increase in output and to the peripheral blood vessels, causing them to constrict.

In addition, changes in blood flow to the kidneys affect the production of an enzyme, called renin, by the kidneys. This enzyme acts to produce an inactive protein (Angiotensin I) which is converted in the lungs to a very powerful vasoconstrictor (Angiotensin II) which also causes the release of aldosterone from the adrenal glands which acts on the kidneys to retain salt and water, thus increasing the blood volume. Renin release is activated by a reduced blood supply to the kidneys which can be caused by narrowing of arteries and thus a vicious circle is set up in patients with raised blood pressure because they have narrowing of the peripheral arteries.

Heart muscle and muscles in blood vessels can also exert their own control; for example, an increase in blood volume in the heart increases the force of contraction of heart muscle. Similarly, a rise in blood volume in arteries causes their muscle walls to contract and increase the peripheral resistance. Both these mechanisms can affect the blood pressure.

Drugs used to treat high blood pressure are complex chemicals with many actions and effects upon the body; if used appropriately they prolong life, but when wrongly used and when given in wrong dosage they may be dangerous as well as useless.

The aim of using drugs is to try to limit or reverse the damage which occurs in blood vessels of patients with raised blood pressure. This is attempted by lowering the blood pressure with drugs to a level just above the accepted 'normal' and by balancing their desired effects with a minimum of tolerable adverse effects. Adverse drug effects include faint feelings on standing up after sitting or lying down (*postural hypotension*), failure to ejaculate in men, diarrhoea, mood changes, blurred vision, drowsiness, stuffy nose, and changes in libido.

With appropriate drug treatment patients with severe blood pressure now have a far better chance of living much longer than they did, say, ten years ago. Many symptoms disappear and the risk of heart failure, angina and stroke may be impressively reduced. The effects of high blood pressure upon the blood vessels in the eyes may also be decreased. The drug treatment of moderate blood pressure also produces much benefit, and in early middle and middle-aged patients life can be prolonged by the treatment of mild or moderate blood pressure even though they may be without symptoms of raised blood pressure. Because of greater risks men need treatment more than women.

Drugs Used to Treat Raised Blood Pressure

Drugs used to treat raised blood pressure affect principally the blood volume and/or peripheral resistance.

Diuretics

These drugs cause a fall in blood pressure associated with a fall in circulating blood volume and cardiac output. However, during long-term use the blood volume returns to 'normal' and yet there is a continuing reduction in blood pressure with a reduction in peripheral resistance. Doses required to produce a fall in blood pressure seldom produce a troublesome fall in blood potassium and only a few patients may require potassium supplements if they are on long-term diuretic treatment for their hypertension (see p. 185). The **thiazide diuretics** are the most effective (see p. 181).

Centrally Acting Drugs

Drugs in this group affect both the central (the brain) and peripheral (the nerves) components of the sympathetic nervous system but the central effects predominate. Thus they rarely cause postural hypotension but may produce drowsiness, depression and excessive dreaming.

Methyldopa (Aldomet, Dopamet, Hydromet, Medomet) is thought to produce a false nerve transmitter which stimulates adrenaline receptors in the blood pressure control centre in the brain which responds by reducing the constriction of arteries causing a reduction in resistance to the flow of blood and a fall in blood pressure.

Reserpine-like drugs deplete the central and peripheral nerve endings of noradrenaline and thus reduce sympathetic control of blood vessels, producing dilatation. They can cause severe depression and are seldom used to treat hypertension.

Clonidone (Catapres) acts in a similar way to methyldopa.

Adrenergic Neurone Blockers

The **guanethidine group of drugs** prevent the release of noradrenaline from sympathetic nerve endings producing dilatation of blood vessels. They produce dry mouth, nasal stuffiness, impotence, failure to ejaculate, diarrhoea, fluid retention, postural hypotension and muscle weakness. They are used to treat severe hypertension and the group includes **guanethidine (Ismelin), bethanidine (Bendogen, Esbatal)** and **debrisoquine (Declinax)**.

Ganglion Blockers

These drugs block acetylcholine in the autonomic ganglia (rather like switchboxes), thus reducing sympathetic activity generally. This causes heart rate and peripheral resistance to fall, lowers the output from the heart and reduces the blood pressure. Their many adverse effects include rapid beating of the heart, blurred vision, dry mouth, constipation, difficulty in passing urine, impotence and failure to ejaculate. A severe adverse effect is a fall in blood on standing (postural hypotension). This group of drugs includes **hexamethonium, pempidine, mecamylamine** and **pentolinium**. They are now obsolete.

Vasodilators

Hydralazine (Apresoline) lowers both lying and standing blood pressures. It causes vasodilatation by a direct action on the muscles of the blood vessels, thus producing a decrease in peripheral resistance and a fall in blood pressure. It causes headache, nasal stuffiness, flushing, gastro-intestinal upsets, tachycardia and in certain patients who break the drug down slowly, it produces systemic lupus erythematosus (SLE) (a disorder like rheuma-toid arthritis with skin rashes).

Other direct acting vasodilators include **diazoxide (Eudemine), sodium nitroprusside (Nipride)** and **minoxidil (Loniten)**.

Alpha Adreno-receptor Blockers

These drugs block alpha receptors (see p. 96). Those that are not selective may produce tachycardia, a severe fall in blood pressure, and they may precipitate angina because they reduce the blood supply to the heart. They are not used in the routine management of hypertension but may be used in a crisis and in the diagnosis and pre-operative treatment of patients with a phaeochromocytoma. They include **phenoxybenzamine (Dibenyline), phentolamine (Rogitine)** and **indoramin (Baratol)**. Selective alpha-blockers include **prazosin (Hypovase)** and **terazosin (Hytrin)**. They produce fewer adverse effects than the non-selective ones.

Beta Adreno-receptor Blockers (Beta-blockers)

These are discussed in detail on p. 152. They cause a fall in blood pressure but their mode of action is not understood. They reduce heart output, alter the sensitivity of baroreceptors (p. 162), block peripheral adrenoreceptors (p. 162) and some of them depress renin production (p. 162).

Angiotensin-converting enzyme inhibitors

Captopril (Acepril, Capoten) and **enalapril (Innovace)** inhibit the conversion of angiotensin I to angiotensin II (see p. 162), reduce constriction of arteries and reduce blood volume.

Calcium-channel Blockers

Nicardipine (Cardene); nifedipine (Adalat) and **verapamil (Berkatens; Cordilox; Securon; Univer)** reduce constriction of arteries, cause a fall in resistance to the flow of blood and reduce blood pressure. They are being used increasingly to treat raised blood pressure.

Other Drugs

Metirosine (Demser) affects the production of adrenaline-like chemicals in the body and is used in the pre-operative treatment of phaeochromocytoma. It should not be used to treat essential hypertension. **Calcium antagonists** (see p. 154) are being used increasingly to treat hypertension.

Treatment of hypertension

General measures should include stopping smoking, reducing salt intake (no added salt with meals), reducing weight if you are overweight, reducing the amount of alcohol you drink if you are a moderate to heavy drinker, eating a well-balanced diet and taking adequate rest and exercise.

The drug treatment of hypertension involves using a diuretic with or without a beta-blocker. If this combination does not work then a vasodilator should be added and/or one of the drugs which act on the sympathetic system.

26 Drugs Used to Treat Atherosclerosis of the Arteries

Atherosclerosis refers to the thickening of the walls of arteries caused by deposits of fats and other substances. This causes the vessels to become narrow and the lining surface roughened. This narrowing produces serious impairment of blood flow. Atherosclerosis of the coronary arteries has been directly related to angina and to deaths from heart attacks due to coronary thrombosis. When it affects the arteries supplying the brain it may cause impairment of mental function and thrombosis leading to paralysis. In the legs it may cause pains in the muscles on exercise, poor circulation to the skin and many other serious consequences.

In recent years it has become apparent that there are many factors which cause coronary artery disease. We should all know the risks of smoking, overeating and not taking enough exercise. One fairly constant factor which has been discussed is the relationship between high 'blood fat levels' and coronary artery disease in some patients. I use 'blood fat levels' to cover a complex group of fats (which includes cholesterol) and other chemicals which are called lipoproteins. The importance of the relationship between 'blood fat' levels and atherosclerosis is continually being examined. In families who suffer from high blood fat levels and in patients with such disorders as diabetes (in which the blood fat levels are increased) the incidence of coronary artery disease is markedly increased. In countries where diets are different from many Western countries and where it has been found that blood fat levels are lower, the incidence of coronary artery disease is less: it dropped during the Second World War in some European countries, probably because of changes in diet (e.g., less animal fats in food). Animal experiments have also shown this relationship between diet and atherosclerosis.

Drugs are available which lower 'blood fat' levels but the need to use these drugs is not clear. Different drugs lower different 'blood fats' and yet the part played by each is not fully understood. Certain high-risk patients may benefit from the use of these drugs – patients in whom high blood fat levels run in the family; patients with high blood fat levels and high blood pressure; and patients who have survived a coronary thrombosis. But, obviously, the most sensible approach to treatment of a high 'blood fat' is to control the diet.

Obesity may be associated with a high 'blood fat' level, so may the amounts of carbohydrates or fats in the diet. The type and ratio of different fats in the diet can also influence the 'blood fat' levels, particularly the ratio of what are called unsaturated fatty acids (in vegetable and fish oils) to saturated fatty acids (in animal fats and dairy produce). A source of unsaturated fatty acids was shown, many years ago, to be beneficial in preventing coronary artery disease. However, although there has been an increased consumption of vegetable oils over this period there is still some confusion; for example, coconut oil is high in saturated fatty acids and is less desirable than animal fats and dairy produce whereas sunflower oil is a good source of unsaturated fatty acids.

The answer is to eat a well-balanced diet, take regular exercise, keep your weight down and cut out smoking. If you are diet-conscious then eat margarine instead of butter and fry in vegetable oil instead of lard and so on. And just to make it more difficult refined sugar is also suspected of being a contributory factor in causing coronary artery disease.

Drugs which Lower Blood Fat Levels

Clofibrate (Atromid-S) and bezafibrate (Bezalip) are effective in lowering certain of the 'blood fats', although their mode of action is not fully understood. They affect enzymes in the body and prevent the formation of cholesterol. They produce a group of symptoms which include muscle cramps, stiffness, weakness and muscle tenderness. They should not be given to patients with impaired kidney or liver function or during pregnancy. Their long-term use has been shown to be associated with severe complications and they are only recommended in patients with signs of eye damage (exudative retinopathy), fatty deposits in the skin (xanthomata) and high blood fat levels (hyperlipoproteinaemias) and where careful investigations have been carried out by the doctors to define the type and severity of the underlying disorders – gemfibrozil (Lopid) is also used to reduce blood fat levels, and Maxepa (a mixture of fish oils, see Part Three) is used to reduce certain blood fats (triglycerides).

Nicotinic acid and related drugs (e.g., nicofuranose (Bradilan)) may reduce 'blood fat' levels but may produce flushing and itching, which usually clears after a few weeks in most patients. Such large doses may however cause liver damage and jaundice. Acipimox (Olbetam) is related to nicotinic acid but is more active and longer lasting.

Cholestyramine (Questran) also reduces blood fat levels. It works in the gut by exchanging chloride ions for bile salts (which are formed in part from 'blood fats') which it binds into an insoluble complex that is excreted in the faeces, so preventing the reabsorption of bile salts and cholesterol. This causes further conversion of 'fats' to bile salts, which eventually may lead to a reduction in blood 'fat levels'. It may also interfere with the absorption of other drugs (chlorothiazide, phenobarbitone, tetracyclines, thyroid hormones and many others). High doses interfere with the absorption of fat and fat-soluble vitamins such as vitamins A and D. Therefore, any other drug should not be taken within one hour of a dose of cholestyramine. Extra vitamin A and D should be taken, of a type that can be mixed with water; patients on prolonged treatment should also take vitamin K. **Colestipol (Colestid)** produces similar effects.

Probucol (Lurselle) lowers blood fat levels by increasing the breakdown of cholesterol to bile salts.

Blood fat levels are low in patients with disorders which cause overworking of the thyroid gland and they are high in patients with disorders which cause underworking of the gland. Although drugs related to thyroid hormones lower blood fat levels (e.g., **dextrothyroxine; Choloxin**), they also push up the frequency and severity of anginal attacks in patients suffering from coronary artery disease. They may, in addition, produce disorders of heart rhythm and other adverse effects, and are therefore not suitable for lowering blood fat levels.

Oestrogens (female sex hormones) when given to males reduce their blood fat levels, but high doses are needed, which make them develop breasts, become impotent, lose their libido and, not surprisingly, become depressed.

The Use of Blood Fat Lowering Drugs

Obviously the future must lie in attempting to prevent atherosclerosis by controlling our diet, taking more exercise and cutting out smoking. In the meantime these drugs are of use in treating selected patients who have been shown to have raised blood fat levels, although as yet conclusive proof of their long-term value is needed. The three drugs discussed – clofibrate, nicotinic acid and cholestyramine – work on different 'blood fats'. The decision to use one or the other must depend upon detailed and repeated tests of blood fat levels, careful examination and the rigorous selection of at-risk patients for treatment.

27 Drugs Used to Treat Disorders of the Circulation

The Use of Drugs to Increase Circulation to the Limbs

The blood supply to the arms and legs may be affected by anything which obstructs the flow of blood through the arteries. This may be caused by a blockage within the artery; for example, a thrombosis which if recognized very quickly may sometimes be treated by surgical removal. However, most thromboses are treated with drugs which stop the blood from clotting. The flow of blood may also be reduced by narrowing of arteries, which may be caused by hardening and loss of elasticity of the artery walls (arteriosclerosis). This process occurs with advancing age, especially in those patients with high blood pressure, where such changes may be found not only in medium-sized and large arteries but also in the smaller arteries which supply the various tissues and organs of the body. Medium and large arteries may also be affected by atherosclerosis which is a process of 'furring up' on the inside walls of arteries. This narrows the artery and reduces the blood flow. It may affect the coronary arteries supplying the heart, the circulation to the brain or the circulation to the limbs. It appears to be related to blood fat levels (see p. 167). The artery walls may also be affected by inflammation (e.g., syphilis) or by allergic reactions. An obscure disorder called Buerger's disease (thrombo-angitis-obliterans) occasionally affects the arteries of the legs in middle-aged men who are heavy smokers.

The amount of blood flowing through an artery may also be reduced because its walls close up (go into spasm) due to some fault in the control mechanisms which normally govern the supply of blood to a particular tissue or organ. Blood flow to any part of the body (e.g., skin, muscle) is controlled by a balance between the pressure of blood within the arteries and the amount of resistance the flow meets when it gets to the blood vessels which supply the tissues. This resistance can vary and is delicately controlled by the body. It is produced by controlling the degree of spasm of the terminal vessels and smaller arteries. This spasm is under continuous monitoring by nerves in the vessel walls which respond to three mechanisms. Firstly, stimulation of the nerves releases a chemical called noradrenaline which produces constriction. Secondly, the muscles of these blood vessels have a natural tone which makes them 'want' to constrict. Thirdly, a variety of chemicals produced by the body in response to certain reactions may cause them to open up or close down.

There are two types of nerve receptors in blood vessels which are simply called alpha-receptors and beta-receptors (p. 171). The alpha-receptors cause constriction and beta-receptors cause dilatation of the vessels.

Drugs which improve the circulation act by either blocking the stimulation of the alpha-receptors; by stimulating the beta-receptors; or by acting directly upon muscles in the vessel walls. Unfortunately, most disorders of circulation are due to changes in the artery walls (arteriosclerosis, atherosclerosis) which make the walls harden and unresponsive to stimulation. Also, if a medium or large artery supplying an arm or leg is hardened and narrowed, the branch arteries (collateral circulation) are usually working to maximum capacity and cannot be further stimulated to dilate. In such cases the use of drugs may be harmful; for example, it may divert an already poor blood supply from the skin to the muscles instead, leading to further damage to the skin.

Drugs used to improve circulation are often referred to as **vasodilator drugs** and the patients who may benefit from the use of these drugs are those with disorders due to spasm of arteries (vasospasm). For example, there is a vasospastic disorder called Raynaud's disease which usually affects women under fifty. In these patients exposure to cold, and sometimes emotion, may cause the fingers to 'go dead'. All fingers are affected and sometimes the toes. The patient experiences pins and needles, numbness, burning and pain. The fingers go pale, bluish and then red. Vasodilator drugs may benefit those patients with mild symptoms but severe and long-standing symptoms are usually associated with irreversible changes in the vessels which may make vasodilator drugs ineffective.

Vasodilator drugs are of limited value in other vasospastic disorders. Their benefit to patients with chilblains is very doubtful and their use to prevent frostbite has been disappointing. This is because exposure to low temperatures closes up the blood vessels supplying local areas of skin and makes them unresponsive to vasodilator drugs. Other conditions such as acrocyanosis (blueness of the fingers, hands, ears and nose on exposure to cold) and erythrocyanosis (a bluish-red discoloration of the legs) are not helped by such drugs. A disorder characterized by red, burning feet (erythromelalgia) may occasionally be helped by vasodilator drugs.

In patients with disease of artery walls (arteriosclerosis, atherosclerosis, Buerger's disease) vasodilator drugs may not work, but they may increase blood flow to the skin and be of use in treating ulcers of the skin caused by poor circulation. They may also be of use in treating gangrene.

Poor circulation may cause pain in the muscles on exercise (intermittent claudication), but, unfortunately, this is not much helped by vasodilator drugs. 'Rest pains' in the limbs (a warning that gangrene may be developing) may be helped.

Vasodilator drugs relax the muscles in vessels either directly or indirectly through adrenergic nerves. The ones used to treat peripheral vascular disorders and disorders of cerebral arteries include alpha-adrenergic receptor blockers, beta-adrenergic stimulants and drugs which act directly on the vessels as a muscle relaxant.

1. Alpha-adrenergic Receptor Blocking Drugs

These drugs block the alpha-receptors and, therefore, cause the peripheral blood vessels to dilate. Their effects are most marked in the blood vessels in the skin of the arms and legs. The blood vessels supplying muscles are affected much less. The selective alpha-blockers **prazosin (Hypovase)** and **thymoxamine (Opilon)** have been used to treat Raynaud's disease.

Phenoxybenzamine and thymoxamine should be given with caution to patients with high blood pressure, impaired kidney function, or coronary artery disease and not to any patient in whom a fall in blood pressure may be harmful.

2. Beta-adrenergic Receptor Stimulant Drugs

These cause dilatation of the arteries by stimulating the beta-receptors. Since beta-receptors are mainly present in blood vessels supplying muscles, these drugs are principally used to improve the blood circulation to muscles. They stimulate the heart, increase its rate and output and are likely to cause a fall in blood pressure. The most commonly used is **isoxsuprine (Duvadilan)**. It should be given with caution to patients with low blood pressure or to those with a fast heart rate.

3. Nicotinic acid derivatives

These drugs cause arteries to dilate by a direct unknown action upon the artery walls. They cause vasodilatation and increase the blood flow to muscles and skin. The changes in the skin circulation are more marked in the face and neck (where you blush) than in the arms and legs. They include nicotinic acid (in Pernivit), nicofuranose (Bradilan), inositol nicotinate (Hexopal) and nicotinyl alcohol (Ronicol).

4. Other drugs

Calcium-channel blockers (p. 154) such as **nifedipine**, dilate peripheral arteries and have been used to treat Raynaud's disease.

Cyclandelate (Cyclobral, Cyclospasmol) which affects calcium metabolism in the muscle walls of arteries causing them to dilate is used to treat circulatory disorders.

The so-called cellular activators improve oxygen and glucose use by cells and are used to treat circulatory disorders. They include **co-dergocrine (Hydergine)** from ergot and **naftidrofuryl (Praxilene)**.

The antihistamine **cinnarizine (Stugeron)** is also beneficial in some people as is **oxpentifylline (Trental)** which is a xanthine derivative (see caffeine, p. 81).

The Use of Vasodilator Drugs

Mild adverse effects with vasodilator drugs are common, and when given in effective dose they usually cause rapid beating of the heart and a fall in blood pressure. You may develop flushing of the face and stuffiness of the nose. Some of the drugs may cause gastro-intestinal symptoms – nausea, vomiting, diarrhoea. Some patients complain of feeling excitable. Vasodilator drugs should not be used in patients with coronary artery disease, congestive heart failure, peptic ulcers, overworking of the thyroid or with glaucoma. They should be used with caution by patients with impaired heart function, diabetes or impaired kidney function.

They may be of some use in disorders of arterial spasm but their use in arterial diseases which damage vessel walls is doubtful. There is no one drug which may be recommended over the others in the various groups. They are sometimes prescribed for chilblains, but warm surroundings (e.g., central heating), warm clothes and exercise will be of more benefit than any drug available.

Drugs Used to Increase the Circulation to the Brain

No drug has a special effect upon the blood vessels which supply the brain. Those that are used are general vasodilators. Their effectiveness in treating disorders produced by changes in the arteries supplying the brain, though of help in some patients, has never been clearly evaluated because of the complexities involved. Furthermore, there are risks involved in the use of such drugs – fall in blood pressure and redistribution of blood supply away from areas that may require more oxygen as the result of an already diminished blood supply.

Cyclandelate (Cyclobral, Cyclospasmol), **isoxsuprine (Defencin*, Duvadilan)** and **naftidrofuryl (Praxilene)** are principally used for this purpose. **Ergot alkaloids** (as, for example, in **Hydergine**) may also be tried. **Nimodipine (Nimotop)** is a new calcium-channel blocker used to dilate the arteries of the brain in order to improve the blood supply following spasm of the arteries which may occur as a result of bleeding between the membranes of the brain (subarachnoid haemorrhage).

28 Drugs Used to Prevent Blood from Clotting

Drugs used to prevent blood from clotting are called anticoagulants. We do not completely understand how these drugs work, partly because of the complexities involved in the process of clotting. There are a series of clotting factors which have been recognized as contributing to the eventual formation of a blood clot. Anticoagulant drugs interfere with this process.

Anticoagulant drugs interfere with blood clotting and yet they are principally used to treat patients who have developed a clot. A thrombosis is a clot of blood which develops on the inside wall of a blood vessel and may be related to damage or changes in the surface lining and also to changes in the blood. The relationship between blood clotting (as tested outside in the laboratory) and the development of a thrombosis inside a blood vessel is not known. Even so, prolonged clinical experience of the use of anticoagulant drugs in thousands of patients has shown that they are of great benefit in treating thromboses – if used appropriately.

Anticoagulants are used to treat a thrombosis (e.g., deep leg vein thrombosis) in which they may reduce further thrombosis. They may also prevent pieces of the thrombus (clot) coming loose and being carried by the flow of blood to other organs – if these are the lungs or brain, the consequence may be serious and sometimes fatal. This process of a clot loosening and passing along the blood-stream is called embolism. The piece of clot which ends up wedged in and blocking a blood vessel is called an embolus. This process is one of the great dangers of thrombosis, particularly if the thrombosis affects the veins in the abdomen or legs after injury, surgical operations or childbirth.

Anticoagulants greatly reduce the risk of death in patients with thrombosis affecting deep veins of the legs or abdomen and in those patients who have developed an embolus in their lungs. They may also help to prevent deep vein thrombosis, particularly in elderly patients confined to bed after a surgical operation. Anticoagulant drugs are also used to treat thrombosis of the vessels supplying the eyes and to treat thrombosis occurring in other arteries. They are used to treat patients with rheumatic heart disease who develop irregularities of heart rhythm and who run the risk of shooting off an embolus when the heart rate is controlled by drugs. Anticoagulants are also used after heart operations and in kidney dialysis.

Anticoagulants are more effective in preventing thrombus formation or the extension of an existing thrombus in the veins where blood flows more slowly and the thrombus consists of a fibrin web enmeshed with platelets and red blood cells. They are less effective in the arteries where the blood flows much faster and the thrombus is formed mainly of platelets with little fibrin.

Anticoagulant Drugs

Anticoagulant drugs may be divided into two groups: those that act directly by interfering with the process of blood clotting and have to be given by injection (e.g., heparin, which prevents blood from clotting even in a test tube); and those that act indirectly and may be given by mouth. The latter act only inside the body by interfering with the production of factors involved in blood clotting. Those drugs which act directly like heparin are rapidly effective whereas those that act indirectly are slow to work (up to three days).

Direct-acting Anticoagulants (heparin and ancrod)

Heparin preparations for intravenous use include **heparin injections, Monoparin, Multiparin, Pump-Hep** and **Unihep**. For subcutaneous use they include **heparin injection, Calciparine, Minihep, Minihep Calcium, Monoparin, Monoparin Calcium, Uniparin, Uniparin Calcium, Uniparin Forte. Heparin flushes** for keeping catheters and cannulas open include **Hep-Flush, Heplok** and **Hepsal**.

Heparin acts directly in the blood by preventing thrombin formation, by inhibiting thrombin activity and reducing platelet stickiness. It does not work when given by mouth; it is best given by injection into a vein. It works immediately, but its effects quickly wear off and it has to be given every four or six hours. It may also be given by injection under the skin. The normal time taken for the blood to clot on glass (known as the clotting time) is about five to seven minutes. If heparin is to be effective the dose should be adjusted to keep the clotting-time above fifteen minutes. The test usually used is the activated thromboplastin time (a measure of clotting time). Adverse effects to heparin therapy are bleeding into various sites and, in rare cases, fever and allergic reactions. Signs of overdose are nose bleeds, bruising, and red blood cells in the urine. Slight bleeding due to overdosage can usually be treated by stopping the drug. Severe bleeding may be reduced by giving a slow intravenous injection of protamine sulphate.

Ancrod is a purified extract from the venom of the Malayan pit-viper and it prevents the formation of fibrin. It may cause bleeding, skin rashes, and swelling and redness at the site of the injection. Some patients show resistance to a second course of treatment, particularly after intramuscular injections. Its effects may be reversed by a specific anti-venom or by giving fibrinogen (a blood-clotting factor) or an infusion of plasma.

Indirect-acting Anticoagulants (Oral Anticoagulants, Vitamin K Antagonists)

Oral anticoagulants antagonize the effects of vitamin K which is essential for the development of four clotting factors by cells in the liver. They include two main groups:

Coumarin derivatives. These include **nicoumalone (Sinthrome)** and **warfarin sodium (Marevan, Warfarin WBP)**. They may be taken by mouth and are slow to act. **Nicoumalone** works within 36 to 48 hours and its effects wear off within 36 to 48 hours of the last dose. **Warfarin sodium** works in 36 to 72 hours and its effects may last up to 4 to 5 days after stopping the drug. It is also used as a rat poison.

Indanedione derivatives. **Phenindione (Dindevan)** is the most frequently used of this group. It takes up to 24 to 48 hours to reach its desired effect and this wears off within 1 to 4 days of stopping the drug. Its metabolites colour the urine reddish-orange. Early signs of over-dosage are bleeding from the gums or elsewhere and red blood cells in the urine. Deaths have occurred in people allergic to phenindione; it is therefore used less frequently than the coumarins.

The Use of Oral Anticoagulants

Because of the delayed action an initial loading dose was given in the past. This technique has been largely discontinued because of the danger of haemorrhage. Therefore, in order to start patients off on a course of anticoagulants in emergency situations heparin is given at the same time, usually for the first two days. Maintenance doses of oral anticoagulants are calculated according to a blood-clotting test called the prothrombin-time. This is carried out in a laboratory and the aim of treatment should be to keep the prothrombin-time at two to three times the normal value of twelve seconds. (A ratio of patient's time over a control time (i.e., blood from a normal person) is sometimes used and this ratio should be kept between 1·8 and 3.) Daily estimates should be made initially and once a steady prothrombin-time is achieved the frequency of tests may be reduced. Since these drugs are accumulative, the dose should not be changed more frequently than every five or seven days. Bleeding is the most common adverse effect (e.g. bruising, bleeding gums, blood in the urine); it may be reduced by administering vitamin K – in about four hours by intravenous injection, or by mouth in about twelve hours. Massive bleeding will require the transfusion of fresh frozen plasma. Before using these drugs a knowledge of other drugs which interact with them is necessary.

Because of the risk of severe hypersensitivity reactions from phenindione and other indanedione derivatives it is better to use one of the coumarin derivatives – e.g., warfarin sodium or nicoumalone.

Precautions in the Use of Oral Anticoagulants

Oral anticoagulants should be used with caution in patients with impaired kidney or liver function and in patients in whom there is a risk of haemorrhage (they may be used during menstruation). They should not be used within three days of childbirth or of a surgical operation. Mothers on these drugs should not breast feed unless blood-monitoring facilities are available, and the drugs should not be taken in the first three months and last few weeks of pregnancy.

Many drugs interact with oral anticoagulants. For example, the effects of phenindione are increased by clofibrate, and by anabolic steroids (see p. 226). The effect of warfarin sodium is increased by, for example, aspirin and other salicylates, clofibrate, dextrothyroxine, disulfiram and possibly by anabolic steroids, certain antibiotics, quinidine, chloral hydrate, amiodarone and cimetidine. Effects are decreased by barbiturates, glutethimide, vitamin K, griseofulvin and rifampicin.

If you are on an oral anticoagulant drug you should carry a warning card and carefully check the list of drugs which may interact with anticoagulants. If there is an unexpected change in your prothrombin-time then check on any drug you have been taking to see if it interferes with the effects of the anticoagulant drug you are on.

Antiplatelet Drugs

When the lining (endothelium) of blood vessels is injured, platelets stick to the damaged wall. This stimulates them to release several chemicals including a prostaglandin which is converted to thromboxane which stimulates the platelets to stick together. This mass of sticky platelets can then stimulate the formation of a clot (thrombus). There are drugs available which help to reduce this platelet stickiness:

Aspirin inhibits the production of thromboxane (a chemical which produces platelet stickiness) and helps to reduce thrombus formation. A single dose of aspirin has an effect on platelet stickiness and the bleeding time for up to five days. It has now been found of value in the treatment of disorders produced by transient reduction in blood flow to the brain (transient cerebral ischaemia) and in preventing a recurrence of coronary thrombosis if taken regularly in a small dosage. Used daily for three weeks preceding surgery it may reduce the incidence of post-operative deep vein thrombosis and pulmonary embolism.

Sulphinpyrazone (Anturan) is used to treat gout (see p. 202). It also inhibits prostaglandin synthesis and is used to treat and prevent thrombosis. However, unlike aspirin, it only works for as long as it is in the circulation.

Dipyridamole (Persantin) in high doses has been claimed to have some effect in reducing platelet stickiness and has been used along with an aspirin in order to prevent thrombus formation on heart valves, but it is probably no better than aspirin alone.

Other antiplatelet drugs include **clofibrate** (p. 168) and **dextran**.

Antifibrinolytic drugs

Tranexamic acid (Cyclokapron) impairs the breakdown of fibrin in thrombi and is used to treat bleeding caused by excessive breakdown of fibrin. It blocks the activation of plasminogen to plasmin. **Aprotinin (Trasylol)** is another antifibrinolytic, it prevents plasmin from being dissolved.

Other drugs

Ethamsylate (Dicynene) prevents bleeding from small capillaries by improving the function of their lining and improving the stickiness of platelets.

Fibrinolytic Drugs

These drugs activate plasminogen to form plasmin which breaks down the fibrin in thrombus. They include **streptokinase (Kabikinase, Streptase)** which is an enzyme produced by bacteria (haemolytic streptococci) and **urokinase (Ukidan, Urokinase)** obtained from human urine. Both drugs are given intravenously to treat massive thromboses. Adverse reactions may occur with streptokinase; these include rashes, bronchospasm and anaphylaxis. Severe bleeding may occur with both drugs.

The term diuretic refers to a drug which acts upon the kidneys to produce an increased output of sodium salt and water in the urine. These drugs are used to treat disorders of the heart, kidneys or liver which result in an excessive retention of fluids in the body, so much so that swelling may be visible – this is called oedema or what used to be called dropsy. Swelling of the tissues is usually more obvious in the feet and ankles because of the effect of gravity. In a patient confined to bed the fluid gravitates to the lower part of the back which may then be swollen. Excessive fluid inside the abdominal cavity is called ascites. Diuretics are also used to treat disorders in which fluid accumulates in the lung tissue (pulmonary oedema) – this may be a serious medical emergency.

Some weak diuretics are used to decrease the fluid pressure inside the eyeball, as in the treatment of glaucoma, where the drainage of the eye fluid is impaired. But, it must be remembered that the underlying disease process in all of these disorders is not affected by diuretic treatment. In addition, diuretics are used to counter the salt and water retention produced by other drugs, and to treat overdose with certain drugs that are excreted by the kidneys, by increasing output of urine. However, their most common use is in the treatment of raised blood pressure.

The kidneys exercise a most delicate and complex control over the body's salt and water balance. Salt at first enters the urine but is subsequently reabsorbed into the blood-stream according to body needs. The amount of salt in the urine governs the amount of water passed out by the process known as osmosis (water moves from the weaker solution to the stronger when separated by a partially permeable membrane). The process of osmosis takes the direction from the weaker to the stronger solution so that if there is a lot of salt in the urine, a lot of water will pass out and be excreted in the urine. In addition, there are other rather complex chemical and hormonal processes which affect the amount of salt and water passed out in the urine.

The great majority of diuretics in use today act directly upon the kidneys by depressing the reabsorption of salt from the urine back into the blood-stream, thus producing an increased output of salt and water from the body (**diuresis**) – the increase in water excretion is therefore a secondary result of decreased salt reabsorption. Sodium is the important electrolyte – when this is not reabsorbed, water will also not be reabsorbed and diuresis (increased volume of urine) is produced. Some diuretics as well as affecting the reabsorption of sodium also interfere with the reabsorption of potassium. This produces a low blood potassium level which may produce muscle weakness, constipation, loss of appetite and, more seriously, a low blood potassium affects the heart. It also sensitizes the heart to digitalis drugs which are frequently used to treat heart failure and disorders of heart rhythm (see p. 160).

There are four main groups of diuretics – thiazides and related drugs, loop diuretics, aldosterone antagonists and potassium sparing diuretics. Other diuretics include mild diuretics used to treat glaucoma, osmotic diuretics and xanthine diuretics.

Thiazide Diuretics and Related Drugs

Thiazides comprise the largest group of diuretic drugs. They act on the tubules in the kidneys (proximal segment of the distal convoluted tubule) preventing salt reabsorption. These drugs are of moderate potency and vary in their duration of effect. When used in effective dosage they all increase the excretion of potassium. They are used to treat disorders where fluid is retained in the body, as in heart failure. They are also used alone or in combination with other drugs to treat raised blood pressure (see p. 163).

They include:

bendrofluazide (Aprinox, Berkozide, Centyl, Centyl-K, Neo-Naclex, Neo-Naclex K)
benzthiazide (Dytide (with triamterene))
chlorothiazide (Saluric)
chlorthalidone (Hygroton, Hygroton-K and Kalspare (with triamterene))
clopamide (Brinaldix-K)
cyclopenthiazide (Navidrex, Navidrex-K)
hydrochlorothiazide (Esidrex, Esidrex-K, Hydrosaluric and in **Amilco, Hypertane, Moduretic, Moduret, Normetic, Synuretic** and **Triamco (with added amiloride) and in Dyazide (with added triamterene)** and **Acezide** and **Caposide (with captopril))**
hydroflumethiazide (Hydrenox and Aldactide (with spironolactone))
indapamide (Natrilix)
mefruside (Baycaron)
methyclothiazide (Enduron)
metolazone (Metenix)
polythiazide (Nephril)
xipamide (Diurexan).

All thiazide diuretics have similar effects and adverse effects to chlorothiazide; they may rarely cause nausea, dizzinesss, weakness, numbness and pins and needles, skin rashes, allergic reactions, blood disorders and sensitivity of the skin to sunlight.

Thiazide diuretics reduce sodium and potassium blood levels* and sometimes increase blood calcium. They may send up the blood sugar and cause sugar to appear in the urine in diabetics and other susceptible individuals. They may also cause an increase in blood uric acid level and trigger off an attack of gout in some people. They should be used with caution in patients with impaired kidney or liver function or with diabetes.

A restricted salt intake (no added salt at the table) is helpful to patients being treated for fluid retention. A diet rich in potassium (e.g. fresh fruit) can help to compensate for the loss of potassium produced by diuretics. Some patients, however, will need to take potassium supplements as well. However, these are not very pleasant to take; they may irritate the stomach and may produce ulcers in the gut.

Including potassium in diuretic tablets has never been convincingly shown to be of any benefit in preventing a fall in body potassium levels. It is better to use the diuretic intermittently (every other day or twice a week), and maintain a good diet. If potassium levels fall then the addition of a potassium-sparing diuretic (p. 184) or supplements of potassium salts given separately from the diuretics will help. Potassium chloride is the best salt to use because of the loss of chloride which diuretics produce. **Effervescent potassium chloride** tablets (**Sando-K, Kloref**) are satisfactory. **Slow-release potassium chloride (Slow-K)** tablets may cause ulcers of the gut. *Liquid preparations of potassium chloride are safest.*

Because of the effect of thiazide diuretics on blood sugar, they may sometimes trigger off an attack of diabetes in a person predisposed to develop diabetes. If you are on long-term treatment with one of these drugs you ought to get your urine tested for sugar periodically. Similarly if you have a family history of gout it may be worth asking your doctor to check your blood uric acid level at intervals. Your blood salt levels should also be checked at intervals.

Diuretic drugs are not prescribed with the respect they deserve. They are valuable drugs and have revolutionized the treatment of congestive heart failure and raised blood pressure. Yet they are often prescribed in inappropriate dosage for too long a time and without sufficient advice to the patient about frequency of dosage and diet and warnings of adverse effects.

---

* The reduction in body potassium may increase the toxicity of digoxin and related drugs on the heart.

Loop Diuretics

These include **frusemide (Aluzine, Diumide-K, Diuresal, Dryptal, Frumil** and **Lasoride (with amiloride), Frusene (with triamterene), Frusetic, Frusid, Lasikal, Lasilactone (with spironolactone), Lasix, Lasix+K), ethacrynic acid (Edecrin)** and **bumetanide (Burinex, Burinex K)** also **piretanide (Arelix)**. They inhibit salt reabsorption in the ascending limb of the loop of Henle in the kidneys and are therefore known as loop diuretics. These are more potent than the thiazide diuretics and although they are chemically different they have similar effects. They act quickly when given by injection and the duration of their effect is short. Dosage must be controlled with caution since high doses may produce a massive output of urine leading to a fall in blood pressure, which may result in a decreased production of urine by the kidneys. They are of use where urgent diuresis is required – e.g., oedema of the lungs – and where thiazide diuretics have failed. They should be used with caution in elderly patients with enlarged prostate glands since the increased production of urine may cause retention of urine. These drugs may cause potassium loss* and some patients may require potassium supplements. They may produce skin rashes, tinnitus (ringing in the ears) and deafness in patients with impaired kidney function.

Aldosterone Antagonists

Aldosterone is a hormone produced by the adrenal glands. It plays a role in the body's salt and water balancing mechanisms. An excess of it may be produced by a tumour of the adrenal glands or in response to certain disorders such as severe congestive heart failure or cirrhosis of the liver associated with the collection of increased fluid in the abdomen (ascites). It works on the kidneys where it increases the reabsorption of sodium and the excretion of potassium. There are drugs which block these effects thus increasing the excretion of sodium (which takes water with it) and reducing the excretion of potassium.

Spironolactone (in **Aldactide, Aldactone, Diatensec, Laractone,** in **Lasilactone, Spiretic, Spiroctan, Spirolone**) is such a drug. It is of some use in treating ascites due to cirrhosis of the liver, but in treating other disorders not primarily due to hyperaldosteronism (increased production of aldosterone) it is best combined with a thiazide diuretic. It is absorbed from the gut, is slow to act (up to three days) and it is excreted slowly. Because of the risk of causing a high blood potassium, spironolactone should be given with caution to patients with impaired kidney function. **Potassium canrenoate**

---

* See note on p. 182.

(**Spiroctan-M**) has similar uses to spironolactone but it can be given by injection. It is broken down in the liver to canrenone, which is a breakdown product of spironolactone.

Potassium-sparing Diuretics

Triamterene (in Dyazide (with hydrochlorothiazide), Dytac, Dytide (with added benzthiazide) in Frusene (with frusemide), Triamcol (with hydro-chlorothiazide)) reduces sodium reabsorption in the distal renal tubules and thus reduces potassium loss in the urine. It was originally thought that it blocked the effects of aldosterone on the kidneys like spironolactone but animal experiments have not shown this. Triamterene is not a very potent diuretic and it is usually combined with a thiazide diuretic. It should be used with caution in patients with impaired liver or kidney function and in those with diabetes. **Amiloride (Midamor)** has effects and uses similar to triamterene.

The principal use of triamterene and amiloride is in combination with a thiazide diuretic in order to reduce potassium loss in the urine. Occasionally the use of such combinations, particularly in patients with impaired kidney function, can cause dangerously high blood potassium levels. Therefore, blood potassium levels should be regularly monitored in these patients.

Mild Diuretics Used to Treat Glaucoma

In the early 1950s a group of diuretics was introduced which blocked the action of an enzyme (an organic catalyst) which is involved in the kidneys' control of water and salt balance. The enzyme is responsible for exchanging hydrogen ions for sodium ions in the urine so that body sodium is conserved. The diuretics block this action and cause the sodium not to be reabsorbed. This group of drugs includes **acetazolamide (Diamox)** and **dichlorphenamide (Daranide)**. Acetazolamide causes mild adverse effects fairly frequently. The body's potassium and sodium level may fall after prolonged use and patients with impaired liver function may become confused and disoriented. Acetazolamide may rarely damage the kidneys and bone marrow producing blood disorders. Dichlorphenamide produces similar adverse effects but no blood disorders or kidney damage have been reported.

In the treatment of glaucoma they reduce the formation of fluid inside the eye and reduce the pressure. Tolerance quickly develops to the diuretic effects, and they should only be given intermittently, although some eye specialists seem to go on using them indefinitely.

Osmotic Diuretics

Any substance which passes out of the blood in the kidneys and into the urine may interfere with salt reabsorption, resulting in an increase in urine volume and the excretion of larger amounts of sodium and potassium. The ones used for this purpose are called osmotic diuretics and they should produce no other action in the body. They include **mannitol, urea, glucose** and **sucrose**.

Mannitol is a type of alcohol which is excreted by the kidneys and because it is not reabsorbed it causes diuresis. It has to be given by intravenous injection. Glucose and sucrose are sugars and act in a similar way.

Urea (Carbamide) is rarely used as an osmotic diuretic.

Osmotic diuretics may be used to keep urine flow going after severe injury, in order to prevent kidney damage, to eliminate certain drugs after overdose (e.g., aspirin, barbiturates) and to reduce the pressure due to fluid accumulation inside the eyes in glaucoma and inside the skull after head injury. They are rarely used to treat oedema.

Xanthine Diuretics

This group includes **caffeine, theophylline** and **theobromine**. They are present in tea, coffee, cola and cocoa. They are mild diuretics and work both directly and indirectly on the kidneys to produce a diuresis.

Use of Diuretics

Thiazide diuretics are taken by mouth and are useful for long-term treatment and the choice is not critical. Potassium loss may be reduced by taking them every other day or twice a week and by taking a diet containing foods high in potassium (e.g., fruit) or by taking potassium supplements and by not adding salt to the diet. In urgent cases of oedema, **bumetanide**, **frusemide** or **ethacrynic acid** by injection is indicated but opinion is divided about their prolonged use by mouth once the patient has got over the acute episode. A milder diuretic (e.g. a thiazide) should be substituted. **Spironolactone** is of use in treating disorders where there is considered to be an increased production of aldosterone hormone. The combination of a potassium sparing diuretic (**triamterene, amiloride**) with a thiazide diuretic may be helpful in certain patients. But remember, any combination of diuretics should be used with caution because of the risks produced by an increase or decrease in body potassium level.

Potassium Salts

Supplementary potassium salts should be taken when drugs which may produce potassium loss in the urine are taken over long periods of time. These drugs include the corticosteroids (p. 216), diuretics (p. 180) (particularly potent ones such as frusemide) and carbenoxolone (p. 140). With these drugs it is important to take potassium supplements if you are elderly, if you are on digoxin or a related drug (see p. 156) or if you have a chronic diarrhoea disorder. Potassium supplements may be unnecessary when thiazide diuretics are used to lower blood pressure in the absence of heart failure. Potassium sparing diuretics (e.g., triamterene, amiloride) help to avoid the need for potassium supplements, as does intermittent treatment (e.g., every other day) with thiazide diuretics. See comment on dietary potassium p. 182.

Potassium salts are best taken in liquid form, e.g., **effervescent potassium tablets**. Available brand preparations include **Kay-Cee-L** syrup, **Kloref** effervescent tablets, **Kloref-S** effervescent granules and **Sando-K** effervescent tablets.

30 Morphine and Related Pain Relievers

The Relief of Pain

We all experience pain at some time or another and each of us varies in the amount of pain we can tolerate. Severe, continuous or unusual pain needs explaining and relief. If we have sprained an ankle, we can understand the cause of the pain and it is reasonable to take a pain reliever. But all too often we take pain relievers for pain, particularly headaches, without attempting to identify the cause. Pain is only a symptom and, therefore, you should always try to determine the cause. If you have toothache, do not just take pain relievers – go to your dentist. If you get recurrent headaches try to think what brings them on – noise, smoking, worry, something in the diet, and so on. Very often pain produces fear and anxiety – somebody with chest pain may worry that he has a bad heart and somebody with headache may worry about a brain tumour. If you have a pain that is continuous or unusual for you or if you find yourself becoming anxious or worrying about pain then these are sufficient reasons to consult your doctor. We are not all stoics and continuous pain can make some of us depressed and irritable. By far the most common pains are headaches and those from muscles and joints (e.g., rheumatic and arthritic disorders). Drugs which are taken to relieve the pain of such disorders are amongst the most frequently taken drugs.

Nerve endings, highly sensitive to pain, are widely distributed throughout various tissues of the body. These respond to pressure or stretching which produces the sensation of pain. They are also very sensitive to chemical stimulation (e.g., a burn). The area of pain can usually be identified: in the skin or subcutaneous tissue, in muscles or joints, or in an internal organ, e.g., heart or lungs, gall-bladder, stomach or bowels. The relief of these pains need not necessarily rely on pain-relieving drugs – cold water applied to a skin burn may relieve the pain, heat or massage may relieve muscle pain, and an alkali mixture may relieve the pain of a peptic ulcer. It must be obvious, therefore, that the best way to treat pain is to attempt to relieve the underlying cause. Where the cause of the pain cannot be removed then pain relievers should be used.

There are two main types of pain-relieving drugs – those that work at the site of the pain and those that work on the brain. For example, a local anaesthetic injected into a nerve in your finger will 'freeze' that finger and cut off the transmission of painful stimuli up the nerve to the brain so that you will not feel the pain, whereas a general anaesthetic reduces your brain function so that you are unaware of the pain. Those pain relievers that work at the site of pain block painful impulses; those that work on the brain interfere with perception of pain and alter the appreciation of pain by the brain centres. There are thus two non-specific approaches to the relief of pain which may be used in combination.

Drugs which depress the brain are often called narcotics. The term may also cover general anaesthetics, hypnotics and opiates. Others use the term narcotic when talking about derivatives of opium and morphine-like drugs. Many consider the term narcotic to be equivalent to 'addiction-producing' and legally, narcotics can cover all sorts of drugs including cocaine. When discussing pain relievers (analgesics) it is usual to talk about **narcotic analgesics** (those analgesics of natural or synthetic origin with actions like morphine) and **non-narcotic analgesics** (e.g., aspirin). Narcotic analgesics act principally on the brain and may produce drug dependence; non-narcotic analgesics act principally at the site of the pain.* The former are used frequently and effectively to relieve severe pain usually from internal organs but also from other parts of the body and the latter are used to relieve skin, muscle, joint, bone or tooth pains.

Numerous factors make us feel pain more at one time than at another. A soldier in war time who has an injured leg may need fewer pain relievers than a factory worker in peace time. This is because as a soldier he can see that his injury will get him sent home, away from the area of combat: whereas if he were a factory worker he can see his injury resulting in loss of work and therefore income. We feel pain much more if we are tense, anxious, worried or depressed and, of course, the reverse applies too.

For these reasons, the testing of pain relievers in animals and on volunteer 'patients' under laboratory conditions often gives no real indication of the pain-relieving potential of a drug on 'real' patients. The marked individual variations in response to drugs are further influenced by weight, sex, physical and psychological disorders, time of treatment and place of treatment. Further, about two in five patients can get relief of pain from placebo (dummy) tablets or injections. This is an interesting phenomenon but the placebo effect soon wears off with repeated doses of dummy drugs. A pain-relieving drug must therefore be tested on patients suffering from pain. Morphine-type drugs are usually tested on post-operative pain after abdominal surgery and aspirin-like drugs are tested on rheumatic or arthritic pain.

* By blocking prostaglandins which cause inflammation.

Morphine and Related Drugs Used to Relieve Severe Pain

alfentanil (Rapifen)
buprenorphine (Temgesic)
dextromoramide (Palfium)
diamorphine (heroin)
dipipanone (Diconal)
fentanyl (Sublimaze, Thalamonal)
levorphanol (Dromoran)
morphine (Cyclimorph, Duromorph, MST Continus, Nepenthe,
    Oramorph Solution)
methadone hydrochloride (Physeptone)
nalbuphine (Nubain)
opium (raw opium)
papaveretum (Omnopon; opium concentrate)
pethidine (in Pamergan P100)
phenazocine (Narphen)
phenoperidine (Operidine)

Opium has been used since prehistoric times. It is obtained from the opium poppy and contains many drugs called opium alkaloids. **Morphine** as a pain reliever is the most widely used opium alkaloid. Concentrated preparations of opium are also available (e.g., **papaveretum: Omnopon**) for the relief of pain. Papaveretum is about 50 per cent **morphine** but it also contains **codeine** (used to treat pain, cough and diarrhoea), **noscapine** (used to treat cough), and **papaverine** (which is not related chemically to the other opium alkaloids) which is used to treat spasm of smooth muscle, e.g. broncospasm (as in asthma) and intestinal colic.

Morphine produces its main effects upon the brain, heart and circulation, and the bowel. Its actions on the brain cause relief of pain, suppression of the cough centre and stimulation of the vomiting centre; drowsiness, a relaxed mood and sleep may occur. It may sometimes produce the opposite effect and cause mild anxiety and fear. Mental clouding with inability to concentrate may occur. It also causes constriction of the pupils and sweating. With increased doses these effects increase and the patient may develop nausea, vomiting, and depression of respiration.

Morphine has to be used with caution in patients with chest disorders such as asthma and chronic bronchitis, and after operations, because not only does it discourage deep breathing, it also suppresses cough, with the result that the patient may get a collapsed lung through accumulation of bronchial secretions. Also morphine-induced vomiting can be harmful in patients recovering from an operation on their stomachs or who have just had a coronary thrombosis or a cataract operation. For this reason it is sometimes combined with an anti-vomiting drug **(cyclizine)**.

Morphine also acts on the muscles of the gut causing constipation and should preferably not be given for gut pain (phenazocine is more suitable). It causes a rise in pressure in the gall-bladder and should not be used for gall-bladder pain since it may make it worse. It may cause a fall in blood pressure and dilatation of the blood vessels in the skin (probably by releasing histamine). It should, therefore, be used with caution in patients who are shocked through loss of blood. Rarely patients may develop delirium and insomnia. Increased pain sensitivity may occur after the effects of the drug have worn off.

Tolerance and drug dependence may develop to morphine (see p. 189). When it is stopped, patients may experience mild withdrawal symptoms which include sweating, nausea, weakness, headache and restlessness.

However, patients in pain (e.g., those dying from cancer) should be given a sufficient dose to keep them free from pain and at regular intervals (every four hours) throughout the day and night.

Diamorphine (heroin) is a powerful pain reliever. It produces more euphoria than morphine but less nausea, constipation and fall in blood pressure.

Methadone is a synthetic drug with actions identical to those of morphine. It is an effective drug for the relief of moderate to severe pain. It has an extended duration of action. It is used to treat heroin addicts (see p. 50). Vomiting is as common as with morphine but sedation is less. It is effective when taken by mouth. It is also used to suppress coughs (e.g., **Physeptone** linctus). **Levorphanol** like methadone is less sedating than morphine, and has a prolonged action.

Pethidine is a synthetic pain reliever with similar effects to morphine. It does not constrict the pupils but like morphine it may cause vomiting. Pethidine is used to relieve moderate to severe pain, it is more powerful than codeine but less powerful than morphine. It is used to relieve pain in head injury and in childbirth.

Dipipanone may be given by mouth with an anti-vomiting drug (e.g., **Diconal**). **Phenazocine** by mouth is a moderate pain reliever and by injection is an effective severe pain reliever. It is of particular use in relief of pain from gall-bladder disease because it has less tendency to increase pressure inside the gall-bladder. **Dihydrocodeine (D F 118, D H Continus)** relieves moderate pain, suppresses cough and is effective by mouth. It produces adverse effects like those of morphine but these are usually less severe. It produces dependence of the morphine type. **Dextromoramide** is used to treat moderate pain. It is as effective by mouth as by injection. It should not be used in women in labour. **Fentanyl levorphanol, nalbuphine and phenoperidine** are used during anaesthesia and to relieve post-operative pain.

Morphine Antagonists

In 1953 a morphine antagonist – **nalorphine** – was found to bring on acute withdrawal-like effects in patients who had been on morphine or heroin for long periods. In addition it was found to have good pain-relieving properties. However, it was unsuitable for use because of its bad effects on mood and because it also produced vivid daydreams, hallucinations, difficulty in focusing the eyes, sweating, nausea and feelings of being drunk.

Nalorphine in high doses has the ability to prevent or abolish many of the actions of morphine and the precipitation of withdrawal symptoms in patients who are physically dependent upon morphine or related narcotics. It is described as a partial agonist. **Naloxone (Narcan)** is related to nalorphine but has no respiratory depressing effects. It is now the preferred treatment for depression of respiration caused by narcotic overdose.

The discovery of these drugs led to research for pain relievers with less risk of dependence than morphine. One of these, **pentazocine (Fortral)**, is a partial antagonist with pain-relieving properties between those of codeine and morphine. It is more effective when given by injection than by mouth. It is mildly sedative and produces less respiratory depression than morphine. The incidence of nausea and vomiting is about the same as with morphine. The drug rarely causes constipation. In high doses it may cause a rise in blood pressure and heart rate. Cases of physical drug dependence of the morphine type have been reported in patients taking pentazocine over a long term. It may also cause hallucinations.

Buprenorphine (Temgesic) has mixed morphine agonist/antagonist properties and is useful for relieving pain but it may produce vomiting. It is longer acting than morphine and may be taken under the tongue (sublingually) or by injection. Unlike most morphine-related drugs its respiratory depressant effects are only partially reversed by naloxone. **Meptazinol (Meptid)** is a partial agonist; it produces nausea and vomiting and is claimed to produce a low incidence of respiratory depression.

Warning: Those narcotics that relieve moderate to severe pain differ markedly in structure and yet have similar actions and effects. Their adverse effects include nausea, vomiting, drowsiness, dizziness, constipation and respiratory depression. They differ in their onset and duration of action, in whether they are effective by mouth and in the way that individuals respond to them. They may all cause tolerance and physical dependence, and are potential drugs of abuse. They increase the effects of alcohol and other depressant drugs and they should not be taken by patients who drive motor vehicles and/or who operate machinery.

Morphine-related Drugs Used to Relieve Mild to Moderate Pain

Codeine is obtained from opium and is present in numerous preparations. It produces less mood change and is not as effective as morphine in relieving pain. It is used to relieve mild to moderate pain (often in combination with aspirin, paracetamol or some other pain reliever). It causes constipation. It is also used in cough medicines and diarrhoea mixtures. **Dihydrocodeine Dextropropoxyphene (Doloxene)** has effects and uses similar to codeine. It is slightly less effective and is usually given in combination with other pain relievers by mouth – for example, with paracetamol (as in Distalgesic). **Ethoheptazine** is structurally related to pethidine, but it is only a mild pain reliever.

Warning: **Codeine, dihydrocodeine, dextropropoxyphene** and **ethoheptazine** may produce dependence. They are related to morphine. Read pp. 189 and 190 and note the warning on p. 191.

Combinations of dextropropoxyphene with paracetamol and with aspirin can be more dangerous in overdose than aspirin or paracetamol on their own.

Nefopam (Acupan) is unrelated to morphine. It relieves moderate pain. It should not be used in patients taking paracetamol because of the risk of liver damage.

31 Aspirin and Paracetamol

Aspirin and Related Drugs

Preparations of **aspirin** include **Anadin, Aspergum, Aspro, Bayer Aspirin,** in **Codis, Caprin, Claradin, Laboprin, Levius, Nu-Seals Aspirin, Palaprin Forte (aloxiprin), Paynocil** and **Solprin**

Benorylate (Benoral) is a combined form of aspirin and paracetamol

Diflunisal (Dolobid) is a close relative of aspirin

Salicylic acid – in numerous preparations

Salsalate (Disalcid) and **choline magnesium trisalicylate (Trilisate)** are salicylates like aspirin

Aspirin

Aspirin is one of the most widely used drugs. It relieves mild pain, particularly such pains as toothache and pains in muscles, ligaments and joints. Its long-term use does not lead to tolerance or physical dependence. It brings down the temperature and relieves inflammation. It stimulates respiration, causes a fall in blood sugar and if taken regularly it reduces certain blood fat levels. Aspirin in high doses makes the kidneys pass out urates (see drug treatment of gout), but in low doses it can cause retention of urates. It antagonizes all drugs which cause a fall in blood uric acid levels. It is therefore of no use in treating gout. Aspirin alters the blood salts (acid/base balance) and interferes with some of the processes involved in blood clotting. It also causes water retention when given in high doses and it increases the body's metabolic rate (rate of burning up energy).

Aspirin in mild overdosage may produce 'salicylism' – deafness, noises in the ears, nausea and dull headache. These are related to dose and disappear if the drug is stopped. It is irritant and can cause pain in the stomach, with nausea and vomiting. It also produces superficial ulcers in the stomach which may bleed and lead to iron-deficiency anaemia. This may occur without indigestion symptoms and may be a real danger in elderly patients on poor diets low in iron, in women with heavy periods, and in debilitated patients.

It helps not to take aspirin on an empty stomach and to take only the soluble form with plenty of fluids. It may also help to take a buffered or enteric coated preparation if you are on regular aspirin treatment. If you have a peptic ulcer or hiatus hernia you should *not* take aspirin. It is considered to be a causative factor in many patients admitted to hospital with bleeding from the stomach or duodenum, especially when taken after alcohol. For long-term use a specially coated aspirin (enteric coated) that does not dissolve until it enters the small intestine is available, but it takes up to six hours to work.

A dose of aspirin every four to six hours is sufficient to maintain effective blood levels. It dissolves in the stomach faster and is absorbed more quickly if it is taken with large drinks of warm water or an alkali mixture (the basis of some commercial preparations which contain sodium bicarbonate and fizz in water).

As it is used so indiscriminately it is not surprising that adverse effects occur. You should be aware of its dangers in elderly and debilitated patients and in patients with impaired function of their kidneys, liver or blood-clotting mechanisms. Aspirin should not be given to children under the age of 12 years because of the risk of producing brain and liver damage resulting in severe vomiting, impaired consciousness, delirium and coma (Reye's Syndrome). This can occur after a viral infection such as influenza or chicken pox. Fifty per cent of those affected die and some survivors have brain damage.

Warning: **Allergy to aspirin:** Patients can become intolerant to aspirin and develop vasomotor rhinitis (allergic runny nose), sinusitis, nasal polyps, bronchial asthma, swelling of the throat and nettle rash. Low blood pressure and collapse may rarely occur. There is cross sensitivity with tartrazine (an orange dye in food and drinks) and with indomethacin and some other drugs used to treat rheumatoid arthritis and related disorders.

Aspirin overdose can be serious – always take the patient to the nearest hospital. Remember aspirin is present in hundreds of compound preparations; always read the contents and note that aspirin may be called acetyl salicylic acid, acid acetylsal, or acetylsalicylicum.

Salicylamide has effects and uses like aspirin but is not as effective.

Benorylate relieves pain, reduces inflammation and brings down temperature. It is a chemically combined form of aspirin and paracetamol and may cause less irritation of the stomach.

Diflunisal has similar effects to aspirin but appears to produce less damage to the stomach.

Paracetamol (Acetominophen)

Preparations of **paracetamol** include **Calpol, Disprol, Hedex, Paldesic, Pameton, Panadol, Panasorb, Salzone**.

Paracetamol is an effective mild pain reliever and anti-pyretic (lowers a raised temperature). It is a suitable alternative for patients sensitive to aspirin. It has no anti-inflammatory or anti-rheumatic properties. Regular and prolonged use is dangerous because it may cause liver and kidney damage. Paracetamol should not be used indiscriminately just because it produces less stomach upset than aspirin.

Overdose with paracetamol may cause serious liver damage which can be fatal.

Combined Pain Relievers

There are many preparations on the market which contain mixtures of mild pain relievers. These usually contain two or more of the following – **aspirin, paracetamol, codeine, dihydrocodeine, dextropropoxyphene, ethoheptazine** or **pentazocine**. Many also contain **caffeine** which is said to improve their effectiveness. There is much disagreement as to whether these combined preparations work any better than the single drug but there is no doubt that you can become dependent on any preparation that contains one or more of the following drugs – **codeine, dihydrocodeine, dextropropoxyphene, ethoheptazine** or **pentazocine**. They are also more expensive and may complicate the treatment of overdose.

Chronic Poisoning with Mixtures of Pain Relievers

Mixtures of **phenacetin** with **aspirin, caffeine** and/or **codeine** were widely available in various combinations and doses. The prolonged daily use of those containing phenacetin caused severe kidney damage and should not be used. Other mixtures containing aspirin, paracetamol, codeine and caffeine should be used with caution, i.e., avoid prolonged regular daily use.

32   Drugs Used to Treat Rheumatoid Arthritis and Related Disorders

There are three major groups of drugs used to treat rheumatoid arthritis and related disorders. These are:
1. Non-steroidal anti-inflammatory drugs (N S A I drugs)
2. Corticosteroids
3. Drugs which may affect the disease process.

Non-steroidal anti-inflammatory (N S A I) drugs:
aspirin and related drugs
azapropazone (Rheumox)
diclofenac sodium (Rhumalgan, Voltarol)
diflunisal (Dolobid)
etodolac (Lodine, Ramodar)
fenbufen (Lederfen)
fenoprofen (Fenopron, Progesic)
flurbiprofen (Froben)
ibuprofen (Apsifen, Brufen, Ebufac, Famefen, Fenbid, Hedamol, Ibular, Ibumetin, Ibu-Sio, Inabrin, Librofem, Maxagesic, Motrin, Novaprin, Nurofen, Paxofen, Proflex, Relofen, Sinitol, Supren, Uniprofen)
indomethacin (Artracin, Flexin Continus, Imbrilon, Indocid, Indocid-R, Indoflex, Indolar S R, Indomod, Mobilan, Rheumacin L A, Slo-Indo)
ketoprofen (Alrheumat, Orudis, Oruvail)
mefenamic acid (Ponstan, Ponstan Dispersible)
nabumetone (Relifex)
naproxen (Laraflex, Naprosyn, Synflex)
piroxicam (Feldene, Larapam)
sulindac (Clinoril)
tiaprofenic acid (Surgam, Surgam S A)
tolmetin (Tolectin, Tolectin D S)

1.   Non-steroidal Anti-inflammatory Drugs (N S A I D)

Aspirin is an excellent anti-inflammatory drug but needs to be given regularly in fairly high doses to relieve the pain of rheumatoid arthritis and related disorders. Aspirin produces adverse effects such as stomach upsets and gastric bleeding which may be reduced by taking aspirin after meals and/or by taking a special preparation such as **aloxiprin (Palaprin Forte)** or special intestinal release preparations **(Caprin, Levius, Nu-Seals Aspirin)**. **Benorylate (Benoral)** is an aspirin/paracetamol compound and produces less damage to the stomach than aspirin. **Choline magnesium trisalicylate (Trilisate)** and **salsalate (Disalcid)** are salicylates (i.e., aspirin related); they are also claimed to produce fewer adverse effects.

The non-steroidal anti-inflammatory drugs other than aspirin and salicylates are a complex group of drugs which share the ability to relieve inflammation by blocking prostaglandin production (p. 308). They also share similar adverse effects, such as gastro-intestinal upsets and gastric bleeding, and each one needs using with caution, particularly in the elderly and in anyone with impaired liver or kidney function or with peptic ulcers. They should preferably not be used in early pregnancy and they should be used in the minimum dose possible. They do not cure rheumatoid arthritis or related diseases, they merely reduce inflammation and therefore relieve pain and swelling of joints. The choice of drug is whatever suits you – the selection is not critical. But you must read about a particular drug in Part Three of this book.

Warning: Patients sensitive to aspirin (i.e. those patients who develop skin rashes and wheezing if they take aspirin, see p. 194) may also produce similar sensitivity reactions to any one of this group of drugs (refer to the list on opposite page).

2. Corticosteroids (e.g., Prednisolone) and Corticotrophins (e.g., ACTH)

These drugs reduce inflammation and are discussed in Chapter 37 on corticosteroids. They are not curative and joint destruction may progress even though the symptoms are relieved. They should be used as reserve drugs when other treatments fail to produce relief. Preferably they should be used for only one or two months at a time, although some doctors continue treatment indefinitely because when the drugs are reduced and stopped symptoms flare up and make life for the patient intolerable again. There are very important precautions which should be applied to the use of these drugs – read corticosteroids, p. 216.

3. Drugs which May Affect the Disease Process

Certain drugs have been used for many years and are thought by some doctors to produce improvement in joints and other tissues affected by rheumatoid arthritis and related diseases. They take many months to work and are used only when N S A I drugs have failed or when there is evidence of progressive joint damage or general complications, e.g. affecting the eyes and/or skin. They include **gold**, **chloroquine** and **penicillamine**. Look up each drug in Part Three.

Gold

Gold is often most effective in active, progressive rheumatoid arthritis. It should not be used if at all possible in pregnant women, in elderly and debilitated patients, and in patients with high blood pressure.

Gold is usually given by intramuscular injection (**sodium aurothiomalate, Myocrisin**) and has to be stopped in one third of patients because of intolerance. **Auranofin (Ridaura)** is a gold preparation which can be taken by mouth.

For adverse effects see relevant entry in Part Three. Frequent medical check-ups, including blood and urine tests, are necessary because skin rashes and blood and kidney damage are quite common.

Chloroquine

Chloroquine (Avloclor, Malarivon, Nivaquine) is an anti-malaria drug but it is sometimes used in high doses to treat rheumatoid arthritis. Prolonged use of these high doses may lead to the development of corneal opacities causing misty vision, and irreversible damage to the retina of the eye resulting in blindness. Symptoms may come on long after the drug has been stopped. Regular examinations of the eye by a specialist are necessary. **Hydroxychloroquine (Plaquenil)** is an alternative. For adverse effects see entry in Part Three.

Penicillamine

Penicillamine (Distamine, Pendramine) aids the elimination of toxic metals from the body. It is used in lead poisoning and to treat certain disorders of copper metabolism. Occasionally it is used as a reserve drug in the treatment of severe rheumatoid arthritis that has not responded to other treatments. For adverse effects see entry in Part Three. Regular medical check-ups, including blood and urine tests, are necessary.

Immunosuppressants

These drugs are often used along with corticosteroids to treat severe rheumatoid and related disorders. The ones used include **azathioprine (Azamune, Imuran), chlorambucil (Leukeran)** and **methotrexate (Emtexate, Maxtrex)**. Look up each drug in Part Three.

The Use of Drugs in the Treatment of Rheumatic and Arthritic Disorders

I have used the vague terms 'rheumatic' or 'arthritic' to cover a multitude of disorders which may vary from a 'rheumatic' condition causing mild pain and swelling in one joint to the serious disease called rheumatoid arthritis which may affect one or more joints and be associated with other serious disorders affecting arteries and various internal organs. Therefore treatment will of course vary, and reserve drugs such as corticosteroids, gold and chloroquine will only be used in serious cases and under specialist care.

Of the commonly used anti-rheumatic drugs, the choice is a matter of balancing adverse effects of stomach irritation and bleeding with the beneficial effects. Other adverse effects such as salt retention, bone-marrow damage and potential risks of interaction with other drugs should be considered. And so the selection of the most appropriate drug will require skill and patience depending on the severity of the disorder being treated. You as a patient should be aware of these problems and check the various adverse effects of individual drugs in Part Three of this book.

None of these drugs cure. Their actions are non-specific and they are used to relieve pain and swelling, and to reduce inflammation.

Aspirin is the drug of first choice. But for rheumatic disorders it must be given in high doses. If aspirin does not work **ibuprofen** or a related drug may be tried in those patients not sensitive to aspirin. If these are not effective then **indomethacin** may be tried. For early morning stiffness and pain a suppository preparation may be useful.

Depending on the severity of your symptoms a moderate pain reliever may have to be used in addition (particularly at night) – for example, **dihydrocodeine (DF 118), pentazocine (Fortral), dextropropoxyphene (Doloxene)**.

Corticosteroids (e.g., prednisolone) by mouth and **adrenocorticotrophin (ACTH)** by injection are reserve drugs for pain associated with chronic inflammatory conditions if other treatments fail to produce relief. Local injection of hydrocortisone into a joint may help but has been criticized by some experts because repeated use may damage the joints.

Gold, chloroquine or penicillamine, although not usually used in the first few months of treatment, are sometimes tried in order to prevent irreversible joint damage developing. But these drugs including corticosteroids and ACTH should only be used by specialists experienced in treating rheumatic disorders. If you require these drugs you should preferably be under surveillance in a hospital out-patients' department.

Osteoarthritis

Aspirin, indomethacin, ibuprofen and related drugs may relieve some pain and stiffness in osteoarthritis. **Paracetamol and codeine compounds** relieve mild pain. **Phenylbutazone** (only available in hospitals) **or indomethacin** are said to be superior to aspirin in the treatment of ankylosing spondylitis.

Rheumatic Liniments and Balms

These are principally rubefacients and are discussed on p. 275.

Note: Drug treatment of rheumatoid arthritis and related disorders is only a part of overall treatment which should include physiotherapy, hydrotherapy, wax baths, surgery and splints and diet where appropriate.

33 Drugs Used to Treat Gout

Gout is a relatively uncommon disease which causes recurrent attacks of acute pain and swelling, at first affecting one joint (usually the big toe) but later many joints. The *primary* form of gout is a hereditary disease, rare in women, and usually comes on in the over-forties. It is more common in temperate climates and sometimes diet may bring on an acute attack. In gout there is an increased production of uric acid, or a decreased excretion of uric acid or a combination of both. Uric salts (urates) are deposited in the tissues around joints and in the kidneys. *Secondary* gout can occur in certain blood disorders, in kidney failure and be brought on by drugs such as thiazide diuretics.

Drugs Used in the Treatment of Gout

Drugs are used to treat patients with gout in order to relieve pain and inflammation in an acute attack. They are also used to increase the elimination of urates by the kidneys or to block the production of uric acid in order to prevent attacks coming on.

Acute Attacks

Acute attacks of gout are usually treated with a non-steroidal anti-inflammatory (NSAI) drug such as **indomethacin** or **naproxen**. The choice is not critical. You should not use aspirin. If the attack does not respond to an NSAI drug, a **corticosteroid** is often of value, e.g., corticotrophin 80 unit IM daily for two days.

Colchicine obtained from the autumn crocus relieves the pain and inflammation of gout within a few hours. It is absorbed from the gut and broken down in the liver. Some is excreted unchanged in the bile and goes back into the gut which increases the abdominal pain, vomiting and diarrhoea which it causes. It should be used with caution in elderly or debilitated patients and in those with liver or kidney disease.

Recurrent Gout

With recurrent attacks of gout you can aim at increasing the excretion of uric acid in the urine with drugs such as **probenecid** or **sulphinpyrazone** or you can reduce the formation of uric acid from purines with a xanthine-oxidase inhibitor such as **allopurinol**.

Probenecid (Benemid) promotes the excretion of urates by reducing their reabsorption from the urine by the kidneys. It has no pain-relieving properties and is of no use in an acute attack of gout. It may set off an acute attack of gout in the first few weeks of treatment so the patient must be warned. **Sulphinpyrazone (Anturan)** causes excretion of urates. It may also trigger off an acute attack of gout in the first few weeks of treatment. **Azapropazone (Rheumox)** is an NSAID (p. 196) which may be used to treat an acute attack of gout and also to prevent gout because it increases the excretion of uric acid in the urine.

Warning: Drugs which increase the excretion of uric acid (uricosuric drugs) may cause crystals of urate in the urine, therefore it is very important to drink plenty of fluids if you are taking these drugs.

Allopurinol (Aloral, Aluline, Caplenal, Cosuric, Hamarin, Zyloric) affects uric acid production and reduces the concentration of uric acid in the blood. Acute attacks of gout may be triggered off in the early stages of treatment but after a few weeks to months acute attacks stop and deposits of uric acid salts in cartilage get smaller (these are often visible in the cartilage of the ear lobes and are known as tophi). It may prevent kidney damage in gout and stops the formation of uric acid stones in the kidneys. Allopurinol is therefore useful for treating gout in patients with kidney disorders whereas other anti-gout drugs may not be effective or may not be advisable to use. It also prevents a rise in blood uric acid levels in patients being treated for heart failure with diuretics. Some of these diuretics, called thiazides (see pp. 181–2), may cause a rise in blood uric acid, and allopurinol stops this.

It is often difficult to differentiate between migraine and headache. Some doctors label one-sided headache as migraine, particularly if it is accompanied by nausea and vomiting. Others look for all the classical symptoms of migraine – one-sided headache associated with nausea and vomiting and preceded by visual symptoms (e.g., flashing lights), speech disturbances, or disturbances of sensation (e.g., pins and needles in a foot or hand).

Migraine is uncommon under the age of five years and then its incidence increases with advancing age until it levels off in middle age. The incidence declines in old age. It is more common in women than in men and it may be associated with menstruation. There are many myths about migraine sufferers; for example, there is not sufficient evidence to indicate that they are more tense, neurotic or obsessional than non-sufferers. Nor is there evidence to suggest that more professional people suffer from migraine than other groups, or that migraine sufferers are more intelligent, that they suffer more from high blood pressure or visual disturbances or that they are more involved in work which involves close vision. There is limited evidence that it runs in families.

Many statements about migraine sufferers are made by doctors who only see a small self-selected group – those who have decided to consult a doctor. They cannot be assumed to be representative of migraine sufferers in general.

An attack of migraine is associated with changes in the calibre of the blood vessels supplying the head and brain. It is thought that these changes occur in response to certain chemicals which are produced by the body and which are also present in various foods such as cheese. Underlying constitutional factors, which may be biochemical, possibly cause a predisposition to develop migraine in response to certain external factors.

Factors which may trigger off a migraine attack include:

Psychological – e.g., anxiety, tension, worry, emotion, depression, shock, excitement.
Physical – e.g., over-exertion, lifting, straining, bending, heading a football.

External factors – e.g., sunlight, weather, travelling, change of routine, staying in bed, watching television, noise, smells, smoking, drugs.

Dietary – e.g., irregular meals, fasting, certain foods such as cheese, onion, cucumber, bananas, chocolate, fried foods, pastry, cured meats which contain sodium nitrates and nitrites (e.g., hot dogs, ham, bacon), alcohol.

Treatment of Migraine

The most important part of treatment is to try and prevent an attack coming on. This means attempting to identify the trigger factors which bring on your attack. (See, for example, the list above.) If you develop migraine always go through a check list of trigger factors – cross off the ones which you cannot directly relate to your attack. Try to avoid obvious trigger factors – it may be something simple like having to avoid cheese, or it may be very difficult like trying not to get tense or anxious and learning to relax. This will take time and patience but it will be worth it. Some migraine clinics teach relaxation and other useful methods of preventing an attack, but on the whole the vast majority of sufferers manage very well without ever seeing a doctor. Many learn how to cope with an attack but they should also try to prevent attacks coming on.

Drugs

Drug Treatment of an Acute Attack

The principle is to anticipate the onset of an attack and to take medication as soon as there is any indication that an attack is pending.

Since gastric absorption is poor in migraine, **metoclopramide** (10 mg) by mouth at the first sign of an attack followed by a mild analgesic (**aspirin** 600 mg or **paracetamol** 1 g) in about 10 minutes can be very effective. The metoclopramide delays emptying of the stomach and improves absorption of the analgesic which is best given in liquid form. In severe cases, metoclopramide may be given by injection.

The claimed benefit of combination preparations such as **Migravess** and **Paramax** needs careful assessment. Combinations of paracetamol with an antihistamine plus codeine and a laxative as in **Migraleve** and **Migralift**, or with a sympathomimetic and a sedative as in **Migril** have not been convincingly shown to be better than an analgesic alone.

Instead of the above, **ergotamine** and **dihydroergotamine** may help patients who experience several attacks. **Ergotamine** (e.g., **Cafergot**) may be dissolved in the mouth, inhaled through the mouth or taken as tablets or capsules, suppositories or injections. **Dihydroergotamine** produces less vomiting and a reduced risk of adverse effects but is less effective.

Note: Doses of ergotamine are cumulative and can induce chronic background headache for which the patient may take more ergotamine risking further adverse reaction (see ergotamine, in Part Three).

Ergotamine preparations include **oral ergotamine (Cafergot, Migril), sublingual (Lingraine), inhaler (Medihaler-Ergotamine)** and **suppositories (Cafergot). Dihydroergotamine mesylate (Dihydergot)** is available as an injection. **Isometheptene (Midrid)** is an alternative to ergometrine preparations.

Phenothiazine anti-emetics (e.g., **chlorpromazine (Largactil), prochlorperazine (Stemetil)** and **trifluoperazine (Stelazine))** are frequently used to prevent nausea and vomiting (by suppository or injection) but **metoclopramide (Gastrobid Continus, Gastromax, Maxolon, Metox, Metramid, Mygdalon, Parmid, Primperan)** is more effective.

Non-steroidal anti-inflammatory drugs such as **mefenamic acid (Ponstan)** appear to provide useful relief to some sufferers.

Prevention of Attacks

If migraine attacks are occurring frequently (e.g., one or more attacks every two weeks) then it is helpful to try to prevent these attacks by taking a suitable drug regularly, but only for a few months at a time and providing general measures have also been taken (see p. 204).

Drugs used include: analgesics (e.g. the regular daily use of **aspirin** or **ibuprofen**), beta-blockers (**propranolol** and **atenolol** have been shown to be moderately effective in preventing attacks) and **clonidine (Dixarit)**, which is helpful in those patients where attacks are clearly linked to constituents in the diet. It may make depression worse and produce insomnia. **Pizotifen (Sanomigran)** may be effective in some patients and **methysergide (Desiril)** may be used in patients resistant to all other forms of therapy. **Amitriptyline** (a tricyclic antidepressant) or **phenelzine** (an MAOI) may be of use in depressed patients, and **diazepam** in anxious patients.

Read up about each drug in Part Three.

A Biochemical Perspective

Several complex biochemical changes are thought to occur in migraine. There is a rise in noradrenaline in the blood, the blood platelets become more sticky and aggregate, and chemicals such as serotonin are released. Serotonin causes constriction of arteries and dilatation of capillaries which may contribute to early symptoms of migraine (e.g., visual disturbances). In addition, aggregated platelets and other cells (mast cells) are thought to release chemicals (neurokinins and prostaglandins) which make the pain receptors in the blood vessels more sensitive to pain. With such observations it is possible to rationalize some of the drug treatments of migraine.

Beta adreno-receptor blockers (e.g., **propranolol, atenolol**) may be used to reduce the effects of noradrenaline. **Aspirin** blocks prostaglandins and discourages platelet aggregation and therefore lessens the release of serotonin. **Dipyridamole** produces similar effects. **Clonidine** reduces the effects of serotonin as does **methysergide** and **pizotifen**. The latter drug also blocks histamine, tyramine and other chemicals. In an acute attack the release of prostaglandins contributes to the pain and their blocking with **aspirin**, **ibuprofen** or **mefenamic acid** may be helpful. A herbal remedy – the plant **feverfew** (*Chrysanthemum parthenium*) is claimed to work in some patients. It blocks prostaglandin production and relieves the stickiness of platelets, both of which are thought to be involved in migraine.

Non-drug treatments are clearly desirable and include relaxation, yoga, biofeedback and acupuncture. The avoidance of foods and activities which trigger off an attack is very important.

35 Iron

Iron is necessary for the manufacture of blood; its deficiency leads to anaemia. There are many causes of anaemia other than iron deficiency, but it is by far the commonest cause and the easiest to treat. Iron-deficiency anaemia is not uncommon in women, infants and elderly people. The deficiency may be caused by a poor diet lacking foods rich in iron – these include liver, meat, eggs, wholemeal cereals, oatmeal, peas, beans and lentils. Poor iron intake is likely to occur because of faulty feeding in babies and infants and in the elderly who live alone. **Blood loss is a principal cause of iron-deficiency anaemia**, e.g., menstruation (particularly at the menopause when menstruation may be heavy and frequent), bleeding from a peptic ulcer, bleeding from the stomach due to the regular taking of aspirin and other anti-rheumatic drugs, and bleeding at childbirth. Worm infections of the gut may produce iron deficiency, as may disorders of the stomach (e.g., surgical removal of part of the stomach in the treatment of duodenal ulcer) and intestine (e.g., ulcerative colitis). Thus treatment will require special attention to the cause of the iron-deficiency anaemia as well as the giving of iron. For this reason you should not diagnose iron deficiency just by your appearance or your symptoms. It really is quite impossible to estimate the degree and type of anaemia without special blood tests which will indicate the type of anaemia. And if it is an iron-deficiency anaemia it will indicate whether it is due to blood loss or some other cause.

The symptoms produced by anaemia may be produced by many disorders – some physical, some psychological, some mild and some serious. If you develop symptoms (e.g., tiredness, breathlessness and weakness) and feel that you are anaemic then consult your doctor, who may arrange for a blood test.

Unfortunately doctors use iron preparations quite indiscriminately – as tonics or as a placebo. This reflects badly upon them because the appropriate use of iron produces beneficial effects for the sufferer from iron deficiency. But as with other drug treatments, patients who do not require iron are often given it and many patients who are anaemic and would benefit do not receive it.

Iron is essential for the formation of the pigment in red blood cells called haemoglobin, which is responsible for carrying oxygen to the tissues from the lungs and carbon dioxide from the tissues back to the lungs. Two thirds of the body's iron is present in the haemoglobin of the red blood cells. The rest is stored in the bone marrow, spleen and muscles. Absorption of iron from food takes place principally through the duodenum and upper part of the small intestine. Its absorption is helped by acid from the stomach and it is more easily absorbed in the inorganic ferrous state. Only a small proportion of iron in food is absorbed. Even so the iron content of the average diet in the Western world is sufficient for our needs. Obviously, you will need more if you are pregnant, breast feeding, having heavy periods and so on. The mechanisms for controlling the body's iron content exercise a careful control over the absorption of iron from the gut – if you are iron deficient, absorption is increased. If you are not, then absorption is decreased. Because of menstruation women need to absorb about twice as much iron as men each day.

Iron Treatment

Iron-deficiency anaemia responds well to iron treatment but, as stated earlier, the underlying cause must be diagnosed and treated, and of course this must include advice on diet. In iron deficiency, absorption is increased but in order to produce a suitable response it is necessary to take a large amount of iron each day – about 200 mg. A good response will increase the haemoglobin level (an indication of the degree of anaemia) by about one per cent per day. However, in order to ensure a satisfactory level and to replenish the body's stores, treatment should continue for at least three to six months. Remember it is no use being told that you have got iron-deficiency anaemia and then only remembering to take tablets for a few weeks.

Iron may be given by mouth or by injection into a vein or muscle. Iron by mouth may irritate the stomach and gut to produce nausea, vomiting, diarrhoea or constipation and abdominal pains.

There are numerous oral iron preparations on the market; the cheapest effective preparations are **ferrous sulphate, ferrous gluconate, ferrous succinate, ferrous fumarate**. Stomach upset or diarrhoea may be avoided by taking the drug with meals (although absorption is not as good as before meals) and by starting on a small daily dose – one tablet daily – and then increasing the daily dose up to two or three tablets over a period of one to two weeks. If these attempts fail then more expensive preparations of **slow-release iron** may be of use, and many have the added advantage that you only need to take one daily dose. However, some may release insufficient quantities of iron, because slow-release tablets and capsules of iron are designed to release iron slowly, but before they release their iron they may pass through the first part of the duodenum, where iron absorption is good, and down into a lower part of the gut, where iron absorption is poor.

Injections of iron may be necessary if iron cannot be absorbed from the gut and in certain emergencies, e.g., severe anaemia in late pregnancy. Response to injected iron takes about fourteen days and the dose and interval between doses should be calculated from the patient's haemoglobin level and body-weight. However, it is important to remember that the speed of response is no faster after injected iron than after oral iron in the individual who can absorb iron from the gut. Because of the risk it should only be used where absolutely necessary.

Iron sorbitol (Jectofer) is an iron sorbitol citric acid complex which is given by deep intramuscular injection. Injections can be painful, cause temporary staining of the skin at the site, produce headache, blurred vision, painful muscles, disorientation, flushing, nausea and vomiting and a metallic taste in the mouth and loss of taste. About 30 per cent of the dose is excreted by the kidneys, turning the urine black. Intramuscular iron sorbitol injections should not be given to patients with kidney disorders or infections.

Iron dextran solution (Imferon) has been widely used. It is absorbed more slowly from deep intramuscular injections and it may leave a residue. Repeated use of deep injections of iron dextran solutions has been shown to produce sarcoma (a type of cancer) at the injection sites in rats but no such change has been shown in man. Injections of iron dextran solution may cause pain and staining of the skin at the site of the injection, making a special injection technique necessary; after deep intramuscular injections, fever and rapid beating of the heart may occur. Iron dextran solution may also produce allergic reactions and a small test dose should be given (although not 100 per cent reliable). Infusion into a vein may cause venous thrombosis, fever and rapid beating of the heart and allergic reactions to intravenous infusion may occasionally cause death. Iron dextran solution should not be given to patients with severe liver damage or with bone-marrow depression. It should be given with utmost caution to anyone who has previously suffered from any drug reaction and the patient should be kept under close observation for at least one hour after intravenous infusion. Local inflammatory reactions are much less frequent with intravenous than with intramuscular administration; shock and adverse effects on the heart, however, are more common (although rare).

Finally, iron is a drug which may produce adverse effects. Overdose may cause liver and kidney damage, collapse and death. Iron preparations, like any drug, must be kept out of the reach of children.

The combination of **iron and folic acid** is of use in preventing anaemia in pregnancy. Several preparations to be taken are available which contain the equivalent of about 100 mg of iron and 200–500 micrograms of folic acid.

Vitamins are substances which are essential for the maintenance of normal body function but they are not manufactured by the body. We therefore have to rely upon an outside source, which in a healthy individual is found in a normal well-balanced diet.

When vitamins are taken, not as part of a well-balanced diet, but in highly concentrated forms they must be regarded as drugs and as such they may produce adverse drug effects. Those vitamins that are soluble in water (the B vitamins and vitamin C), if taken in excess of the body's requirements, are quickly excreted. They thus do little harm but their use is often unnecessary and wasteful. However, the fat-soluble vitamins (vitamins A, D, K and E) if taken in excess of daily requirements become stored in the body fat, where they may accumulate until toxic concentrations are reached.

Vitamins may be used to treat recognized disorders produced by vitamin deficiencies, and in such cases doctors often use incredibly high doses. They are also used to prevent vitamin-deficiency disorders developing – as supplements to the individual's diet. Much confusion has, therefore, arisen between the doses used to treat established vitamin-deficiency disorders and the doses used in supplementary treatment. Supplementary dosage need only be at the level of recommended daily intake and there is no merit in taking in more than this. Unfortunately, many over-the-counter preparations contain vitamins and these are the subject of intense marketing. The clear, but wrong and misleading, message which is being given by the manufacturers and promoters is that if 100 units of a vitamin do you good then 1,000 units will do you even better. They are promoted as giving you vitality and zest – you don't really 'live' until you take added vitamins. Yet most people who take supplementary vitamins can afford a well-balanced diet and therefore do not need added vitamins. Still, if people think they will feel better then they probably will, but they ought to know the hazards of overdosage.

Doctors are equally guilty in their indiscriminate use of vitamins. Many patients who might benefit from them never receive them (e.g., elderly people living alone), whereas they are frequenty prescribed as 'tonics' to the well-nourished. Supplementary vitamins may be of great value to those people whose diet is inadequate, e.g., those who are poor, isolated, elderly, or debilitated; those who are faddy about their food; those on diets, e.g., slimming diets; and alcoholics and others who take in too little food. Similarly, some disorders of the stomach and gut may produce inadequate vitamin intake and people with such disorders will require supplementary vitamins. Pregnant women and women who are breast feeding need supplementary vitamins, and so may babies, and children at puberty, during debilitating illness and in certain glandular disorders. But, of course, they are no substitute for a good nutritious diet. After all vitamins are only a small part of food. There is no evidence that minor deficiencies of vitamins cause debility or increased risk of getting colds and other infections.

Since deficiency of a single vitamin is rarely encountered it is best to supplement with several vitamins in doses not larger than the recommended daily requirements which are contained in a 'normal' diet.

Vitamin A

Carotene (pro-vitamin A) and vitamin A are present in dairy produce (milk, eggs, butter, cheese), in green vegetables and carrots, in liver and fish liver oils. Margarine has added vitamin A. Deficiency causes defective vision in dim light and thickening and hardening of the skin (hyperkeratosis) – this also affects the cornea of the eyes. It is fat soluble and if large amounts are taken adverse effects are produced which include loss of appetite, itching, skin disorders, loss of weight, enlargement of the liver and spleen, debility and painful swellings of bone and joints.

Vitamin B Complex

This includes:

vitamin B_1 – thiamine, aneurine
vitamin B_2 – riboflavine
vitamin B_6 – pyridoxine
nicotinamide – nicotinic acid (niacin)
                nicotinic acid amide, niacinamide
folic acid   – pteroylglutamic acid
vitamin B_{12} – cyanocobalamin

Vitamin B_1 (thiamine, aneurine). Vitamin B_1 is present in wheat germ, eggs, liver, peas, beans and other vegetables. Deficiency causes inflammation of nerves (peripheral neuritis), heart failure, oedema, nausea and vomiting. This group of disorders is known as beri-beri. Vitamin B_1 deficiency may also damage the brain (Werniche's encephalopathy) and cause mental confusion (Korsakow's syndrome). These disorders may occur in alcoholics on poor diets deficient in vitamins.

Vitamin B₂ (riboflavine). Vitamin B_2 is present in yeast, milk, liver and green vegetables. Deficiency produces sore lips (angular stomatitis), ulcers of the mouth, a sore magenta-coloured tongue, skin rashes (seborrhoeic dermatitis) and blood vessels on the cornea of the eye (vascularization of the cornea).

Vitamin B₆ (pyridoxine). Vitamin B_6 is present in liver, yeasts and cereals. Deficiency may produce anaemia, nerve damage and skin disorders.

Nicotinamide. Nicotinamide and nicotinic acid (which is converted into nicotinamide in the body) are present in liver, yeast, milk, vegetables and unpolished rice. Deficiency produces pellagra (which affects the mouth, stomach and gut, producing a sore tongue, stomatitis, gastritis and diarrhoea), the brain (causing dementia) and the skin (producing dermatitis).

Folic acid (pteroylglutamic acid). Folic acid is present in green vegetables, yeast and liver. Deficiency produces anaemia and may be caused by poor diet, disorders of the gut which interfere with the absorption of folic acid from the small intestine, and by pregnancy. Anti-convulsant drugs (e.g., phenytoin, primidone, phenobarbitone) may produce anaemia which responds to folic acid. Anti-malarial drugs and nitrofurantoin may also cause anaemia by interfering with the folic acid metabolism.

Vitamin B₁₂ (cyanocobalamin). Vitamin B_{12} is present in meat, milk and eggs. To be absorbed into the blood-stream it has to combine with a substance secreted by the stomach known as the intrinsic factor. Vitamin B_{12} is known as the extrinsic factor and the combination of intrinsic with extrinsic factor is absorbed through the small intestine. Vitamin B_{12} is stored in the liver. Its main action is upon blood formation by the bone marrow. Deficiency produces a special type of anaemia called pernicious anaemia which is usually due to lack of the intrinsic factor in the stomach. It may also be produced after surgical removal of large parts of the stomach, in disorders of the small intestine and, rarely, by dietary deficiency of vitamin B_{12} in strict vegetarians or in those living in the tropics.

Vitamin C (Ascorbic Acid)

Vitamin C is present in citrus fruits, rose hips and green vegetables. Cooking reduces the vitamin C content of food. Deficiency causes scurvy – anaemia, haemorrhage into the skin and gums, bruising and bone pains. In children vitamin C deficiency may delay bone growth. Large daily doses of vitamin C (1,000 mg) may possibly reduce some individuals' chances of getting the common cold, and reduce the severity of an attack.

214 of 672 Drugs Used to Treat Specific Disorders

Vitamin D

Vitamin D is present in dairy produce and fish oils. It is also produced by the body after exposure of the skin to sunshine. The average diet of babies and some children may not provide sufficient vitamin D, particularly if they are not exposed to sufficient sunshine. Vitamin D deficiency produces rickets in children (by interfering with calcium absorption) and osteomalacia (bone softening) in adults. Excessive dosage produces a rise in blood calcium which causes debility, drowsiness, nausea, abdominal pains, thirst, constipation, loss of appetite, deposits of calcium in various tissues and organs, kidney damage and kidney stones.

Vitamin K

Vitamin K_1 is present in greens and vegetables, and vitamin K_2 is produced by bacteria in the gut. Vitamin K is necessary for the production of various blood-clotting factors by the liver. Vitamin K_1 is fat soluble and requires bile salts for its absorption from the gut. Deficiency causes a reduction in blood-clotting factors resulting in bleeding and delayed blood clotting. It may be caused by disorders of the gut which interfere with its absorption; obstruction to the production of bile (obstructive jaundice); and by some drugs (e.g., sulphonamides and tetracyclines) which affect the bacteria in the gut which produce vitamin K_2.

Vitamin E

Vitamin E is present in the oil from soya bean, wheat germ, rice germ, cotton seed, maize and green leaves (e.g., lettuce). Opinion on the importance of vitamin E is divided. In animals deficiency of vitamin E has been claimed to produce numerous effects on the reproduction system, muscular system, heart and circulation and blood. Because deficiency in rats was found to produce adverse changes in early pregnancy in females and wasting of the testes in males it quickly became known as the 'anti-sterility vitamin' and was widely promoted for its effects on virility. But there is no unequivocal evidence to suggest that it is of use.

Recommended Daily Requirements

Tables of recommended daily requirements are easily found in books on nutrition, human biology, medicine and so on. However, they specifically refer to nutrition and indicate that your food should contain the stated amounts. Unfortunately, the manufacturers give the impression that these amounts are to be *added* to a normal diet. Do not be misled: vitamins may be required to supplement an inadequate diet but never to complement a diet. High-dose vitamin preparations should be avoided – do not be attracted because they are called 'super vitamins' or any other name that indicates that the dose is above what is normally required.

37   Corticosteroids

The metabolic function of the body is under the control of several glands whose internal secretions (or hormones) are released into the blood-stream to act upon various tissues and organs. These glands include the master gland (the pituitary), the thyroid and parathyroid glands, the pancreas, the adrenal glands and the sex organs (gonads) – testes or ovaries. The effect of these hormones is to stimulate certain body processes.

Under complex control from the brain, the front part (anterior lobe) of the pituitary gland exercises control over the thyroid gland, the cortical part of the adrenal glands and the sex glands. It produces stimulating hormones which act on these organs (often known as target glands) to produce their own secretion of hormones. In addition there is a feedback mechanism so that the production of a stimulating hormone by the pituitary is controlled by the circulating level of hormone from the target gland. For example, if the level of adrenal hormones increases in the blood then the adrenal stimulating hormone decreases, and vice versa. Thus the adrenal glands may be stimulated by giving the patient a hormone obtained from the pituitary glands of slaughtered animals, or the effects of the adrenal glands may be 'mimicked' by giving adrenal cortex extract or synthetic adrenal hormones.

There are two adrenal glands which lie above the upper ends of each kidney. Each consists of a centre (medulla) which produces adrenaline and noradrenaline (see p. 95) and an outer layer known as the cortex. Over thirty hormones have been isolated from the adrenal cortex, the two most important ones being hydrocortisone and aldosterone. The adrenals (from now on this will be used to indicate the adrenal cortex) produce three groups of hormones (known as adrenocortical hormones) which are grouped according to their main function – glucocorticoids act on sugar, protein and calcium metabolism; mineralocorticoids act on salt and water metabolism; and sex hormones. Their production (except aldosterone) is under control of adrenocorticotrophic hormone from the pituitary gland – this may be referred to as ACTH or corticotrophin. Except for aldosterone there is an overlap in the actions and effects produced by these hormones.

The glucocorticoids (and there are many synthetic preparations available) became acclaimed as wonder drugs because they reduce inflammatory, and allergic reactions. They are, therefore, often referred to as anti-inflammatory hormones, *corticosteroids*, or just simply as steroids (since they belong to a chemical group known as steroids). They may also affect salt metabolism, but to different extents than the mineralocorticoids (e.g., aldosterone) which control retention of sodium and excretion of potassium by the kidneys. Aldosterone is discussed in the section on diuretics, p. 183. The sex hormones produced by the adrenals include male sex hormones (androgens) and female sex hormones (oestrogens and progestogens). Before puberty the balance of the two affects the degree of femininity and masculinity of the body. Their major sources in the body, however, are the testes and ovaries – see sections on female sex hormones (pp. 227–34), male sex hormones (pp. 223–5), and anabolic (body-building) steroids (p. 226).

Corticosteroids

The glucocorticosteroids are important drugs which have become widely used for their anti-inflammatory effects, but it must be remembered that these bear no clear relationship to their metabolic effects. In fact, the latter may limit their use. The general term corticosteroid is now applied not only to adrenocortical hormones, but also to a huge number of synthetic preparations which are related and produce similar effects. The principal aim in manufacturing these products has been to try and separate the anti-inflammatory and anti-allergic effects from their metabolic effects on sugar, protein salts and water. Modifications of the basic cortisone structure have produced drugs with greatly increased anti-inflammatory properties, particularly when applied to the skin. Betamethasone, dexamethasone, hydrocortisone, prednisolone and prednisone are used for their anti-inflammatory effects. Prednisolone is the most commonly used by mouth. Prednisone is converted to prednisolone in the liver. Cortisone is not used because it causes fluid retention. Hydrocortisone hemisuccinate and hydrocortisone sodium phosphate can be given by intravenous injection, e.g., in the treatment of shock and bronchial asthma. Mineralocorticoid effects (e.g., fluid retention etc.) are most marked with fludrocortisone and deoxycortone and negligible with betamethasone, dexamethasone, methyl prednisolone and triamcinolone. They occur only slightly with prednisone and prednisolone.

Available preparations are listed on pp. 220–22.

To produce desired anti-inflammatory and other effects corticosteroids have to be given in doses far in excess of the body's needs, which greatly increase the risks of adverse effects. In these doses their effects on metabolism are complex: for example, hydrocortisone affects salt and water balance producing salt and water retention (causing raised blood pressure) and potassium loss; sugar and carbohydrate metabolism is affected, producing a raised blood sugar and sugar in the urine (glycosuria); protein metabolism is affected, producing muscle weakness: calcium metabolism is affected producing softening of bones (osteoporosis); retarded bone growth in children, wasting of the skin with appearance of stripes (striae) and delayed wound healing occur; fat metabolism is affected resulting in fat being laid down on the face (moon face), shoulders (buffalo hump) and on the abdomen; the effect on calcium metabolism produces increased calcium excretion in the urine and the risk of kidney stones; and uric acid excretion is increased. Other effects include indigestion and aggravation of peptic ulcers (see p. 136) and effects on the blood vessels contributing to a raised blood pressure. In addition, hydrocortisone reduces the inflammatory response which may mask symptoms and signs of infections, e.g., tuberculosis. It also reduces the allergic response, interferes with the processes which produce immunity and decreases the ability of the white blood cells to fight infection. It may cause mood changes and it suppresses the complex nervous and hormonal response to stress (the hypothalamic–pituitary–adrenocortical system), which may produce collapse and death.

The various corticosteroids used to treat inflammatory, allergic and rheumatic disorders produce the same effects as hydrocortisone but to very different degrees so that their net effect may vary quite markedly. This depends upon their chemical structure and dosage. The general term corticosteroid, whilst convenient, is really so broad as to rob it of much of its meaning particularly since it is usually applied to those chemical variations which have been developed specifically for their anti-inflammatory effects.

Hydrocortisone is the corticosteroid most commonly used for injection and **prednisolone** is the most popular preparation by mouth. Injections of hydrocortisone are used in emergencies (e.g., severe asthma attacks, status asthmaticus). Short tapered courses of prednisolone are given by mouth in the treatment of bronchial asthma, allergies and other disorders. Long-term daily maintenance doses of prednisolone are used in such disorders as asthma, rheumatic disorders, skin disease and blood disorders.

If you are on long-term corticosteroids this means that, as well as continuing to see the specialist at intervals, you should visit your own doctor on a regular basis in between times. Long-term treatment with high doses of steroids can cause a number of adverse effects, which should be reported to your doctor. Medication with any other drug must only be carried out after consultation with your doctor.

Warning: in the individual with normally functioning adrenal glands the production of corticosteroid hormones is increased at times of stress, e.g., injury, surgery and infections. This problem of increased need during stress is exaggerated in patients in whom corticosteroids are being used. The amount of circulating corticosteroids in the blood suppresses the production of ACTH by the pituitary gland, which leads to 'disuse' changes in the adrenal glands and failure of the stress mechanism. If these drugs have been used for more than a few weeks the body will fail to react in the normal way to physical stress, with the result that the patient may collapse and even die. For this reason their daily dose needs increasing three- or four-fold during such episodes, and corticosteroid drugs should never be stopped suddenly. They should be tapered off very slowly over many weeks (depending, of course, upon how long the patient has been on them). These dangers mean that every patient on corticosteroids should carry a warning card, and if they have received them for one month or more in any two-year period they should continue to carry a steroid warning card because collapse can occur during a surgical operation up to two years after stopping them.

In order to minimize most of the above adverse effects corticosteroid preparations (e.g., **prednisolone**) should wherever possible be administered on alternate days in the morning in the smallest effective dose for the shortest period of treatment possible. This is possible with many of the diseases treated with corticosteroids.

Adrenocorticotrophic Hormone (ACTH: Corticotrophin)

This is a very complex chemical produced by the anterior lobes of the pituitary gland, which respond rapidly (within minutes) to the body's requirements. The pure substance was isolated from the pituitary glands of slaughtered animals in the 1940s and it was first synthesized twenty years later. The synthetic preparations are less likely to cause allergic reactions because they are not contaminated with animal protein. ACTH stimulates the adrenals to produce corticosteroids (the most important of which is hydrocortisone) and to a lesser extent male sex hormones (androgens).

The principal effects produced by ACTH are those produced by corticosteroids. Therefore, it should not be used, although it often is, with the idea that it will produce selective anti-inflammatory effects – it will *always* produce disturbances of salt and water balance. ACTH is inactive when given by mouth and has to be given by injection. When given by intravenous injection it produces rapid effects which quickly wear off. Its effects may be prolonged by giving the injection under the skin or into a muscle but even then these only last for about six hours. Long-acting ACTH preparations are available – these contain, for example, gelatin which delays the release of ACTH so that its effects may last for 24 to 72 hours or zinc hydroxide which makes the injection effective for about 48 hours. With the exception of adrenal deficiency disorders (e.g., Addison's disease) and over-activity disorders of the adrenals, it is used to treat disorders which also respond to corticosteroids. Because it does not produce disuse changes in the adrenals, it is easier to withdraw ACTH than corticosteroids and therefore it may be of use in short-term therapy. However, over the long term it is not as useful because it is not as selective as oral anti-inflammatory corticosteroids, and it has to be given by injection. It may produce the adverse effects described under corticosteroids, and in particular, diabetes may be made worse and insulin dosage may have to be increased. High blood pressure and acne occur more frequently but stomach troubles occur less frequently. It may produce allergic reactions and increase skin pigmentation, and long-term use may cause the adrenal glands to undergo changes of 'over-use' and the pituitary changes of 'under-use' – it should always be slowly withdrawn after long-term use. The use of ACTH on alternate days in children is sometimes used to try to reduce the possibility of growth retardation which can occur on regular daily use of corticosteroids.

A quick-acting ACTH injection is available (**Acthar injection**) and also a long-acting one (**Acthar Gel injection**). **Tetracosactrin (Synacthen** and **Synacthen Depot)**, a synthetic polypeptide resembling ACTH, is widely used for diagnosis and treatment.

Corticosteroid Preparations

Corticosteroid mouth preparations
triamcinolone (Adcortyl in **Orabase** oral paste)
hydrocortisone (Corlan)

Corticosteroid enemas
hydrocortisone (Colifoam, Cortenema)
prednisolone (Predenema, Predfoam, Predsol)

Corticosteroid ear preparations
betamethasone (Betnesol, in **Betnesol N, Vista-methasone,** in **Vista-methasone N)**
hydrocortisone (in Neo-cortef, in Framycort)
prednisolone (Predsol, in Predsol-N)

Corticosteroid local injections
dexamethasone (Decadron, Oradexon)
hydrocortisone (Hydrocortistab)

methylprednisolone (Depo-Medrone)
prednisolone (Deltastab, Codelsol)
triamcinolone (Adcortyl, Kenalog, Lederspan)

Corticosteroid eye preparations
betamethasone (Betnesol, Betnesol N, Vista-methasone, Vista-methasone N)
clobetasone (Eumovate, Eumovate N)
dexamethasone (Maxidex, Maxitrol, Sofradex)
fluorometholone (FML suspension, in FML-Neo)
hydrocortisone (Neo-Cortef, in Cortucid, in Framycort)
prednisolone (Predsol, in Predsol-N)

Corticosteroid rectal preparations
betamethasone (Betnovate cream, suppositories)
fluocortolone (in Ultraproct ointment and suppositories)
hydrocortisone cream, ointment and suppositories (in Anugesic HC, in Anusol HC, in Proctofoam HC, in Proctosedyl, in Uniroid, in Xyloproct)
prednisolone (Predsol suppositories, in Anacal, in Scheriproct)

Corticosteroid nasal preparations
beclomethasone (Beconase nasal aerosol, Beconase aqueous nasal spray)
betamethasone (Betnesol drops, Vista-methasone drops)
budesonide (Rhinocort nasal aerosol)
flunisolide (Syntaris nasal spray)

Corticosteroid tablets and injections
betamethasone (Betnelan, Betnesol)
cortisone (Cortelan, Cortistab, Cortisyl)
dexamethasone (Decadron, Oradexon)
fludrocortisone (Florinef)
deoxycortone (Percorten M crystules*)
hydrocortisone (Efcortelan, Efcortesol, Hydrocortistab, Hydrocortone, Solu-Cortef)
methylprednisolone (Depo-Medrone, Medrone, Min-I-Mix Methylprednisolone, Solu-Medrone)
prednisolone (Codelsol, Delta-Phoricol, Deltacortril Enteric, Deltastab, Precortisyl, Prednesol, Sintisone)
prednisone (Decortisyl, Econosone)
triamcinolone (Adcortyl, Kenalog, Ledercort)

Corticosteroid inhalers
beclomethasone (Becloforte, Becotide, in **Ventide)**
betamethasone (Bextasol)
budesonide (Pulmicort)

Corticosteroid skin applications
alclometasone (Modrasone)
beclomethasone (Propaderm)
betamethasone (Betnovate, Diprosalic, Diprosone)
clobetasol (Dermovate)
clobetasone (Eumovate, in Trimovate)
desonide (Tridesilon)
desoxymethasone (Stiedex)
diflucortolone (Nerisone, Temetex)
fluclorolone (Topilar)
fluocortolone (Ultradil Plain, Ultralanum Plain)
fluocinolone (Synalar)
fluocinonide (Metosyn)
flurandrenolone (Haelan, Haelan–x)
hydrocortisone (in numerous creams, lotions and dressings)
methylprednisolone (in **Neo-Medrone)**
triamcinolone (Adcortyl, Ledercort)

The development and maintenance of reproductive organs is under the control of chemicals known as steroid hormones. These hormones are produced by the male and female sex glands, the adrenal glands and the placenta (afterbirth). The hormones concerned with the development and maintenance of the male reproductive system are called androgens. Several androgens are produced by the testes and adrenal glands. The most powerful of these is known as testosterone.

The master gland (the pituitary) produces a hormone called gonado-trophin, which stimulates the testes to make these male sex hormones. At puberty they are made in sufficient amounts to produce changes usually known as secondary sexual characteristics (or masculinization effects or androgenic effects). The voice-box enlarges and the voice gets deeper, the genitals get bigger and hair begins to appear in various parts of the body. They are responsible for the growth and development of the testicles to produce sperm. At puberty there is also a spurt in growth; body protein builds up, muscles develop and bones grow. The latter effects may be separated from the effects upon the sex organs, and because they are related to protein build-up they are called anabolic effects. Male sex hormones (androgens), therefore, have two principal effects: (1) **androgenic** – they affect the development and maintenance of reproductive organs and function; (2) **anabolic** – they affect growth, muscle bulk and protein build-up.

However, those male sex hormones which produce predominantly androgenic effects will also produce some anabolic effects and those which have principally anabolic effects will also produce some androgenic effects. Testosterone is the natural androgenic hormone produced by the testes but there are several synthetic preparations available. Similarly much attention has been directed to manufacturing synthetic anabolic steroids. Those with marked androgenic properties and also some anabolic properties include: **Mesterolone (Pro-Viron), methyltestosterone, testosterone (Primoteston Depot, Restandol, Sustanon, Virormone)**.

Male sex hormones with mainly anabolic properties and relatively weak androgenic effects are discussed in the section on anabolic (body-building) steroids.

Androgenic male sex hormones are used principally to treat disorders produced by failure of the testes to make these hormones. This failure may be primary, due to lack of development or under-development of the testes, or secondary, due to failure of the pituitary gland to produce sufficient gonadotrophin. In under-development or if used in adolescent males, they produce development of the secondary sexual characteristics. They stimulate growth, but may produce stunting of growth because they also close off the growing ends of the long bones in the body.

In small doses they stimulate the production of sperms but in high doses they suppress the production of gonadotrophin by the pituitary, thus causing suppression of sperm production.

Male sex hormones are of no use in treating male sterility unless this is due to under-development of the testes and they are of no use in treating impotence unless this is due to testicular failure. However, in primary failure they rarely reverse sterility and in secondary failure gonadotrophin therapy is used. They were previously used in women to treat abnormal menstruation and painful periods, and to suppress milk production after childbirth. They may be used to treat certain patients with breast cancer. Small doses combined with female sex hormones (oestrogens) have been used to treat menopausal symptoms.

They may all be taken by mouth but because testosterone is rapidly broken down in the liver it is given by depot intramuscular injection. The adverse effects produced by testosterone and other androgens may be related to their androgenic and anabolic effects. They include increase in skeletal weight, salt and water retention, oedema, increased number of blood vessels in the skin, increased blood calcium levels and increased bone growth. In women they may affect gonadotrophin production by the pituitary and lead to suppression of the ovaries and menstruation. Large and continued doses cause masculinization in women – deep voice, acne, the male pattern of baldness, hairiness, shrinking of the breasts, and increase in size of the clitoris with an increase in libido. Androgenic steroids should not be given to patients with cancer of the prostate gland and they should not be used in pregnancy because the unborn baby may be affected. They should be used with caution by patients who would be made worse by salt and water retention, e.g., patients with heart failure, impaired kidney function or epilepsy. Phenobarbitone may reduce the effects of testosterone by increasing its breakdown in the liver. Dose-related jaundice may occur with methyltestosterone. Isolated cases of cancer of the liver have been reported for certain anabolic and androgenic steroids used for prolonged periods.

An anti-androgenic drug (**cyproterone; Androcur**) is used to treat severe hypersexuality and sexual deviation in males. It inhibits sperm production and produces reversible infertility. It has also been used to treat severe and excessive hair growth (hirsutism) in women. **Goserelin (Zoladex)** mimics the action of the gonadotrophin releasing hormone (see part III).

39 Anabolic (Body-building) Steroids

We have seen that male sex hormones may produce two main effects – androgenic and anabolic. Many anabolic compounds have been developed and vigorously marketed as body builders. All produce some androgenic effects but they cause less virilization than the androgenic hormones in women. These products have been widely promoted for the treatment of disorders where there is an increase in breakdown of body protein, e.g., after major surgery or a severe accident and for treating patients with long-standing debilitating diseases. The giving of an anabolic steroid is not a good idea in these disorders; it is much more important to ensure that the patient takes a nourishing diet (high in protein) so that the body's own mechanisms control the required build-up of protein.

The anabolic steroids which are available are all derivatives of testosterone. They include:

drostanolone (Masteril)
nandrolone (Deca-Durabolin, Durabolin)
oxymetholone (Anapolon)
stanozolol (Stromba).

All anabolic steroids produce adverse effects similar to those produced by testosterone (see section on male sex hormones, pp. 223–5). They may be given by mouth or injection. Those which may be taken by mouth may cause jaundice when taken over a prolonged period of time. These should not be used in patients with impaired liver function and they may increase the effects of some anticoagulant drugs. The main adverse effects of anabolic steroids are fluid retention and masculinization. They should not be used in patients suffering from cancer of the prostate gland and in pregnancy.

Whilst doctors have slowly moved along their typical path of drug use – enthusiastic and widespread use followed by more cautious assessment – these drugs are used for non-medical purposes by athletes without any evidence that the benefits outweigh the risks of their use. They are used in the treatment of breast cancer and aplastic anaemias.

The new-born baby girl's ovaries contain thousands of eggs or ova. Each ovum is in a fluid-filled sac called a follicle. Before puberty many of these follicles enlarge but then shrink.

Puberty

At puberty the ovaries begin to undergo cyclical changes under stimulation from hormones produced by the master gland (the pituitary). The uterus and vagina enlarge, the breasts develop, fat is laid down in certain areas giving the characteristic female figure, and hair starts to grow under the arms and on the pubes.

Menstruation

The anterior pituitary gland produces two hormones which affect the growth of the ovaries. These are called gonadotrophins because they make the gonads (ovaries) grow. One is called follicle-stimulating hormone (FSH) which stimulates the development of follicles around the ova in the ovaries. This makes the follicles grow and as one of them starts to grow more than the others it starts to produce its own female sex hormones, called oestrogens. These oestrogens then start to work on the lining of the uterus making it grow thicker. As the blood concentration of oestrogens increases the pituitary's production of FSH decreases. The other gonadotrophic hormone is called luteinizing hormone (LH) and it acts on the follicle, making it rupture and release the ovum. This process is known as ovulation. LH also ensures the continuing development of the follicle after it has released the ovum and converts it into a yellowish body (corpus luteum) producing a different female sex hormone called progesterone, which belongs to the group of female sex hormones known as progestogens. This also acts on the lining of the uterus making it ready to receive a fertilized ovum.

The first change in the uterus when its lining thickens under the influence of oestrogens is called the proliferative phase (phase of growth). The subsequent phase, after ovulation, when progesterone makes it undergo special changes in preparation for receiving a fertilized egg (ovum) is called the secretory phase (because cells develop which will be ready to secrete nutritious fluids if conception occurs and the fertilized egg settles on the lining of the uterus). Doctors, by taking a scraping (or biopsy) from the lining of the uterus, are able to tell whether the lining has undergone both changes, proliferative and secretory, and so are able to tell whether the patient has ovulated. They are also able to determine whether oestrogens and progesterone have been made in sufficient quantities to produce the changes.

Progesterone inhibits the production of LH by the pituitary whereas oestrogens stimulate its production, and so it can be seen that there is a delicate balance between FSH and LH production by the pituitary gland and the production of oestrogens and progesterone by the developing follicle and the corpus luteum respectively.

Before puberty the production of FSH and LH by the pituitary is not enough to stimulate the development of a follicle around an ovum and only small quantities of oestrogens and progesterone are produced by the ovaries. Two or three years before the development of menstruation puberty changes are already taking place. This is thought to be due to the growth and development of the pituitary gland and also part of the brain known as the hypothalamus which exerts control over the nervous and hormonal activity in the body. As the pituitary gland develops it starts to increase its production of FSH and LH. These get to work on the ovaries and cause groups of follicles to develop. As they grow they start to produce more and more oestrogens. These oestrogens work on various tissues in the body producing the secondary sexual characteristics and in addition the lining of the uterus starts to thicken and the first menstrual period develops (the menarche).

During the time after the first menstrual period the pituitary and hypothalamus are also developing and at times produce too little gonado-trophic hormone to affect the production of oestrogens by the ovaries. Thus the lining of the uterus does not thicken and a young girl may go several months without a period or having irregular periods. As the pituitary settles down the periods will become more regular and menstruation will start to occur approximately every twenty-eight days.

During these first few months, ovulation does not usually occur because the pituitary does not produce sufficient LH hormone. But as the cycles without ovulation continue (usually known as anovulatory cycles) more and more oestrogens are produced by the follicles and LH production increases, eventually causing ovulation (release of the ovum).

At the time of ovulation, the lining of the uterus is ready to receive the ovum, which after ovulation leaves the ovary and passes down a fallopian tube into the cavity of the uterus. If the ovum is not fertilized by a male sperm (and this often takes place as the ovum passes down the tube) it slowly disintegrates as it passes down the cavity of the uterus.

If the ovum is not fertilized, LH production falls and the corpus luteum shrinks, resulting in a decreasing production of progesterone and oestrogens. As the level drops the blood vessels supplying the lining of the uterus close off, the lining disintegrates and menstrual bleeding starts. When progesterone production by the shrinking corpus luteum declines the pituitary responds by producing more LH. In response to a decreased production of oestrogens the pituitary starts to produce more FSH and the cycle starts all over again. The increase of FSH and LH starts to work on the ovaries, a new group of follicles starts to develop and the whole sequence of changes is repeated.

Pregnancy

If the ovum is fertilized it burrows into the lining of the uterus and becomes anchored. It develops a layer of cells around it (the trophoblast) which multiply and eventually form the placenta (afterbirth). At this early stage the trophoblast cells surrounding the developing fertilized ovum (now called an embryo) start to produce chorionic gonadotrophin hormone (chorionic because it is produced by the cells which go to form part of the placenta called the chorion and gonadotrophin because it works on the gonads, or ovaries). Chorionic gonadotrophin, like LH, works on the corpus luteum in the ovary and maintains its development. This results in an increased production of progesterone by the corpus luteum, despite the fall-off in LH production by the pituitary.

Under stimulation from progesterone, the lining of the uterus continues to provide nutrition for the developing embryo until the placenta is developed. This then takes over essential duties – supplying nutrients, carrying away unwanted products, and supplying oxygen and other gases to the developing baby and carrying away carbon dioxide. In addition the placenta (which links the baby's blood supply directly to the mother's) continues to produce chorionic gonadotrophin but also starts to produce its own oestrogens and progesterone.

This delicate and complex balance of hormones ensures that the pregnancy becomes established. After about twelve weeks the chorionic gonadotrophin production by the placenta starts to fall off, the corpus luteum shrinks at about sixteen to eighteen weeks, and production of chorionic gonadotrophin reaches a low level which lasts throughout the pregnancy. At the same time production of oestrogens and progesterone by the placenta continues to increase throughout the pregnancy, falling abruptly after delivery. The fall in oestrogens then stimulates the pituitary to produce FSH, a group of follicles gradually starts to develop in an ovary and the menstrual cycle is set in motion again. The high oestrogen and progesterone levels in pregnancy are responsible for breast development. Some chorionic gonadotrophin hormone is excreted in the urine and gives a positive urine pregnancy test early in pregnancy.

After childbirth the sucking of the baby at the breast stimulates production of a milk-producing hormone (prolactin) by the pituitary gland. This stimulates further milk production (supply meets demand). At the same time prolactin serves a useful purpose by stopping the production of FSH by the pituitary and thus preventing the development of follicles in the ovaries. This prevents the breast-feeding mother from menstruating for several months after delivery, depending, of course, on how long she breast feeds. However it does not necessarily mean that a breast-feeding mother cannot get pregnant.

Menopause

As the ovaries get older the follicles start responding less and less to FSH. This results in a decreased production of oestrogens and for a time an increased production of FSH. Also LH production falls and ovulation fails to occur during some cycles. As ovarian function continues to decline, ovulation stops altogether. Oestrogen and progesterone production fall right off and eventually menstrual periods stop. The rise in FSH production may affect other pituitary hormone production which may cause various menopausal changes; these include increase in weight, hot flushes, bone changes and psychological symptoms. The lack of oestrogens produces shrinking of the secondary sex organs – the breasts become smaller, the vulva and vagina undergo changes and the ovaries and uterus shrink.

From this brief description of the hormonal control of puberty, menstruation, pregnancy and the menopause it can be seen that there are two groups of hormones which control numerous functions in the female body – these are oestrogens and progestogens. Many synthetic preparations of these hormones are available and they are used for a wide variety of disorders.

Oestrogens

The main sources of oestrogens are the ovaries and the placenta. They are also produced in small amounts by the adrenal glands and by the testes in the male. Over twenty different oestrogens have been isolated from the urine of pregnant women. The three main oestrogens produced by the ovaries and placenta are **oestrone, oestradiol** and **oestriol**. The most potent natural oestrogen is oestradiol. Oestriol is produced in large quantities by the placenta during pregnancy.

Oestrogen Preparations

The preparations available for use include naturally occurring oestrogens such as oestradiol and oestrogens obtained from the urine of mares. Oestrogens are steroid chemicals and there are numerous synthetic steroid oestrogens available which resemble oestradiol in structure. These are broken down more slowly in the body than naturally occurring oestrogens and so their effects last for a longer time – the two main synthetic oestrogens are **ethinyloestradiol** and **mestranol**. They are present in many female hormone preparations, particularly oral contraceptive drugs. Other chemicals are available, which, although not steroids, have oestrogenic effects – the main one in this group is **stilboestrol**.

The various oestrogen preparations available include **ethinyloestradiol, mestranol, oestradiol (Benztrone, Estraderm, Hormonin, Progynova), oestriol (Ortho-Gynest, Ovestin), piperazine oestrone (Harmogen), stilboestrol and conjugated oestrogens (Premarin)**.

Many preparations of female sex hormones contain both oestrogens and progestogens. **Ethinyloestradiol** is present in many combination products; so too is **mestranol**.

Oestrogens are used as replacement treatment in patients who have deficient oestrogen production due to underdevelopment of the ovaries, which causes delayed puberty and absence of periods (primary amenorrhoea); to treat menstrual irregularities; to treat menopausal symptoms; cancer of the prostate gland in men; softening of bones (osteoporosis) in post-menopausal women; in sub-fertility; to treat cancers of the breast and prostate in selected cases; and in oral contraceptive preparations.

Adverse effects from oestrogens include nausea and vomiting, which are directly related to dose, tenderness and enlargement of the breasts, headache, dizziness, irregular vaginal bleeding, fluid and salt retention, and growth of breasts in men. Low doses of oestrogen may stimulate growth of cancer of the breast and uterus. The oestrogens in oral contraceptive preparations may be responsible for changes in blood clotting leading, rarely, to the risk of venous thrombosis, and the use of high doses of oestrogens to stop milk production just after childbirth may be associated with an increased risk of thrombosis. They are not now used for this purpose and have been replaced by bromocriptine.

Oestrogens should not be used in patients with a family or personal history of cancer of the breast, uterus or genital tract. They should not be used in patients with a history of thrombosis and they should not be used post-operatively. They should be used with caution in patients with varicose veins, obesity or diabetes. They should preferably not be used to stop milk production just after childbirth.

Progestogens

Following ovulation, progesterone is responsible for the secretory changes in the lining of the uterus during the last two weeks of the menstrual cycle. It is also necessary for maintaining pregnancy. In addition it has many other effects. It plays an important role in the development of the placenta and it stops movements of the uterine muscle. It stops ovulation during pregnancy and plays a part in further breast development. It is produced by the corpus luteum and acts only on tissues which have been previously subjected to the actions of oestrogens. Progesterone increases the use of energy by the body and the body temperature rises at ovulation and stays up until menstruation (i.e., during the secretory phase). This is a test for fertility, as it shows whether the patient ovulates. It is also a test to determine the time of ovulation – when pregnancy is more likely to occur – and from this the 'safe period' may also be worked out, that is, the time of the month when the risk of pregnancy is reduced. Progesterone also affects salt excretion by the kidneys.

Progesterone and Progestogen Preparations

Progesterone (Cyclogest, Gestone) is rapidly broken down in the liver to pregnanediol. It is, therefore, inactive by mouth and has to be given by suppository, intramuscular injection or by implanting a pellet under the skin. It is insoluble and cannot be injected into a vein.

There are two groups of synthetic progestogens: those related to progesterone **(allyloestrenol (Gestanin), dydrogesterone (Duphaston), hydroxyprogesterone (Proluton Depot) and medroxyprogesterone (Depo-Provera, Provera))** and those related to the male sex hormone testosterone: **norethisterone (Primolut N, Utovlan)** and **gestodene** (in **Femodene**). The synthetic progestogens are mostly broken down in the body to testosterone and oestrogen. The progesterone derivatives obviously have less virilizing effects than the testosterone derivatives. Progesterone does not produce virilizing effects.

Progestogens are used in oral contraceptive preparations. They are also used, combined with oestrogens, to control heavy and irregular periods. Painful periods may be reduced by stopping ovulation with an oral contraceptive agent which contains a progestogen. They may also be helped by a progestogen called **dydrogesterone (Duphaston)**, which does not stop ovulation and has no oestrogenic and androgenic properties. Similarly, such a non-oestrogenic progestogen may be of use in treating pre-menstrual symptoms such as tension, headaches, and breast fullness and pain which comes on during the week preceding a period. Synthetic progestogens were previously used in treating threatened miscarriage (abortion) and in recurrent miscarriages (habitual abortion) but were of no real value. **Progesterone (Cyclogest, Gestone)** should preferably be used to treat these disorders.

Synthetic progestogens may produce greasy hair, acne, breast tenderness and depression of mood before a period. Those used in oral contraceptives may also produce increase of appetite and weight, cramps in the legs and abdomen, changes in libido, fluid retention, white vaginal discharge, reduced menstrual loss and dry vagina. Breakthrough bleeding (bleeding between periods) whilst on progestogens is another adverse effect.

Those progestogens with some androgenic properties should be avoided during pregnancy because they may cause masculinization of an unborn baby girl. They should not be used by patients who have had jaundice or any other liver disease and they should be used with caution in patients with impaired kidney function and in those with Addison's disease. They should not be used in patients with epilepsy.

Oestrogen and progestogen combination products are widely prescribed for a variety of conditions, often without sufficient understanding of the disorder being treated. However, the most common use of such combinations is in oral contraceptives.

Dysmenorrhoea (Period Pain)

Because it stops ovulation the pill (combined oestrogen/progestogen) is very effective in relieving period pains and so is progestogen on its own (e.g., dydrogesterone).

With period pains it has been shown that prostaglandins are released (see p. 308) and a drug which blocks these is often helpful, e.g., **aspirin** or one of the non-steroidal anti-inflammatory (NSAI) drugs such as **ibuprofen** or **mefenamic acid** – see p. 196. **Vitamin B$_6$ (pyridoxine)** is claimed to be of use in some women. Over-the-counter medicines, except those that contain **aspirin** or **paracetamol** in an appropriate dose, have not been subjected to satisfactory tests of their effectiveness.

Oestrogen Replacement Therapy for the Menopause

The term *menopause* refers to the stopping of the menstrual periods and the term *climacteric* refers to the longer-term effects produced when ovarian function gradually ceases. The whole process is usually referred to as 'the menopause'.

The only symptoms of the menopause that are unequivocally due to **oestrogen deficiency** are hot flushes and atrophic changes in the vagina. These respond to oestrogen therapy. Oestrogens are also helpful in osteoporosis (bone-softening). The use of oestrogens to improve psychological symptoms has not been clearly demonstrated. They should not be used in patients with oestrogen-dependent cancer of the breast and womb, with a past history of thrombosis or liver disease. They should be used in the smallest dose for the shortest period of time and on a cyclical basis (e.g., 25 days in every month). They should be given along with a progestogen for ten days of the cycle in those patients who have not had a hysterectomy.

Premenstrual Syndrome

Synthetic progestogens have long been tried in this disorder without much success, and it is now argued by some that natural **progesterone** should be used. In premenstrual syndrome, cyclical, physical and mental symptoms occur in relationship to times of periods and it is suggested that in this disorder the body fails to produce sufficient progesterone in the last two weeks of the menstrual cycle (the luteal phase) and therefore the treatment is to give the naturally occurring progesterone. It is suggested that the use of synthetic progestogens merely damps down the little progesterone the patient is making, which makes the condition worse, as does the use of the combined oestrogen/progestogen pill in these patients. As stated earlier, because progesterone is rapidly absorbed from the gut and broken down in the liver it has to be given by a route which avoids this 'first pass' through the liver. The routes available are by injection (**Gestone**), by suppository (**Cyclogest**) or by implant.

41 Oral Contraceptive Drugs

To understand the use of oral contraceptives read the section on female sex hormones. It is most important that you should understand the hormonal control of the menstrual cycle and in particular the parts played by the female sex hormones, oestrogens and progestogens.

There are three types of oral contraceptives: combined oestrogen/progestogen preparations (usually known as 'the pill'), sequential preparations containing oestrogens and progestogens, and progestogen-only preparations.

The **progestogens** used in oral contraceptives belong to two groups. Those chemically related to the male sex hormone testosterone, and having some oestrogenic, androgenic and anabolic activities as well as progestogenic, e.g., **norethisterone, lynoestrenol** and **ethynodiol**. The other groups are more closely related to the naturally occurring progesterone and include **megestrol**. Progestogens make the mucus at the entrance of the womb sticky (the 'mucus plug') which prevents sperm from entering. They also help to stop ovulation by blocking L H production.

The **oestrogens** used in oral contraceptives are **ethinyloestradiol** and **mestranol**. Mestranol is converted into ethinyloestradiol in the body (i.e., it is a precursor of ethinyloestradiol), so when we talk about the oestrogens in oral contraceptives we are usually talking about ethinyloestradiol and its precursor mestranol. Oestrogens stop the production of FSH and therefore the follicle does not develop and ovulation is prevented. However – and this is very important – the production of FSH is related to the circulating level of oestrogen so that a small dose of oestrogen may actually lead to increased FSH production and therefore stimulation of the follicle producing ovulation. An equally important point to remember is that a medium dose of oestrogen may merely delay ovulation. But as we shall see later the principal risks of the pill are thought to be due to its oestrogen content and so the smallest effective dose has to be used, which may not be enough to stop some women ovulating. The safest dose now seems to be 0·05 mg or less of ethinyloestradiol or mestranol – so take note. The name of the oestrogen and progestogen in your pills will be entered in small type on the packet – look for these.

The Combination Pill – 'The Pill'

In these the dose of **oestrogen** is usually below 0·05 mg.* Many go below this to 0·03 mg. With low oestrogen pills (0·030 to 0·035 mg) the margin of safety is reduced and it is very important not to miss one. Below 0·030 mg they are even less safe. The dose of **progestogen** also varies but there is a much wider margin of safety and since progestogens also stop ovulation, affect the lining of the uterus and alter the stickiness of the mucus in the cervical canal (all useful ways of stopping conception) they introduce a large additional safety factor against you getting pregnant. The combined effect of the oestrogen and progestogen in the pill also affects the lining of the womb so that the implantation of the fertilized egg is discouraged.

Low-dose oestrogen ('mini-pills' or 'micro-pills') and low-dose progestogen pills may cause breakthrough bleeding. Ovulation may also occur in these cases and so there is a risk of pregnancy if you are on a pill which gives you breakthrough bleeding – get your doctor to switch you on to a higher-dose progestogen pill. Also high-dose progestogen combination pills give a wider margin of safety if you happen to forget to take one, but note the risks, p. 246.

Triphasic Oral Contraceptives

It makes sense to try to reduce the dose of both drugs in the pill and to try to 'mimic' the pattern of oestrogen and progestogen production by the body (see p. 227). The triphasic pills try to do this – the **progestogen** is given incrementally – 0·05 mg for the first six days, 0·075 mg for the next five days and 0·125 mg for the last ten days. The dose of **oestrogen** (ethinyloestradiol) is 0·03 mg daily except during the middle five days when it is 0·04 mg. However, the chemical changes that take place in the blood in response to other forms of pill can also occur with the triphasic pill. They are more complex to take and there is a greater margin of error if tablets are omitted. They may produce 'premenstrual syndrome' and painful periods. Vaginal discharges are more common. They include **Trinordiol** and **Logynon E D** (the pack contains seven inactive pills to reduce error). They should be used by smokers in their early thirties, possibly by women over 45 years of age and by women with absent periods on the 'ordinary' pill.

Progestogen-only Preparations

These are started on the first day of the cycle and then taken every day right through without missing a day. They may be used before the periods start

* 1·0 mg = 1000 micrograms (0·05 mg = 50 micrograms)

after childbirth. The progestogen makes the mucus in the cervical canal sticky, thus preventing sperm from entering the uterus. There is, therefore, a much greater risk if you forget to take one of these pills and have sexual intercourse that day. They may produce heavy and irregular periods and breakthrough bleeding. With these progestogen-only pills there is also a risk of pregnancy even if you do not forget to take one every day. However, they produce fewer adverse effects than the combination preparations because of the absence of oestrogens. For patients over 35 years of age who smoke and for patients who cannot tolerate combination pills the progestogen-only pill forms an alternative, and they are also of use in patients due to have a surgical operation since oestrogens should not be taken at these times – but remember there *is* a risk of pregnancy. If you miss out a dose by 3 hours or more, there will be a risk of pregnancy. You should complete the course as usual, but take additional precautions for 14 days. Similar precautions should be taken when switching from a combined pill to a progestogen only one.

Progestogen-only pills may produce irregular menstrual bleeding (which can be heavy), breast tenderness, skin flushing, an acne-like rash, headaches and migraine.

Depot progestogen injections (medroxyprogesterone: Depo-Provera). This is a long-acting preparation given by intramuscular injection. One injection provides contraception for three months. It produces similar problems to oral preparations, particularly irregular and sometimes heavy periods, and transient infertility or irregular periods after stopping treatment.

Morning-after Pills

There are two methods of post-coital contraception: hormone pills or intra-uterine devices.

To be effective, hormonal therapy should be started within 72 hours of unprotected intercourse, thereafter the failure rate rises substantially above the claimed 1 per cent. **High-dose oestrogen** has been used (5 mg of ethinyloestradiol daily for five days); this produces severe nausea and vomiting in 20 per cent of patients and there is a risk of ectopic pregnancy in 10 per cent of patients in whom the method fails. The use of stilboestrol in the first three months of an established pregnancy may produce abnormalities in the baby and has been associated with the production of vaginal cancer in girl offspring during their teens. High-dose oestrogen regimens have therefore fallen out of favour. Current methods now involve the use of **oestrogen/progestogen** preparations to be taken in two doses, twelve hours apart (e.g., **Eugynon 50** or **Ovran**: two pills immediately and two in twelve hours). Nausea occurs in 50–60 per cent and vomiting in 30 per cent but these symptoms are short-lived and rarely severe. Other adverse effects such as headaches, dizziness, breast tenderness and withdrawal bleeding may occur.

Note that if this method fails 2·5 per cent of babies have some degree of congenital abnormality.

The pills must be taken *within* the first 72 hours (i.e., before implantation of the fertilized ovum).

If the morning-after pill (post-coital pill) is contra-indicated then the insertion of an intra-uterine device within the first 72 hours is an alternative. With post-coital I U Ds, pain and abnormal bleeding may occur and there is always a risk of infection. They should not be used in young women who have not had a baby.

How to Take the Combined Pill ('The Pill')

For convenience the term 'the pill' refers only to the most commonly used oral contraceptive – the oestrogen/progestogen combination. The first course may be started on the first or fifth day of the menstrual period taking the day that the period started as the first day. You then take a pill daily for twenty, twenty-one or twenty-two days or for whatever number of days it states in the instructions on the packet, preferably at the same time each day. The different number of days recommended for different preparations does not really matter; what does matter is that you take yours daily on the recommended number of days. The number of days is adjusted so that you have a menstrual cycle of twenty-eight days, because this is what most women are used to and perhaps feel happier with. When you have finished the first month's course of twenty-one days or whatever it is, you will get a period in one to five days. You then start the next course according to the instructions – for ease many preparations contain twenty-one pills in a packet so that in a twenty-eight-day cycle you take the pill for three weeks and stop it for one week. The packets are push-out types and the days of the week are often marked so that it is easy for you to remember when you stopped and need to re-start. If you have not got a good memory there are preparations available which contain seven dummy tablets. The dummy tablets are a different colour from the contraceptive pills but all you have to do, having started the first course, is to take one pill every day – you do not have to remember when to stop and when to start.

Because intercourse is more common at night a lot of women take the pill before going to bed. This is fine, but it does not really matter what time of day you take it so long as you take it every day (i.e., every twenty-four hours), preferably at the same time. Avoid any risk of getting pregnant during the first two weeks of your first month's course on the pill,* by using additional contraceptive methods – with subsequent courses you will be safe. Also, when changing from one contraceptive preparation to another, particularly from a high-dose to a low-dose oestrogen preparation, do not run the risk of getting pregnant during the first two weeks (some say four weeks) on the new pill. If you forget to take the pill on one day take it as soon as you remember (certainly within twelve hours of the right time), and then take that day's pill at your usual time. If you forget to take the pill for two days (36 hours or more) ovulation may occur. Read your instructions carefully: some say take a double dose for the next two days and then carry on with your normal routine; others say carry on as normal but do not run the risk of getting pregnant. If you miss three days, stop, wait seven days (during which time you should have a period) and start a new course but avoid the risk of getting pregnant for the first two weeks. If you think you may have got pregnant during the days when you forgot to take the pill, or if you are scared or worried that you have got pregnant then stop the pill. If you have a 'normal' period then start the new course *but* if you are at all suspicious and particularly if your period is scanty or does not start, do *not* start a new month's course. *Wait* until forty days from the first day of your previous period and get a urine pregnancy test done (you may get a false negative before this time). Advise your doctor or pharmacist of any other drugs you are taking, as some may interfere with the test. If the test is negative use extra contraception when starting your next course on the fifth day of your next period and in the first two weeks on the pill because this will be like starting a new course.

Remember if you have an episode of diarrhoea or vomiting whilst on the pill it may interfere with its absorption – take extra precautions for the rest of that month.

If you do not have a period, carry on as normal. If you miss two periods, stop the pill and have a urine pregnancy test done. If you have been on the pill for some time and then get breakthrough bleeding between periods, stop the pill and consult your doctor.

Adverse Effects from the Pill

The commonly used oestrogens in the pill are **mestranol** and **ethinyl-oestradiol** and the commonly used progestogens include **norethisterone, norgestrel, ethynodiol, lynoestrenol, desogestrel** and **levonorgesterel**.

If you read the section on female sex hormones, which you should have

---

* You can get protection by starting the pill on the first day but this will alter your menstrual cycle (i.e., you will be one week early).

done before reading this section, you will have noted the adverse effects produced by **oestrogens**. These adverse effects are related to dose and may occur to a varying degree in different individuals. And so patients on the pill may experience adverse effects of oestrogens. In addition, they may also experience adverse effects of progestogens. The dose-related adverse effects of progestogens and oestrogens taken together are depressed mood, increased appetite, cramps in the legs and abdomen, changes in libido, fluid retention, white vaginal discharge, reduced menstrual loss, dry vagina and increased weight. In addition, there are other adverse effects produced by such combinations. In some they may affect the circulation, producing headaches, migraine, flushing, dizziness and changes in blood pressure, swelling of the ankles and thrombophlebitis. These tend to occur with high-dose oestrogen and medium-dose progestogen preparations. Blood clotting may be affected by high-dose synthetic oestrogen preparations which may therefore increase the risk of thrombosis. Some of these adverse effects need to be discussed more fully.

The **progestogen*** in the pill may cause a depressed mood in some, but it is not the progestogen alone – it seems to require oestrogen as well to produce this unpleasant adverse effect, and so it is the combination which causes the trouble. Norethisterone particularly seems to be related to depression of mood (so check which pill you are on if you are depressed). There is a suggestion that **vitamin B₆ (pyridoxine)** may help to control this depression.

The greatest risk from the pill is the development of a thrombosis in a vein and the shooting off of part of this clot into the lungs leading to death. This process is called *thromboembolism* and the thrombosis usually occurs in the *deep veins* of the legs or pelvis. It may also occur in the vessels supplying the brain (cerebral thrombosis), producing a stroke.

This very rare risk of thrombosis is not related to how long you have been on the pill, but it is thought to be roughly proportional to the dose of synthetic oestrogen in a preparation. There is also a greater risk if you are over 35 years of age and you smoke. There is no obvious difference between mestranol and ethinyloestradiol. The safety level for oestrogen appears to be about 0·05 mg and the majority of pills do not now go above this level.

There has been no proved association between taking the pill and developing a coronary thrombosis. Of course, there may be an added risk in high-risk patients – those with raised blood pressure who are also heavy smokers, or those with high blood fat levels and a family history of a parent or brother or sister dying from a coronary thrombosis under the age of about sixty.

* See warnings on the risk of cancer of the breast and uterus on p. 246.

The pill has many effects upon the body's metabolism – over fifty have been recorded affecting various functions. For example, blood sugar and fat levels may be raised, liver function tests changed, blood-clotting factors altered and thyroid function tests affected. They may predispose to infections of the cervix particularly by thrush (candida) and cause loss of periods in someone who has previously had irregular or scanty periods. Itching vagina (pruritus vulvae) may be produced by the pill; vaginal discharge and pruritus vulvae are more likely to occur if you are given a tetracycline or other such broad-spectrum antibiotic as well, for some other infection (e.g., bronchitis). Itching of the skin may occur and some women get a brownish colour on their face (chloasma, as seen in pregnancy). A blistering skin rash (porphyria) on exposure to the sun may rarely occur, and some women's hair goes thin for a few months after stopping the pill.

After stopping the pill some women fail to have a period. This is more common in women with late puberty who previously had irregular periods. It is caused by failure of the pituitary to recover from its suppression by the high blood levels of oestrogens and progestogens whilst on the pill. The hypothalamus may also not recover its full function. The lining of the uterus in these women may not respond to oestrogens produced by their own ovaries because they have been under daily influence for many months of the oestrogen and progestogen in the pill they have been taking. Loss of periods does not appear to be harmful and if a woman does not want to get pregnant there is no need to give a drug to stimulate ovulation. Remember also that after being on the pill it may take some women a few months to get pregnant but this is not related to the length of time that they were taking the pill.

The possible long-term risk of cancer of the breast, uterus, cervix or vagina needs to be considered. The study of these risks is made more difficult by the frequently prolonged delay in the development of cancer and the complicating socioeconomic factors known to influence the incidence of cancers of this kind. Women taking oral contraceptives should have regular medical examinations.

Precautions

To reduce the risk of thrombosis it is better to use a pill that contains 0·05 mg or less of an oestrogen.

To reduce the risk of depression it is better to use a low-dose progestogen pill.

It is best not to use the pill if you have a high blood fat level.

You should not take the pill if you have had a previous deep vein thrombosis or embolism. Previous superficial thrombophlebitis is not a reason for not taking the pill, but regular medical supervision is necessary.

Do not take the pill within one month of a surgical operation or within one month after childbirth. A progestogen-only pill has fewer adverse effects if you are breast feeding and may be taken during this time.

Do not take the pill if you have had an attack of jaundice or severe itching of the skin during pregnancy.

Do not take the pill if you have or have had a cancer of a breast.

Do not take the pill if you have an acute or severe long-standing liver disorder, if you have angina or have had a heart attack or stroke.

Do not take the pill if you have attacks of severe migraine (e.g., associated with pins and needles in hands and/or feet). An increase in the frequency or severity of headaches indicates that a medical examination is required.

If you are at the menopause (and being on the pill will not affect your symptoms) stop the pill for two or three months to see if a period comes on, and if it does go back on the pill for two or three months. If you do not have a period do not go back on to the pill. But take alternative contraceptive precautions for two years if you are under fifty years of age, for one year if you are over fifty.

If you have a family history of diabetes then you should be cautious. But having diabetes need not stop you going on the pill, although it may increase your insulin requirements.

If you are due to have thyroid tests then stop the pill for two months before – it interferes with tests for thyroid functions.

Be cautious when using corticosteroids (e.g., prednisolone) – they may send your blood pressure up.

Remember certain drugs can speed up the breakdown of the pill in the liver (e.g., rifampicin, phenytoin and phenobarbitone). Check with your doctor, pharmacist or local drug information centre. During treatment with any of these drugs you should take additional precautions.

Remember if you have a bout of diarrhoea or vomiting you may not have absorbed sufficient drug to be effective, and you should use additional precautions for the rest of the month. Antibiotics such as ampicillin interfere with absorption from the gut.

If ever you are in doubt, always continue to take the pill as directed but take additional precautions until the end of the month.

Varicose veins are not considered to be a reason for not taking the pill – but check carefully with your doctor.

Piles (haemorrhoids) are not a reason for not taking the pill.

If you have a raised blood pressure your doctor should keep you under regular observation and also if you have epilepsy, otosclerosis (a type of

Oral Contraceptive Drugs 243

progressive deafness), multiple sclerosis, or any disease which is likely to get worse during pregnancy.

It may be best not to take the pill if you have had previous episodes of severe mental depression but discuss this with your doctors.

Remember – you may get depressed if you change from a high- to a low-dose oestrogen pill.

Remember there may be a need to use additional contraceptive methods if you change pills (e.g., from high-dose to low-dose). Check with your doctor or pharmacist.

If you are over thirty-five and on the pill you should not smoke.

Read about breakthrough bleeding, spotting and scanty or absent periods.

Read what to do if you forget to take a pill.

Check when to avoid the risk of getting pregnant.

Young girls (under sixteen years of age) should not go on the pill until their periods have started and are occurring regularly.

Young girls on the pill for more than nine months should stop their pill for one month and have their daily temperatures checked to see if they are ovulating. If they are then they can carry on with the pill. If they are not ovulating they should not be on the pill and should be referred to a gynaecologist.

When to Stop the Pill Immediately

If you get pregnant.

If your blood pressure rises.

Four weeks before a surgical operation or when confined to bed after an accident or an illness.

If you get jaundice.

At the first signs of a thrombosis.

If you get migraine and have never previously had an attack.

If you have had migraine before and develop a very severe attack.

Any severe or unusual headaches.

Any disturbance of vision.

The risk of thrombosis or heart failure is increased if you are overweight, smoke and are aged thirty-five or over. Diabetes, raised blood pressure and a family history of high blood fat levels add to these dangers.

Changes in Menstruation

'Spotting', which is a very slight show of blood between periods, is usually of no significance. Carry on with the pill since it usually clears up. If it recurs the next month consult your doctor.

    'Breakthrough bleeding', which is bleeding in between periods like a small period, may be stopped by taking two pills a day for two or three days and then going back on the normal course. Alternatively, you may carry on the course and see how things are with the next month's course. If it recurs consult your doctor. Another way is to stop the pill for seven days and then re-start another course. Whichever you choose, if breakthrough bleeding occurs two months running you must see your doctor and have a gynaecological examination which will usually include a cervical smear test. Such an examination is also necessary if spotting or breakthrough bleeding occurs for the first time after prolonged use of the pill or if it recurs at irregular intervals. Decreased menstrual flow is nothing to worry about.

The Choice of Pill

Progestogens act on the uterus which has been subjected (primed) to the effects of **oestrogens**. Various preparations may therefore be compared by how long they can delay a period when given in equally effective doses. In this way oestrogens may also be compared and from such studies we have learnt that ethinyloestradiol is about twice as potent as mestranol. Similarly, the progestogens can be ranked in order of potency (from strongest to weakest): **norgestrel, ethynodiol, lynoestrenol, norethisterone, megestrol**. What is more, different chemical structures of the same drug can vary; for example, levonorgestrel is about twice as potent as norgestrel.

In the body the ratio of oestrogens to progestogens is delicately balanced to produce optimum chances of getting pregnant. Some women may produce too much oestrogen and therefore have heavy, frequent periods whereas others may produce too much progestogen and suffer from scanty and irregular periods. Both these groups of women do not produce the ideal balance of hormones to encourage conception and they may therefore be sub-fertile. It follows, therefore, that if an oestrogen is given to some women it may produce heavier periods whereas progestogens, in some women, may produce scanty periods or even absent periods if given in sufficient dosage (the principle of preparations used to delay the onset of menstruation). When the drugs are stopped, withdrawal bleeding will occur. Now it can be seen that effects produced by oestrogens can be balanced by adding progestogens. As the doses of these increase the risk of pregnancy gets less. But, unfortunately, adverse effects start to increase. High doses of oestrogens will produce the adverse effects mentioned earlier, as will increasing the dosage of progestogens. Thus there is a spectrum of effects and adverse effects produced by the various combination oestrogen/progestogen pills. Therefore, a pill should be chosen for you which takes into account how regular and heavy your periods were and its potential for producing adverse effects in *you*. Re-read this section and the section on female sex hormones and make a note of the facts which apply particularly to *you*; for example, whether you previously had scanty periods or heavy periods, whether you are overweight or smoke, whether you have a raised blood pressure or have had a previous thrombosis, whether you have previously had some episodes of depressed mood, what adverse effects you have felt on certain contraceptive preparations, and so on. Remember, you may be on the pill for many years; it is most important for you and your doctor to choose the pill which suits *you* and it is no use your doctor fixing in his mind one particular brand-named product and prescribing it for everybody who wishes to take an oral contraceptive.

Oral Contraceptive Drugs

Combined Oestrogen and Progestogen pills – Fixed Doses

Name	Oestrogen: Dose		Progestogen: Dose	
Eugynon 50	ethinyloestradiol	(0·05 mg)	norgestrel	(0·5 mg)
Gynovlar 21	ethinyloestradiol	(0·05 mg)	norethisterone	(3·0 mg)
Minilyn	ethinyloestradiol	(0·05 mg)	lynoestrenol	(2·5 mg)
Minovlar	ethinyloestradiol	(0·05 mg)	norethisterone	(1·0 mg)
Minovlar ED	ethinyloestradiol	(0·05 mg)	norethisterone	(1·0 mg)
Ovran	ethinyloestradiol	(0·05 mg)	levonorgestrel	(0·25 mg)
Ovulen 50	ethinyloestradiol	(0·05 mg)	ethynodiol	(1·0 mg)
Norinyl-1	mestranol	(0·05 mg)	norethisterone	(1·0 mg)
Ortho-Novin 1/50	mestranol	(0·05 mg)	norethisterone	(1·0 mg)
BiNovum	ethinyloestradiol	(0·035 mg)	norethisterone	(0·5 and 1·0 mg)
Brevinor	ethinyloestradiol	(0·035 mg)	norethisterone	(0·5 mg)
Neocon 1/35	ethinyloestradiol	(0·035 mg)	norethisterone	(1·0 mg)
Norimin	ethinyloestradiol	(0·035 mg)	norethisterone	(1·0 mg)
Ovysmen	ethinyloestradiol	(0·035 mg)	norethisterone	(0·5 mg)
Synphase	ethinyloestradiol	(0·035 mg)	norethisterone	(0·5 and 1·0 mg)
TriNovum	ethinyloestradiol	(0·035 mg)	norethisterone	(0·5/0·75/ 1·0 mg)
Conova 30	ethinyloestradiol	(0·03 mg)	ethynodiol	(2·0 mg)
Eugynon 30	ethinyloestradiol	(0·03 mg)	levonorgestrel	(0·25 mg)
Femodene	ethinyloestradiol	(0·03 mg)	gestodene	(0·075 mg)
Loestrin 20	ethinyloestradiol	(0·02 mg)	norethisterone	(1·0 mg)
Loestrin 30	ethinyloestradiol	(0·03 mg)	norethisterone	(1·5 mg)
Marvelon	ethinyloestradiol	(0·03 mg)	desogestrel	(0·15 mg)
Mercilon	ethinyloestradiol	(0·03 mg)	desogestrel	(0·15 mg)
Microgynon 30	ethinyloestradiol	(0·03 mg)	levonorgestrel	(0·15 mg)
Minulet	ethinyloestradiol	(0·03 mg)	desogestrel	(0·075 mg)
Ovran 30	ethinyloestradiol	(0·03 mg)	levonorgestrel	(0·25 mg)
Ovranette	ethinyloestradiol	(0·03 mg)	levonorgestrel	(0·15 mg)

Combined Oestrogen and Progestogen – **Biphasic and Triphasic Doses**

Name	Oestrogen: Dose		Progestogen: Dose		
BiNovum	ethinyloestradiol	0·035 mg	norethisterone	0·5 mg	– 7 tablets
	ethinyloestradiol	0·035 mg	norethisterone	1·00 mg	– 14 tablets
Synphase	ethinyloestradiol	0.035 mg	norethisterone	0·5 mg	– 7 tablets
	ethinyloestradiol	0·035 mg	norethisterone	1·00 mg	– 9 tablets
	ethinyloestradiol	0·035 mg	norethisterone	0·5 mg	– 5 tablets
Trinovum	ethinyloestradiol	0·035 mg	norethisterone	0·5 mg	– 7 tablets
		0·035 mg	norethisterone	0·75 mg	– 7 tablets
		0·035 mg	norethisterone	1·00 mg	– 7 tablets
Logynon*	ethinyloestradiol	0·030 mg	Levonorgestrel	0·05 mg	– 6 tablets
		0·040 mg	Levonorgestrel	0·075 mg	– 5 tablets
		0·030 mg	Levonorgestrel	0·125 mg	– 10 tablets
Trinordiol	ethinyloestradiol	0·030 mg	Levonorgestrel	0·05 mg	– 6 tablets
		0·040 mg	Levonorgestrel	0·075 mg	– 5 tablets
		0·030 mg	Levonorgestrel	0·125 mg	– 10 tablets

* Logynon E D as for Logynon – 21 active tablets plus 7 dummy tablets – take one each day for 28 days.

Progestogen-only Preparations

Name	Progestogen	Dose
Depo-Provera	medroxyprogesterone	50 mg and 150 mg/1 ml injection
Femulen	ethynodiol	0·5 mg
Micronor	norethisterone	0·35 mg
Microval	levonorgestrel	0·03 mg
Neogest	norgestrel	0·075 mg
Norgeston	levonorgestrel	0·03 mg
Noriday	norethisterone	0·35 mg
Noristerat	norethisterone	200 mg/1 ml injection

Warning: there has been a reported association between the progestogen content of the combined pill ('the pill') and cancer of the breast and cancer of the cervix. It is clearly best to avoid the high potency progestogens (see p. 244).

Post Coital Contraceptive

Eugynon 50, Ovran, Schering PC$_4$ ethinyloestradiol (0·05 mg) levonorgestrel (0·025 mg).

The Combined Oral Contraceptive ('The Pill')

Summary of Precautions and Adverse Effects

Use with caution if you suffer from: obesity, diabetes, raised blood pressure, heart or kidney disease, migraine, epilepsy, depression, asthma, multiple sclerosis, if you wear contact lenses, have varicose veins, smoke, if you are over thirty-five years of age, or if you are breast feeding.

Do not use if you are: pregnant, have a history of thrombosis or jaundice, if you have liver disease, sickle cell anaemia, high blood fat levels, cancer of the breast or womb, severe migraine, undiagnosed bleeding from the vagina, history of severe itching (pruritus) in pregnancy or deteriorating otosclerosis. *Adverse effects include:* nausea, vomiting, headache, tenderness of the breasts, changes in body-weight, thrombosis, change in libido, depression, brown pigmentation on the face (chloasma), raised blood pressure, impairment of liver function, reduced menstrual loss, 'spotting' early in cycle, loss of periods and rarely photosensitivity (sensitivity of the skin to sunlight).

Diabetes is the term used to refer to diabetes mellitus, which is a disorder characterized by a deficiency or diminished effectiveness of insulin, a hormone produced by the pancreas and responsible for lowering the blood sugar level by encouraging the burning up of sugar in the tissues to produce energy. Insulin is also responsible for converting glucose into a substance called glycogen for storage in muscles and in the liver for future use, and for the formation of fat for storage. It also influences protein build-up.

There are many factors which contribute to these processes but, very simply, diabetes may be regarded as either a disorder which results in too little insulin production by the pancreas for the body's requirements or a disorder in which the insulin it produces is not effective in carrying out these processes, or both. The results are that glucose removal from the blood is reduced and the release of glucose into the blood by the liver is increased. Thus glucose is over-produced and under-used, resulting in a high blood sugar level – hyperglycaemia. Diabetes may therefore be caused by a disorder of the pancreas, resulting in its failure to produce insulin; by the presence of body chemicals which block the effects of insulin; or by increased production of glucose by the liver (for example, adrenaline increases the breakdown of liver glycogen and pushes up the blood sugar levels).

High blood sugar levels (hyperglycaemia) may result in sugar appearing in the urine because the kidneys cannot cope with the high concentrations; this results in an increased volume of urine leading to salt and water loss and thirst. Because the diabetic patient is unable to use the glucose in the blood, fat is mobilized and used for energy. This results in an increased amount of fat breakdown products accumulating in the blood producing what is called ketosis and an alteration in the acidity of the blood. These chemical changes may cause coma and death if untreated. In addition, protein is also broken down, which produces wasting of muscles and loss of weight.

Many factors influence the development and progress of diabetes; for example, hereditary factors, age, sex, weight, infections, stress, and physical disorders. Its treatment is difficult but rewarding and should always be in the hands of experts. Successful treatment of diabetes should be a joint effort between doctor and patient; this gives a good example of how important it is for the patient to know what is wrong with him, to know about the drugs he is taking, to know the effects and adverse effects of these drugs, to know when to adjust the dosage, and to know what other drugs to take and not to take.

The Drug Treatment of Diabetes

In addition to diet, there are two main approaches to the treatment of diabetes – insulin by injection or blood sugar lowering drugs by mouth. The latter are called oral anti-diabetic drugs or oral hypoglycaemic drugs (hypoglycaemia meaning low blood sugar).

Insulin

Insulin is a hormone produced and stored by the beta cells of the pancreas. As a drug its principal source is from slaughtered animals. Pork and beef insulins are the ones used routinely; the choice is not critical except that some patients may, rarely, become allergic to one type. Insulin must be given by injection because it is inactivated when given by mouth. In everyday treatment it is injected under the skin (into different sites). Insulin pumps are available to provide continuous subcutaneous (under the skin) injections. In an emergency (e.g., diabetic coma) insulin is injected into a vein or muscle. An enzyme called insulinase, found mainly in the liver, is responsible for its breakdown in the body.

Insulin production by the pancreas is principally regulated by the blood sugar level but many other factors may also affect its production and breakdown. For example, many diabetic patients require doses far in excess of 'normal' output in order to control their symptoms. It is suggested that insulin antagonists may account for this by interfering with its effects.

Insulin is used to treat diabetes in young patients and diabetes developing in older individuals in whom no improvement has been obtained in response to diet control and oral anti-diabetic drugs. Insulin is also necessary in pregnancy and in elderly patients (who normally do well on diet and oral anti-diabetic drugs) when they have a severe infection or are undergoing surgery. At these times – during infections, injury or surgery – the body normally requires more insulin.

Initial treatment with insulin should always be carried out in hospital, where repeated estimations of blood sugar levels may be made. Where appropriate, patients are shown how to give themselves their own injections of insulin and they should be allowed to experience the effects of an underdose and overdose and how to correct these. This process is known as stabilization: it is most important and should not be hurried. The patient is ready for discharge when the most appropriate dosage regimen of insulin for controlling his symptoms, blood sugar levels and the amount of sugar in his urine has been worked out. But he should not be discharged until he understands his diet, how to give himself his injection (if appropriate), test his blood and/or urine for sugar and knows when and how to increase the dose as required.

The choice of insulin preparation will depend on many factors and in particular on the duration of action of the various preparations available.

Injected insulin is rapidly inactivated by the liver, and therefore much work has gone into making insulin injections long acting by ensuring their slow absorption into the blood-stream from their injection sites. Because most insulins are obtained from animals they may cause allergic reactions in some patients.

Beef and pork insulins are available as insulin injections (**soluble insulin injections, ordinary insulin, regular insulin, unmodified insulin**).

Soluble insulin is acidic and it was suggested that a neutral solution would be more easily absorbed into the blood-stream. **Neutral insulin (neutral insulin injections)** is such a neutralized preparation, which is said to act more rapidly than soluble insulin and also to have a more prolonged effect. **Biphasic insulin** is a mixture of beef insulin crystals in a neutralized solution of pork insulin.

By altering the acidity and adding zinc to insulin suspensions zinc combines with the insulin to produce larger particles which, after injection, act as a depot to produce a slow release of insulin. These preparations are called **insulin zinc suspensions (I.Z.S.)** or **lente insulins** (*lente* meaning 'slow'). The size of particles determines the speed of action. **Amorphous I.Z.S.** has a rapid onset of action and acts for a moderate duration of time (**semilente**). **Crystalline I.Z.S.** has a slower onset of action and a prolonged duration of action (**ultralente**). When the two types are mixed a preparation with an intermediate duration of action is produced (**lente insulin**).

Another method of making insulin act over a longer period is to add protamine (a protein obtained from fish sperm) to a suspension of insulin. The **protamine** and **insulin** form a complex which is much less soluble and from which insulin is slowly released after injection. The duration of action of this complex may be further prolonged by adding zinc to form **Protamine Zinc Insulin**. However, its use is complicated by the hazard that if the blood sugar is controlled through the daytime it may fall too low during the night and early morning. Attempts to balance this effect lead to the combined use of Protamine Zinc Insulin and soluble insulin. The combined effects provide sufficient cover during the day without too high a dose of Protamine Zinc Insulin working on through the night. This should not be mixed in the same syringe because excess protamine in the P.Z.I. may attach itself to the soluble insulin. Such a combination is still needed in some severe diabetics but its use has generally been replaced by the lente insulins. Some patients may be allergic to protamine and an alternative protein preparation is available – **Globin Zinc Suspension** – but this also causes allergic reactions. A preparation containing less protamine and zinc called **Isophane Insulin** is also available.

By means of chromatographical separation, impurities from the pancreas are removed from insulin preparations, thus reducing the risk of antibody formation against the insulin which has hitherto greatly impaired its effectiveness. These are called **highly purified insulins**.

Care should be taken when changing a patient from conventional insulins on to highly purified insulins since there is usually a reduced insulin need.

Human insulins are available and are useful where problems of immunity have developed to animal insulins. They may be **biosynthetic** (crb) or similar to human insulin in structure and prepared from **pork material** (emp).

In treating diabetes expert advice is needed on the choice of insulin preparation, the dose and timing of injections, and the time of meals. In addition a patient needs expert advice on diet, weight, smoking and exercise. The commonest adverse effect of insulin treatment is hypoglycaemia or low blood sugar. This happens when a patient receives too much insulin. This may occasionally occur if a patient misses out a meal or eats a diet lacking sufficient carbohydrates. The early symptoms are weakness, giddiness, pallor, sweating, increased production of saliva in the mouth, sinking feeling in the stomach, palpitations, irritability and trembling. If these are not immediately relieved by taking a glucose sweet or sugar the patient may develop changes in mood, be unable to concentrate, lack judgement and lose self-control. Loss of memory, paralysis, double vision, pins and needles in the hands and feet, unconsciousness, convulsions and death may occur. Every diabetic patient should be allowed to experience the early warning effects of hypoglycaemia and then be taught the correct treatment to prevent an attack coming on. If a patient is unable to understand these effects and instructions then the nearest relative or friend should be instructed.

Other adverse effects from insulin include allergic reactions – skin rashes, itching and swelling of the face and throat. These may sometimes be controlled by changing the preparation – for example one patient may be allergic to beef insulin but not to pork insulin and vice versa. Nettle-rash and other local reactions may occur at the site of injections resulting in wasting of the fatty tissue under the skin; alternatively fatty swellings (lipomata) may rarely occur. Rotation of injection sites can help prevent these complications.

An immune reaction to insulin may rarely occur resulting in a dramatic increase in the amount of insulin required. The insulin becomes 'neutralized' and less effective. This reaction is more common with beef insulin than with pork insulin. Certain glandular disorders may increase sensitivity to insulin (e.g., underworking of the pituitary gland or adrenal gland) resulting in low blood sugar levels. Oral contraceptive agents and thiazide diuretics may make diabetics worse by lessening the effects of insulin so that more insulin will be required when taking such drugs.

If you are on insulin you should carry a warning card saying that you are a diabetic and giving the name and dose of the insulin preparation you are taking. The card should state that if you are found behaving strangely you should be given sugar by mouth.

Short-acting Insulins

Acid insulin
   Hypurin Soluble (beef, highly purified)
Neutral insulin
   Neutral insulin (beef, highly purified)
   Human Actrapid (highly purified – emp)
   Human Velosulin (human, highly purified – prb)
   Humulin S (human, highly purified – prb)
   Hypurin Neutral (beef, highly purified)
   Neusulin (beef, highly purified)
   Quicksol (beef, highly purified)
   Velosulin (pork, highly purified)

Intermediate-acting Insulins

Biphasic insulin
   Human Actraphane
   Human Initard 50/50 (emp)
   Human Mixtard 30/70 (emp)
   Humulin M1, M2, M3, M4 (human prb and isophane insulins in varying concentrations)
   Initard 50/50 (50% pork isophane, highly purified and 50% pork neutral, highly purified)
   Mixtard 30/70 (isophane insulin; pork, highly purified 70%, neutral insulin; pork, highly purified 30%)
   Rapitard M C (crystalline insulin; beef, highly purified 75% with neutral insulin pork, highly purified 25%)
   Insulin Zinc Suspension (amorphous)

Semitard M C (pork, highly purified)
Isophane insulins
  Human Insulatard (isophane human – emp)
  Human Protaphane (emp)
  Humulin I (prb)
  Hypurin Isophane (beef, highly purified)
  Insulatard (pork, highly purified)
  Monophane (beef, highly purified)
  Neuphane (beef, highly purified)

Long-acting Insulins

Insulin zinc suspension (mixed)
  Insulin zinc suspension; mixed; I.Z.S., Lente
  Human Monotard (highly purified – emp)
  Humulin Lente (highly purified – emp)
  Hypurin Lente (beef, highly purified)
  Lentard M C (beef and pork, highly purified)
  Monotard M C (pork, highly purified)
  Neulente (beef, highly purified)
  Tempulin (beef, highly purified)
Insulin zinc suspension (crystalline)
  Human Ultratard (emp)
  Human Zn (crb)
Protamine zinc insulin
  Hypurin Protamine Zinc (beef, highly purified)

Oral Hypoglycaemic Drugs

Oral hypoglycaemic drugs are drugs which may be taken by mouth to produce a fall in blood sugar. There are two main groups – the sulphonyl-ureas and the biguanides.

The Sulphonylureas and Related Drugs

It is thought that these drugs lower blood sugar levels by acting on the pancreas to secrete more insulin. They also have a direct effect upon the liver and potentiate the action of insulin throughout the body. They are only effective in the presence of some pancreatic function and they do not affect the take-up and release of glucose by muscles. But their action may be much more complicated than is generally thought. Their rate of breakdown in the body varies and this affects their duration of action.

The sulphonylureas include **acetohexamide (Dimelor), chlorpropamide**

(Diabinese, Glymese), glibenclamide (Daonil, Euglucon, Libanil, Malix, Semi-Daonil), gliclazide (Diamicron), glipizide (Glibenese, Minodiab), gliquidone (Glurenorm), tolazamide (Tolanase) and tolbutamide (Glyconon, Rastinon). Any of these drugs may produce hypoglycaemia (fall in blood sugar) particularly in the elderly and those with impaired kidney or liver function. They should be used with caution in these patients and also in patients with serious thyroid disorders, because they may affect thyroid function. Glymidine (Gondafon) is closely related to the sulphonylureas.

Sulphonylureas tend to encourage an increase in weight. They should not be used in obese diabetics unless they have been on a strict diet and lost weight nearly down to the normal weight for their sex and age (at least within 15 per cent of that weight). They should be used with caution in breast-feeding mothers, the elderly and in patients with impaired function of their kidneys, liver, thyroid or adrenal glands. Those sulphonylureas that are principally broken down in the liver should be used in patients with impaired kidney function, e.g., gliquidone, gliclazide or a short-acting one such as tolbutamide should be used. Adverse effects include discomfort in the stomach, nausea, vomiting and loss of appetite. Nerve damage may occur, producing weakness and pins and needles. Sensitivity reactions may occur in the first two months of treatment and include skin rashes, fever and jaundice. Blood disorders have been reported and chlorpropamide has rarely produced photosensitivity (skin rashes on exposure to sunlight).

Biguanides

The only available biguanide is metformin (Glucophage, Orabet). It increases glucose uptake by muscles in the presence of insulin and it reduces the release of glucose by the liver. It may reduce absorption of carbohydrates from the gut and therefore its effects may modify insulin requirements in diabetics and it also produces a loss of weight in overweight diabetics.

Deaths have been reported due to alterations in the acidity of the blood (lactic acidosis) in patients taking phenformin and it has been withdrawn from the market. Metformin should not be given to patients with congestive heart failure or to those patients with impaired kidney or liver function. It should not be used in pregnancy. Alcohol should be used with caution by patients taking metformin. Lactic acidosis may also be produced by metformin and therefore it should not be used in patients with impaired function of their kidneys or liver or in the elderly. Metformin may produce nausea, diarrhoea, vomiting, loss of appetite, and decreased absorption of vitamin B_{12}.

Warning: the blood sugar lowering effects of oral hypoglycaemic drugs may be increased by alcohol, aspirin, phenylbutazone, sulphonamides and monoamine oxidase inhibitors. Corticosteroid drugs may increase blood sugar levels, so may oral contraceptive drugs and thiazide diuretics. Caution is therefore necessary when using these drugs in patients who are receiving oral hypoglycaemic drugs.

Many patients taking chlorpropamide suffer from facial burning and flushing very shortly after drinking alcohol. This reaction to alcohol may be inherited. It also occurs with tolbutamide and rarely with glibenclamide.

A major long-term study in the U.S.A. and additional studies elsewhere have indicated that oral hypoglycaemic drugs are no more effective than diet alone in prolonging life in diabetic patients. Instead, they have suggested an increased incidence of abnormalities in electrical activity of the heart, heart attacks (myocardial infarction) and death.

While these findings are not uniformly accepted by the medical community, they have led to more stringent guidelines for the use of oral hypoglycaemic drugs. They should be used only in patients with diabetes of the maturity-onset type who cannot be treated with diet alone or who are unwilling or unable to take insulin if weight reduction and dietary control fail.

The sometimes high incidence of 'secondary failure', whereby an initially successful oral hypoglycaemic agent subsequently fails to maintain a low blood sugar, often responds to the addition of a different chemical class of oral hypoglycaemic drug. However, in the light of the toxicities discussed earlier, this practice has become questionable. These drugs should not be used in pregnancy or in a diabetic emergency (as before surgery). Concurrent alcohol use should be avoided since it could produce nausea and possibly potentiate the hypoglycaemic effects of the sulphonylureas.

Guar Gum

Guar gum (**Glucotard, Guarem, Guarina**) if taken in large enough quantities can result in some reduction of plasma glucose concentrations. It probably works by retarding carbohydrate absorption from the gastrointestinal tract. Because it needs water to work it is important to maintain an adequate intake of fluid.

Drugs Used to Treat Thyroid Disorders

The thyroid gland lies in the neck in front of and on both sides of the wind-pipe (trachea). It produces two hormones called thyroxine and tri-iodothyronine. These hormones are responsible for increasing the metabolism (use of energy) of the cells in the body. The thyroid gland is under control of the master gland (pituitary gland) which produces a thyroid stimulating hormone (thyrotropic hormone). If there is a deficiency of thyroid hormones in the blood, the pituitary increases its stimulation of the thyroid gland. The reverse happens if there is an increase of thyroid hormones in the blood.

Thyroid hormones are available for treatment either in extracts of thyroid glands obtained from slaughtered animals or as synthetic preparations of thyroxine or tri-iodothyronine. Thyroid extracts were previously used but because of their unpredictable strengths and problems with standardization their use has now largely given way to synthetic preparations which are highly purified and standardized.

There are several disorders of the thyroid gland for which drug treatments are used – these include goitre, underworking of the gland (hypothyroidism, myxoedema), overworking of the gland (hyperthyroidism or thyrotoxicosis) and other rare disorders such as thyroiditis (inflammation of the thyroid gland).

Goitre

A simple enlargement of the thyroid gland is called a goitre and it is the body's response to a deficiency of thyroid hormone production. This deficiency, as stated previously, results in the pituitary gland producing an increased amount of thyroid stimulating hormone which causes the thyroid gland to enlarge in an attempt to produce more hormone. Because iodine is necessary for the production of thyroid hormones, enlargement may occur (goitre) if the diet is deficient in iodine. This may occur in certain areas well away from the sea, where water supplies lack iodine and sea foods rich in iodine are scarce. Excessive calcium in hard water may interfere with the absorption of iodine from the gut and, rarely, there are genetic factors which interfere with the thyroid gland's manufacture of hormones. Some drugs may also interfere with thyroid hormone production, e.g., para-amino-salicylic acid and sulphonamides. Iodine mixtures taken for coughs may produce thyroid enlargement and the gland may enlarge during certain periods of increased demand, e.g., puberty, pregnancy, breast feeding. Whatever the cause of simple goitre the deficiency of thyroid hormone leads to an increase in size of the gland.

The treatment of goitre is to give synthetic thyroid hormone in order to reduce the amount of thyroid stimulating hormone being produced by the pituitary, and therefore to reduce the size of the gland.

Underworking of the Thyroid Gland

Underworking of the thyroid gland or hypothyroidism may be congenital. The baby is born with some defect of the thyroid gland and the lack of thyroid hormones affects the baby's mental and physical development, producing a group of characteristics called cretinism. Rarely, underworking of the thyroid gland may occur during childhood, more frequently it occurs in adult life. Hypothyroidism results in a slowing down of all metabolic processes in the body. It may be associated with a thick, pale swelling of the skin which is called myxoedema.

Disorders of the thyroid gland associated with under-production of thyroid hormones include cretinism, juvenile myxoedema, adult hypothyroidism, adult myxoedema. The treatment of these disorders is to give synthetic thyroid hormones in order to replace the hormones which the gland is incapable of producing.

Thyroid (Thyroid Extract, Desiccated Thyroid)

Despite its variable composition, clinical results with thyroid are remarkably uniform and it is widely used, being the least expensive of the different thyroid preparations. It contains variable amounts of thyroxine and tri-iodothyronine; the extract is somewhat unstable and loses potency upon prolonged exposure to the air.

Thyroxine Sodium (Eltroxin)

The sodium salt of thyroxine is soluble and may be given by mouth. It is considered to be the drug of choice in most thyroid deficiency disorders. Because of its delayed effects, the starting dose must be small and the dose then slowly increased at two-weekly intervals until the required response is obtained. At the start of treatment thyroxine may produce rapid beating of the heart, anginal pain in patients with coronary artery disease and muscle cramps. Too large a dose may cause restlessness, excitement, irregular heart rhythm, headache, flushing, sweating, diarrhoea, excessive loss of weight and muscle weakness, and may affect the heart. These symptoms are usually temporary and related to dose. Large *initial* doses may cause death in patients with myxoedema and heart disease. Thyroxine should, therefore, be used with caution in patients with heart disease. It may increase the effects of anticoagulants and upset the stability of patients receiving anti-diabetic drugs. Phenytoin may affect laboratory tests for thyroxine, giving low results.

Liothyronine Sodium (Tertroxin, Tri-iodothyronine)

This produces similar adverse effects to thyroxine. These disappear when the dose is reduced or the drug is stopped. It is used when a slightly more rapid effect is required. It should not be given to patients with angina or heart disorders. In emergencies it can be given by intravenous injection.

Overworking of the Thyroid Gland (Hyperthyroidism, Thyrotoxicosis)

This occurs more frequently in women than in men, and usually in early adult life. But it is not uncommon in later life when its features differ from those seen in the younger person. The cause is unknown. It produces many symptoms which include nervousness, tiredness, sweating, trembling, diarrhoea, breathlessness, enlargement of the thyroid gland in some patients but not in others, prominence of the eyes, heart disorders, increase of appetite and yet loss of weight.

The treatment is to give antithyroid drugs, or to remove part of the gland by surgery, or to knock it out using radioactive iodine. None of these treatments has any effect upon the underlying cause of the disorder but they do effectively prevent the consequences of over-stimulation of the gland (and therefore the body) until a natural remission occurs.

Antithyroid Drugs

Drugs are of particular use in children, young adults, pregnant women and patients with mild overworking of their thyroid glands. Treatment should continue for up to two years and there is a need for constant supervision by a specialist in thyroid disorders.

Antithyroid drugs interfere with the production of thyroid hormones by the thyroid gland and control may be achieved by observing changes in the patient's symptoms and by measuring the pulse rate and body-weight. It is customary to start with high doses and then slowly reduce the daily dose to a satisfactory maintenance level. There are three groups of drugs used to suppress thyroid function:

(1) Thiocarbamines which include the thiouracils (e.g., **propylthioura-cil**) and the imidazoles (e.g., **carbimazole (Neo-Mercazole)**). These inhibit thyroxine production.

(2) **Potassium perchlorate** which blocks iodine uptake by the thyroid.

(3) **Iodine** and **iodides** which increase the storage and diminish the release of thyroid hormones.

Potassium perchlorate may produce blood disorders and is used occa-sionally when adverse effects develop to other antithyroid drugs. **Methyl-thiouracil** should not be used because the incidence of adverse effects is greater than with propylthiouracil or carbimazole. The choice is between **carbimazole** and **propylthiouracil**. Cross-sensitivity between the two drugs is uncommon so that one of them may be substituted for the other if the patient develops a skin rash.

Iodine and **iodides** cause shrinking of overworking goitres (toxic goitres) but this effect is transient and is only used before surgery and in emerg-encies. Iodine is of no use in the treatment of hyperthyroidism. Iodine should not be given to patients who are receiving potassium perchlorate since it can cause the thyrotoxicosis to flare up.

Antithyroid drugs should be stopped immediately if you develop a sore throat and/or skin rashes, fever and swollen glands. Blood disorders usually clear up on stopping the drug. These adverse effects usually occur within the first month of treatment.

The dose of antithyroid drugs should be given once daily. It takes up to two months before the patient feels the benefit of treatment. In too large a dose they can produce hypothyroidism which may cause enlargement of the gland. They also increase the blood supply to the gland, which may produce problems if the gland is surgically removed.

Antithyroid drugs do not alter the disease process; they simply control symptoms until natural remission occurs.

Propranolol and related drugs are of value in relieving the symptoms of thyrotoxicosis (tremor, rapid heart beat, etc.), in preparation for surgery, whilst awaiting the effects of radioactive iodine therapy, and in the treat-ment of thyrotoxic crises when it is given intravenously.

Radioactive Iodine Therapy

Radioactive iodine (I_{131}) is absorbed from the gut and concentrates in the thyroid gland where it emits primary beta radiation causing local destruction of the thyroid gland. It is the treatment of choice in patients over about 45 years of age, in patients who have relapsed after surgery and in those patients in whom surgery or the prolonged use of anti-thyroid drugs is contraindicated. It should not be used for the treatment of children and women of childbearing age. There is no evidence of an increased risk of thyroid cancer or leukaemia after radioactive iodine therapy. The dose is difficult to predict, response is variable, and there is a high incidence of hypothyroidism (underworking) produced by treatment.

Surgery (Partial Thyroidectomy)

Indications for surgery vary between countries and between individual doctors. It is the treatment of choice for a toxic nodule, a large goitre, and in patients under the age of 45 years who relapse after drug therapy.

44 Local Anaesthetics

Local anaesthetics are drugs which block the transmission of sensory impulses in nerve tissues when applied locally in appropriate concentrations. Their effects are reversible and they are used to produce loss of pain without loss of nervous control – they could be called local pain relievers. However, they can produce loss of nervous control (paralysis) if injected directly into a nerve fibre. Those local anaesthetics in common use have been selected because they do not irritate the tissues to which they are applied and they cause no permanent nerve damage. They are soluble in water and the solutions can be sterilized. Their choice depends upon the speed with which they work, their duration of action and their potential adverse effects when absorbed into the blood-stream. The latter is important since they may affect all nervous tissues including the brain.

Local anaesthetics block the physio-chemical processes which are responsible for nerve impulses developing and passing along nerves to the brain. Their effects quickly wear off when removed from their site of action and for this reason it is customary to mix a local anaesthetic with a drug which closes off the blood supply (vasoconstrictor drug) thus delaying the 'washing' of the local anaesthetic into the blood-stream. The drugs used for this purpose are adrenaline and noradenaline. Their use is not without danger; for example, if the mixtures are used to block pain in a finger, the constriction of blood vessels may so affect the circulation as to cause gangrene. Therefore, they should not be used near terminal arteries as in the fingers, toes, ears, nose and penis.

Local anaesthetics may be absorbed into the blood-stream and produce stimulation and then depression of the brain. This may cause anxiety, restlessness, yawning, nausea, vomiting, twitching, convulsions, coma and death. Pallor, sweating, a fall in blood pressure, irregular heart rhythm, heart failure and respiratory failure may also occur, producing sudden collapse and death. Repeated local use may cause allergic reactions producing skin rashes, asthma and anaphylactic shock. They should be given with utmost caution to patients with impaired heart or liver function. Adverse effects are reduced by adding vasoconstrictor drugs. When applied to the eye, the protective blink reflex is lost and particles blown into the eye can damage the cornea, therefore a protection (for half a day) should always be worn over an eye that has had anaesthetic drops applied.

Local anaesthetics may be administered in several different ways according to the drug being used. *Surface* or *topical anaesthesia* (as a solution, jelly or lozenge) blocks pain in nerve endings in the skin or mucous membranes and to do this the local anaesthetic must have good powers of penetration. *Local* or *infiltration anaesthesia* is produced by *injection* into the area. To be effective the drug must not be absorbed too quickly into the blood-stream otherwise its effects wear off.

Injections of local anaesthetics are also used to produce *regional nerve block* to cut off pain sensation in an area, e.g., a *nerve block* as used by dentists. *Epidural anaesthesia* is a nerve block produced by injecting the anaesthetic into the space between the lining membranes of the spinal cord (used in childbirth). *Caudal anaesthesia* is an injection into the space between the lining membranes at the lower end of the spinal cord where the main nerves from the spinal cord run together before leaving the spine to supply the pelvis and legs.

Spinal anaesthesia is produced by injecting the local anaesthetic inside the covering membrane of the spinal cord, causing temporary paralysis of the nerves with which it comes into contact. The area affected is determined by the specific gravity of the drug (i.e., the rate at which it drops down the fluid inside the spinal cord) and by tipping the patient up or down according to the area which is to be anaesthetized. It can be used in patients who are not suitable for a general anaesthetic.

The choice of local anaesthetic depends upon many factors but in particular upon the risk of absorption and the production of dangerous adverse effects.

Injectable local anaesthetics in common use include **bupivacaine (Marcain)**, **lignocaine (Xylocaine)**, and **prilocaine (Citanest)**. **Procaine** is seldom used. **Amethocaine** is principally used as a surface anaesthetic in solution (e.g., eye drops) and in lozenges for the throat. **Benzocaine** is used in lozenges for sore throats and in ointments used to treat haemorrhoids. **Cinchocaine (Nupercainal)** is also used as a surface anaesthetic. **Cocaine** solutions are used for application to the nose, throat, eyes and larynx before local surgery. Other local anaesthetics included in eye drops are **lignocaine, oxybuprocaine** and **proxymetacaine**.

45 Drugs Used to Treat Skin Disorders

Drugs Used in Skin Applications

We know surprisingly little about the causes of many common skin disorders, for example, eczema, psoriasis, acne, warts, dandruff. Against such a background of ignorance it is not surprising that there are many myths about treatment. As I have said previously in this book, where there are many claimed treatments for a particular disorder there often is no specific treatment – otherwise we would all know about it and use it. This applies particularly to skin disorders.

Thanks to the pharmaceutical industry we have seen great advances in the specific and effective cure of many infective skin disorders (see antibiotic and antifungal drugs). We have also seen the introduction of the corticosteroids, which has revolutionized the relief of many skin disorders. Other old-fashioned treatments continue, for example, tar, dithranol, resorcinol, etc., and others such as the antihistamines have not produced the results that we hoped for, except in their specific and effective use by mouth in allergic rashes, particularly those due to drugs. Most skin treatments remain non-specific and at the very least they should not make the disorder worse. Yet the widespread uses of antihistamines, local anaesthetics, antibiotics and antiseptics in skin applications have led to the production of allergic rashes and the inappropriate use of corticosteroids has led to other problems (p. 270).

In the treatment of skin disorders the danger is that skin preparations containing too many potent drugs may be applied in too large a quantity to too large an area too often and over too long a period of time; even base creams may produce allergies. You should be as sensible about applying drugs to the skin as you should be about taking drugs by mouth. Know what you are treating, know what you are applying and know the benefits and risks. With long-standing skin disorders you can always ring the changes by using different recommended preparations but do not be conned into paying huge sums of money to private hair and skin clinics – if they really had a specific and effective treatment for a disorder would we not all know about it and use it?

There are numerous skin applications available – creams, ointments, lotions, dusting powders, sprays, pastes. They are used for treating skin disorders in different stages of severity and in different areas of the body. For example, *lotions* (watery solutions) are used in acute skin conditions and where the skin is unbroken. Watery lotions act by evaporation and cool the skin. When used, they should be applied frequently. The addition of alcohol to a skin lotion increases its cooling effects. They are useful for applying a drug in a thin layer over a large surface or on hairy areas of the skin. When the skin is broken an *astringent* (p. 278) may be included, as it helps to seal the weeping surface of the skin. *Shake lotions* are used for scabbed and dried skin disorders. They cool by evaporation and deposit a powder on the surface. *Dusting powders* (e.g., talc) are useful for treating skin disorders which affect skin folds – under the arms, in the groin, under the breasts. *Creams* moisten the skin more than ointments and cosmetically are more acceptable. *Ointments* are greasy and give more covering than creams; this occlusiveness helps to maintain the hydration of the skin. Ointments are more suitable for chronic, dry, scaly lesions. *Pastes* are stiff preparations and are useful for dry scaly patches.

The choice of the base for creams and ointments and other skin applications is often of equal importance to the choice of 'active' drug in the preparations. The base of a skin application (vehicle) can affect the degree of hydration of the skin and the ability of the active drug to penetrate the skin. Because of the complexity of formulation of many skin preparations it is important to be most careful about dilution which can not only affect the effectiveness of a preparation but also affect its effective life.

The groups of drugs most frequently included in skin applications and which I discuss in this section are:

1. Soothing skin applications – demulcents and emollients. These usually form the base or vehicle in which other drugs are included.
2. Protective skin applications
3. Sunscreen and anti-sunburn skin applications
4. Corticosteroid skin applications
5. Antibiotic skin applications
6. Antifungal skin applications
7. Anti-parasitic skin applications
8. Antiseptics and disinfectants
9. Rheumatic liniments, rubefacients and counter-irritants
10. Anti-itching skin applications and drugs
11. Antihistamine skin applications
12. Local anaesthetic skin applications
13. Caustic and keratolytic skin applications
14. Astringent skin applications

15. Anti-perspirant skin applications
16. Deodorant skin applications
17. Other drugs used in skin applications

1. Soothing Skin Applications

Demulcents

These are usually gums from stems, roots, and branches of various plants, for example, gum arabic, gum tragacanth, liquorice root, agar and sodium alginate (from algae). Synthetic drugs like methylcellulose are also used. **Glycerin** is a common constituent of skin applications and mixed with starch it forms a jelly base called starch glycerite. Glycerin should only be used in low concentrations because it can be irritant. Propylene glycol is related to glycerin and is used in lotions and ointments because it mixes with water (hydrophilic) and also dissolves in oils. Many other glycols are used to make water-soluble bases for ointments.

Demulcents are soothing because they coat the surface of the skin or mucous membranes (mouth, gums and throat) and protect the underlying area from the air and other irritating agents.

Emollients

Emollients are fats and oils which are soothing when applied to the skin. They soften the skin and are chiefly used as a base to which other active drugs (e.g., antibiotics) are added. They soften the skin by forming an oily film over the surface of the skin, thus preventing water from evaporating from the surface cells and so keeping them moist.

Emollient skin applications contain vegetable oils, animal fats, paraffin and related chemicals, and waxes.

The vegetable oils are usually cotton-seed oil, corn oil, peanut oil, almond oil and cocoa-bean oil. Animal fats are wool fats from the wool of sheep. These are of two types – wool fat (**anhydrous lanolin**) and hydrous wool fat (known just as **lanolin**) which is wool fat mixed with 20 to 30 per cent of water. Wool fat can produce skin allergies. It is not used as often as it used to be and yet the message is still given that there is something magical about preparations that contain lanolin.

Paraffin-related preparations include mineral oil (liquid paraffin), white petroleum, and yellow petroleum (e.g., **Vaseline** is a brand preparation of white and yellow petroleum jellies). Waxes are principally obtained from beeswax (yellow wax). White wax is bleached beeswax. Spermaceti* is a

---

* Spermaceti was replaced by jojoba oil in 1982 in E.E.C. countries. It comes from the beans of the jojoba bush, a native of Northern Mexico and Southern California.

waxy substance from the head of the sperm whale which was used to raise the melting point of ointments to stop them melting too easily when applied to warm skin (**cold creams**) particularly in hot climates. Spermaceti is present in rosewater ointment along with white wax, almond oil, rose water and rose oil. This mixture forms the basis of most commonly used cold creams.

2. Protective Skin Applications

Protectives are applications used to cover the skin and mucous membranes in order to protect them from contact with an irritating agent. They are by definition insoluble and inactive and cover the skin physically rather than having any chemical effect. They include *dusting powders* which are used to protect the skin in certain areas (e.g., skin folds) and on the surfaces of ulcers and wounds. They are smooth and prevent friction, and some absorb moisture from the surface of the area to which they are applied. Those that do this help to decrease friction and prevent infection (for example, ones containing **zinc oxide** or **starch**). On open wounds they make a crust and those containing starch have to have an antiseptic added to stop the starch fermenting. Dusting powders often contain **talc** (which is mainly magnesium silicate) and of course talc is widely available as talcum powders.

Mechanical protectives such as **collodion** were used to close off small wounds but it is now considered better to let the air get to a wound. **Petroleum gauze** and **gauzes impregnated with antibiotics** are useful as protective dressings to wounds although the tendency now is to use dry non-adherent dressings. **Barrier creams** are used to protect the skin against irritants which are water soluble. They usually contain **dimethicone (silicone)** or a related silicone oil. These adhere to the skin and have water-repellent properties. They are available as ointments and sprays as well as creams. They provide protection against the irritating effects of soap, water, skin cleansing agents and breakdown products from urine. They may be useful in preventing bed-sores and nappy rash. They should not be used on inflamed or damaged skin or near the eyes because they may produce irritation. There are numerous preparations containing silicone available (e.g., **Rikospray silicone, Siopel, Vasogen**). It is worth trying one of these preparations in order to prevent bed-sores or nappy rash but their use is less effective in preventing industrial dermatitis. Barrier creams may produce allergic skin reactions.

3. Sunscreen and Anti-sunburn Skin Applications

The health-promoting properties of sunlight have long been recognized but it is only in the past fifty years that sunbathing for cosmetic reasons has become fashionable. And it is only in more recent years that the harmful effects of solar radiation and ultra-violet light from artificial sources have become recognized. Excessive exposure to the sun's rays without appropriate protection is harmful: it causes burning and ageing of the skin, cancer of the skin and cataracts.

Sunburn and suntan are caused by ultra-violet rays (UVR). The shorter ultra-violet light waves cause the burning and the longer waves cause the tanning. Tanning results from migration of the brown pigment, **melanin**, from the base layer of the skin up into the surface cells. This provides some protection against sunburn but the main protection comes from a thickening of the surface layer of cells.

The acute effects (sunburn) and the chronic effects of sunlight on the skin are directly related to the total dose of UVR received by the skin, i.e., by the intensity, duration and frequency of exposure. Protection is offered by the melanin content of the skin and the capacity of the skin to produce new protective melanin on the skin surface (i.e., to tan). **Sunscreening** preparations have an important function insofar as they can protect the structure and function of the skin from damaging rays. They are chemicals in the form of clear or milky solutions, gels, creams or ointments which reduce (filter out) the harmful rays. They work by absorbing, reflecting or scattering the rays. The selection of a skin application should therefore depend upon your liability to sunburn and to tan.

Sunscreening Preparations

Sunscreen preparations may be grouped into two broad categories: those applied to the skin and those taken by mouth.

Sunscreens for application to the skin are either **chemical sunscreens** or **physical sunscreens. Chemical sunscreens** contain one or more UV-absorbing chemicals which filter off the harmful rays. They are usually colourless and must be non-irritant and non-staining. Frequently used products include **aminobenzoic acid, padimate, benzyl salicylate, mexenone, methyl salicylate**.

Physical sunscreens are usually opaque formulations and contain particles which reflect and scatter the harmful rays. They include **titanium dioxide (Metanium), talc, zinc oxide, kaolin, ferric chloride** and **ichthyol**. They are usually messy and not acceptable but they may be essential for patients who are ultrasensitive to the sun's rays. Physical sunscreens tend to melt in the heat of the sun.

In recent years preparations containing **methoxypsoralen (bergapten)** or **bergamot oil** (which contains **methoxypsoralen**) have been heavily promoted. The application of these formulations actually stimulates tanning (melanogenesis) which may provide improved protection but they can produce sunlight sensitivity with subsequent pigmentation. Their association with an increased risk of skin cancer has not been proved.

Sun Protection Factor (SPF)

This is a measure of the effectiveness of a sunscreen preparation. It is the ratio of the amount of harmful rays required to produce redness of the skin through a sunscreen preparation to the amount required to produce redness without any sunscreen application.

Categories of Sunscreen Products

	SPF
Minimal sun protection	2–4
Moderate sun protection	4–6
Extra sun protection	6–8
Maximal sun protection	8–15
Ultra sun protection	15 and over

Factors that Influence the Sun Protection Factor (SPF)

These include the subject (skin type, age, amount of sweating, skin site), the UV intensity (season, weather, reflection), radiation source (the sun, type and age of lamp), concentration of sunscreen application, the base (vehicle) used in the preparation, the thickness of the application, effect of water (e.g., after swimming), environment (temperature, humidity, wind) and sweating. In addition the testing procedure is very important because the effectiveness of a sunscreen preparation out of doors may not be related to its performance indoors (i.e., under laboratory conditions).

The most important consideration when purchasing a sunscreen preparation is how *you* react to sunlight. Buy a preparation that suits *your requirements* and one that is manufactured by a reputable company. Most sunscreens should be re-applied after swimming and during prolonged sunbathing.

Sunscreens do not stimulate tanning. Increased tanning is caused by the activation and proliferation of the pigment cells in the skin (melanocytes). This process is decreased by the application of effective sunscreens.

Patients suffering from sensitivity to sunlight (photosensitivity) often require combination therapy with two sunscreen preparations, the first application in an alcoholic solution which evaporates and then a second application of a cream on top.

Adverse Effects of Sunscreens

Certain sunscreen formulations containing **aminobenzoic acid** may cause selective burning (smarting) and occasionally contact or photo-dermatitis. Patients allergic to sulphonamides and certain local anaesthetics (benzocaine and procaine) may have allergic reactions to aminobenzoic acid. Patients on sulphonamides or thiazide diuretics may cross-react with aminobenzoic acid and develop dermatitis.

Oral Treatment of Photosensitivity (Sensitivity to Sunlight)

The effectiveness of most orally taken drugs for protection against sunlight has never been proven. Those with limited effectiveness include **beta-carotene** (a precursor of Vitamin A) which is a natural constituent of many plants including oranges, carrots and tomatoes. It is used to colour foods. Its use should be monitored by measuring the blood carotene levels, which are related to the degree of protection. The anti-malarial drugs (e.g., **chloroquine**) have been used for many years to provide protection in patients sensitive to sunlight.

Quick Tanning Preparations

These applications, which contain drugs such as **dihydroxyacetone (DHA)**, do not stimulate the production of the tanning pigment in the skin; rather they stain the skin yellow-brown. This can be washed off with soap and water or with solvents. It offers no protection to sunlight. Similarly the use of tanning tablets which contain **canthaxanthin** merely colour the skin and underlying fat orangey-brown. It is used to colour foods and medicines. All products containing **canthaxanthin** have been withdrawn because of the risk of eye damage.

Sunburn

There are several treatments for sunburn; amongst the most common are **calamine lotion** and **zinc lotion**. Applications containing a **corticosteroid** (see p. 218) can be very effective. Most experts say do not use applications containing an **antihistamine** because they may produce sensitivity and usually in sunburn there is a fairly large area of skin to be treated.

Drug Induced Sunlight Sensitivity (Photosensitivity)

This means the skin is excessively sensitive to sunlight and goes red and burns very easily. It may be due to a drug. For example, tetracyclines and sulphonamides, antibiotics, griseofulvin, phenothiazine major tranquillizers, oral anti-diabetic drugs; thiazide diuretics; nalidixic acid, used to treat urinary infections; oral contraceptive drugs and gold; diphenhydramine (an antihistamine) and, rarely, saccharin.

Drugs applied to the skin may also sensitize it to sunlight, for example, **tar** (the basis of tar and ultra-violet ray treatment of psoriasis) and **hexachlorophane**, an antiseptic present in numerous skin applications and toiletries. Various **deodorants** may also sensitize the skin, and so too may sunscreen applications (e.g., **aminobenzoic acid**).

The important thing to remember is that if you burn more quickly than usual for you then always think – is it a drug I am taking or a skin application I am using? Stop any of these immediately and check whether they produce sunlight sensitivity.

Some people are actually allergic to sunlight and can develop severe dermatitis on exposed parts of their skin. Certain disorders may produce sunlight allergy, for example, porphyria (a disorder of metabolism). If you develop a rash on the exposed parts of your skin always consult your doctor.

4. Corticosteroid Skin Applications

If you read about corticosteroids on pp. 216–22, you will learn that they reduce inflammatory and allergic reactions. For these reasons they are widely used to treat many skin disorders, in order to reduce the redness, soreness, swelling, pain and irritation which often characterize such conditions. **Corticosteroids** are present alone or in combination with other drugs in numerous skin, eye and ear applications prescribed by doctors. They are very effective, particularly where there is an allergic factor present. However, they do not cure but only suppress the symptoms, so that if the underlying skin disorder is not self-limiting, or if the causative agent is not removed (for example, contact dermatitis caused by an article worn on the body), it will flare up again when the corticosteroid preparation is stopped. This is known as a rebound effect.

Corticosteroids available for use on the skin are listed on p. 222. These vary in potency and so concentrations included in skin preparations vary from 0·001 per cent for triamcinolone up to 2·5 per cent for hydrocortisone. The popularity of any particular preparation may reflect more on the results of vigorous sales promotion rather than on any clear differences in effectiveness.

In using corticosteroid skin preparations it must be remembered that when inflammation is reduced the resistance to infection is lowered and secondary infection may occur. This is particularly likely to happen when corticosteroids are used under occlusive (e.g., plastic) dressings. This may cause boils, thrush and other infections to develop. Allergies may also occur to corticosteroid applications and this should always be considered if there is a poor response to treatment.

Long continued use of corticosteroids under plastic dressings may produce a local wasting of the deep layers of the skin to produce a flattened, depressed stripy-looking area. This may take many years to go away. Some corticosteroids applied to the skin may enter the blood circulation and have an effect upon the pituitary gland (p. 217). This is particularly likely to happen with children (who may also lick the ointment off the skin) and in adults using very large amounts. Very rarely hair may grow at the site of repeated applications of corticosteroids.

Some skin disorders can get infected and become soggy with pus (e.g., infected eczema). In these infected skin disorders the use of an application containing a corticosteroid and an anti-infective drug (e.g., an antibiotic) may be very effective. Such a combination is also useful on skin rashes in areas where infection is likely to occur, for example, in the groin or around the anus. But do not forget that there is a slight risk that an anti-infective drug may produce an allergic reaction which the corticosteroid will mask. Remember this if a skin rash seems to be getting worse despite the fact that initially it improved with such a preparation.

The wrong use of such combinations in primary infective skin disorders may produce very severe effects. For example, if used to treat impetigo (a bacterial infection of the skin) a small localized patch may be turned into a serious widespread skin infection; a simple fungus infection (e.g., athlete's foot) may spread over a large area; and herpes simplex (cold sores) may produce nasty ulcers.

Do not forget also that corticosteroids can delay the healing of ulcers (particularly leg ulcers). Finally, it is important that you should not borrow skin ointments containing a corticosteroid or anti-infective drug from a neighbour or friend – different disorders and different people respond differently.

Corticosteroid skin preparations are not curative and if treatment is suddenly stopped the skin condition may flare up. They are of no use in treating nettle-rash (urticaria). Prolonged use may produce wasting of the deep layer of the skin particularly when used on the face, flexures (knees and elbows) and on moist parts of the skin. They may also produce soreness and irritation at the site of application, irreversible 'stretch marks', increase growth of hair, acne, mild depigmentation and sometimes a dermatitis around the mouth in young women. They should not be used in patients with acne rosacea of the face and in patients (usually children) with eczema of the flexures.

Corticosteroids mixed with an antibiotic, antifungal drug, or an antiseptic, may be used where the primary skin condition would be expected to respond to corticosteroids but where there is an added infection (e.g., infected eczema). To repeat my warning, such combinations should not be used where the skin disorder is primarily infective. The choice of preparation is not critical. Such simple principles as not too much for too long should apply and if the disorder gets worse stop the treatment and see your doctor.

5.   Antibacterial Applications

When a skin infection is superficial (e.g., impetigo) an antibiotic skin application can be dramatically effective. If the infection is deep under the skin surface (e.g., an abscess) then local applications of an antibiotic will be useless and you will need an antibiotic by mouth or injection.

When the sulphonamides and penicillin were introduced doctors used them liberally in skin applications and produced many allergic reactions in their patients. Not only were these allergic reactions inconvenient for the patients, they were positively dangerous for some. They sensitized the patient to the drug, with the consequent risk of a severe allergic reaction if that patient had to be given a sulphonamide or a penicillin by mouth for some more serious infection. Another problem was the development of resistant organisms.

Because of these risks, apply the general principle of not using an antibiotic skin application which is known to produce allergic reactions and is also used by mouth or by injection to treat other infections. There are numerous antibiotic skin applications on the market containing antibiotics which are only used topically: **colistin, framycetin, gramicidin, mafenide, neomycin, nitrofurazone, polymyxin B** and **silver sulphadiazine**. Other antibiotics used to treat skin infections but which are also taken by mouth include **chlortetracycline, fusidic acid, gentamicin tetracycline** and **chloramphenicol**.

Antibiotic skin applications should be used for as short a period as possible over as small an area as possible and if the disorder gets worse they should be stopped immediately.

6.   Antifungal Skin Applications

Before reading this section it is useful to read the section on antifungal antibiotics (pp. 296–7). Here you will learn about the antifungal drugs which may be used locally and by mouth. Some of these have revolutionized the treatment of fungus and yeast infections.

These include such drugs as: **griseofulvin (Fulcin, Grisovin)** used by mouth to treat fungus infections of the hair, skin and nails (e.g., favus, ringworm, athlete's foot); **amphotericin (Fungilin)** given by mouth to treat severe fungus infections affecting internal organs but also applied to the skin to treat fungus infections of the groin and nail beds; **clotrimazole (Canesten)** used to treat fungal infections of the skin and vagina in local applications. **Chlorphenesin (Mycil)** also has antibacterial effects and is used in ointments and powders to treat athlete's foot and other fungal infections. **Natamycin (Pimafucin)** is used topically to treat fungal and yeast infections of the skin and vagina. **Nystatin (Nystan)** is used to treat thrush and is used in powders, drops, ointments, pessaries and tablets. **Propionic acid** (which is also used as a food preservative) and **sodium propionate** are used in ointments to treat fungal skin infections (tinea). **Tolnaftate (Tinaderm)** is available in cream, solution and powder to treat fungal skin infections. **Undecenoic acid (Mycota spray)** and **zinc undecenoate (Mycota)** cream and powder are also used. **Econazole (Ecostatin, Pevaryl)** and **miconazole (Daktarin, Dermonistat, Monistat)** are broad-spectrum anti-fungal drugs.

7. Anti-parasitic Skin Applications

Benzyl benzoate (Ascabiol), monosulfiram (Tetmosol) and **lindane (Lorexane, Quellada)** are useful for treating scabies. The applications should be applied all over the body (below the head) after a bath; the whole household should be treated and all clothes should be washed. Three successive treatments at about twelve-hourly intervals should be applied. Benzyl benzoate may produce transient burning of the skin and rashes. The severe itching produced by scabies may be relieved by **crotamiton (Eurax)**.

Head lice and body lice have become resistant to dicophane (DDT), gamma benzene hexachloride and lindane. Other more effective preparations contain **carbaryl (Carylderm, Clinicide, Derbac-C, Suleo C)** or **malathion (Derbac-M, Prioderm, Suleo-M)**. Everyone in a household with lice must be treated and all clothes and bed-clothes must be washed. Lice are now becoming resistant to these preparations.

8. Antiseptics and Disinfectants

There is quite a mix-up between the terms antiseptic and disinfectant. In general we usually use the term *antiseptic* to describe those drugs applied to the skin or other parts of the body in an attempt to prevent infection. We use *disinfectant* to describe a chemical applied to objects in order to destroy germs. Antiseptic preparations applied to the skin are sometimes called *germicides*. Antiseptics may kill or prevent the growth of bacteria, fungi

274 Drugs Used to Treat Specific Disorders

and viruses. Some disinfectants are used as antiseptics in reduced strengths but some are too irritant and some antiseptics are not strong enough to use as disinfectants.

Antiseptics and disinfectants belong to various chemical groups which can make the choice look very complex and confusing. In fact most doctors learn to use one or two preparations (often by their brand name) and I think this is the best advice I can give you. The choice is not critical and the need to use such preparations is greatly overemphasized in the advertising media.

Some Main Chemical Groups to which Antiseptics and Disinfectants Belong

Chlorine and chlorine-releasing substances. Chlorine kills germs and the most commonly used chlorine-releasing chemical is **sodium hypochlorite**. This is present in commonly used preparations such as **Domestos** and **Milton**. Others include **chlorinated soda solution (Dakin's solution)** and **chlorinated lime** (this is often mixed with boric acid solution as in **Eusol**).

Detergents. These include complex ammonia compounds such as **benzalkonium (Roccal)**, **cetylpyridinium** and **domiphen**. These last two are used as antiseptics in throat lozenges, e.g., **Merocet** and **Bradosol**, respectively (see p. 104). The most commonly used antiseptic detergent is **cetrimide (Cetavlon)** which is present in numerous preparations (e.g., **Savlon** cream) and **Drapoline** which contains benzalkonium and cetrimide. An important point to remember about these preparations is that soap can reduce their activity. They are also prescribed as shampoos by doctors for the treatment of scurfy disorders of the scalp.

Phenol and related drugs. These lose their effects fairly quickly when diluted. They include **phenol**, **cresol** and **thymol**. Solutions of these should not be applied to large wounds since they can be absorbed into the blood-stream and can be very toxic.

Chlorinated phenols. The two most widely used of these include a mixture of **chlorinated phenols (Dettol)**, and **hexachlorophane** (e.g., **Ster-Zac**). Hexachlorophane was widely used in the sixties and it was included in numerous skin applications and toilet preparations, even in toothpaste. An indication to the inclusion of an antiseptic in a preparation is given by the title 'medicated'. Most of this 'medication' is totally unnecessary. Following reports that hexachlorophane produced brain damage when applied extensively to the skin of premature babies, its use became restricted and its concentration in skin preparations was reduced. It may produce skin sensitivity and also make the skin sensitive to sunlight. **Chlorocresol** is another example of a chlorinated phenol.

Iodine compounds include **weak iodine solution (Iodine Tincture)** and **povidone-iodine (Betadine, Disadine D P, Videne)**. These preparations may produce skin sensitivity and interfere with the function of the thyroid gland.

Dyes. There are two types of dyes used as antiseptics:

(1) Acridines, which include **acriflavine, aminacrine** and **proflavine**. These are slow acting but work in the presence of pus and damaged tissues, which inhibit the effects of some antiseptics. In high concentration they may delay wound healing and they may produce skin sensitivity.

(2) Dyes such as **brilliant green, gentian violet** and **malachite green**. These are derivatives of triphenylmethane and were widely used before the introduction of antibiotics and antifungal drugs.

Formaldehyde. **Formaldehyde** and related drugs may be used as disinfectants, but not as antiseptics because they irritate the skin.

Chlorhexidine. **Chlorhexidine** (e.g., **Hibitane**) is frequently used as an antiseptic. It may occasionally cause skin sensitivity and it is inactivated by soap and by cork (so it should not be kept in a corked bottle).

Other chemical groups. These include alcohols (e.g., **ethyl alcohol, benzyl alcohol**), oxidizing compounds (e.g., **hydrogen peroxide**), salts of heavy metals (e.g., **mercury** and **silver**) and acids (e.g., **acetic acid**).

Choice of Antiseptic and Disinfectant

Chlorine-releasing substances such as sodium hypochlorite (e.g., **Domestos, Milton**) or chlorinated phenols (e.g., **Dettol**) are perfectly suitable as disinfectants, but do not forget that chlorine acts as a bleach (e.g., Domestos). For cleaning the skin a detergent such as cetrimide (**Cetavlon, Savlon**) is useful and so are chlorinated phenols (e.g., **Dettol**, hexachlorophane (**Ster-Zac**) and chlorhexidine (e.g., **Hibitane**)). Mixtures of cetrimide and chlorhexidine are also available (**Savlon** liquid antiseptic) and providone-iodone (**Betadine**) is useful.

9. Rheumatic Liniments – Rubefacients and Counter-irritants

Rubefacients are drugs which are applied to the skin to produce 'inflammation' – dilatation of the blood vessels in the skin, causing redness and warmth. This reaction is used to bring relief from a deep-seated pain by the process known as *counter-irritation*. For example, applying a counter-irritant to the abdominal wall may relieve underlying gut pain; on the same principle was the old-fashioned treatment of pleurisy – a hot poultice.

A commonly used counter-irritant is heat from a hot-water bottle, or from a heat lamp or diathermy machine. Many drugs are also used as counter-irritants in **rheumatic liniments**, rubs and other applications. They include **methyl salicylate** (related to aspirin), **camphor oil, menthol** and

methyl nicotinate. Rheumatic liniments also have various aromatic oils added to make their smell distinctive.

The choice of a rheumatic liniment is not critical; one may smell nicer than another. The rubbing and massaging is more important.

10.   Anti-itching Skin Applications and Drugs

There are many causes of itching (pruritis). These may be in the skin, such as allergic skin rashes, eczema, nervous rashes, scabies and body lice. In these disorders scratching may give relief but often leads to the skin being damaged and further itching. In elderly patients the skin may degenerate producing itching. Some drugs, e.g. morphine, may produce itching. Kidney disorders, liver and gall-bladder disorders and diabetes may also produce itching. It is therefore important for you to be examined by your doctor if you have an itching disorder because it is better to treat the cause than to treat the itch. There are two main approaches to the drug treatment of itching but generally treatment is disappointing.

1.   Skin Applications

These may contain **antiseptics** (p. 273) in very low concentrations, for example **phenol, benzyl alcohol, balsam of Peru, chlorbutol.** These may however irritate the skin and produce allergic rashes. **Local anaesthetics** (p. 278) are often used in low concentrations in skin applications, but again these may irritate the skin and produce skin allergies. **Antihistamine** creams (p. 277) are useful for small areas (e.g., insect bites) but are not recommended for large areas because they too may produce allergic skin rashes. Other drugs such as menthol and camphor are also used.

Crotamiton (Eurax) may be useful in some patients, but it should be applied with caution to inflamed skin because it may make it worse. **Calamine lotion** is probably just as effective. **Corticosteroid** skin applications (p. 270) are now probably the most widely used and most effective, particularly in treating itching and inflamed skin disorders. The **fluorinated corticosteroids** are the most effective for relieving itching. Other drugs used to treat itching include **titanium dioxide (Metanium)** which is also used as a suntan application (p. 267). It is present in some face powders and cosmetics.

2.   Drugs by Mouth

There are two main groups of drugs which are taken by mouth to relieve itching. There are the **antihistamines** and the **major tranquillizers.**

One commonly used drug from the antihistamine group is **trimeprazine (Vallergan)**.

The severe itching which accompanies obstructed gall-bladder disease may be relieved by a male sex hormone, for example testosterone (p. 223), which may also be helpful in senile pruritus and obstructive jaundice. **Cholestyramine** (p. 168) may help in liver and gall-bladder disease because it reduces the blood level of bile salts, which is high in these disorders; it is thought that they are the cause of the itching.

Sedatives or anti-anxiety drugs (e.g., a benzodiapezine such as **diazepam**) are also used, but these must be given with caution to the elderly with pruritus. The same caution should apply to the use of antihistamines and major tranquillizers in the elderly, because they can quickly become confused under an apparently 'normal' dose of any of these drugs. Simple skin applications should be tried first, such as a small volume of **liquefied phenol added to calamine lotion** or some other mixture – discuss this with your doctor or pharmacist.

Pruritus Ani and Vulvae

Irritation of the anus and vaginal area is not uncommon and may be caused by diabetes, thread worms, vaginal discharge, athlete's foot fungus and thrush (particularly after a course of antibiotics by mouth). Vaginal deodorant sprays and wipes may also produce vaginal irritation. As with general itching it is important to attempt to diagnose the cause and treat it. Sometimes this is difficult because of complex social, psychological and sexual factors. The most effective applications to use in the treatment of pruritus ani and/or vulvae are those which contain a **corticosteroid** combined with an **antifungal drug**, and an **antiseptic**.

Oestrogen creams may help the elderly woman with pruritus vulvae.

11. Antihistamine Skin Applications

There are numerous skin applications available which contain antihistamines. These are sometimes of use in treating small, acute, irritating and painful skin lesions such as an insect bite or nettle-rash. Their regular use and their use on large areas should be avoided because they can produce allergic skin rashes. Antihistamine skin applications available include **mepyramine (Anthisan, Anthical); diphenhydramine (Caladryl); antazoline (R.B.C.)**.

The choice of antihistamine preparation is not critical but their use is very limited; always read the instructions on the package.

12.   Local Anaesthetic Skin Applications

There are numerous skin applications which contain a local anaesthetic. Their widespread or regular use is not recommended because of the risk of producing irritation of the skin and allergic rashes.

Preparations available include **cinchocaine (Nupercainal), benzocaine** (in **Dermogesic**), and **amylocaine** (in **Locan** which also contains **amethocaine** and **cinchocaine**).

Choice of preparation is not critical but it is very important always to read the instructions on the package.

13.   Caustic and Keratolytic Skin Applications

Caustics are drugs which are used to destroy tissue at the site of application. If it causes a scab by precipitating protein from the damaged cells then it is also called a *cauterizant* or an *escharotic*. Surgeons use electric needles to burn (or cauterize) the ends of small bleeding blood vessels.

Some commonly used caustics are **acetic acid, phenol, podophyllum, trichloroacetic acid** and **silver nitrate**. They are used to treat warts and corns.

Keratolytics are included in some skin applications because they loosen the surface cells of the skin and cause them to swell and go soft so that they can easily be cut off. They are used to treat warts, corns and acne and include **benzoic acid, salicylic acid, acetic acid** and **resorcinol**.

14.   Astringent Skin Applications

Astringents are drugs which act on the surface of cells to precipitate protein. They do not enter the cell and therefore they do not kill the cell but they make its surface less permeable to water, etc., and so it dries up and shrinks. They are included in skin applications and have the effect of hardening the skin, drying up soggy areas of damaged skin and reducing minor bleeding from skin abrasions. Astringents in various dilutions may be used in throat lozenges, mouth washes, eye drops, ear drops and in preparations used to treat haemorrhoids; as caustics (for burning off dead tissue, etc.) and in the past they have been used to treat diarrhoea and other disorders of the gut. They are now widely used in anti-perspirant sprays and applications (see below). The main ones used are **salts of zinc and aluminium** and **tannins**.

Alum (potassium aluminium sulphate powder) is used as an astringent to treat sweating sore feet, to shrink the stump of the umbilical cord and to treat skin abrasions, small cuts and ulcers. **Dried alum (burned alum)** is even more astringent than alum. **Aluminium acetate solution** is a useful astringent lotion and is also used in ear drops. **Aluminium sulphate** is a strong astringent and may be used as a mild caustic; so may **silver nitrate**. **Gall** is used as an astringent to shrink haemorrhoids; it is the main source of **tannic acid**, which was widely used as an astringent in gargles, mouth washes, anti-diarrhoeal remedies and to treat burns. It is now seldom used because on damaged skin it produces a thick scab and can be absorbed to produce serious toxic effects, including liver damage. **Hamamelis** is another astringent used to shrink haemorrhoids and **hamamelis water (witch hazel)** is used as a cooling application on sprains and bruises. **Krameria** is also used to shrink haemorrhoids and is included in some throat lozenges. **Zinc chloride** is used as a caustic, astringent and deodorant. **Zinc sulphate** is used as an astringent, particularly in eye drops. **Calamine** is used as a mild astringent.

Aluminium acetate and **zinc acetate** are mild astringents of choice but it really depends on what is being treated – sweating feet or a small abrasion, haemorrhoids or a leg ulcer. If in doubt always consult your doctor or pharmacist.

15. Anti-perspirant Skin Applications

These are available in every size, shape and colour of container, as pads, sprays, roll-ons and creams; and with every possible smell to be applied to an ever-increasing number of parts of our bodies (male and female).

The drugs most commonly used as anti-perspirants include **salts of aluminium and zinc**. Some may stain fabric, some are acidic and irritate the skin, and some are soluble in alcohol and may be used in sprays and aerosols. Those anti-perspirants which contain an aluminium salt may produce an allergic skin rash in sensitive skins. The mechanism of action of anti-perspirants is unknown but they are considered by some experts to be astringents.

16. Deodorant Skin Applications

Like anti-perspirants the market is flooded with deodorant preparations. They reduce the number of bacteria that live on the skin. Since these bacteria break down sweat their reduction produces a reduction in body odour. **Antiseptics** such as **hexachlorophane** and **benzalkonium** are frequently used in deodorant preparations. Hexachlorophane may produce allergic skin rashes on sensitive skins, and benzalkonium and related complex ammonia compounds are inactivated by soap and can irritate the skin in concentrations above 1 per cent. Some deodorants contain **anti-**

biotics which can also cause allergic reactions and sensitize the individual to their future use. In addition people may become allergic to the perfume used in these preparations.

Remember if you develop a rash in the areas where you apply a deodorant or anti-perspirant consider that it may be an allergic reaction and stop the application immediately.

It is a sad consequence of contemporary marketing that women (particularly young women) are persuaded to feel unclean if they do not use vaginal deodorants (feminine sprays and wipes). And yet they may mask uncleanliness and are potentially harmful. There is gathering evidence that pregnant women may run a risk from such applications. Drugs enter the bloodstream more easily from mucous surfaces such as the mouth, rectum and vagina than they do from the skin. In pregnant women these drugs can enter the developing baby, and experiments have shown that **hexachlorophane** applied to rats' vaginas can damage unborn rats. Vaginal deodorants are best avoided – stick to soap and water – because in addition they may cause irritation and bladder trouble (urethritis and cystitis), particularly sprays. Furthermore, we do not know about the long-term effects of the propellants used in such sprays.

17.   Other Drugs Used in Skin Applications

Allantoin is used in preparations to treat psoriasis; e.g., **Alphosyl lotion** contains **allantoin** and **coal-tar extract** in a non-greasy base. It is also used to treat cracked nipples and nappy rash in **Massé cream**.

Cade oil is used in preparations to treat eczema and psoriasis.

Calamine is used as a mild astringent in creams and lotions, and in dusting powder.

Dithranol kills parasites and is used in small concentrations in ointments and pastes to treat psoriasis and other long-standing skin disorders. It can burn and stain the skin brown and cause allergic rashes in sensitized patients.

Ichthammol is slightly antibacterial and it irritates the skin. It has been used in skin applications to treat chronic skin disorders (e.g., eczema), and mixed with glycerin it was often used as an application on superficial thrombophlebitis, on abscesses and in infections of the ears.

Potassium hydroxyquinoline is used to treat bacterial and fungal infections of the skin. It has been used as a deodorant and appears in **Quinoderm** cream, used to treat acne.

Salicylic acid is used to treat hardened skin and corns.

Selenium sulphide is used to treat dandruff and other scalp disorders.

Starch is used in dusting powders.

Sulphur is a mild antiseptic and has been used to treat acne and other disorders.

Talc is used as a dusting powder.

Tar is used to treat eczema and psoriasis.

Zinc oxide is used as a mild astringent (p. 278) and as a soothing agent and protective (p. 266).

These drugs appear in numerous proprietary preparations for the treatment of many skin disorders. Read details about them in Part Three.

Antibiotics

The term antibiotic means destroying life and is applied to drugs obtained from micro-organisms (e.g., moulds) and used to kill another group of micro-organisms. Antibiotics may be antibacterial and/or antifungal. They are chemicals which stop the growth of micro-organisms (bacteriostatic) and/or eventually kill them (bactericidal). There are numerous antibiotics available and they vary in their structure, action, effects and the type of bacteria which are sensitive to them. They are produced by various micro-organisms such as fungi and bacteria and have been obtained from moulds, soil and other sources. Those produced from moulds may be called biosynthetic and those whose structure is modified by the addition of other chemicals to the growing medium are called semi-synthetic.

An antibiotic may be tested by inoculating micro-organisms into a liquid culture medium which contains varying dilutions of the drug. Antibiotics are not effective against all micro-organisms; some are effective against bacteria, others against fungi, some against many bacteria and some against only a few. The number of types of bacteria against which a particular antibiotic is effective is called its antibacterial (or antifungal) spectrum. If it is active against many types of bacteria it is called a broad-spectrum antibiotic.

Bacteria may become resistant to an antibiotic (even when it is used correctly) by several very complex mechanisms, and generally if resistance develops to one antibiotic from a group of antibiotics then there is cross-resistance to other antibiotics in that group. The use of two or more antibiotics together may help to prevent or delay the development of resistance. This is a technique frequently used in the treatment of tuberculosis but not normally recommended in treating other disorders except where two drugs act synergistically. Drug resistance may also be developed by micro-organisms because of improper treatment. This may be due to giving inappropriate doses, inappropriate intervals between doses, inadequate lengths of treatment or inappropriate antibiotic combinations.

Delay in starting antibiotics may affect response and so will the response of the body to the infecting micro-organism and to the drug. For example, pus cells may destroy the antibiotic effects, the acidity of the urine may change the effectiveness of certain antibiotics given to treat urinary infections, an abscess with tough walls will prevent antibiotics from getting into the abscess, and antibiotics may not be able to pass certain barriers (e.g., into the eye). They may not be absorbed from the gut. The 'condition' of the patient may affect the choice of drug as will the risk of allergic reactions in certain individuals. Patient (host) factors such as age, genetic characteristics, general physical condition (e.g., liver and kidney function), pregnancy, and other infections present may also affect the choice of an antibiotic drug. Furthermore, the patient's response to treatment and in particular his 'defence mechanisms' against infections are very important, because even when the antibiotics work, the body has got to get rid of the micro-organisms.

Antibiotics may be used effectively to prevent the development of an infection if given just after exposure (e.g., high doses of penicillin after running the risk of getting gonorrhoea (providing tests have excluded syphilis)) or if given to prevent recurrence of infection with a particular organism (e.g., to prevent certain types of tonsillitis). However, they have often been used for wrong reasons and have caused many complications, when used to sterilize the gut before abdominal surgery, for example, or to 'prevent' bacterial infections in patients with virus infections.

Adverse effects produced by antibiotics are on the increase. This is related to the increasing number of preparations available and the increasing number of patients being treated. Antibiotics may produce specific adverse effects (e.g., chloramphenicol may damage the bone marrow, neomycin may damage the kidneys) but in addition all antibiotics share two major adverse effects – the risk of allergic reactions and the risk of super-added infections with other micro-organisms.

Allergic reactions include anaphylactic shock, skin rashes, swollen face, fever and painful joints, bone-marrow damage and jaundice. Superinfections occur because many micro-organisms live together in a balanced community in many parts of our bodies (nose, mouth, gut, skin, lungs, bladder, vagina). Any disturbance in this balance (i.e., an antibiotic, which may knock out one group of organisms) may lead to an over-growth (superinfection) of other micro-organisms, for example, yeasts, fungi, and bacteria. These are usually minor but may occasionally be very serious and, rarely, fatal. They are difficult to treat and are more likely to occur with broad-spectrum antibiotics, in children under three years of age, in elderly and/or debilitated patients and in patients with disorders such as diabetes and pulmonary infections.

Remember antibiotics are valuable drugs if used appropriately but because they are very effective in treating some infections they should not

284 Drugs Used to Treat Specific Disorders

be used to treat all infections (e.g., virus infections). They should not be used for minor infections. They should be used in appropriate doses at appropriate intervals and for an appropriate length of time. They should not be used just because they are new, particularly when effective established alternatives are available. Finally, they should never be taken without medical supervision. Never take antibiotics because 'there were a few left in the house', or 'because they did my neighbour good'. Unless you and your doctor have decided that self-treatment with an antibiotic is appropriate for you, do not take them without advice and do not always expect them from your doctor.

Penicillins

Penicillin was the first antibiotic to be produced by growing *penicillium* mould on broth. It became available for use in 1941. The original crude extracts of the fermentation of the mould contained several penicillins. By adding various chemicals to the fermentation, a number of naturally produced penicillins have been developed; these include **benethamine penicillin, benzathine penicillin, benzylpenicillin** and **phenoxymethylpenicillin (penicillin V)**. In addition the chemical structure of the penicillin may be altered to produce what are called semi-synthetic penicillins. They are not wholly synthetic; the basic penicillin structure is still obtained from moulds by fermentation.

These products are all known as peniicillins and **benzylpenicillin** is often taken as the main example. The semi-synthetic penicillins have advantages over benzylpenicillin because most of them are more resistant to the acid in the stomach and are more effective by mouth, some of them are active against many more types of bacteria (*broad-spectrum*) and some are effective against bacteria which have developed a resistance to benzylpenicillin. However, it is important to remember that when bacteria *are* sensitive to **benzylpenicillin** or **phenoxymethylpenicillin (penicillin V)**, the other penicillins are *not* usually as effective.

Penicillins damage the developing cell walls of multiplying bacteria, making them burst. They therefore kill bacteria (*bactericidal*) but only when they are multiplying. Now other antibiotics (e.g., tetracyclines) interfere with bacterial growth (multiplication) and are called *bacteriostatic*. It follows that, if a tetracycline and a penicillin are given together, they will *antagonize* each other, theoretically making each other less effective. However, depending on its concentration, any penicillin or other antibiotic may be both bacteriostatic and bactericidal.

Bacteria may become resistant to the effects of penicillins in two ways. They may produce enzymes which inactivate the penicillin – the best known of these is called *penicillinase* which disrupts the chemical structure (the beta-lactam ring) of the penicillin nucleus, making it inactive. In addition, some bacteria develop a tolerance to penicillin (resistance) and they just go on multiplying in the presence of doses which would previously have killed them. Development of resistance has often been related to the indiscriminate use of penicillins and it is a serious risk, particularly in surgical wards in hospital. Fortunately, some of the semi-synthetic penicillins are resistant to penicillinase, e.g., methicillin, cloxacillin, flucloxacillin.

Allergic reactions to penicillins are not uncommon and when given to a patient who has become hypersensitive, an allergic reaction may occur, producing skin rashes, swelling of the face and throat, fever and swollen joints. Anaphylactic shock (see p. 126), which is very rare, may be followed by death. It is more common after injections and in patients who have previously had an allergic reaction to penicillin. Penicillin sensitivity may be produced by skin ointments, ear drops, eye drops, and throat lozenges. It may also follow the handling of penicillin (e.g., nurses drawing up injections), breathing it in and drinking milk from cows treated with penicillin for mastitis. For these reasons penicillin should not be used in topical applications and throat lozenges. The latter may produce a sore tongue, mouth and lips and also a black furring of the tongue. Ampicillin may produce a skin rash in patients suffering from glandular fever or chronic lymphatic leukaemia. This is different from the usual penicillin rash and is specific to ampicillin. It is probably a toxic reaction and penicillins can be used in future in these patients. All penicillins may cause diarrhoea, nausea, heartburn and pruritus ani. Diarrhoea is commonest with ampicillin which can cause severe colitis.

Apart from allergy, penicillins are safe drugs. Adverse effects are more likely to occur because of errors in prescribing than from any other cause. Remember cross-allergy to penicillin occurs: if you are allergic to one (say penicillin V) you may be allergic to another (e.g., ampicillin). Skin testing for allergy is not too useful because allergy is thought (in some cases) to be due to the breakdown products of penicillin in the body rather than to the penicillin drug. Also some people consider the products developed during manufacturing (and included in the preparation) to be a cause of allergy to a penicillin preparation. The proper combination of skin tests is probably useful in detecting those patients who are likely to have a life-threatening anaphylactic reaction. Interference with the balance of bacteria in the gut may produce diarrhoea. Manufacturing-process contaminants may also account for other symptoms such as diarrhoea. A rare adverse effect of the penicillins is irritation of the brain producing disorders of brain function (encephalopathy). This occurs when very high doses are used intravenously or intramuscularly or when normal doses are used in patients with impaired kidney function. Injection of penicillin into the spinal fluid in high doses can cause convulsions and should be avoided.

Penicillins should not be taken for trivial infections or by patients who have had a previous allergic reaction. They should be taken with caution by patients who have had an allergic reaction to any other drug. They provide us with a range of very valuable antibiotics, which, if used appropriately, are very effective.

The dosage varies according to the penicillin used, the route of administration, the disorder being treated and the patient. **Benzylpenicillin** is best given by injection, **procaine penicillin**, which is long acting, is given by intramuscular injection and **penicillin V** is useful by mouth. **Methicillin, cloxacillin** and **flucloxacillin** are active against penicillinase producing resistant bacteria; they may be given by injection (cloxacillin and flucloxacillin may be given by mouth) but should be strictly reserved for treating such infections. **Ampicillin** is usually taken by mouth, except in serious infections, when it is given intravenously. It has become widely prescribed for upper and lower respiratory infections, urinary infections (e.g., cystitis) and other infections. It is often used inappropriately – for the wrong disorder, in the wrong dosage, and for the wrong length of time. Frequently it is used for disorders which would improve better on benzylpenicillin or penicillin V. **Amoxycillin** is very effective and need only be given every eight hours by mouth. It has the same spectrum of activity as ampicillin but it is better absorbed.

Penicillinase-sensitive Penicillins

benzylpenicillin (Crystapen)
benethamine penicillin (in Triplopen)
benzathine penicillin (Penidural)
penamecillin (Havapen)
phenethicillin (Broxil)
phenoxymethylpenicillin (Penicillin V; Apsin VK, Crystapen, Distaquaine
   V-K, Econocil VK, Stabillin V-K, V-Cil-K)
procaine penicillin (Bicillin, Depocillin)

Penicillinase-resistant Penicillins

cloxacillin (Orbenin)
flucloxallin (Floxapen, Ladropen, Stafoxil, Staphlipen)
methicillin sodium (Celbenin)

Broad-spectrum Penicillins

amoxycillin (Amoxidin, Amoxil)
ampicillin (Amfipen, Ampilar, Penbritin, Vidopen)

bacampicillin (Ambaxin)
ciclacillin (Calthor)
mezlocillin (Baypen)
piperacillin (Pipril)
pivampicillin (Miraxid, Pondocillin, Pondocillin Plus (with pivmecillinam))
talampicillin (Talpen)

Augmentin contains **amoxycillin** with a beta-lactamase inhibitor (**clavulanic acid**) which inhibits penicillinase. Preparations containing a broad-spectrum penicillin and a penicillinase-resistant penicillin include **Ampiclox** (**ampicillin** and **cloxacillin**), **Magnapen** (**ampicillin** and **flucloxacillin**) and **Flu-Amp** (**ampicillin** and **flucloxacillin**).

Azlocillin (Securopen), carbenicillin (Pyopen), carfecillin (Uticillin), piperacillin (Pipril) and ticarcillin (Ticar) are active against certain gram-negative bacteria of the *Pseudomonas* and *Proteus* species. **Mecillinam** (**Selexidin**) is effective against certain gram-negative infections of the gut. **Pivmecillinam** (**Selexid**) is broken down in the body to mecillinam. **Timentin** contains clavulanic acid and tircacillin.

Cephalosporins and Cephamycins

The **cephalosporins** are broad-spectrum semi-synthetic antibiotics produced from a natural mould antibiotic (cephalosporin C). They act on much the same groups of bacteria as the natural penicillins but so far they are relatively resistant to penicillinase but not to an enzyme (beta-lactamase) produced by some bacteria which makes cephalosporins inactive by damaging the chemical structure (the beta-lactam rings). They also act on a broad spectrum of bacteria in the same way as ampicillin and are effective against some bacteria which are resistant to ampicillin. They may produce allergic reactions and cross-allergy may occur between cephalosporins and some penicillins in some patients. About 10 per cent of patients allergic to penicillin will be allergic to cephalosporins. Cross-resistance may be shown to cephalosporins by bacteria resistant to methicillin and cloxacillin. Cephalosporins may produce bleeding in elderly and debilitated patients. **Cephaloridine** can produce kidney damage which is made worse by high doses (over 6 g per day) and by the additional use of diuretics such as frusemide and ethacrynic acid.

The **cephalosporin group** includes cefaclor (Distaclor), cefadroxil (Baxan), cefotaxime (Claforan), cefoxitin (Mefoxin), cefsulodin sodium (Monaspor), ceftazidime (Fortum), ceftizoxime (Cefizox), cefuroxime (Zinacef, Zinnat), cephalexin (Ceporex, Keflex-C), cephalothin (Keflin), cephamandole (Kefadol), cephazolin (Kefzol), cephradine (Velosef) and lata-moxef (Moxalactam).

Other beta-lactam antibiotics include aztreonam (Azactam) which has a wide spectrum of activity against bacteria, including beta-lactamase producing bacteria.

Macrolide antibiotics

This group includes erythromycin (Arpimycin, Erycen, Erymax, Erythro-cin, Erythromid, Erythroped, Ilosone, Ilotycin, Retcin).

Erythromycin is active against a narrow group of bacteria similar to those sensitive to the natural penicillins. It is bacteriostatic. It may be of use in treating tissue infections caused by bacteria resistant to the natural penicil-lins or if the patient is allergic to penicillins. It has been widely used but bacteria quickly become resistant to it, especially if it is given for more than one week. Its use has been replaced by other antibiotics in many cases. It is inactivated by the acid in the stomach and has to be given in acid-resistant capsules, or specially covered tablets (enteric-coated) as one of its esters (e.g., erythromycin oleate or stearate). Erythromycin estolate (Ilosone) may cause liver damage with jaundice and fever if a second or subsequent course is given, particularly if it is given for more than two weeks. This is thought to be an allergic reaction and clears up when the drug is stopped.

Lincosamide antibiotics

This group includes clindamycin (Dalacin C) and lincomycin (Lincosin). They may cause severe diarrhoea and colitis (particularly lincomycin and clindamycin), liver damage and allergy (fever and skin rashes). Lincomycin and clindamycin are particularly known for causing a potentially life-threatening inflammation of the bowel (pseudomembranous colitis). While this occurs with other antibiotics as well, the incidence appears higher with these two and their use should be restricted to the limited number of infections where they are clearly the drugs of choice. Taken orally, lincomycin is poorly absorbed, unlike clindamycin, which is almost completely absorbed.

Tetracyclines

The first tetracycline to be discovered was Aureomycin, in 1948; it was grown from moulds. Another one, called Terramycin, was discovered in

1950. Two years later their chemical structure was determined and it was found to consist of a basic structure of four rings (tetra-cyclic). The antibiotics were therefore called tetracyclines and the generic name of chlortetracycline was given to Aureomycin and oxytetracycline to Terramycin. The names Aureomycin and Terramycin remained as brand names. **Oxytetracycline (Terramycin)** is also available under other brand names: **Berkmycen, Imperacin, Oxymycin, Terramycin** and **Unimycin**. Since the fifties numerous tetracyclines have been produced and tested but only a few have proved to be of value. These include **demeclocycline (Ledermycin), tetracycline (Achromycin, Sustamycin, Tetrabid, Tetrachel, Tetrex), chlortetracycline (Aureomycin)**, a lysine complex of a tetracycline called **lymecycline (Tetralysal), doxycycline (Nordox, Vibramycin), methacycline (Rondomycin), clomocycline (Megaclor)** and **minocycline (Minocin)**.

One of the problems with the tetracyclines is that they are only partially absorbed from the gut and enough reaches the lower bowel to affect the normal organisms which live there. This may alter the balance between bacteria and fungi and lead to a superinfection with thrush (*Candida*), which can infect the mouth, bowel, anus and vulva, producing soreness and irritation. A more serious risk in hospitals is a super-added infection with resistant bacteria such as *pseudomonas* or *proteus* which may cause severe enteritis and very rarely death. This is more likely to follow the use of tetracycline during abdominal operations. These super-added infections may also affect the lungs.

Absorption of tetracyclines from the gut may be decreased by interaction with calcium, iron and magnesium salts when these are taken at the same time. Milk, antacids, and salts of calcium, magnesium and iron have the same effect – none of these should be taken at the same time as a tetracycline or its absorption will be decreased and the desired therapeutic effects will not be achieved. Absorption is similarly reduced by food, with the exception of doxycycline and minocycline. *Every container of tetracyclines should carry a date beyond which the capsules should not be used*, because of the toxicity of tetracycline breakdown products.

Demeclocycline (demethylchlortetracycline), doxycycline and **minocycline** are better absorbed than the other tetracyclines. Tetracyclines are excreted in the urine and in the bile. **Doxycycline** is excreted primarily via the bile and hence is the safest tetracycline in kidney failure. Since its excretory products are largely inactive, it has less effect on natural bowel bacteria than other tetracyclines, and accordingly a lower incidence of superinfection.

Very rarely tetracyclines given by injection may produce severe liver damage (sometimes fatal) when given to pregnant women with infections of their kidneys. Tetracyclines are deposited in growing teeth producing discoloration and staining in young children. It is not only the first set of teeth which is affected – the adult teeth may also be stained for life and there is an added risk of tooth decay. They are also deposited in bone and bone growth stops during tetracycline treatment. These effects on teeth and bone may occur before the baby is born (if the mother is given tetracyclines) and right on into childhood. They should therefore be avoided in pregnancy and preferably not given to children under seven (some say eight or twelve) years of age. They may discolour nails at any age if taken over a prolonged period. **Doxycycline** is said to cause less staining than the other tetracyclines. Allergic reactions to tetracycline drugs are rare. Sensitivity of the skin to sunlight may occur in patients receiving **demeclocycline** or **doxycycline**; this is less likely with the others.

Tetracyclines may affect protein production in the body and also kidney function. These may be indicated by a rise in the blood levels of breakdown products of proteins (as estimated by blood urea levels for example). Urea and other waste products are excreted by the kidneys and this may have no consequence if the kidneys are healthy. However, if their function is impaired these waste products may rise in the blood, producing loss of appetite, vomiting and weakness. This is called kidney failure and may occur unexpectedly in elderly patients who are given tetracyclines, usually for a chest infection. Doxycycline, which needs to be given only once a day, is said to affect patients with impaired kidneys less than other tetracyclines, because it has no effect on protein production and is excreted mainly via the gut.

Because of increased bacterial resistance, the tetracyclines are used much less than previously. Their uses include the treatment of chronic bronchitis, certain atypical pneumonias and acne.

Streptomycin and Other Aminoglycosides

Streptomycin was discovered in soil in 1944. Other chemically related antibiotics have since been discovered. They include **gentamicin (Cidomycin, Genticin, Lugacin), amikacin (Amikin), framycetin sulphate (Soframycin), kanamycin (Kannasyn), neomycin sulphate (Mycifradin, Nivemycin), netilmicin (Netillin), tobramycin (Nebcin)**. They are bactericidal against a wide sprectrum of bacteria responsible for serious infections. Bacteria quickly develop resistance to streptomycin and less quickly to the others.

They are poorly absorbed from the gut and have to be given by intramuscular or intravenous injection. They are quickly excreted by the kidneys and impaired kidney function may lead to dangerously high blood levels. They are painful when given by injection and their principal adverse effects include deafness (which may be permanent) and disorders of the organ of balance due to damage to the main nerve which supplies the ear and organ of balance. They may also damage the kidneys and affect nerve-muscle junctions, producing muscle weakness and depression of respiration.

These adverse effects are more likely to occur with high doses, prolonged courses of treatment, in patients over middle age and in patients with impaired kidney function. Allergic reactions may occur, particularly with streptomycin, which may also cause severe allergic skin reactions in those handling the drug (e.g., nurses). Anyone handling the drug should be very cautious and wear gloves. They should, where possible, not be used in pregnancy since they can damage the baby's hearing. Their use along with certain diuretics which can damage hearing (e.g., frusemide, ethacrynic acid) should be avoided and their use should always be monitored using blood level measurements.

Streptomycin is used to treat tuberculosis in combination with other drugs such as isoniazid. It is also used to treat plague. **Neomycin** is too toxic for systematic use. It is not absorbed from the gut and can be used to sterilize the bowel before surgery. Its main use is in applications for the skin, eyes and ears. Patients can become hypersensitive to neomycin.

Framycetin is similar to neomycin and is only used in topical applications. It is very toxic to hearing and balance and also to the kidneys.

Gentamicin is related to neomycin; it is active against a wide spectrum of bacteria, has to be given by injection and it may damage the kidneys and the main nerves to the ear, causing disorders of balance. It is used to treat severe infections. **Tobramycin** has similar actions to gentamicin. **Amikacin** is useful against bacteria resistant to gentamicin but it may damage hearing. **Kanamycin** is rarely used except in serious infections resistant to gentamicin.

Polymyxins and Related Antibiotics

The polymyxins are a group of antibiotics which includes **polymyxin A, B, C, D** and **E**. Two are principally in use, **polymyxin B (Aerosporin, Polybactrin)** and **colistin (Colomycin)**. They are used to treat very severe infections and colistin is used in skin applications. Polymyxins are poorly absorbed from the gut and even with injections it is difficult to get a high blood level, therefore large doses have to be used. They may produce kidney damage and, rarely, damage to nerve–muscle junctions, producing muscle weakness and depression of respiration. After injection, polymyxin B may produce mild adverse effects upon the nervous system – dizziness and sensory disturbances over the face, hands and feet.

Some Other Antibacterial Drugs

Chloramphenicol (Chloromycetin, Kemicetine) was the first broad-spectrum antibiotic to be discovered. It was introduced in 1947 and soon became widely promoted and prescribed. Its indiscriminate use for minor infections has often led to unnecessary deaths due to bone-marrow damage. It is a valuable drug for treating typhoid fever and a certain type of meningitis. Its potentially fatal toxicity precludes its use in all but serious infections resistant to other less toxic antibiotics. It is also used in eye, ear and skin applications.

Sodium fusidate (Fucidin) is the sodium salt of fusidic acid and is chemically related to cephalosporin P. It is well absorbed from the gut, broken down in the liver and excreted in the urine and bile. It is active against penicillinase-producing bacteria and should be reserved specifically for treating these infections. It penetrates bone and is used to treat bone infection (osteomyelitis). Bacteria readily develop resistance. It may be given in combination with other antibiotics such as flucloxacillin.

4-Quinolones are effective antibacterial drugs. **Acrosoxacin (Eradacin)** is only used to treat gonorrhoea in patients allergic to penicillins or if the infection is resistant to penicillins or other antibiotics. **Nalidixic acid (Mictral, Negram, Uriben)** and **cinoxacin (Cinobac)** are used to treat infections of the urinary tract. **Ciprofloxacin (Ciproxin)** is active against a wide range of organisms and is useful for treating bacterial diarrhoea infections, certain lung infections, gonorrhoea, urinary tract infections and certain blood poisonings (septicaemia).

The **rifamycins** are related to streptomycin. Several have been produced and one of them is used. **Rifampicin (Rifadin, Rimactane)** is used to treat certain infections, particularly tuberculosis, and also leprosy. Adverse effects include nausea and occasionally jaundice, blood disorders and allergic reactions. It should not be used during the first three months of pregnancy. It turns the urine pink, and affects the breakdown in the liver of other drugs (e.g., oral contraceptives and anticoagulants). Repeated tests of liver function should be carried out before and during treatment.

Vancomycin (Vancocin) is too toxic to be used for routine use and should be reserved for treating infections resistant to other antibiotics or patients with colitis caused by other antibiotics. It is not absorbed from the gut and has to be given by intravenous injections, which may be painful and produce thrombophlebitis. Average doses may produce fever and skin rashes. Large doses or prolonged use may produce irreversible deafness. When given to treat pseudo-membranous colitis (a severe type of colitis produced by antibiotics) it is given by mouth, and because it is not absorbed it does not produce systemic effects.

Spectinomycin (Trobicin) is used to treat gonorrhoea in patients allergic to penicillins or in patients whose infections are resistant to penicillins and other antibiotics.

Nitroimidazoles

Metronidazole (Elyzol, Flagyl, Metrolyl, Nizadol, Vaginyl, Zadstat) and **tinidazole (Fasigyn)** are active against anaerobic bacteria and protozoa. They are of particular use in preventing and treating abdominal surgical infections and in treating infections of the vagina or mouth (acute ulcerative gingivitis). They are also used to treat amoebiasis and giardiasis.

Sulphonamides

In 1935 it was found that the red dye, **prontosil rubra**, protected mice from streptococcal infections and that the active antibacterial agent in the body was a breakdown product of the red dye called sulphanilamide. Following this discovery hundreds of similar drugs have been produced and tested for antibacterial activity. They belong to the sulphonamide group and they stop bacteria from multiplying (bacteriostatic) by affecting (competing with) the use of a vitamin called folic acid, which is essential for their cell nutrition.

These drugs were used extensively in the past but because of increasing bacterial resistance and the availability of other more effective and less toxic antibiotics their use has significantly decreased. One use is in the treatment of urinary tract infections caused by bacteria sensitive to the sulphonamides; for this purpose *sulphamethizole* is recommended.

Adverse effects to sulphonamide drugs are relatively common and vary according to the particular sulphonamide used and the susceptibility of the patient. Those patients who break down certain drugs slowly (slow acetylators) may be more at risk. Generally, adverse effects are mild and often related to the length of treatment and not always to the dose. Common adverse effects with the earlier sulphonamides included nausea, vomiting, diarrhoea, headache, dizziness, drug fever and skin rashes. Cyanosis (blueness) occurred with some of the drugs due to their action on haemoglobin in the red blood cells. Other adverse effects included kidney damage, nerve damage, mood changes, confusion, joint pains, disorders of the arteries (polyarteritis nodosa), kidney damage, liver damage and blood disorders. Allergic reactions occur with the sulphonamides and direct exposure to sunlight should be avoided since it can trigger off a sensitization dermatitis. Very rarely they may produce a severe disorder of the skin and mucus membranes characterized by red swellings and ulcers. This is called Stevens–Johnsons syndrome which may be fatal in 25 per cent of cases.

Sulphonamides should not be used in pregnancy, in infants under 6 weeks of age, in patients with kidney or liver failure, in patients who are jaundiced or who have anaemia or other blood disorders. They should be used with caution in patients who are breast feeding, sensitive to sunlight or with impaired kidney function. Patients should drink adequate fluids and have regular blood counts. The sulphonamides in use include:

calcium sulphaloxate (Enteromide)
sulfametopyrazine (Kelfizine W)
sulphadiazine
sulphadimidine (Sulphamezathine)
sulphaguanidine
sulphaurea (Uromide)

The long acting sulphonamides (sulfametopyrazine, sulphadimethoxine, sulphamethoxypyridazine) need to be used in less frequent doses but they accumulate in the body and are more likely to produce adverse effects. Those sulphonamides that are poorly absorbed from the gut (calcium sulphaloxate, phthalylsulphathiazole and sulphaguanidine) were previously used to treat infections of the gut and to prepare the bowel before abdominal surgery. They should not be used for these purposes. In the treatment of intestinal infections they prolong rather than shorten the time to control diarrhoea by masking bacterial diarrhoea and carrier states or pseudo-membranous colitis (a severe colitis produced by antibiotics). They should not be used in skin applications.

Combinations of Sulphonamides with Trimethoprim

Trimethoprim is a wide-spectrum antibacterial drug which interferes with the metabolism of bacterial cells at a stage just after the one which sulphonamides block. The use of **trimethoprim (Ipral, Monotrim, Syraprim, Tiempe, Trimogal, Trimopan)** and a sulphonamide together, therefore, successfully blocks vital processes in the cellular development of bacteria. This is an example of one drug potentiating the action of another by acting *synergistically*. Whilst sulphonamides alone are bacteriostatic this combination is bactericidal. **Co-trimoxazole (Bactrim, Chemotrim, Comox, Fectrim, Laratrim, Septrin)** contains 400 mg of **sulphamethoxazole** and 80 mg of **trimethoprim**. Trimethoprim is well absorbed when taken by mouth and sulphamethoxazole was selected because it is absorbed and excreted at a similar rate to trimethoprim, so that after a few days the ratio of the two drugs in the blood-stream and urine is kept relatively constant at about 20:1

which was thought optimal for synergism (i.e. working together). The combination reaches satisfactory blood levels in about one hour after absorption, reaching a peak in two to four hours, which lasts for up to seven or eight hours and then tapers off by about twenty-four hours.

Co-trimoxazole may produce any of the adverse effects already discussed under the sulphonamides; it therefore needs prescribing responsibly and rationally if we are not to see an outbreak of sulphonamide adverse reactions. Also, since it contains two drugs, bacterial sensitivity to *each* drug should be tested and it should only be used if the bacteria are sensitive to *both* drugs, when it obviously has a wider spectrum of activity than sulphonamides alone.

Co-trimoxazole and co-trifamole may produce nausea, vomiting, skin rashes (which may be severe) and blood disorders. These drugs should not be given in pregnancy, to infants under the age of six weeks, to patients with kidney or liver failure, jaundice or anaemia (and other blood disorders). They should be given with caution to breast-feeding mothers and patients who are sensitive to sunlight. Adequate fluids should be taken and regular blood counts should be carried out on patients who are on prolonged treatment. Trimethoprim on its own may produce nausea, vomiting, itching, skin rashes and depressed blood production.

Warning: These drugs affect folic acid metabolism in bacterial cells and they can also affect folic acid metabolism in the body producing anaemia, therefore they should be used with caution in the elderly and chronic sick. They should not be used in pregnancy.

47 Antifungal Drugs

Most fungi in and on the body are harmless but sometimes they may increase and spread to cause infections. For example, *Candida albicans* (which causes thrush in the mouth) lives 'normally' on the skin, in the mouth and in the gut, alongside bacteria, without causing any trouble unless the bacteria are killed off by antibiotics (e.g., if taken by mouth for some infection of the body). Under these circumstances the fungus multiplies and the patient may develop thrush of the mouth, gut, anus and vagina. Occasionally in severely ill patients this can spread to the lungs. Other factors, such as an infection, debility, diabetes, alcoholism and the use of corticosteroids and X-ray treatment, may help to trigger off fungus infections.

Airborne spores may infect the lungs (e.g., *aspergillosis*) and very rarely fungi may affect other organs. More commonly they may infect the scalp (scalp ringworm), groin (*Tinea cruris*), feet (athlete's foot, *Tinea pedis*), nails and the skin (ringworm, *Tinea circinata*).

A few antibiotics have antifungal effects. The three in common use are nystatin (Nystan, Nystatin-Dome), griseofulvin (Fulcin, Grisovin), and amphotericin (Fungilin, Fungizone). Nystatin stops the growth of fungi and is particularly effective against thrush, but it has no effect on bacteria. Natamycin (Pimafucin) is also very useful against thrush infections. Griseofulvin is given by mouth in a fine powdered form (in tablets) when it is fairly well absorbed from the gut. After absorption it is deposited in skin, hair and nails and is effective in treating fungal infections of these tissues (particularly ringworm). Since it does not kill but stops growth, to treat infections of hair and nails it has to be given for prolonged periods (up to several months in some cases). It may cause headache, vomiting, skin rashes and sensitivity of the skin to sunlight. It should not be taken by patients with latent porphyria and it is important to remember that it may increase the effects of alcohol. It can antagonize the effects of phenobarbitone.

Amphotericin is used in lozenges to treat thrush infections of the mouth and throat. For general infections it may be given intravenously but it is very toxic and is reserved for severe systemic fungal infections. Adverse effects are common and include fever, anorexia, nausea, vomiting, low blood potassium, kidney damage and tinnitis (noises in the ears). The injection site should be changed frequently and tests of kidney function should be carried out at frequent intervals. It may be used in ointments which occasionally cause irritation, itching and skin rash.

Flucytosine (Alcobon tablets and IV infusions) is a synthetic antifungal drug active mainly against yeasts such as candida. It can be used intravenously to treat systemic infections.

The imidazole group of antifungal drugs are active against a wide range of fungal and yeast infections. They are used principally to treat fungal infections of the skin and vagina. They include **clotrimazole (Canesten)** cream, solution, spray and dusting powder, used to treat fungal skin infections, **econazole (Ecostatin, Gyno-Pevaryl, Pevaryl)** cream, spray, powder, lotion, and dusting powder, used to treat fungal skin and nail infections, **ketoconazole (Nizoral)** tablets, used to treat skin and systemic fungus infections and as a prophylaxis in patients receiving immunosuppressive drugs, and **miconazole (Daktarin, Dermonistat, Gyno-Daktarin, Monistat)** tablets, cream, dusting powders, used to treat skin, vaginal and systemic fungus infections.

Other antifungal drugs include **chlorphenesin (Mycil)**, **pecilocin** and **propionic acid** (used in foods as a preservative), **sodium propionate, tolnaftate (Timoped)**, **undecenoic acid** and **zinc undecenoate (Mycota)**. These are all mainly used for local applications as powders, sprays, creams, drops and pessaries.

Idoxuridine may be of use in some patients in the treatment of herpes simplex affecting the skin, eyes and genitals. It may also be of use in treating herpes zoster (shingles) where it is said to reduce the duration of pain and the incidence of neuralgia which may follow an attack of shingles (postherpetic neuralgia). It is too toxic to take by mouth and has to be applied locally. Available preparations include **idoxuridine in dimethyl sulphoxide (Herpid solution, Iduridin application)** for the treatment of herpes simplex and zoster affecting the skin; **idoxuridine** in **Dendrid** eye drops, **Idoxene** eye ointment, **Kerecid** eye drops, **Ophthalmadine** eye drops and ointment, and **idoxuridine 0·1% paint** for mouth lesions. It may be used to treat severe **cold sores** (herpes simplex of the lips) in some patients, but it must be applied early and frequently.

Vidarabine (Vira A) is used to treat shingles and chicken pox. **Acyclovir (Zovirax)** is used to treat shingles and herpes simplex infections in patients who are immune dificient. Both **vidarabine (Vira A)** and **acyclovir (Zovirax)** as eye ointments may be used to treat herpes simplex infections of the eyes.

Zidovudine (Retrovir) is an antiviral drug used in the treatment of AIDS.

Amantadine (Symmetrel) is given by mouth to prevent influenza infections and also to treat shingles. It is also used to treat Parkinsonism (see p. 122).

Ribavirin (Virazid) is an antiviral drug used to treat virus chest infections in infants and children (see part III).

A wide range of bacteria may infect the urinary tract to produce infection of the kidneys **(pyelitis)**, the bladder **(cystitis)** and the outlet from the bladder **(urethritis)**. Equally, there is a wide range of effective drugs available to treat these infections, e.g., **sulphonamides, co-trimoxazole, cephalosporins, tetracyclines** and **semi-synthetic penicillins** like **ampicillin**. For infections resistant to these there are the other reserve antibiotics discussed earlier. The dose will depend on many factors: the severity of infection, the type of infecting bacteria, the condition of the patient and in particular on the state of the patient's kidney function.

With urinary tract infections it helps to drink plenty of fluids (one and a half litres a day) and pass urine often. Also the acidity of the urine may affect the effectiveness of an antibiotic. It is worth making the urine acid if you are taking tetracyclines, nitrofurantoin, sodium fusidate or semi-synthetic penicillins. It should preferably be made alkaline if you are taking, for example, erythromycin, lincomycin, gentamicin or cephalosporins. The decision to make your urine acid or alkaline (by taking certain acid or alkaline salts) depends upon how well your kidneys are functioning and this is a decision for your doctor.

Pain on passing urine can be relieved by making the urine alkaline by taking **sodium bicarbonate** (5–10 g daily in divided doses), or by taking **sodium or potassium citrate** (3–6 g every six hours). However they produce nausea and a potassium salt is dangerous in a patient with impaired kidney function. **Hyoscine (hyoscyamus)**, an atropine-like drug, was often combined with potassium citrate to treat urinary symptoms; it was available as mist Pot Cit and hyoscyamus.

Much trouble is caused through inadequate treatment of urinary infections. With first attacks a full course of appropriate antibiotic should be taken after the urine has been examined. With the second and all subsequent attacks, the urine should be re-examined to determine the infecting organism and the appropriate antibiotic should be selected and taken. With recurrent attacks (chronic cystitis) full investigations are necessary, as well as eliminating obvious things like vaginal deodorants which can irritate the lining of the urethra (particularly sprays). Infections of the urinary tract can be due to many causes including anatomical abnormalities, and surgical procedures or catheterization. They can occur in pregnancy and be symptomless and yet require treatment because the kidneys can become infected and be associated with anaemia, prematurity and stillbirth. In chronic cystitis, treatment after relief of acute symptoms should continue probably for up to three months or more, usually at a reduced maintenance dose of the antibiotic used to treat the acute attack or, in selected cases, by using one of the following drugs:

carfecillin sodium (Ulticillin)
cinoxacin (Cinobac)
hexamine (Hiprex)
nalidixic acid (Mictral, Negram, Uriben)
nitrofurantoin (Furadantin, Macrodantin, Urantoin)
noxythiolin (Noxyflex, Noxyflex S) (used as a bladder washout)
potassium citrate (alkalinizes the urine in mild infections)
trimethoprim (Ipral, Monotrim, Syraprim, Tiempe, Trimogal, Trimopan)

Sulphonamides, co-trimoxazole, nalidixic acid and **tetracyclines** should not be used in pregnancy. **Penicillins, cephalosporins** or **nitrofurantoin** are safe to use.

In kidney failure, impairment of function can lead to high blood levels of antibiotics and adverse drug reactions. Tetracyclines and nitrofurantoin should be avoided. Aminoglycosides (see p. 290) should be used with caution.

Bed-wetting (Nocturnal Enuresis)

Drugs are best avoided although some doctors use **tricyclic antidepressants** (p. 77), **ephedrine-like drugs** (p. 95) or **atropine-like drugs** (p. 94) and **desmopressin** (see part III).

Urinary Frequency, Incontinence

This is usually treated with **atropine-like drugs** (p. 94). They include **flavoxate (Urispas), propantheline (Pro-Banthine)** and **terodiline (Terolin)**.

Drugs Used to Relieve Urinary Pain

Potassium citrate mixture, sodium bicarbonate and **sodium citrate (Urisal)**, which make the urine more alkaline, may relieve the discomfort of cystitis. A local anaesthetic gel (e.g., **lignocaine**) may help if the urethra is painful. A **terpene mixture (Rowatinex)** helps to relieve the pain of passing a kidney stone out in the urine and an injection of the NSAI drug **diclofenac** is also effective at relieving the pain produced by a kidney stone.

The drug treatment of tuberculosis has taught doctors a lot about how to use antibiotics and other anti-infective drugs. Specialists in the treatment of tuberculosis have set many excellent examples of how to test for effectiveness and dangers of drugs over the short and long term. In particular, through their efforts and mistakes, we have learned much about how infecting organisms can develop resistance to drugs and how individuals and groups of people can vary in their response to drug treatment.

Because of the very real problem that the bacteria which cause tuberculosis can easily develop resistance to anti-tuberculosis drugs, treatment is now anticipated at two stages – before and after the development of bacterial resistance. Some drugs are therefore used for *first line treatment* and reserve drugs are kept for *second line treatment*, to be used if there is evidence of resistance developing to the initial drugs.

The drugs used in first line treatment are often referred to as primary anti-tuberculosis drugs. Because resistance develops to all anti-tuberculosis drugs if they are given singly, initial treatment always involves the use of three drugs in combination followed by two drugs in combination for continuing long-term treatment. Two-drug-combination treatment is possible once tests have shown which two drugs are most effective against the particular organisms involved. But these tests of *sensitivity* may take up to three months and, for safety, during this period three drugs in combination are nearly always used.

Second line (reserve) drug treatment of tuberculosis is necessary when evidence appears that the infecting organisms are developing, or have developed, resistance to the primary drugs. Since secondary drugs usually produce more adverse effects than the primary ones the decision which ones to use requires great knowledge about the patient, the stage of his illness and the drugs to be used.

Initial-phase treatment now includes the daily use of **isoniazid (Rimifon)** and **rifampicin (Rifadin, Rifater (rifampicin with isoniazid** and **pyrazinamide), Rifinah (rifampicin and isoniazid), Rimactane, Rimactazid (rifampicin** and **isoniazid))** supplemented by **ethambutol (Myambutol, Mynah (ethambutol** and **isoniazid))** or **streptomycin** with the addition of **pyrazina-**

mide (Zinamide), if necessary. These drugs should be continued for at least eight weeks and preferably until the results of the drug-sensitivity tests are available.

Continuing-phase treatment should follow the initial phase and include two drugs one of which is usually the primary drug isoniazid. The other drugs may be rifampicin, ethambutol or streptomycin. Alternative reserve drugs include capreomycin (Capastat), cycloserine, or pyrazinamide.

The *duration* of treatment may vary from nine to eighteen months according to the drugs used and the patient's response.

For adverse effects of each of these drugs see Part Three.

51   Drugs Used to Treat Cancer

Cancer is a disorder of autonomous cell growth which may affect any tissue or organ. Treatment of cancer is aimed at reducing or stopping this disordered growth. Drugs are becoming increasingly useful for this purpose because not only is it possible to prolong the life of many patients suffering from various types of cancer, but drugs can also make life much more comfortable. Because of the many different types and stages of cancer it is difficult to generalize. Furthermore the drugs used are very complex and treatment is always changing as different advances are made.

Drugs used to treat cancer are usually termed *cytotoxic* drugs because they kill cells. Anti-cancer drug therapy is also referred to as chemotherapy. The majority of cytotoxic drugs interfere with cell division and will therefore damage *all* rapidly dividing cells whether normal or cancerous. Areas of rapidly growing normal cells in the body include bone marrow, the lining of the gut, skin and hair. Cytotoxic drugs can therefore produce short-term and reversible damage to these tissues producing anaemia due to damage to red cell production, susceptibility to infection due to damage to white cell production, bleeding due to damage to platelets which produce clotting; nausea, vomiting and diarrhoea due to damage to the lining of the gut, and loss of hair (alopecia).

Cytotoxic drugs are used to treat those primary or secondary cancers which have been shown to respond to drug therapy. They are also used as adjunctive therapy in order to prevent relapse in patients who have had surgery and/or radiotherapy. In addition, some are used to suppress the immune response of the body in patients suffering from auto-immune disorders (a sensitivity of the body to some of its own cells) or in patients who have had an organ transplant where there may be problems of rejection.

Different groups of cytotoxic drugs act differently upon the cellular growth cycle of cancer cells. Some may kill cells whether they are resting or multiplying, some may kill only those cells which are multiplying and some may kill only at a specific time in a particular phase of growth. These are important factors in considering treatment because the combination of drugs which act at different stages can have greater killing effect on cancer cells than drugs used alone. Important regimes of anti-cancer drug therapy therefore include *combined* drug treatments, *intermittent* treatments and also *sequential* treatments in order to achieve a maximum killing effect on the cancer cells for minimum effects upon the normal cells in the body.

Because of the risks from treatment, special facilities for extra support may also be needed, e.g., blood transfusion if blood production gets affected and special precautions against infection if the drugs being used damage the production of white blood cells which are normally involved in the body's protection against infection. This means that, in addition to anti-cancer drugs, several other drugs (e.g., antibiotics) and treatments may be used, which indicates the need for highly specialized care. There are five main groups of cytotoxic drugs.

(1)   Alkylating Agents

These damage DNA and therefore interfere with the cells' ability to multiply (replicate). They may produce infertility which may be permanent and they may damage white cell production in patients who have had continuous and prolonged treatment with these drugs for conditions such as cancer of the ovary.

Alkylating agents

busulphan (Myleran)
carmustine (BiCNU)
chlorambucil (Leukeran)
cyclophosphamide (Endoxana)
estramustine (Estracyt)
ethoglucid (Epodyl)
ifosfamide (Mitoxana)
lomustine (CCNU)
melphalan (Alkeran)
mitobronitol (Myelobromol)
mustine (Mustine Hydrochloride)
thiotepa (Thiopeta)
treosulfan Treosulfan)

(2)   Antimetabolites

These interfere with normal chemical processes inside dividing cells by affecting enzymes (chemicals inside living cells which promote chemical change) thus preventing normal chemical processes from occurring.

Drugs are available which stop the effect of any one of three enzymes that use folic acid, purine or pyrimidine as building blocks. They are therefore known as **folic acid antagonists, purine antagonists** and **pyrimidine antagonists**. They are used to treat leukaemias and have produced dramatic and long-lasting cures in the treatment of choriocarcinoma (a cancer which develops from the tissues of an unborn baby inside the uterus). Pyrimidine antagonists may damage the nails and the lining of the mouth, and produce loss of hair. Folic acid antagonists may interfere with the body's immune response to infection and foreign tissues (e.g., kidney transplants). They include:

cytarabine (Alexan, Cytosar)
fluorouracil (Efudix, Fluoro-uracil)
mercaptopurine (Puri-Nethol)
methotrexate (Emtexate, Maxtvex, Methotrexate)
thioguanine (Lanvis)

(3) Cytotoxic Antibiotics

These interfere with D N A replication and protein synthesis. They include:

actinomycin D (Cosmegen Lyovac)
bleomycin (Bleomycin)
doxorubicin (Adriamycin)
epirubicin (Pharmorubicin)
mitomycin (Mitomycin C K yowa)
plicamycin (Mithracin)

(4) Vinca Alkaloids

These are alkaloids extracted from periwinkle (*Vinca rosea*) which stop cell division. They include:

etoposide (Vepesid)
vinblastine (Velbe)
vincristine (Oncovin)
vindesine (Eldisine)

(5) Immunosuppressants

Some cytotoxic drugs are used to suppress the immune response in patients suffering from auto-immune disease or to prevent rejection of a transplanted organ (e.g., a kidney). They include:

azathioprine (Azamune, Imuran)
chlorambucil (Leukeran)
cyclophosphamide (Endoxana)

Other drugs used to suppress immunity include the **corticosteroids, cyclosporin A (Sandimmun)** a fungal metabolite which inhibits the multiplication of T-lymphocytes and **antilymphocyte immunoglobulin (Pressimmune)** obtained from immunized horses.

A miscellaneous group of cytotoxic drugs includes:

amsacrine (Amsidine)
carboplatin (Paraplatin)
cisplatin (Platinex) – a platinum drug with an alkylating action
corynebacterium parvum (Coparvax) – an immunostimulant
dacarbazine (D T I C-Dome)
hydroxyurea (Hydrea)
mitozantrone (Novantrone)
procarbazine (Natulan)
razoxane (Razoxin)
aminoglutethimide (Orimeten) – blocks conversion of androgens to
    oestrogens and blocks adrenal steroid production
cyproterone acetate (Cyprostat) – blocks actions of androgens
tamoxifen (Noltam, Nolvadex, Tamofen) – blocks actions of oestrogens

Other drugs used to treat cancer include **corticosteroids** (p. 216) and **sex hormones** (p. 223 and 227).

See entries for each drug in Part Three.

Interferons

For many years it had been known that infection with one virus could protect animals against infection with another virus, when it was discovered in 1957 that cells infected with a virus produce a substance which protects other cells from virus infection. These substances (highly active glycoproteins) are known as *interferons*. They act on the surface of cells causing the cell to produce proteins which protect the cell against damage from viruses.

Interferons act specifically on cells from a specific animal, e.g., mouse interferon is inactive in human cells. There are three major types of human interferon and they are standardized by their ability to reduce the replication of viruses in tissue culture – one unit of interferon is roughly the amount which reduces virus replications in tissue culture by half. The three sources of interferon are human white blood cells, fibroblasts and lymphocytes.

Interferons have been tried in the prevention of certain virus infections (e.g., herpes simplex: cold sores) and influenza, to treat viral infections of the eyes and to treat herpes zoster (shingles). Some of these results are encouraging but there is need for much more research.

In the treatment of cancer, interferons have been shown to be of benefit in some experimental tumours in mice but there need to be many well-controlled studies of the effects of interferons in human cancer. Interferons possess actions which obviously could have a beneficial effect. They can stop replication of DNA and RNA tumour viruses; they have been shown to inhibit growth of cancer cells, increase activity of protective white cells (phagocytosis), and increase the effects of killer-cells – both activities leading to destruction of cancer cells; they also affect the immune system by inhibiting (and increasing in some cases) antibody production and therefore may be able to reduce the number of tumour-protecting antibodies which are known to block the body's natural immune response to tumours. See **Intron A**, **Roferon-A** and **Wellferon** in part III.

52 Prostaglandins

Prostaglandins are made by most tissues in the body. There are several types and they are grouped according to their chemical structure. They are used to treat a variety of conditions and the potential for their use appears great. They are used to bring on labour in childbirth and in therapeutic abortion because they cause the uterus to contract. Certain prostaglandins produce dilatation of peripheral blood vessels and have been used to treat disorders of the peripheral circulation (e.g., Raynaud's disease) but their use needs further evaluation. They relax smooth muscle and are to be found in lung tissues where some of them cause constriction of the bronchi and others cause dilatation. They may be involved in producing bronchoconstriction in asthma and their use in its treatment is being investigated. Prostaglandins in the kidneys can affect kidney blood flow and hence the blood pressure (see p. 162).

Prostaglandins are present in the lining of the stomach and provide a protective effect against gastric juice (p. 135). Certain drugs (e.g., aspirin and non-steroidal anti-inflammatory drugs) block the production of prostaglandins and reduce this protective mechanism which may contribute to the development of peptic ulceration, a principal adverse effect of these drugs.

Prostaglandins are also involved in inflammation, in the body's immune response and in tissue damage – e.g., in rheumatoid arthritis. If their production is blocked then the inflammatory process is reduced producing a relief from pain and swelling of joints or other involved tissues. This is the basis for the use of aspirin and non-steroidal anti-inflammatory drugs in the treatment of rheumatoid arthritis and related disorders (see p. 196).

The release of prostaglandins is also thought to contribute to vascular headaches (e.g., migraine) which explains one effect of aspirin (which blocks prostaglandin production) in relieving headache. Paracetamol is a less effective prostaglandin blocker and is of less use than aspirin in relieving vascular headaches. Both drugs can bring down the temperature in fever. In painful periods (spasmodic dysmenorrhoea) the release of prostaglandins in the uterus is thought to produce the painful spasms which can be relieved by a prostaglandin blocking drug, such as ibuprofen.

53 Vaccines

Active Immunity

Vaccines stimulate the production of protective antibodies and other mechanisms involved in the body's protection against disease (i.e., they produce active immunity).

A vaccine may contain inactivated viruses (e.g., influenza vaccine) or inactivated bacteria (e.g., whooping cough or typhoid vaccines). It may contain a toxin produced by a micro-organism (e.g., tetanus vaccine) or it may contain attenuated (weakened) viruses (e.g., polio or measles vaccine) or attenuated bacteria (e.g., BCG vaccine used against tuberculosis).

They are usually given by injection except poliomyelitis vaccine, which is given by mouth, and smallpox vaccine which is injected into the skin (intradermally).

Live micro-organisms multiply in the body and produce a long-standing immunity whereas inactivated vaccines need a series of injections initially and then booster injections at intervals.

Passive Immunity

If plasma from an individual immune to a specific disease is given to a patient who is not immune, then the plasma injected will provide the second individual with immediate protection against that disease. This is called *passive immunity*. The plasma contains *antibodies* against the disease. Another name for these antibodies from humans is *immunoglobulins*. An individual may also be given plasma containing antibodies from a horse and this is usually referred to as *anti-serum*. These preparations from horses can produce severe reactions (serum sickness) because the body reacts to foreign horse proteins in the plasma. Therefore, when possible, anti-serum from horses is not now used and most injections contain immunoglobulins which are human and which rarely produce a reaction, for example, anti-tetanus injections. Diphtheria antitoxin is still prepared in horses and can give rise to serum sickness.

Indications for Vaccination

Anthrax. Anyone exposed to infected hides and carcases or to imported feeding-stuff, bonemeal and fishmeal.

Cholera. Consult the Department of Health and Social Security about the requirements when travelling to certain countries. Booster injections are required every six months for those living in an area where cholera is prevalent.

Diphtheria. See schedule, p. 312.

Hepatitis B. In short supply. Should be given to patients at risk, i.e., those who work in contact with human blood (blood banks, renal dialysis units, etc.) or who are in direct contact with a carrier. Routes of infection include inoculation into a wound, incision, needle prick (note 'main-line' drug abuse) or abrasion.

Influenza. Grown on eggs, therefore should not be given to patients sensitive to eggs or feathers. Use in high-risk patients – elderly, debilitated and those with chronic heart and/or lung disease. Also use in doctors and nurses and those resident in institutions.

Measles. Should be offered to all children in the second year of life. See schedule, p. 312. May be associated with a mild attack of 'measles' with a rash and a raised temperature about one week after injection of the vaccine. Convulsions and brain and nerve complications may occur very rarely. Children with a history of convulsions should be given diluted normal immunoglobulin along with the vaccine. Children with partial or total impairment of their immune system should not be given the vaccine but should be given immunoglobulin if they have been in contact with measles.

Whooping cough (*Pertussis*. See schedule, p. 312). It may produce soreness at the injection-site, a raised temperature and irritability. Screaming and collapse occurred in some infants with the vaccines used in the sixties. Convulsions and brain disorder may very rarely occur. Vaccination should be postponed if a child has a temperature from a respiratory or other infection. Vaccination should *not* be continued in children who have a local or general reaction to the first injection. It should not be given to any child with a history of fits, convulsions or brain damage. It should be used with the utmost caution in children with a history of epilepsy in their family (parents or brothers or sisters) and in children with any evidence of disease of the nervous system. Allergy (e.g., a history of asthma, eczema ~or hay-fever) is not an absolute contraindication to whooping cough vaccination.

Pneumococcal pneumonia. This is used in patients who run a risk of developing pneumococcal pneumonia, e.g., patients who have had their spleen removed. It should not be given to pregnant patients, children under the age of two years, nor when an infection is present. It should be given with caution to patients suffering from heart or lung disease. Hypersensitivity reactions may occur to the vaccine.

Poliomyelitis. See schedule, p. 312. Young parents should receive the vaccine at the same time as their babies in order to prevent contact vaccine-associated poliomyelitis which nonetheless is very rare. It should not be given to anyone who has diarrhoea or to anyone with hypogammaglobulinaemia which is associated with excretion of excessive amounts of live vaccine. *Inactivated* vaccine should be given to pregnant women and to patients on immunosuppressive therapy.

Rabies. The new vaccine (human diploid vaccine) has been shown to be life-saving. Advice on rabies vaccination should be obtained from the Department of Health and Social Security.

Rubella (German measles). Rubella in pregnancy can result in a malformed baby. Immunization is recommended for pre-pubertal girls (age ten to thirteen years) and should not be given in pregnancy. See schedule, p. 312. It is also recommended for those in contact with pregnant women (doctors and nurses) and in patients who wish to become pregnant but who do not show evidence of previous infection (i.e., they do not have antibodies to the rubella virus). Women offered the vaccine should *not* become pregnant for *three months* after immunization. It should also be offered to women just after childbirth to prevent future complications, since about 60 per cent of abnormalities in babies due to rubella occur in women who have had more than one baby. It is responsible for 1 per cent of congenital abnormalities.

Smallpox. Worldwide eradication of smallpox has now been achieved and vaccination is not necessary except in special cases.

Tetanus. See schedule, p. 312. A booster injection is required for a dirty wound; with a clean wound it is not necessary unless five years or more have expired since the last injection. An anti-tetanus immunoglobulin injection should be given for serious dirty wounds along with tetanus vaccination and antibiotics.

Tuberculosis. BCG (Bacillus Calmette-Guérin) is a live bovine vaccine which stimulates hypersensitivity to tuberculosis bacteria. It is offered to children who have not previously had an infection of TB (tuberculin-negative). It should be given (after tuberculin testing) to people living in crowded and poor conditions and to immigrants from countries where there is a high incidence of TB. New-born babies should be inoculated in those communities.

Typhoid. Sensible precautions include not eating green salads, uncooked vegetables and not drinking tap-water in a country where typhoid is present. A local reaction to the vaccine consists of redness, swelling and pain which occurs in about six to eight hours and is followed by headache, fever and malaise for about forty-eight hours.

Typhus. Vaccination is only required when visiting certain countries. Seek advice from the Department of Health and Social Security.

Yellow fever. This should not be given to children under nine months of age since it may cause encephalitis. It should be given neither in pregnancy nor to patients who are sensitive to eggs. Immunization lasts for about ten years.

Schedule of Vaccination and Immunization Procedures (Children and Adults)

During the first year of life. At three months of age, the *first dose* of diphtheria, tetanus and pertussis (whooping cough) vaccine (adsorbed) by injection and poliomyelitis vaccine by mouth should be given. The *second dose* of diphtheria, tetanus and pertussis vaccine (adsorbed) and poliomyelitis vaccine should be given, preferably after an interval of 6 to 8 weeks. The *third dose* of diphtheria, tetanus and pertussis vaccine (adsorbed) and poliomyelitis vaccine should be given, preferably after an interval of 4 to 6 months.

Note: If pertussis vaccine is contra-indicated or the parents decline, diphtheria and tetanus vaccine (adsorbed) should be given by injection in place of the triple vaccine (diphtheria, tetanus and pertussis).

During the second year of life. Live measles vaccine should be given by injection.

At school entry or entry to nursery school. An injection of diphtheria and tetanus vaccine (adsorbed) and poliomyelitis by mouth should be given. There should be an interval of at least 3 years after completing the basic pre-nursery school course.

Between 10 and 13 years of age. Tuberculosis vaccine (BCG. Bacillus Calmette-Guérin) should be given to tuberculin-negative children and to tuberculin-negative contacts at any age. There should be an interval of not less than 3 weeks between BCG and rubella (German measles) vaccination.

Between 10 and 13 years of age. Girls should be given an injection of live rubella (German measles) vaccine regardless of a past history of an attack of rubella.

On leaving school, before employment, or on entering further education. A booster dose of live poliomyelitis vaccine should be given by mouth or inactivated poliomyelitis vaccine by injection, also an injection of tetanus vaccine (adsorbed) should be given.

In adult life. Live poliomyelitis vaccine by mouth or inactivated poliomyelitis by injection should be given to previously unvaccinated adults. Three doses with an interval of 6 to 8 weeks between the first and second doses and of 4 to 6 months between the second and third. A course of live poliomyelitis vaccine by mouth should be offered to travellers to countries where polio is endemic, also to unvaccinated parents of a child being given oral vaccine.

Adult females of child-bearing age should be tested for rubella antibodies and those who are negative should be offered live rubella vaccination by injection. Pregnancy must first be excluded and the patients warned not to become pregnant for 3 months after immunization.

An injection of tetanus vaccine (adsorbed) should be offered to previously unvaccinated adults against tetanus. For adults, 2 doses at an interval of 6 to 8 weeks followed by a third dose 6 months later.

54 Over-the-Counter Medicines and the Treatment of Some Commonly Occurring Disorders

To treat common symptoms there are numerous drug preparations which can be bought over the counter which no doctor would ever prescribe or be allowed to prescribe. Many of them are combinations of drugs given a brand name and sold at a much higher price than the separate drugs would cost. Often these combinations contain doses of drugs which are too small to be effective and some contain drugs which are considered useless or obsolete. The same drugs, in the same doses, under different brand names, may be widely advertised for the treatment of many different disorders. Furthermore, extravagant claims are often made for the benefits of some over-the-counter drugs without any real supportive evidence.

To treat yourself you need to be able to select a drug preparation which will give you the most benefits for the least risks and the smallest expense.

Where appropriate the best guide is to choose over-the-counter preparations which contain drugs which doctors prescribe and in doses which are likely to be effective. Where effective drugs are available only on prescription you need to consult your doctor with a clear idea of what is available to help your particular disorder. You can find out which drugs doctors prescribe for all sorts of different conditions by reading Part Two of this book. Having decided that your disorder can probably be best treated with a particular drug, you can then find out more about it, its effects and adverse effects and recommended dosage, by looking it up under its generic name in the pharmacopoeia in Part Three.

Remember that most symptoms are self-limiting and no treatment is often better than taking medicines.

Drugs Used to Treat Some Commonly Occurring Disorders

Acne (Acne vulgaris). There is no specific treatment for acne and it is best to use what suits you or to keep trying different preparations at intervals. Doctors often prescribe acne treatments which contain keratolytics (p. 278) to peel off the skin, e.g., sulphur, resorcinol, salicylic acid. Ultra-violet light may be used for this purpose and some applications contain an abrasive (e.g., Brasivol). Many acne applications contain detergent antiseptics such as cetrimide and benzalkonium (see p. 274). These have been recommended for cleaning the face at night, as has hexachlorophane (p. 274). Topical antibiotics (e.g., chloramphenicol and neomycin) are also used but not recommended (p. 272) and a corticosteroid (p. 267) mixed with an antibiotic. **Dalacin T** solution contains **clindamycin** (see part III). A daily dose of a tetracycline antibiotic (p. 288) by mouth for several weeks is said to help and co-trimoxazole has also been tried in a similar way. Applications of **tretinoin (Retin-A)** may be useful in some patients but may produce redness and peeling for several days. **Cyproterone**, an anti-androgen (anti-male sex hormone) with **ethinyloestradiol** (a female sex hormone) has been tried in a preparation called **Dianette** with some success in women with severe acne. **Isotretinoin (Roaccutane)** is being tried by mouth but it is only available in hospitals. Remember, where there is no specific treatment for a disorder there are many treatments. Do not waste your money purchasing special preparations, attending private skin clinics or seeing private specialists – they can do no more for you than your own doctor.

Allergies. These are difficult to treat. Avoidance of precipitating factors is important. Drug therapy is often disappointing. Read the chapter on antihistamine drugs, pp. 125–30. Do not waste money on purchasing over-the-counter remedies etc. Consult your doctor if the problem is recurrent or persistent but do not be too optimistic unless an obvious cause can be identified and eliminated.

Allergic drug rashes. Antihistamines by mouth (p. 129) are effective with eruptions of the nettle-rash (urticaria) type. If the rash is severe cortico-steroids by mouth (p. 216) are indicated. Soothing applications (p. 265) and cooling lotions are all that should be applied to the skin. Of course any drug should be stopped immediately a skin rash develops but consult your doctor straight away if you are on any long-term drug medication.

Alopecia (loss of hair). There is *no* specific treatment, therefore do *not* waste your money on purchasing special skin preparations, attending hair clinics or seeing private specialists. The majority of patients get better regardless of treatment and for the ones that do not there is no treatment. For bald patches (alopecia areata) and complete baldness there is no specific treatment. For male-type baldness see **Regaine (minoxidil)** in part III.

Anaemia. Deficiency of iron is the commonest cause of anaemia and blood loss (e.g., heavy periods) is the commonest cause of iron deficiency. If you think you are anaemic consult your doctor and ask for a blood test to be carried out. Do not purchase over-the-counter iron preparations.

Appetite. A persistent change in appetite (e.g., loss of appetite) is a symptom of an underlying disorder which may be physical or psychological. Do not purchase over-the-counter remedies: consult your doctor.

Asthma. Over-the-counter remedies are not effective: consult your doctor. Read about drugs used to treat asthma, pp. 111–16.

Athlete's foot (Tinea pedis). Read section on antifungal skin applications (p. 272) and, depending on how severe it is, discuss the treatment with your doctor. Athlete's foot can sometimes develop like an acute eczema and in this case it needs treating initially as if it were an infected eczema (see p. 317).

Bath salts. Forget the bath salts: have a hot, soothing, relaxing *bath*.

Body odour. See deodorants, p. 279, and note warnings on vaginal deodorants.

Boils. Apply local heat (e.g., magnesium sulphate paste), do not squeeze (it helps to spread the infection) and do not put a plaster over it. If multiple or recurrent, see your doctor for an antibiotic (local and/or by mouth) and to test your urine for sugar.

Bruises. It is claimed that several drugs can dissolve bruising and swelling following injury by removing clotted blood, exudate or dead tissue. They include bromelains (Ananase Forte tablets), chymotrypsin (Chymar injection, Chymoral tablets, Deanase DC tablets), deoxyribonuclease as an aerosol, intramuscular injection, local injection, also as Deanase powder, hyaluronidase (Hylase injection), streptokinase-streptodornase (Varidase tablets, Varidase Topical powder) and trypsin (Trypure powder). Their effectiveness is doubtful. A cold compress is useful.

Burns. For the self-treatment of small burns use no ointment or creams etc.: just cool the area in ordinary cold water and cover with a clean, dry dressing.

Catarrh. Steam inhalations are the best treatment. See p. 102.

Change-of-life symptoms. See menopause, p. 234.

Chilblains. Drugs used to increase the circulation (p. 170) are often not effective and not indicated. Local ointments containing irritants (p. 275) are of very doubtful value; so too are high doses of calcium and high doses of calciferol. Warm clothing is important. The best treatment has been preventative: central heating. It is not worth purchasing an over-the-counter remedy.

Cold remedies. There is no such thing as a 'cold-cure'. See p. 99.

Cold sores (Herpes simplex). Treatment is usually disappointing. Local anaesthetics (p. 278) and astringents (p. 278) have been tried. Antibiotics have no effect upon virus infection. Idoxuridine (p. 298) has been claimed to help; it is an antivirus drug and is used to treat eye ulcers. See warning about using corticosteroid applications (p. 271).

Colic. Do not self-treat: consult your doctor.

Constipation. Avoid drug treatment where possible, try bran and read chapter on drugs used to treat constipation, pp. 146–50.

Corns. Applications used to treat corns usually contain a caustic or keratolytic (p. 278) such as salicylic acid, alum or acetic acid. Consult your chiropodist or pharmacist. Avoidance of ill-fitting shoes is important.

Cough. If you smoke, stop smoking. If you have a cough which persists for more than a few days consult your doctor. Read the chapter on drugs used to treat coughs, pp. 103–106.

Cuts and abrasions. Ordinary soap and water is satisfactory but if you wish you may use an antiseptic cleaning preparation (p. 273).

Cystitis. Do not self-treat.

Dandruff. Any detergent shampoo is of use and there is no evidence that 'medication' (p. 273) is of value. Doctors try keratolytics (p. 278) such as coal tar, sulphur, salicylic acid and selenium sulphide (Lenium, Selsun). Detergent antiseptics are also used by doctors – cetrimide (Cetavlon, Seboderm) and benzalkonium (Capitol).

Diarrhoea. Medicines are seldom necessary: rehydration is important. See p. 143–5.

Dizziness. Do not self-treat: consult a doctor.

Dysmenorrhoea. Read about drugs used to treat dysmenorrhoea (painful periods) on p. 233.

Eczema. Depending upon the acuteness, doctors use lotions, ointments, creams or pastes. Soothing applications (p. 265), mild astringents (p. 278), mild keratolytics (p. 278), corticosteroids (p. 270), antibiotics (p. 272) and antifungal drugs (p. 272) may be used.

Disorders of the ears. For the treatment of wax in the ears see p. 110. It is advisable *not* to purchase ear drops etc. If you have discomfort in your ears which you feel needs treating then consult your doctor.

Eye disorders. Do *not* purchase any over-the-counter preparations. If you feel you have an eye disorder which needs treatment then consult your doctor.

Fever. Sponging with tepid water is helpful. Aspirin is very useful in adults and so is paracetamol in adults and children. Read about these drugs on pp. 193–5.

Gum disorders. Over-the-counter remedies are of little use. Consult your dentist.

Haemorrhoids (piles). Never diagnose haemorrhoids yourself: always consult a doctor. Knowing the correct diagnosis use what the doctor prescribes. Never use sprays. Read about astringents and local anaesthetic applications in the section on drugs used to treat disorders of the skin, pp. 261–81.

Hair and scalp disorders. If you have a persistent or recurrent scalp disorder consult your doctor, particularly if it is worrying you. See drugs used to treat dandruff above.

Health salts, rheumatic salts, backache salts, etc. Most of these contain saline laxatives, see p. 148. You do not have to belch and have loose bowel movements in order to keep healthy.

Heartburn. See antacids, p. 136.

Impetigo. This is an acutely infective skin disorder: consult your doctor. See p. 272.

Indigestion, etc. Read the chapter on drugs used to treat indigestion and peptic ulcer, pp. 135–42. Dietary indiscretion, alcohol and smoking are contributory factors. Ask a pharmacist to recommend a suitable antacid (see p. 136) but if the symptoms persist for a week or two consult your doctor. Note warnings on antacids, p. 138.

Infant powders and mixtures. Read about the types of drug which may be included in preparations used to relieve pain (p. 194), indigestion (p. 136) and constipation (p. 146). This will help you decide that the use of such drug preparations in babies and infants is *usually unnecessary and/or ineffective and/or harmful.*

Insect bites and stings. Usually all that is needed is a cooling or soothing application (p. 265). An antihistamine cream (p. 277) may help, and a corticosteroid application (p. 270) is very effective. An antibiotic needs to be given by mouth if infection develops. If you are allergic to insect bites try an insect repellent containing dimethylphthalate or dibutylphthalate and carry antihistamine tablets (p. 125) with you, or you can be immunized (see your doctor).

Insomnia. Insomnia is a symptom of an underlying physical or psychological disorder. If it persists consult your doctor. Read about sleep, pp. 57–64, and do not purchase any over-the-counter remedies.

Itching. It is very important to treat the underlying cause (e.g., scabies), therefore consult your doctor. Read about drugs used to relieve itching on p. 276: do not purchase an over-the-counter remedy.

Leg ulcers. The underlying cause should be treated first (e.g., diabetes). Local treatment of ulcers is aimed at clearing up any infection (see antibiotic skin preparations, p. 272), and getting rid of the slough and clot which may be helped by using an enzyme preparation such as streptokinase-streptodornase (Varidase) or dextranomer (Debrisan). Washing with a diluted antiseptic cleansing solution such as cetrimide (p. 273) may help. The use of oral zinc sulphate (Zincomed) needs evaluating. The type of dressing used is important: it should be non-adherent. Remember that drugs can be easily absorbed from ulcer sites into the blood-stream. They may also produce local dermatitis (e.g., neomycin or lanolin sensitivity).

Lice. There are very effective treatments for body lice, head lice (nits) etc.: consult your doctor or pharmacist and read p. 273.

Liver pills, etc. These contain drastic laxatives and should be avoided. See p. 146.

Migraine. Prevention is better than cure. See p. 203.

Motion sickness. See p. 130.

Mouth ulcers. See p. 107. There are numerous non-specific, ineffective treatments available. Doctors use applications containing a corticosteroid (p. 270) (e.g., hydrocortisone in Corlan pellets), local anaesthetic applications and local antiseptic applications (p. 273). Soothing applications, astringents (p. 278), protectives, antibiotics (p. 272), antiviral drugs (p. 298) and antifungal applications (p. 272) have been tried. For thrush, nystatin is effective, so is amphotericin. For a severe ulcerative condition of the mouth (Vincent's disease) metronidazole (Flagyl) is effective in tablet form. A liquorice derivative (carbenoxolone) has been used, e.g., Bioral gel and Bioral pellets, to treat aphthous ulcer. Convicing evidence of the effectiveness of over-the-counter remedies for mouth ulcers is not available.

Muscle aches and pains. See rheumatic linaments, p. 200, aspirin and paracetamol, p. 193, and non-steroidal anti-inflammatory drugs, p. 196. Heat and massage are more important than applications which always have a strong, pleasant smell which helps you to believe their effectiveness.

Nappy rash. Prevention is better than cure. Wash and rinse nappies well, or use disposables, and periodically expose the baby's bottom to the fresh air for an hour or so. Any protective (p. 266) or soothing application (p. 265) may help prevent nappy rash, e.g., zinc cream and castor oil or a barrier cream containing a silicone (p. 266). Detergent antiseptics, e.g., benzalkonium (p. 274), may help if a rash has developed and for severe cases a preparation containing a corticosteroid and an anti-infective drug is useful (pp. 270–2).

Nausea. Nausea is a symptom of an underlying disorder. Consult your doctor if it keeps recurring or if it persists for a few days. Read chapter on drugs to treat nausea and vomiting, pp. 131–3.

Pain relievers. See aspirin and paracetamol, pp. 193–5, and non-steroidal anti-inflammatory drugs, p. 196.

Perspiration. See anti-perspirants, p. 279.

Pregnancy sickness. Avoid any drugs if at all possible; see p. 132.

Premenstrual tension. See p. 234.

Pruritus vulvae. See p. 277.

Psoriasis. Depending upon the severity, acuteness and extent of the rash, doctors use lotions, ointments, creams and pastes. These may be soothing applications (p. 265), astringents (p. 278), keratolytics (p. 278) and corticosteroids (of the fluorinated type, p. 276). Tar (p. 281) and dithranol (p. 280) are the most commonly used drugs after the corticosteroids. Coal tar sensitizes the skin to ultra-violet light and this is the basis of tar baths and sunray treatment in psoriasis. Occlusive plastic dressings over corticosteroid creams have produced damage to the skin and other complications

(p. 270). Methotrexate or etretinate may be effective in some patients with severe psoriasis and in psoriasis arthritis.

Ringworm. See antifungal drugs, p. 296, and antifungal skin applications, p. 272. If you suspect you have ringworm consult your doctor.

Scabies. See p. 273. If you suspect you have scabies consult your doctor.

Slimming. This is a multi-million-pound industry tied up with the fashion industry. Read about slimming drugs, p. 88.

Smoking. There is no convincingly effective anti-smoking drug and there is no substitute for willpower.

Sore throat. Throat lozenges, etc. are of very limited use: see p. 107.

Sunburn. Avoidance is best. For treatment, see p. 269.

Sunscreen preparations. See p. 267.

Teething preparations. Any soothing application to the gums is quickly washed away in the saliva and therefore teething applications are useless. In the past some have been very dangerous (e.g., those which contained mercury).

Tonics. If you think something will do you good then it will. But consider why you think you need a tonic and then consult your doctor. Read about tonics, p. 85.

Verrucas. These are warts on the soles of the feet and caustics (p. 278) are usually used to treat them. Three per cent formalin solution foot soaks may be useful. Sometimes they need removing surgically.

Vitamins. Read about the use and misuse of vitamins, pp. 211–15, and eat a well-balanced diet instead of taking vitamin preparations.

Vomiting. See drugs used to relieve vomiting on p. 131. Consult your doctor if vomiting becomes recurrent or persistent.

Warts. If you believe a treatment will make a wart go, it may well do so. Most applications contain caustics (p. 278) or keratolytics (p. 278), e.g., acetic acid, salicyclic acid, nitric acid, formaldehyde and podophyllum. Skin specialists freeze them off with liquid nitrogen or solid carbon dioxide and some are removed surgically. Consult your pharmacist or doctor.

Wax in the ear. See p. 110.

Wind. Most carminatives used to treat wind contain essential oils which can irritate the stomach. Some preparations help some patients.

Worms. See piperazine and viprynium in Part Three.

Warnings about Drug Use

1. Always know the name of the drug that you are taking.
2. Always check its main effects and adverse effects.
3. Always tell the doctor about previous drug reactions and other allergies in you or in any member of your family.
4. Always take the drug according to the instructions on the container.
5. Never take a drug daily for more than one or two weeks without checking on the benefits and risks.
6. Never share prescribed drugs with other people.
7. Never use drugs from an unlabelled container.
8. Never keep unwanted or unused drugs in the house – always flush them down the lavatory.
9. Only keep a few household remedies to hand and in small quantities.
10. Keep all drugs in one safety cupboard out of reach of children.
11. Never mix the contents of one drug container with another.
12. Check with your pharmacist if you are not clear about:
    (a) The expiry date of a drug and where you should store it.
    (b) When you should take it (e.g., before or after meals).
    (c) How you should take it (e.g., with or without a drink of milk).
    (d) How frequently you should take it (e.g., four-hourly, six-hourly, four times in the day or four times in twenty-four hours).
    (e) For how many days you should take it (e.g., always finish a course of antibiotics).
13. Always ask the pharmacist for special-instruction leaflets when obtaining medicaments such as eye drops, nose drops, pessaries, etc.
14. Ask what the doctor means when he states 'as before', or 'as directed'. Ask about the maximum amount of one dose and the maximum allowable in twenty-four hours. Ask how often is 'when necessary'.
15. Be especially cautious when giving drugs to babies, debilitated and elderly patients, to those with impaired kidney or liver function, to patients with heart disease, chest disease, blood pressure, glaucoma, enlarged prostate gland, peptic ulcers, history of allergy or history of drug dependence.
16. If you are planning to become pregnant, if you are or think you may be pregnant, then be extremely cautious about any drugs you take,

particularly from around the time of conception to about the twelfth to fourteenth week of your pregnancy.

17. If you are on corticosteroids, anticoagulants, anti-diabetic drugs, monoamine oxidase inhibitor antidepressant drugs or any other special drugs always ask for and carry a warning card with you.

18. Consider the possibility of an adverse drug effect if a new symptom develops whilst on drug treatment (e.g., diarrhoea, skin rash). If it is a prescribed drug stop taking it and consult your doctor. If it is an over-the-counter drug then stop taking it, check its adverse effects and report to your doctor if the symptom does not clear up.

19. Remember the risk of adverse drug interactions between drugs and also between drugs and certain foods – in particular remember the dangers of taking alcohol while taking a drug.

20. Remember that many drugs may affect your ability to operate moving machinery and drive a motor vehicle – always check for this risk.

21. If a patient under your supervision is confused or depressed and/or drinks alcohol regularly, sometimes to excess, then supervise the issue of tablets on a daily basis.

22. Never keep sleeping drugs at your bedside, particularly if you also drink alcohol. You may take an extra dose in the night without knowing it.

Part Three
PHARMACOPOEIA

In this section drug preparations are listed in alphabetical order. Standard doses of commonly used drugs are given as a general guide but always check the dose of any drug preparation (generic or brand) with your doctor or pharmacist, or with the instructions on the packet. Doses for children have purposely been avoided because these need checking for age, weight and other factors – again, read the instructions on the packet.

If every reported adverse effect of each drug were to be listed, this book would run to several volumes. Therefore, only some of the more commonly recognized adverse effects are given. Each list usually starts with mild adverse effects (such as nausea and dizziness). These are often related to dose and frequency of dosage (dose-related), and can be reduced or stopped by reducing the dosage or stopping the drug. Next, moderate to severe adverse effects are mentioned; finally, some serious reported adverse effects are listed.

The purpose of listing adverse effects is not to alarm you but to alert you to the possibility that the development of any new symptom may be due to the drug you are taking. Also it will help you to weigh up the benefits and risks of a particular drug. Do not decide against a prescribed drug just because its list of adverse effects is longer than that of another drug. The important point is the ratio for *you* of benefits to risks. This needs to be discussed with your doctor.

Warning: Since their effects, adverse or otherwise, may be increased in certain individuals, all medicines should be given with the utmost caution, particularly to babies, children, pregnant women (and those wishing to become pregnant), the elderly, patients who are debilitated by illness, and patients who have disorders of the liver, kidneys or heart.

This warning applies to the use of all medicines, whether given by injection, taken by mouth, applied to the eyes, skin or scalp, or inserted in the ears or up the nose, rectum or vagina.

* *Products marked with an asterisk have now been taken off the market.*

A Popular Pharmacopoeia

A A A spray is used to treat sore throat. It contains benzocaine 1·5 mg, cetalkonium chloride 0·04 mg per 100 mg dose. *Dose:* 2 sprays on to the throat two- or three-hourly.

Abdine: Each **Single Strength** powder contains sodium and potassium tartrate 2·75 g, sodium bicarbonate 2·75 g, and tartaric acid 2·5 g; each **Double Strength** powder contains sodium and potassium tartrate 7 g, sodium bicarbonate 3 g, and tartaric acid 2·5 g.

Abicol is used to treat raised blood pressure. Each tablet contains reserpine 0·15 mg and bendrofluazide 2·5 mg. *Dose:* ½ to 2 tablets morning and evening.

Abidec drops and capsules are multivitamin preparations.

Abietis oil ◊ Siberian fir oil.

Abietis pine oil ◊ Siberian fir oil.

ABVD is a combination of four anti-cancer drugs: **doxorubicin** (adriamycin), **bleomycin**, **vinblastine** and **dacarbazine**. Read entries on each individual drug.

acacia ◊ gum arabic.

acebutotol (Sectral, acebutolol hydrochloride) is a beta-receptor blocking drug used to treat disorders of heart rhythm, angina and high blood pressure. *Adverse effects* ◊ propranolol. Acebutotol has less effect upon the beta-receptors in the bronchi and may be used to treat patients who are also suffering from asthma and other obstructive airway disorders. *Dose:* Angina and hypertension: by mouth, 400 to 900 mg daily in divided doses. Disorders of heart rhythm: the dose depends upon the urgency of the treatment and the disorder being treated.

acepifylline (Etophylate) is used to treat asthma. It has similar properties to aminophylline, but is less liable to cause nausea. *Dose:* By mouth, 0·5 to 1 g three times daily after food. Also available as an injection and suppositories.

Acepril ◊ captopril.

acetaminophen ◊ paracetamol.

Acetarsol is an arsenic compound.

acetazolamide (Diamox) is a diuretic. It is used to reduce the pressure inside the eye in the treatment of glaucoma. *Adverse effects:* These are frequent, mild and reversible on stopping or reducing the dose. They include drowsiness, numbness, and tingling of the face, hands and feet. Fatigue, excitement and thirst may occur and, rarely, skin rashes. Liver, kidney and blood disorders have been reported. The water-salt balance of the body may be disturbed. *Precautions:* It should not be given to patients who have a low blood potassium level (e.g., patients with Addison's disease). *Dose:* By mouth, 500 mg initially and then 250 mg every six hours.

Acetest tablets are used to test for ketones in the urine of patients with diabetes.

acetic acid is used in some cough linctuses, it is also used in rheumatic liniments, in antiseptic skin applications, and in a concentrated form to treat warts and corns.

acetohexamide (Dimelor) is an oral anti-diabetic drug. It may produce headaches, stomach upsets, vertigo, nervousness and occasionally it disturbs liver function tests. ◊ chlorpropamide. *Dose:* 250 mg to 1·5 g daily.

acetomenapthone has vitamin K activity and has similar uses to those described under phytomenadione. It has been used to treat chilblains.

acetone is used as a solvent for fats, resins and other chemicals.

AcetOxyl ◊ benzoyl peroxide.

acetylcholine is a chemical messenger in the parasympathetic nervous system.

acetylcysteine Fabrol; Parvolex) is used to dissolve sputum. It may produce bronchospasm, nausea, vomiting, sore lips, runny nose, and fever. It should be used with caution in elderly and/or debilitated patients who have difficulty in breathing and coughing. In eye drops acetylcysteine thins mucous and provides relief from dry eye syndrome. *Dose:* By direct instillation, 1–2 ml every one to four hours. By mouth, 200 mg in water three times daily. It is also given intravenously in the treatment of paracetamol overdosage. Eye drops, 1 or 2 drops daily or 4 times daily.

acetylsalicylic acid ◊ aspirin.

Acezide tablets contain hydrochlorothiazide 25 mg and captopril 50 mg. Used to treat mild to moderate hypertension ◊ hydrochlorothiazide and captopril.

Achromycin ◊ tetracycline.

Acidol-Pepsin is used to increase gastric acidity. Each tablet contains betaine hydrochloride 388 mg and pepsin 97 mg. *Precautions:* The tablets should be dissolved in water and the solution sucked through a straw to protect the teeth from the hydrochloric acid that is produced. *Dose:* 1 to 3 tablets in water three times daily after meals.

Aci-jel contains acetic acid 0·92%. It is used to treat infections of the vagina. *Dose:* 1 applicatorful vaginally twice daily.

acipimox (Olbetam) lowers blood fat levels. It is related to nicotinic acid (◊ nicotinic acid) but it is more active and longer acting and less likely to cause rebound effects if treatment is stopped. *Adverse effects:* Flushing, rash, redness of the face and blush area, stomach upsets, headache, malaise. *Precautions:* Do not use in patients with peptic ulcers, in pregnancy or when breast-feeding. *Dose:* By mouth, 2 or 3 capsules (250 mg) daily in divided doses. Maximum daily dose = 1200 mg.

Acnaid Lotion contains cetrimide 1% salicylic acid 0·05% and alcohol (90%) 30%.

Acnaveen bar is a skin cleanser for acne. Each bar contains salicyclic acid 2% and sulphur 2%.

Acne-Aid Soap contains sulphated surfactant blend 6·3%.

Acnegel ◊ benzoyl peroxide.

Acnidazil cream is used to treat acne. It contains benzoyl peroxide 5% and miconazole nitrate 2%.

aconite is the dried root of *aconitum napellus*. It contains alkaloids which can produce toxic effects upon. the heart and nervous system. It should *not* be used.

acriflavine is used in antiseptic skin applications. It is incompatible with chlorine antiseptics. It may produce sensitivity of the skin to sunlight.

Acriflex cream is an antiseptic containing chlorhexidine gluconate 1·25% ◊ chlorhexidine.

acrosoxacin (Eradacin; Rosoxacin) is an antibiotic used in the treatment of gonorrhoea in patients allergic to penicillin. *Adverse effects:* Dizziness, drowsiness, gastric disturbances. *Precautions:* The patient's ability to drive or operate machinery may be impaired. *Dose:* By mouth, 300 mg as a single dose on an empty stomach.

Actal ◊ alexitol sodium. It is an antacid. *Dose:* Suck one or two as required.

ACTH ◊ corticotrophin.

ACTH gel ◊ corticotrophin.

ACTH/CMC ◊ corticotrophin.

Acthar gel (adrenocorticotrophic hormone) for injections. ◊ corticotrophin.

Actidil ◊ triprolidine.

Actifed is used to treat coughs and colds. It contains triprolidine hydrochloride 2·5 mg and pseudoephedrine hydrochloride 60 mg in each tablet; 1·25 mg and 30 mg respectively in each 5 ml of syrup *Dose:* 1 tablet or 10 ml three times a day.

Actifed Compound (Actifed syrup with added codeine phosphate (10 mg in each 5 ml)). *Dose:* 10 ml three times a day.

Actinac is used to treat acne. It contains chloramphenicol 1%, hydrocortisone acetate 1%, butoxyethyl nicotinate 0·6%, allantoin 0·6% and sulphur 8%.

actinomycin D (Cosmegen) is an anticancer drug. *Adverse effects:* Nausea, vomiting, abdominal pain and diarrhoea may occur during treatment. Injections may be painful and produce local irritation. The skin marks of X-ray therapy may be made worse by actinomycin D. Days or weeks after treatment has stopped the patient may develop blood disorders (due to bone-marrow damage), nausea, vomiting and diarrhoea. *Precautions:* It should probably be avoided during pregnancy. *Dose:* According to condition being treated.

activated attapulgite is a highly absorbent mineral used to treat diarrhoea.

activated charcoal ◊ charcoal.

activated dimethicone (Infacol) is a silicone used in antacids to disperse wind.

Actonorm gel is used to treat peptic ulcer. It contains aluminium hydroxide gel 220 mg, magnesium hydroxide 100 mg, activated dimethicone 25 mg in 5 ml. *Dose:* By mouth, 5 to 20 mg after meals.

Actron tablets contain aspirin 267 mg, paracetamol 133 mg, caffeine 40 mg, sodium bicarbonate 1·606 g, and citric acid 954 mg.

Acupan ◊ nefopam.

acyclovir (Zovirax) is an antiviral drug used in the treatment of herpes infections and herpetic lesions of the eye. *Adverse effects:* Rashes, changes in blood chemistry, neurological reactions. *Precautions:* Dose should be reduced in renal failure. *Dose:* By slow intravenous infusion 5 mg/kg every 8 hours. Also available in tablets, ointment and eye ointment.

Adalat ◊ nifedipine.

Adalat Retard: Each tablet contains 20 mg nifedipine in a sustained-release form ◊ nifedipine.

Adcortyl ◊ triamcinolone.

Adexolin drops is a multivitamin preparation.

adipic acid is used as an acidulating agent in food.

ADH (antidiuretic hormone) ◊ vasopressin.

adrenaline (epinephrine) acts on the nerve endings of the sympathetic nervous system. It produces the sort of effects caused by fear or emotion; blanched skin (caused by constriction of small arteries), dilatation of the pupils, inhibition of the movements of the gut and bladder and the release of glucose by the liver. In addition it increases the blood supply to muscles, stimulates the heart increasing its rate, relaxes the muscles of the uterus and relaxes bronchial muscles. These are stress effects and prepare the body for what may be called 'fight or flight'. Adrenaline is used medically to treat asthma and to treat shock produced in severe allergic reactions. Because adrenaline constricts small blood vessels it is often mixed with injections of a local anaesthetic in order to stop the latter from getting washed away in the blood-stream too quickly, thereby prolonging its effects. *Adverse effects:* These are common and include anxiety, breathlessness, restlessness, palpitations, rapid beating of the heart, trembling, weakness, dizziness, headache and coldness of the hands and feet. These may even occur with small doses used by dentists in local anaesthetic injections. Nervous and tense individuals easily develop these symptoms when given adrenaline and so do patients with overworking of their thyroid glands. Gangrene of the fingers may occur after the injection of a combined solution of adrenaline and local anaesthetic into a finger. *Precautions:* Adrenaline should not be used in patients who have overworking of their thyroid glands, with coronary artery disease, with a disorder of heart rhythm, with high blood pressure or with hardening of the arteries (arteriosclerosis). It may cause a severe irregularity of heart rhythm in patients undergoing an anaesthetic with halothane, chloroform, cyclopropane and in patients being treated with quinidine or digitalis. Dentists should use caution when giving adrenaline to patients on other drugs such as antidepressants. *Dose:* As a single dose by subcutaneous injection – 0·2 to 0·25 mg.

adrenocorticotrophic hormone ◊ corticotrophin.

Adriamycin ◊ doxorubicin.

Adult cough balsam is used to treat coughs, each 5 ml contains morphine hydrochloride 0·825 mg, squill vinegar 0·6 ml, ammonium acetate 0·175 mg, acetic acid 0·167 ml, glycerin 0·5 ml and sucrose 2 g.

Aerolin Auto aerosol ◊ salbutamol.

Aerosporin ◊ polymyxin B.

Aerrane ◊ isoflurane.

Aezodent ointment is used for the relief of pain and discomfort due to denture irritation. It contains benzocaine 4·6%, chlorbutol 2·5%, methyl salicylate 0·9%, eugenol 0·5% and menthol 0·5%.

Afrazine Nasal Spray contains oxymetazole hydrochloride 0·05%.

After-bite liquid contains ammonia 3·5% and mink oil. It is used to treat insect bites and stings.

agar is obtained from algae. It is soluble in boiling water and swells to form a solid jelly-like mass on cooling. It is not absorbed from the gut and absorbs water to swell; it is therefore sometimes used in laxative mixtures. Agar is also used as a thickener in various manufactured foods.

Agarol emulsion contains liquid paraffin 31·9%, phenolphthalein 1·32% and agar 0·21%. It is used to treat constipation. *Dose:* 5 to 15 ml at bedtime.

Agiolax is used to treat constipation. It contains ispaghula 54·2% and sennoside B 0·31%. *Dose:* 5 to 10 ml before breakfast and after supper without chewing and with a drink.

Aidex Cream contains aminacrine hydrochloride 0·1% and benzocaine 0·1%.

Airball Breathe Easy contains eucalyptus oil 11·4%, menthol 0·57%, and thymol 0·47%.

Akrotherm cream is used to treat chilblains. It contains acetylcholine chloride 0·2%, histamine 0·034% and cholesterol 1%.

Alavac is used to treat allergies to pollens. It is prepared from twelve varieties of common grass pollen.

Albay contains bee or wasp venom 100 micrograms/ml. It is injected subcutaneously in the diagnosis and treatment of allergies to bee or wasp stings.

Albucid ◊ sulphacetamide.

Albustix is used to detect protein in the urine.

alclometasone (Modrasone) is available in cream and ointment. It has effects and uses similar to prednisolone.

Alcobon ◊ flucytosine.

Alcoderm ◊ paraffin.

alcohol (ethyl alcohol; ethanol) is used as a solvent and preservative in drug preparations.

Alcopar ◊ bephenium.

Alcos-Anal ointment is used to treat haemorrhoids. It contains sodium oleate 10%, chlorothymol 0·1% and lauromacrogol 400 2%.

alcuronium (Alloferin; alcuronium chloride) is a muscle-relaxant drug similar to tubocurarine.

Aldactide 25 is a diuretic. Each tablet contains 25 mg of hydroflumethiazide and 25 mg of spironolactone; **Aldactide 50**: Each tablet contains 50 mg of each. *Dose:* By mouth. Raised blood pressure: up to 2 higher strength tablets daily. Congestive heart failure: up to 4 higher strength tablets daily.

Aldactone ◊ spironolactone.

Aldioxa is an astringent containing allantoin.

Aldomet ◊ methyldopa.

Aleudrin ◊ isoprenaline.

Alevaire ◊ tyloxapol.

Alexan ◊ cytarabine.

alexitol sodium (Actal) is an antacid.

alfacalcidol (One-Alpha) is a vitamin D derivative used for the treatment of renal bone disease, rickets and osteomalacia ◊ calciferol. *Dose:* 1 microgram daily.

alfentanil (Rapifen) is a short-acting narcotic pain reliever used during surgery. *Adverse effects:* Include respiratory depression, a fall in blood pressure (hypotension), slowing of the heart rate (bradycardia), nausea and vomiting. *Precautions:* It should be used with caution in patients with chronic respiratory disorders, myaesthenia gravis. A reduced dose should be used in the elderly, in patients with impaired liver function or reduced working of their thyroid gland (hypothyroidism). In childbirth it may reduce respiration in the baby. *Dose:* By intravenous injection, 500 micrograms, then 250 micrograms every four to five minutes as required.

Algesal ◊ diethylamine salicylate.

Algicon tablets contain a co-dried gel of aluminium hydroxide and magnesium carbonate 360 mg, magnesium alginate 500 mg, magnesium carbonate 320 mg, potassium bicarbonate 100 mg and sucrose 1·5 g. A low sodium antacid (see p. 136), but high in sugar.

alginic acid is obtained from coastal algae. It is included in tablets to make them break up (disperse) when they enter the stomach. Sodium alginate is one of its salts.

Algipan is a rheumatic balm. It contains methyl nicotinate 1%, glycol salicylate 10%, histamine hydrochloride 0·1% and casein 0·1%.

Algispray contains glycol salicylate 5%, diethylamine salicylate 5%, methyl nicotinate 1%, vehicle to 100%.

Alka-Donna is an antacid. Each tablet contains belladonna alkaloids 80 micrograms, dried aluminium hydroxide 250 mg and magnesium trisilicate 500 mg. *Dose:* 1 to 2 tablets sucked 3 times daily before meals. Suspension contains 60 micrograms, 2·15 ml and 342·5 mg/5ml of each constituent respectively. *Dose:* 5 to 10 ml 3 times daily between meals. **Alka-Donna P** contains phenobarbitone and should not be used.

Alka-Seltzer Tablets contain aspirin 324 mg, citric acid, anhydrous, 965 mg, and sodium bicarbonate 1·625 g.

Alkeran ◊ melphalan.

alkoyl diethanolamide is a derivative of diethanolamine which is used as an emulsifying and dispersing agent.

allantoin occurs in comfrey root but it is manufactured. It has been used to encourage wound healing and it is used in skin preparations to treat psoriasis and other skin disorders.

Allbee with C is a multivitamin preparation. Each capsule contains thiamine mononitrate 15 mg, riboflavine 10 mg, nicotinamide 50 mg, pyridoxine hydrochloride 5 mg, ascorbic acid 300 mg, calcium panthothenate 10 mg. Each 5 ml of elixir contains thiamine mononitrate 6 mg, riboflavine sodium phosphate 4 mg, nicotinamide 20 mg, pyridoxine hydrochloride 2 mg, ascorbic acid 120 mg.

All Clear Shampoo contains pyrithione zinc 1%.

Allegron ◊ nortriptyline.

Aller-eze tablets and elixir are used to treat hay fever and allergic rhinitis. Each tablet or 10 ml of elixir contains clemastine 1 mg ◊ clemastine.

Aller-eze plus tablets are used to treat hay fever and allergic rhinitis. Each tablet contains clemastine 0·5 mg and phenylpropanolamine hydrochloride 25 mg ◊ clemastine ◊ phenylpropanolamine.

Alloferin ◊ alcuronium.

allopurinol (Aloral; Aluline; Caplenal; Cosuric; Hamarin; Zyloric) reduces the formation of uric acid and is used in the treatment of gout. In the early stages of treatment acute attacks of gout may occur but after several weeks of continuous treatment these become less frequent and stop. Deposits of urate crystals in the skin (tophi) diminish in size. Allopurinol reduces the risk of patients with gout developing kidney stones and it may prevent kidney damage. Unlike other drugs used to treat gout it may be used in the presence of kidney damage and it may also be used to prevent a rise in plasma uric acid which may occur in some patients treated with certain diuretics. It may therefore be used along with a diuretic in patients suffering from gout and congestive heart failure. *Adverse effects:* These include nausea, vomiting, diarrhoea, headaches, fever, abdominal pains and skin rashes. Nerve damage (peripheral neuritis) and enlargement of the liver have occasionally been reported. *Dose:* By mouth, 300 mg daily in single or divided doses.

Allpyral-G is used to treat allergy to pollens. It is prepared from five varities of common grass pollen.

allyloestrenol (Gestanin) is a progestogen. *Dose:* By mouth, 5 to 20 mg daily.

almasilate (Malinal) is an aluminium/magnesium antacid.

Almazine ◊ lorazepam.

Almevax is a rubella (German measles) vaccine.

almond oil is used as a demulcent and as an emollient.

aloe is obtained from the cut leaves of various species of aloe. It is an irritant laxative. Large doses may damage the kidneys.

aloin is extracted from aloes. It is an irritant laxative and causes kidney damage.

Alophen is a laxative. Each tablet contains aloin 15 mg, phenolphthalein 30 mg, ipecacuanha 4 mg, belladonna extract 5 mg. *Dose:* By mouth, 1 to 3, at bedtime.

Aloral tablets ◊ allopurinol.

aloxiprin (Palaprin Forte) is a preparation of aluminium oxide and aspirin. It may cause less bleeding and irritation of the stomach than plain aspirin. *Dose:* 600 to 1,200 mg by mouth (600 mg of aloxiprin being equivalent to 325 mg of aspirin). It should be given in divided doses to a total dose of 600 mg per 6.5 kg of body-weight daily.

Alpha Keri is a bath oil. It contains liquid paraffin 91·7% and lanolin oil 3%.

alpha tocopheryl acetate ◊ tocopheryl.

Alphaderm cream contains hydrocortisone 1% and urea 10%.

alphadolone is a constituent of a general anaesthetic agent (Althesin).

alphaxolone is a constituent of a general anaesthetic agent (Althesin).

Alphosyl lotion and **cream** contain allantoin 2% and coal tar extract 5%.

Alphosyl HC also contains 0·5% hydrocortisone.

Alphosyl P C shampoo contains coal tar extract 5% and allantoin 0·2%. It is used to treat dandruff and psoriasis.

alprazolam (Xanax) is a **benzodiazepine** anti-anxiety drug. *Adverse effects* and *Precautions* ◊ diazepam. *Dose:* 0·25 mg to 0·5 mg three times a day.

alprostadil (Prostin VR) is a prosta-glandin used to maintain patency of the ductus arteriosus in neonates prior to corrective surgery for congenital heart defects.

Alrheumat ◊ ketoprofen.

alseroxylon is an extract of rauwolfia and has reserpine-like actions ◊ reser-pine. It is used to treat raised blood pressure. *Dose:* By mouth, 2 to 8 mg daily in divided doses.

Altacaps ◊ hydrotalcite.

Altacite ◊ hydrotalcite.

Altacite Plus is an antacid used to treat flatulence. Each 5 ml of suspension contains hydrotalcite 500 mg and activated dimenthicone 125 mg. Each tablet contains 500 mg and 250 mg respectively.

althaea (marshmallow) is from the dried, peeled root of *Althaea officin-alis* collected in the autumn from plants less than two years old. It is used as a demulcent and emollient.

Alu-Cap ◊ aluminium hydroxide.

Aludrox ◊ aluminium hydroxide.

Aludrox S A is used to treat indigestion and peptic ulcer. It contains alumin-ium hydroxide gel, magnesium hy-droxide and 8 mg of secbutobarbitone and 2·5 mg of ambutonium in each tablet or 5 ml of suspension. *Dose:* 1 or 2 tablets or 5 to 10 ml three to four times daily between meals and at bed-time.

Aluhyde is used to treat indigestion and peptic ulcer. It contains alumin-ium hydroxide gel 245 mg, magnesium trisilicate 245 mg, and belladonna ex-tract 7·8 mg. *Dose:* By mouth, 2 after meals.

Aluline ◊ allopurinol.

Alum is a strong astringent. Its use is limited. It may be used to treat cuts and abrasions, sweaty feet, corns and mixed with zinc dusting powder (paediatric alum) to apply to the stump of the umbilical cord after it has been cut.

aluminium acetate is used as an astrin-gent.

aluminium chlorhydroxide is used as an astringent and antiperspirant.

aluminium chloride (Anhydrol Forte, Driclor) is an astringent and an anti-perspirant. It is used to stop excessive perspiration of axillae, hands and feet. *Dose:* Apply at night when necessary, wash off in the morning.

aluminium glycinate is used as an anta-cid. Prolonged use may cause con-stipation. *Dose:* By mouth, 0·5 to 2 g when necessary.

aluminium-guaiphenesin complex ◊ guaiphenesin.

aluminium hydroxide (Aludrox; alu-minium hydroxide mixture; alumin-ium hydroxide gel; dried aluminium hydroxide gel; aluminium hydroxide tablet) is a useful slow-acting antacid. *Adverse effects:* It may cause consti-pation and it may interfere with the absorption of phosphates and vitamins. Aluminium hydroxide decreases the absorption of tetracycline antibiotics from the gut and therefore reduces their effectiveness. These drugs should not be given together. *Dose:* Aluminium hydroxide gel, 10 to 15 ml as needed; dried aluminium hydroxide gel, 0·5 to 1 g as needed.

aluminium hydroxide-magnesium carbonate is used as an antacid. *Dose:* By mouth, 375 to 750 mg when necessary.

aluminium magnesium silicate is used as a thickening agent and as a binder in various drug preparations.

aluminium oxide is used as an antacid. *Dose:* By mouth, 0·5 to 1 g when necessary.

aluminium phosphate gel is an antacid which is an alternative to aluminium hydroxide and does not interfere with the absorption of phosphates.

aluminium silicate ◊ kaolin.

aluminium sodium sulphate is a mixture of salt (sodium chloride) and aluminium sulphate. It is used as a caustic skin application.

aluminium sulphate solution is used as an astringent.

Alunex ◊ chlorpheniramine.

Alupent ◊ orciprenaline.

Alupent inhaler ◊ orciprenaline.

Alupram ◊ diazepam.

Aluzine ◊ frusemide.

alverine citrate (Spasmonal) is an antispasmodic drug used to relieve gastrointestinal spasm and period pain. *Adverse effects:* Drowsiness, weakness, dry mouth and occasionally low blood pressure may occur. *Dose:* 60 to 120 mg up to three times daily.

Alyrane ◊ enflurane.

amantadine (Symmetrel; amantadine hydrochloride) is an anti-viral drug used to prevent influenza A infections. It is also used to treat Parkinsonism. *Adverse effects:* It may cause indigestion, excitement, dizziness, tremors, slurred speech, ataxia, depressed mood, insomnia, and lethargy. Occasionally it may cause nausea, anorexia, vomiting and skin rash. These effects are dose related. Very high doses may cause convulsions. *Precautions:* It should not be given to patients with epilepsy and it should be given with caution to the elderly and patients receiving stimulants. It may increase the effects of benzhexol, benztropine and orphenadrine. These drugs are also used to treat Parkinsonism and their dose should be reduced if amantadine is also given. *Dose:* 200 mg daily by mouth for ten days following exposure to influenza. For Parkinsonism, 100 mg daily for one week followed by 100 mg twice daily.

Ambaxin ◊ bacampicillin.

ambenonium (ambenonium chloride) has similar effects and adverse effects to neostigmine. *Dose:* 5 to 25 mg three to four times daily.

amber oil is obtained from resins. It has properties similar to turpentine and is used in rheumatic liniment.

ambucetamide is an anti-spasmodic drug used in the treatment of period pain.

ambutonium has atropine-like effects. It is an ingredient of Aludrox-SA.

amethocaine is a local anaesthetic. It is more toxic than procaine by injection and cocaine by local application, but it is relatively safer because its local anaesthetic action is greater and it can, therefore, be used in smaller concentrations. Hypersensitivity and allergic reactions have been reported.

Amfipen ◊ ampicillin.

amikacin (Amikin; Amikacin sulphate) is an aminoglycoside antibiotic similar to kanamycin ◊ kanamycin. *Dose:* By intramuscular or intravenous injection, 15 mg per kg body-weight daily in two divided doses.

Amikin ◊ amikacin.

Amilco is a diuretic. Each tablet contains amiloride 5 mg and hydrochlorothiazide 50 mg. *Dose:* 1 to 2 daily, maximum 4 daily.

amiloride (Midamor; amiloride hydrochloride) is a diuretic drug. It may cause dizziness, rashes, mental confusion and weakness. It should be given with caution to patients with impaired kidney function. *Dose:* By mouth, 10 to 40 mg daily.

aminacrine (aminacrine hydrochloride, aminoacridine hydrochloride) is used as a skin antiseptic. It is related to proflavine but is less staining.

aminoacetic acid (glycine, glycocol) is an amino-acid which is an essential constituent of the diet to form body proteins.

amino acids are constituents of proteins and are essential for health.

aminoacridine hydrochloride ◊ aminacrine.

aminobenzoic acid is used in suntan cream. It is included in the vitamin B group of drugs.

aminoglutethimide (Orimeten) is used in the treatment of certain forms of advanced cancer to help alleviate discomfort. *Precautions:* Because the drug blocks the body's production of cortisone, corticosteroids must be given by mouth. *Dose:* 250 mg up to four times daily.

aminophylline (Phyllocontin; theophylline and ethylenediamine) relaxes involuntary muscles and is used to relieve spasm of the bronchi as in asthma or bronchitis. It also makes you pass more salt and water in the urine (diuretic effect), increases the heart rate and stimulates respiration. *Adverse effects:* It can irritate the lining of the stomach and causes nausea and vomiting. It is, therefore, given by injection or by rectum. Rapid injection of aminophylline may cause nausea, vomiting, restlessness, dizziness, rapid heart rate, fall in blood pressure and disordered heart rhythm. Similar effects occasionally occur with suppositories which may also irritate the rectum. Intramuscular injections are painful. *Precautions:* Injections should be given slowly. *Dose:* By mouth, 100 to 300 mg in one dose;

intravenously, 250 to 500 mg in one dose not more frequently than every eight hours; by rectum, 360 mg once or twice a day.

Aminoplasmal parenteral nutrition fluids provide essential and non-essential amino acids and electrolytes.

aminopyrine ◊ amidopyrine.

amiodarone (Cordarone X; amiodarone hydrochloride) is used to treat disordered rhythms of the heart. *Adverse effects:* Patients on continuous therapy may develop micro-deposits in the cornea of their eyes; these can be identified on slit-lamp examination. Nerve damage and Parkinsonism may also develop. These complications disappear when the drug is stopped. It may cause sensitivity to sunlight in some people and occasionally the skin turns a slate grey colour. Dose-related symptoms include nausea, vomiting, metallic taste in the mouth, nightmares, sleeplessness, fatigue and vertigo. *Precautions:* It should not be used in patients with thyroid dysfunction, heart block or sinus bradycardia (slow heart rate) and in patients with latent heart failure. It may increase the effects of digoxin and it should be used with caution in combination with beta-receptor blockers and calcium antagonists as a tendency to slow the heart rate may be potentiated. It may potentiate the action of warfarin. Thyroid function should be monitored throughout treatment with amiodarone since it may produce either increased or decreased function of the thyroid gland. *Dose:* By mouth, 200 to 600 mg daily in divided doses.

amitriptyline (Domical; Elavil; Lentizol; Tryptizol; amitriptyline embonate; amitriptyline hydrochloride) is a tricyclic antidepressant drug. *Adverse effects:* These are similar to those described under imipramine. In the first few weeks of treatment adverse effects may dominate desired effects. These include dryness of the mouth, blurred vision, drowsiness and constipation. Trembling, rapid beating of the heart and a fall in blood pressure may also occur. *Precautions:* Amitriptyline should be given with utmost caution to patients with glaucoma, patients who might develop urinary retention and to patients who have received M.A.O. inhibitors in the previous ten days and in patients who are already taking these drugs. It should preferably be avoided in patients with heart disease, particularly those with disorders of heart rhythm. *Dose:* Amitriptyline hydrochloride: initial dose, 30 to 150 mg daily (at night or in divided doses); maintenance dose, 20 to 100 mg daily (at night or in divided doses). Amitriptyline embonate is tasteless and is therefore used in mixtures; 1·5 g is equivalent to 1 g of amitriptyline hydrochloride.

Amm-i-dent contains carbamide [urea] 13%.

ammonia (Strong ammonia solution; aromatic ammonia solution) is used in smelling salts and rheumatic liniments. It is very irritant to the skin and its use in cosmetics is restricted. It is said to be useful in relieving stings from Portuguese men-of-war.

ammoniated mercury is included in some ointments. It should not be used in infants and children since mercury can be absorbed from the skin and produce toxic effects ◊ mercury.

ammonium acetate is occasionally used as a mild cough expectorant, and as a diuretic.

ammonium alum is used as an astringent.

ammonium bicarbonate is irritant to the lining of the stomach and is used in some cough expectorants.

ammonium chloride is present in many cough medicines. It is irritant and of doubtful value. It produces a mild diuretic effect.

Amovon Corn Caps are plasters spread with an ointment containing salicyclic acid 40%.

Amoxidin ◊ amoxycillin.

Amoxil ◊ amoxycillin.

amoxycillin (Amoxidin; Amoxil). Similar to ampicillin, ◊ ampicillin. *Dose:* By mouth, 250 mg eight-hourly. Injections are also available.

amphetamine sulphate is a stimulant. It produces increased activity and mental alertness. It lifts mood, diminishes the sense of fatigue and produces wakefulness. Some people develop headache, restlessness and insomnia. Large doses produce a lift in mood followed by a fall when you may feel exhausted and depressed. It was previously widely prescribed for the treatment of depression and obesity. However, because of its abuse potential and risk of dependence the prescribing of amphetamine is restricted to treating narcolepsy and occasionally hyperactivity in children. *Adverse effects:* Include dry mouth, nausea, difficulty in urinating, agitation, restlessness, trembling, loss of appetite and constipation. Rapid beating of the heart with disordered rhythm may also occur. Large doses produce fatigue, depression, fever, hallucinations, convulsions and coma. Amphetamine is a drug of dependence. *Dose:* 5 to 10 mg two to three times daily.

amphotericin (Fungilin; Fungizone) is an antibiotic related to nystatin. It has an antifungal action against a wide range of yeasts and fungi (e.g., thrush). *Adverse effects:* Unpleasant and potentially dangerous adverse effects are common because high doses have to be used. These include headache, loss of appetite and fever which passes off after the first few days. Debility, muscle and joint pains, sweating, flushing, and diarrhoea may occur. Low blood pressure, blurred vision and convulsions have been reported. Application to the skin may produce local irritation, itchiness and skin rash. The most serious adverse effect is kidney damage. *Precautions:* It should be injected slowly into a vein. Tests of kidney function should be frequently carried out and the drug stopped at the first sign of kidney damage. *Dose:* Initially up to 0·25 mg per kg of body-weight daily, increased to 1 mg per kg on alternate days by slow intravenous injection.

ampicillin (Amfipen; Ampilar; Britcin; Penbritin; Vidopen; ampicillin sodium (for injections)) is a semi-synthetic penicillin. *Adverse effects:* Ampicillin may cause diarrhoea, nausea and vomiting. Allergic reactions such as itching skin, fever and swelling of the throat may occur. Ampicillin can cause two types of skin rash: a nettle-rash (urticaria) which is a sign of penicillin allergy and requires the immediate stopping of the drug; the other rash is red and looks a bit like measles, and can develop ten to twenty days after starting the drug (even if the course of treatment has finished). On stopping ampicillin the rash disappears and a subsequent course will not necessarily reproduce the rash. It is not, therefore, a true penicillin allergy like the urticarial rash. This red measles-like rash occurs in about 90% of patients suffering from glandular fever who are treated with ampicillin. This is an interesting observation but it also shows how frequently ampicillin is used to treat non-specific sore throats. *Precautions:* Patients allergic to penicillin must be assumed to be allergic to ampicillin. *Dose:* By mouth, 250 mg to 1 g every six hours; by intramuscular injection, or by intravenous injection, 500 mg to 2 g every six hours.

Ampiclox is an antibiotic. Each vial contains ampicillin 250 mg and cloxacillin 250 mg. *Dose:* 1 or 2 vials by injection every four to six hours.

Ampilar ◊ ampicillin.

amsacrine (Amsidine) is used to treat leukaemia.

Amsidine ◊ amsacrine.

amylacetate is used as a solvent.

amylmetacresol is an antiseptic used chiefly as a mouthwash or gargle, or in lozenges for infections of the mouth and throat.

amyl nitrite is used to relieve angina and may also be used to relieve kidney pain (renal colic) and gall-bladder colic. *Adverse effects:* Include flushing of the face, throbbing headache and faintness. Restlessness, vomiting and a blue coloration of the lips may occur with high doses. *Precautions:* Amyl nitrite should not be used in patients who have had a coronary thrombosis. *Dose:* 0·12 to 0·3 ml by inhalation.

amylobarbitone (Amytal; amobarbital) is an intermediate-acting barbiturate used as a sedative and hypnotic. *Adverse effects, Precautions* and *Drug Dependence* ◊ phenobarbitone. *Dose:* Sleeping dose: 100 to 200 mg at night; sedative dose: 30 to 60 mg three times a day.

amylobarbitone sodium (Sodium Amytal; amobarbital sodium; soluble amylobarbitone) is an intermediate-acting barbiturate used as a sedative and hypnotic. *Adverse effects, Precautions* and *Drug Dependence* ◊ phenobarbitone. *Dose:* Sleeping dose: 100 to 200 mg at night; sedative dose: 60 mg three times daily.

amylocaine (amylocaine hydrochloride) is a local anaesthetic.

Amytal ◊ amylobarbitone.

Anacal is used to treat haemorrhoids. It contains heparinoid 0·2%, prednisolone 0·15%, lauromacrogol 5% and hexachlorophane 0·5%.

Anadin Extra: Each tablet contains aspirin 300 mg, paracetamol 200 mg and caffeine 45 mg. *Dose:* By mouth, 1 or 2 every four hours. Maximum of 6 in a day.

Anadin Maximum Strength Capsules: each contain aspirin 500 mg and caffeine 32 mg.

Anadin Soluble Tablets: Effervescent tablets each containing aspirin 325 mg and caffeine citrate 30 mg.

Anadin Tablets each contain aspirin 325 mg, caffeine 15 mg, and quinine sulphate 1 mg.

Anaflex ◊ polynoxylin.

Anafranil ◊ clomipramine.

Anafranil SR ◊ clomipramine.

Ananase Forte ◊ bromelains.

Anapolon 50 ◊ oxymetholone.

Anbesol contains lignocaine hydrochloride 0·9%, chlorocresol 0·1%, and cetylpyridinium chloride 0·02%.

Ancoloxin is used to treat pregnancy sickness. Each tablet contains meclozine dihydrochloride 25 mg and pyridoxine hydrochloride 50 mg. Pyridoxine is vitamin B_6. *Dose:* 2 at night.

ancrod (Arvin) is a drug used to stop blood from clotting. It is obtained from the venom of the Malayan pitviper. Some patients may show resistance to a second course of ancrod, particularly after intramuscular injections. *Dose:* Initially 2 to 3 units per kg of body-weight intravenously over four to twelve hours, then 2 units per kg.

Andrews Liver Salts contain anhydrous citric acid 19·5%, sodium bicarbonate 22·6%, magnesium sulphate (dihydrate) 17·4%, and sucrose 40·5%.

Andrews Liver Salts for Diabetics contain tartaric acid 40%, sodium bicarbonate 42·33%, magnesium sulphate (dihydrate) 17·63%, and saccharin sodium 0·05%.

Androcur ◊ cyproterone.

Andursil is used to treat indigestion and peptic ulcer. Each tablet contains aluminium hydroxide-magnesium carbonate 750 mg and activated dimethicone 250 mg and each 5 ml contains aluminium oxide 200 mg, magnesium hydroxide 200 mg, aluminium hydroxide-magnesium carbonate 200 mg, activated dimethicone 150 mg. *Dose:* By mouth, 1 or 2 tablets or 5 to 10 ml three to four times daily and at bedtime or when necessary.

Anectine ◊ suxamethonium.

Anestan Tablets: Each tablet contains ephedrine hydrochloride 15 mg, theophylline hydrate 60 mg, and salicylamide 130 mg.

Anethaine ◊ amethocaine.

anethole smells of aniseed and is sweet tasting. It is present in some cough medicines as an expectorant and in some cold remedies. It is also used in some preparations to relieve wind.

aneurine is vitamin B_1.

Aneurone mixture is a tonic containing strychnine 0·25 mg, thiamine 0·5 mg, caffeine 15 mg, compound gentian infusion 1·25 ml and sodium acid phosphate 30 mg in each 5 ml.

Anexate solution for injection ◊ flumazenil.

Anflam cream and ointment contains 1% hydrocortisone ◊ hydrocortisone.

Angiers Junior Aspirin* tablets each contain aspirin 75 mg.

Angilol ◊ propranolol.

Anhydrol Forte ◊ aluminium chloride.

anhydrous citric acid ◊ citric acid.

anhydrous lanolin ◊ wool fat.

anise (aniseed) is used to treat wind (carminative) and in cough remedies. It is used mainly as the oil (aniseed oil) for its smell and taste.

aniseed ◊ anise.

anise oil (anisi oil) is a pale yellow oil from anise (aniseed). It is used as a flavouring agent and is included in cough remedies. It is also used to treat wind (carminative).

Anodesyn Ointment contains ephedrine hydrochloride 0·25%, lignocaine hydrochloride 0·5%, and allantoin 0·5%. **Suppositories** contain in addition bronopol 0·2%.

Anovlar 21 is an oral contraceptive. Each tablet contains norethisterone acetate 4 mg and ethinyloestradiol 0·05 mg.

Anquil ◊ benperidol.

Antabuse ◊ disulfiram.

Antasil is used to treat indigeston and peptic ulcers. Each tablet contains aluminium hydroxide 400 mg, magnesium hydroxide 400 mg and activated dimethicone 250 mg; each 5 ml contains the same ingredients but only 150 mg activated dimethicone. *Dose:* By mouth, 1 or 2 tablets or 5 to 30 ml liquid between meals and at bedtime.

antazoline (antazoline sulphate; antazoline phosphate) is an antihistamine. It is used in nose drops.

Antepar ◊ piperazine.

Antepsin ◊ sucralfate.

Anthical Cream contains mepyramine maleate 1·5% and zinc oxide 15% in a vanishing cream basis.

Anthisan ◊ mepyramine.

Anthranol contains dithranol and salicylic acid ◊ dithranol ◊ salicylic acid.

Antibactic lozenges are used to treat throat infections. Each lozenge contains amylmetacresol 0·5 mg and cetylpyridinium chloride 1·5 mg.

antilymphocyte immunoglobulin (Pressimmune) is a sterile, pyrogen-free, isotonic solution for injection which contains 50 mg horse immunoglobulin (IgG + IgT) in each ml. It contains no preservative. It is used as an immunosuppressive agent in organ and tissue transplant. It is also used to treat some auto-immune diseases. *Adverse effects:* Fever, itching, urticaria, nausea, anaphylactic reactions.

Precautions: Careful tests for sensitivity should be carried out using intracutaneous and conjunctival tests. It is used as a prophylaxic against rejection and is a treatment for rejection crisis. If sensitivity tests are positive then it should be administered with utmost caution.

Antipeol ointment contains zinc oxide 20%, ichthammol 2·8%, urea 0·1% and salicylic acid 0·1%.

antipyrin ◊ phenazone.

Antoin is a pain-reliever. Each tablet contains aspirin 400 mg, codeine phosphate 5 mg and caffeine citrate 15 mg. *Dose:* 1 to 2 in water three or four times daily.

Antraderm ◊ dithranol.

Anturan ◊ sulphinpyrazone.

Antussin Cough Syrup Each 5 ml contains dextromethorphan hydrobromide 5·28 mg, phenylephrine hydrochloride 3·52 mg, ammonium chloride 44 mg, and ipecacuanha liquid extract 0·005 ml.

Anugesic-HC suppositories and cream are used to treat haemorrhoids. It contains pramoxine 1%, hydrocortisone acetate 0·5%, balsam of Peru 1·8%, benzyl benzoate 1·2%, resorcinol 0·87% and bismuth oxide 0·87%.

Anusol cream is used to treat haemorrhoids. It contains benzyl benzoate, bismuth salts, balsam of Peru, resorcin and zinc oxide.

Anusol HC ointment is used to treat haemorrhoids. The HC stands for hydrocortisone. Anusol HC contains balsam of Peru 1·87%, benzyl benzoate 1·25%, bismuth oxide 0·875%, bismuth subgallate 2·25%, boric acid 18%, resorcin 0·875%, zinc oxide 10·75%, hydrocortisone acetate 0·25% and base to 100%.

Anusol HC suppositories are used to treat haemorrhoids. The HC stands for hydrocortisone. They contain balsam of Peru 1·87%, benzyl benzoate 1·2%, bismuth resorcin compounds 1·75%, bismuth subiodide 0·019%, bismuth subgallate 2·25%, boric acid 5%, zinc oxide 11% and hydrocortisone acetate 10 mg, and base to 100%.

Anusol ointment and suppositories for treating haemorrhoids, contain boric acid 18%, zinc oxide 10·75%, kaolin 2·37%, bismuth resorcin 1·75%, bismuth subgallate 2·25%, bismuth subiodide 0·04%, balsam of Peru 1·87%, magnesium stearate 0·5% with added wool fat, cocoa butter, castor oil and soft paraffin.

Anxon ◊ ketazolam.

Apisate sustained-release tablets contain diethylpropion 75 mg and B vitamins. It is a slimming drug.

apomorphine (apomorphine hydrochloride) makes you vomit by stimulating the vomiting centre in the brain. It was used to treat non-corrosive poisonings by mouth. *Precautions:* It should not be used in patients who are unconscious or in patients who have taken corrosive poisons. *Dose:* By injection, 2 to 8 mg under the skin or into a muscle.

APP is used to treat indigestion and peptic ulcers. Each tablet contains papaverine hydrochloride 3 mg, homatropine methylbromide 1·5 mg, calcium carbonate 180·5 mg, magnesium carbonate 180 mg, magnesium trisilicate 92·5 mg, bismuth carbonate 12·5 mg, aluminium hydroxide 15 mg. The powder form contains the same ingredients in different proportions. *Dose:* By mouth, 1 to 2 tablets or 5 ml powder in water three or four times daily.

Apresoline ◊ hydralazine.

Apricot kernel powder contains laetrile.

Aprinox ◊ bendrofluazide.

aprotinin (Trasylol) is an enzyme inhibitor, used in the treatment of pancreatitis. *Dose:* depends on the severity of the condition.

Apsifen ◊ ibuprofen.

Apsin VK ◊ phenoxymethylpenicillin.

Apsolol ◊ propranolol.

Apsolox ◊ oxprenolol.

Aqua-Ban Tablets: Each contains ammonium chloride 325 mg and caffeine 100 mg.

Aquadrate ◊ urea.

Aquasept disinfectant ◊ triclosan.

aqueous cream contains emulsifying wax 9%, white soft paraffin 1·5%, liquid paraffin 6%, phenoxyethanol 1% and water 69%.

aqueous iodine solution (Lugol's solution) contains iodine 5% and potassium iodide 10%. It is used before surgical removal of an overworking thyroid gland.

arachis oil is peanut oil.

Aradolene cream is a rubefacient. It contains diethylamine salicylate 5%, capsicum 0·4%, camphor oil 1·4%, menthol 2·5%.

Aramine ◊ metaraminol.

Arelix ◊ piretanide.

Arfonad ◊ trimetaphan.

argipressin (Pitressin) is synthetic vasopressin ◊ vasopressin.

Arilvax is a vaccine for yellow fever.

arnica flower (extract of) is used as a local application to bruises and sprains. It is of doubtful value. It is used in homeopathic medicine.

Arobon powder is used to treat diarrhoea. It contains ceratonia 80% and starch 15%. *Dose:* 20 to 40 g in water daily.

aromatic chalk powder ◊ chalk.

Arpicolin ◊ procyclidine.

Arpimycin (erythromycin ethyl succinate) ◊ erythromycin.

Arret: Each capsule contains loperamide 2 mg ◊ loperamide.

Artane ◊ benzhexol.

Artificial Suntan Lotion ◊ dihydroxyacetone.

Artracin ◊ indomethacin.

Arvin ◊ ancrod.

Asacol tablets ◊ mesalazine.

Ascabiol ◊ benzyl benzoate.

Ascalix ◊ piperazine.

ascorbic acid is vitamin C.

Aserbine contains malic acid, benzoic acid, salicylic acid and propylene glycol. The solution and cream are used to remove dead tissue around wounds, pressure sores and varicose ulcers.

Ashton and Parsons Powders: Each powder contains matricaria tincture (1 in 10) 4 mg and lactose 126 mg. It is used for infant stomach upsets.

Asilone is used to treat indigestion and peptic ulcers. The suspension contains polymethylsiloxane 125 mg, aluminium hydroxide gel 420 mg, and light magnesium oxide 70 mg. Tablets contain 200 mg of polymethylsiloxane, 500 mg of aluminium hydroxide and sorbitol 5 g. *Dose:* 5 to 10 ml or 1 to 2 tablets before meals and at bedtime.

Askit Powders each contain microfined aspirin 530 mg, aloxiprin 140 mg, caffeine citrate 110 mg, and aluminium glycinate 30 mg. Hot Lemon Askit contains the same active ingredients as Askit powders.

Asmaven ◊ salbutamol.

Asma-Vydrin* is used to treat bronchial asthma. It contains adrenaline 0·55%, atropine methonitrate 0·14% and papaverine hydrochloride 0·88%. *Dose:* 1 or 2 inhalations, repeated after 30 minutes if necessary up to a maximum of 12 inhalations in 24 hours.

Aspav tablets are used to relieve mild pain. Each tablet contains aspirin 400 mg and papaveretum 10 mg.

Aspellin rheumatic liniment contains aspirin 1·2%, menthol 1·4%, camphor 0·6% and methyl salicylate 0·6%.

Aspergum chewing gum tablets contain aspirin 227 mg.

aspirin (preparations include: Claradin, Solprin, sustained-release preparations: Breoprin, Caprin, Levius, Nu-Seals Aspirin; acetylsalicylic acid) is an effective mild pain reliever, it brings down the body's temperature (antipyretic) and it reduces inflammation. *Adverse effects:* Aspirin may produce irritation of the lining of the stomach and may cause nausea, vomiting, pain and bleeding from the stomach. This is not altered by changes in formulation and it may be unaccompanied by indigestion symptoms. Some people are allergic to aspirin and develop skin rashes and symptoms like those seen in hay-fever or asthma. It increases blood-clotting time and it may produce swelling of the throat (angioneurotic oedema) and nettle-rash (urticaria). High doses produce dizziness, noises in the ear (tinnitus), sweating, nausea, vomiting, mental confusion and over-breathing. *Precautions:* Aspirin should not be taken by anyone with a stomach upset or disorder such as peptic ulcer. It should never be taken on an empty stomach or with alcohol. Always take aspirin with a long drink of fluid. Aspirin should not be given to children under 12 years because of the risk of producing brain and liver damage (see warning on p. 194). Aspirin should not be given to people who suffer from haemophilia or to people on anticoagulant drugs. Aspirin may increase the effects of drugs used to treat diabetes, it increases the toxicity of sulphonamides, and it decreases the effects of some drugs used to treat gout. It should be given with caution to the elderly and debilitated who may be anaemic and to people who are anaemic or suffer from impaired kidney function. Its combination with other pain relievers may possibly produce kidney damage if such a mixture is taken regularly for many years. Aspirin is a drug and the consequences of overdose are serious but it is a most valuable drug if used sensibly. *Dose:* By mouth; for pain, 300 to 900 mg in one dose (1 to 3 tablets) up to a maximum of 3 tablets four times daily. Higher doses are used in acute rheumatic disorders.

Aspro: Each tablet contains microfined aspirin 320 mg. **Effervescent Aspro:** Each tablet contains aspirin 300 mg. **Aspro Clear:** Each soluble tablet contains aspirin 300 mg, in an effervescent basis.

astemizole (Hismanal) is an antihistamine. *Adverse effects* and *Precautions:*

See antihistamines (pp. 127–32). Causes less drowsiness. May cause weight gain. Do not take in pregnancy or when breast-feeding. *Dose:* 10 mg *once* daily, before a meal.

AT 10 ◊ dihydrotachysterol.

Atarax ◊ hydroxyzine.

atenolol (Tenormin, Tenormin LS) is a beta-receptor blocking drug used to treat hypertension, angina and cardiac arrhythmias. *Adverse effects* and *Precautions* ◊ propranolol. *Dose:* By mouth, 50 to 100 mg daily.

Atensine ◊ diazepam.

Ativan ◊ lorazepam.

Atkinson & Barker's Infants' Gripe Mixture: Each 5 ml contains light magnesium carbonate 250 mg, sodium bicarbonate 75 mg, sucrose 487·5 mg, alcohol 0·356 ml, fennel oil 0·004 ml, and dill oil 0·004 ml.

Atlas Dermalex cream contains allantoin 0·25%, squalane 3%, and triclosan 0·075% in a water mixable base. It is used to prevent pressure sores and irritation of the skin and also to treat dry skin. Allantoin occurs in comfrey root but it is manufactured. It is said to help wound healing. Squalane is obtained from fish oils (particularly shark oil), and is used in skin applications to aid penetration into the skin. Triclosan is an antibacterial drug that can produce contact dermatitis.

atracurium (Tracrium; atracrium besylate) is a non-depolarizing muscle relaxant. It is used to relax muscles during surgery. It is inactivated by thiopentone and other alkaline solutions. *Dose:* By intravenous injection,

300 to 600 micrograms per kg initially and then 100 to 200 micrograms per kg as required.

Atrixo Hand Cream contains a silicone oil and fatty alcohols with parabens.

Atromid-S ◊ clofibrate.

atropine (atropine methonitrate; atropine sulphate) acts on the brain and nerves. It initially stimulates the brain producing excitement and restlessness. In large doses it causes depression, drowsiness, delirum and coma. It reduces the muscular rigidity and salivation of Parkinsonism. It diminishes the production of saliva by the salivary glands and sweat by the sweat glands. It also reduces secretions produced by the bronchial tubes, stomach and gut. It relaxes involuntary muscles when they are in spasm, increases the heart rate and dilates small blood vessels. Atropine has three effects upon the eyes: it dilates the pupils, paralyses the muscles that help you to focus and increases the pressure of the fluid inside the eye. Atropine and atropine-related drugs are used to dry up secretion in the lungs before a general anaesthetic and to treat renal colic or colic from the gall-bladder, asthma, peptic ulcers, diarrhoea and Parkinsonism. Atropine should not be used to dilate pupils because of its prolonged action – it may trigger off an attack of glaucoma. *Adverse effects:* These include dryness of the mouth, thirst, dilatation of the pupils, dry skin, rapid beating of the heart, flushing, difficulty in urinating and constipation. Dizziness, vomiting and ataxia may occasionally occur. Toxic doses cause rapid beating of the heart, increased breathing, high tempera-

ture, rash, hallucinations, and delirium. Allergy to atropine is common – it causes skin rashes and red eyes (conjunctivitis). *Precautions:* Atropine should not be given to patients with glaucoma (closed angle or narrow angle). It should be given with caution to patients with enlarged prostate glands (it can cause retention of urine) and to patients with heart disorders. Its effects may be increased by other drugs, e.g. major tranquillizers, antidepressants, and antihistamines. It should not be given to patients who have received (in the previous ten days) or are receiving M.A.O. inhibitor antidepressant drugs. *Dose:* Atropine methonitrate is used mainly to treat congenital pyloric stenosis (narrowing of the outlet of the stomach) – 0·2 to 0·6 mg, half an hour before meals. Atropine sulphate: by mouth, 0·25 to 2 mg daily in single or divided doses; by injection, 0·25 to 2 mg (subcutaneous, intramuscular or intravenous).

Atrovent ◊ ipratropium.

Atrovent Forte inhaler is a bronchodilator containing ipratropium bromide 0·04 mg.

attapulgite ◊ activated attapulgite.

Attenuvax is a brand of measles vaccine.

Audax drops for earache contain choline salicylate 20% and macrogol 1·25%.

Audicort ear drops contain neomycin 0·35%, undecenoic acid 0·7%, triamcinolone acetonide 0·1% and benzocaine 5%.

Audinorm ◊ docusate sodium.

Augmentin antibiotic tablets contain clavulanic acid 125 mg and amoxycillin 250 mg. *Dose:* By mouth, 1 or 2 tablets three times a day. Also available as dispersible tablets and as junior suspension (amoxycillin 125 mg and clavulanic acid 62 mg in 5 ml) and paediatric suspension (125 mg and 31 mg in 5 ml respectively).

Auralgan ear drops: Each 1 ml of the drops contains phenazone 54 mg and benzocaine 14 mg. It is used to treat earache and to soften ear wax.

Auralgicin ear drops contain benzocaine 1·4%, ephedrine hydrochloride 1·0%, phenazone 5·5%, chlorbutol 1·0%, potassium hydroxyquinoline sulphate 0·1% and glycerin.

Auraltone ear drops contain phenazone 5% and benzocaine 1%.

auranofin (Ridaura) is an orally active gold compound used to treat rheumatoid arthritis. Its effectiveness is comparable to gold injections. *Adverse effects:* Diarrhoea, nausea, abdominal pain, ulceration of the intestine, rashes, itching, soreness and ulcers in mouth (stomatitis), loss of hair, blood disorders, kidney damage, scarring of the lungs (fibrosis). *Precautions:* Do not use in patients with a history of ulceration of the intestine, fibrosis of the lungs, severe dermatitis, bone marrow damage or severe blood disorders. Do not use in patients with severe kidney or liver disease, or in pregnancy or when breast-feeding. Use with caution in patients with impaired kidney or liver function, inflammatory bowel disease, skin rashes or bone marrow disease. Blood counts and urine tests for protein should be carried out before treatment and at one monthly intervals during treatment. Women of child-bearing age should, where appropriate, use contraceptives during and for six months after treatment. *Dose:* By mouth, 3 mg twice daily or 6 mg once daily initially for 3–6 months, increase if necessary to 3 mg three times dialy for a further three months.

Aureocort cream and ointment contain triamcinolone acetonide 0·1% and chlortetracycline hydrochloride 3%.

Aureomycin ◊ chlortetracycline.

Autan gel, spray and stick are insect-repellants.

Aveeno regular oilated bath additive in sachets is a soothing skin application which contains protein fraction of oats 40% and liquid paraffin 37%.

Aventyl ◊ nortriptyline.

Avloclor ◊ chloroquine.

Avomine ◊ promethazine.

Avrogel contains salicylic acid 1·5%, resorcinol monoacetate 1%, and hexachlorophane 0·2%.

Axid capsules ◊ nizatidine.

Ayds cubes contain liquid glucose with vitamin A 850 units, thiamine 0·425 mg, riboflavine 0·425 mg, nicotinic acid 6·49 mg, calcium 216·5 mg, phosphorus 107·6 mg, and iron 5·41 mg in each ounce.

Ayrtons Antiseptic Cream contains zinc oxide 5%, boric acid 1%, phenol 1%, methyl salicylate 0·5%, anhydrous lanolin 20%, paraffin ointment to 100%.

Ayrtons Bronchial Emulsion contains liquid paraffin 25%, glycerol 5%, sodium hypophosphite 1%, calcium hypophosphite 1%, compound benzoin tincture 2·5%, squill vinegar 5%, acetic acid 1%, and capsicum tincture 0·25%.

Ayrtons Burn Cream contains aminacrine hydrochloride 0·1% in a non-greasy basis.

Ayrtons Children's Cough Syrup Each 5 ml contains blackcurrant syrup 0·75 ml, wild cherry syrup 0·5 ml, tolu syrup 0·835 ml, glycerol 0·25 ml, and ipecacuanha liquid extract 0·00625 ml.

Ayrtons Cold Sore Lotion contains camphor 1·5%, eucalyptus oil 1·5%, flexible collodion 25%, and benzoin tincture to 100%.

Ayrtons Corn and Wart Paint contains salicylic acid 12·5%, zinc chloride 2%, hypophosphorous acid 0·1%, and collodion basis to 100%.

Ayrtons Earache Drops contain camphor 2·5%, cajuput oil 3·12%, rosemary oil 3·12% and safrol 3·12% in arachis oil. It is used to treat earache and to soften earwax.

Ayrtons Heart Shaped Indigestion Tablets Each contains sodium bicarbonate 55 mg, heavy magnesium carbonate 80 mg, calcium carbonate 475 mg, pepsin 1 mg, pancreatin 1 mg, and oleoresin capsicum 5 micrograms.

Ayrtons Insect Bite Cream contains antazoline hydrochloride 2%, benzocaine 3%, and cetrimide 0·5%.

Ayrtons IVY Tablets contain ferrous gluconate 98 mg, dried yeast 195 mg, vitamin B_1 170 micrograms, and ascorbic acid 4 mg.

Azactam ◊ aztreonam.

Azamune ◊ azathioprine.

azapropazone (Rheumox) is an antirheumatic drug. *Adverse effects:* These include gastric irritations and skin rashes. *Precautions:* It should be used with caution in patients with acute gastritis, impaired kidney function, or with gastric or duodenal ulcers. It potentiates the effects of warfarin. *Dose:* By mouth, up to 300 mg four times daily.

azatadine (Optimine; azatadine maleate) is an antihistamine. *Adverse effects* and *Precautions:* Similar to promethazine but azatadine is said to cause less drowsiness. *Dose:* By mouth, 1 to 2 mg twice daily.

azathioprine (Azamune; Imuran) is an immuno-suppressive drug. *Adverse effects:* It may damage the bone marrow, producing blood disorders, and cause muscle wasting and skin rashes. For further adverse effects ◊ mercaptopurine. *Precautions:* It should not be used in patients with impaired liver function and probably not in pregnancy. *Dose:* 2 to 5 mg per kg of body-weight daily according to needs. By mouth or injection.

azlocillin (Securopen) is a broad-spectrum penicillin antibiotic. *Adverse effects* and *Precautions* ◊ benzylpenicillin. It should not be used during the first three months of pregnancy. *Dose:* By intravenous injection (5 g every eight hours) or by intravenous infusion.

aztreonam (Azactam) is a beta-lactam antibiotic (e.g., penicillins and cephalosporins) with a wide spectrum of activity against bacteria, including beta-lactamase producing bacteria. *Adverse effects* include skin rashes, itching, blood disorders, liver damage, allergy, diarrhoea, nausea and/or vomiting, mouth ulcers, altered taste, cramps in the stomach, and pain and inflammation at the site of injection. It may rarely produce a thrush infection, weakness, confusion, dizziness, sweating, headache, muscle aches, fever, sneezing and a blocked nose, a fall in blood pressure, breast tenderness and bad breath. *Precautions:* It should be used with caution in patients sensitive to penicillins and cephalosporins. Breast-feeding mothers should not breast feed during treatment. It should not be used in pregnancy or in patients allergic to the drug. *Dose:* 3 g to 8 g daily in divided doses by intravenous injection or infusion or by intramuscular injection.

azulene is said to have anti-inflammatory properties.

Babelix Baby Cough Syrup Each 5 ml contains dilute acetic acid 0·4165 ml, tolu solution 0·0625 ml, and sucrose 2·225 g.

Baby Chest Rub contains camphor 5%, turpentine oil 5%, menthol 2%, eucalyptus oil 2%, cedar wood oil 0·5%, nutmeg oil 0·1%, and thyme oil 0·1%.

Baby Gripe Mixture Each 5 ml contains dill oil 0·0017 ml, caraway oil 0·0017 ml, and sodium bicarbonate 124 mg.

Baby Gum Lotion contains cetylpyridinium chloride 0·01%.

bacampicillin (Ambaxin; bacampicillin hydrochloride) is a broad-spectrum penicillin. It has effects and uses similar to those described under ampicillin. *Dose:* By mouth, 400 mg 2 to 3 times daily. Doubled in severe infections.

bacitracin is an antibiotic used mainly for application to the skin.

baclofen (Lioresal) is a muscle relaxant used to relieve spasm in conditions such as multiple sclerosis. *Adverse effects:* Include nausea, drowsiness, fatigue, depression and skin rashes. *Precautions:* It should not be used in patients with a history of epilepsy. *Dose:* 5 mg three times daily gradually increasing, if necessary.

Bactrian Antiseptic Cream contains cetrimide 1%.

Bactrim ◊ co-trimoxazole.

Bactroban ointment is used to treat bacterial skin infections, it contains mupirocin 2%.

Balmosa Cream is used to treat rheumatism. It contains menthol 2%, camphor 4%, methylsalicylate 4%, and capsicum 0·035%.

Balneum ◊ soya oil.

Balneum with Tar emolient bath oil is used to treat psoriasis. It contains soya oil 55% and coal tar 30%.

balsam of Peru is used in skin applications as a mild antiseptic. Continued use may cause allergic skin rashes.

Baltar shampoo is used to treat scalp disorders. It contains coal tar distillate (1·5%) in a soap-free shampoo. *Adverse effects:* Very rarely an allergic rash of the skin may occur. *Precautions:* Do not use on broken skin or on weeping or moist skin rashes. *Dose:* Use the shampoo one to three times weekly depending on the severity of the condition.

bamethan (bamethan sulphate) is used to treat disorders of the circulation. *Adverse effects:* Postural hypotension, tachycardia, flushing. *Precautions:* It should be used with caution in patients with angina. *Dose:* By mouth, 12·5 to 25 mg four times daily.

Banish contains benzethonium chloride 0·064%, *N*-(trichloromethylthio) cyclohex-4-ene-1,2-dicarboximide [captan] 0·108%, and sp. meth. indust. 16·7% by weight.

Banish Shampoo contains sodium *o*-phenylphenate tetrahydrate 0·3% and *para*-chloro-*meta*-xylenol 0·2%.

Banocide ◊ diethylcarbamazine.

Bansor Mouth and Throat Antiseptic contains cetrimide 0·01%.

Baratol ◊ indoramin.

barbital sodium ◊ barbitone sodium.

barbitone is a barbiturate sedative.

barbitone sodium (barbital sodium; soluble barbitone) is a long-acting barbiturate.

Barquinol HC cream contains hydrocortisone acetate 0·5% and cliquinol 3%.

basic fuchsin ◊ magenta.

Baxan ◊ cefadroxil.

Baycaron ◊ mefruside.

Bayolin cream is used in rheumatic conditions. It contains benzyl nicotinate, glycol salicylate and heparinoid.

Baypen ◊ mezlocillin.

BC500 is a multivitamin preparation. Each capsule contains thiamine mononitrate 25 mg, riboflavine 12·5 mg, nicotinamide 100 mg, pyridoxine hydrochloride 10 mg, cyanocobalamin 5 micrograms, ascorbic acid 500 mg and calcium pantothenate 20 mg.

BC 500 with iron is a compound iron preparation. Each tablet contains ferrous fumarate 200 mg, thiamine mononitrate 25 mg, riboflavine 12·5 mg, nicotinamide 100 mg, pyridoxine hydrochloride 10 mg, ascorbic acid 500 mg, calcium pantothenate 20 mg.

bearberry is obtained from the dried leaves of the bearberry. It has diuretic and astringent properties. It has been used to treat urethritis and cystitis.

beclamide (Nydrane; benzchlorpropamide) is an anti-convulsant drug used to treat epilepsy. It may cause stomach upsets, dizziness, nervousness and skin rash. *Dose:* By mouth, up to eight 500 mg tablets daily to start with and then reducing.

Becloforte ◊ beclomethasone.

beclomethasone (Propaderm; beclomethasone dipropionate) is a corticosteroid used in skin applications. It is also available as an inhaler (**Becloforte, Becodisks** and **Becotide**) for the treatment of asthma. The maximum daily dose is 20 inhalations. Fungal growth (thrush) in the mouth and throat can occur. A nasal spray (Beconase) is available for the treatment of nasal allergy.

Becodisks ◊ beclomethasone. The disk device has eight blisters on a circular disk. Each blister contains 100 or 200 micrograms of beclomethasone powder mixed with powdered lactose. The particle size of the beclomethasone is small enough to be breathed into the lungs whereas the powdered lactose is deposited in the mouth and throat. To use the device the patient raises the lid which punctures the blister with a needle and the patient inhales the powdered contents of the blister.

Beconase ◊ beclomethasone.

Becosym is a vitamin B complex preparation. The forte tablets contain thiamine hydrochloride 15 mg, riboflavine 15 mg, nicotinamide 50 mg and pyridoxine hydrochloride 10 mg. The syrup contains thiamide hydrochloride 5 mg, riboflavine 2 mg, nicotinamide 20 mg, pyridoxine hydrochloride 2 mg/ 5 ml.

Becotide ◊ beclomethasone.

Bedranol ◊ propranolol.

Beecham's Catarrh Capsules contain aluminium-guaiphenesin complex 127 mg and phenylpropanolamine hydrochloride 25 mg.

Beecham's Pills contain ginger 20·3 mg, coriander 4·4 mg, hard soap 9·7 mg, aloes 42 mg, rosemary oil 700 micrograms, juniper oil 700 micrograms, anise oil 200 micrograms, capsicum oleoresin 100 micrograms, ginger oleoresin 400 micrograms, and light magnesium carbonate 2·5 mg.

Beecham's Powders: Each sachet contains aspirin 600 mg and caffeine 50 mg, in a basis containing cinnamon oil.

Beecham's Powders + Hot Lemon: Each sachet contains aspirin 600 mg, caffeine 50 mg, and ascorbic acid 40 mg, in a basis containing lemon juice and cinnamon.

Beecham's Powders Mentholated: Each sachet contains aspirin 600 mg and caffeine 50 mg with menthol and flavourings.

Beecham's Powders (Tablet Form): Each tablet contains aspirin 300 mg and caffeine 25 mg, in a basis containing cinnamon oil.

Beehive balsam is a cough medicine containing in each 5 ml, purified honey 0·75 g, glycerin 0·5 ml, ipecacuanha liquid extract 0·015 ml and terpeneless lemon oil 0·00025 ml.

beeswax Yellow beeswax is used in skin applications. It may produce allergic reactions. White beeswax is bleached beeswax.

belladonna alkaloids and extracts ◊ atropine.

Bellocarb tablets contain belladonna dry extract 10 mg, magnesium carbonate 300 mg and magnesium trisilicate 300 mg.

Bemax is stabilized wheat germ which contains in each oz carbohydrate 10·1 g, protein 7·2 g, vitamin B_1 400 micrograms, vitamin B_2 160 micrograms, niacin 1·5 mg, vitamin B_6 270 micrograms, vitamin E 6·3 mg, manganese 3·6 mg, iron 1·9 mg, and copper 180 micrograms.

Benadon ◊ pyridoxine.

Benadryl ◊ diphenhydramine.

Bendogen ◊ bethanidine.

bendrofluazide (Aprinox; Berkozide; Centyl; Neo-Naclex; Urizide bendroflumethiazide) is a diuretic. It has effects, uses and adverse effects similar to those described under chlorothiazide. It is long acting (about eighteen hours). *Dose:* By mouth, 5 to 20 mg once a day, reducing to a maintenance dose of 2·5 to 10 mg daily or on alternate days.

bendroflumethiazide ◊ bendrofluazide.

Benemid ◊ probenecid.

Benerva ◊ thiamine.

Benerva compound is a proprietary preparation containing three B vitamins.

benethamine penicillin is a long-acting penicillin given by intramuscular injection. ◊ benzylpenicillin. It is a constituent of Triplopen.

Bengers contains partially dextrinised wheaten flour, sodium bicarbonate, and the pancreatic enzymes amylase and trypsin.

Bengué's Balsam cream and **ointment** contain menthol 20% and methyl salicylate. It is a rubefacient.

Benoral ◊ benorylate.

benorylate (Benoral, Triadol) is a paracetamol-aspirin ester. *Adverse effects:* It may produce nausea, gastric upset, drowsiness, dizziness, noises in the ears and skin rashes. *Precautions:* It should be used with caution in patients with impaired kidney or liver function. It should not be given to patients who are sensitive to aspirin. *Dose:* 10 ml suspension (4 g) twice daily; in tablet form (750 mg), two tablets three times daily.

Benoxinate ◊ oxybuprocaine.

Benoxyl 5, 10 and 20 ◊ benzoyl peroxide.

Benoxyl 5 and 10 with Sulphur is used to treat acne. The cream and lotion contain benzoyl peroxide 5% and sulphur 2%.

benperidol (Anquil) is an antipsychotic drug used to treat sexual deviants. *Adverse effects* and *Precautions* ◊ haloperidol. Parkinsonism, skin rashes and fall in blood pressure have been reported. *Dose:* By mouth, 0·25 to 1·5 mg daily in divided doses.

benserazide blocks the breakdown of levodopa in the body and is used to treat Parkinsonism.

Bentex ◊ benzhexol.

bentonite is a soapy clay used to make suspensions semi-solid.

Benylin Day and Night Cold Treatment contains 15 yellow and 5 blue tablets. Each yellow tablet contains paracetamol 500 mg and phenylpropanolamine hydrochloride 25 mg. Each blue tablet contains paracetamol 500 mg and diphenhydramine hydrochloride 25 mg. *Dose:* By mouth, 3 yellow tablets during the day and 1 blue tablet at night. *Warning:* May cause drowsiness and alcohol should be avoided.

Benylin Decongestant cough syrup contains diphenhydramine hydrochloride 14 mg, menthol 1·1 mg, pseudoephedrine hydrochloride 10 mg and sodium citrate 5 mg in each 5 ml. *Dose:* 10 ml four times a day.

Benylin Expectorant: Each 5 ml contains diphenhydramine hydrochloride 14 mg, ammonium chloride 135 mg, sodium citrate 57 mg, menthol 1·1 mg and alcohol 5%. *Dose:* 5 to 10 ml every two to three hours.

Benylin Fortified is used to treat dry irritating coughs. Each 5 ml contains diphenhydramine hydrochloride 14 mg, dextromethorphan hydrobromide 6·5 mg, sodium citrate 57 mg and menthol 1·1 mg.

Benylin Mentholated is used to treat coughs. It contains in each 5 ml diphenhydramine hydrochloride 14 mg, dextromethorphan hydrobromide 6·5 mg, pseudoephedrine hydrochloride 22·5 mg and menthol 1·75 mg.

Benylin with Codeine: As for Benylin Expectorant but the ammonium chloride is replaced by codeine phosphate 5·7 mg/5ml. *Dose:* 5 to 10 ml every two to three hours.

Benzagel 5 and 10 gel ◊ benzoyl peroxide.

benzalkonium (benzalkonium bromide and benzalkonium chloride) is used as an antiseptic and disinfectant. It is present in numerous skin creams and has effects like cetrimide. It is used as a preservative in eye drops and is present in some throat lozenges. In high concentrations it is used to remove warts.

benzathine penicillin (Penidrual) is a long-acting penicillin given by mouth and by intramuscular injection. *Dose:* Suspension, 10 ml (450 mg/10 ml) every six to eight hours.

benzchlorpropamide ◊ beclamide.

benzethonium (benzethonium chloride) is a detergent disinfectant with effects and uses similar to cetrimide.

benzhexol (Artane; Bentex; Broflex; benzhexol hydrochloride; trihexyphenidyl hydrochloride) is related to atropine. It diminishes salivation, increases heart rate, dilates the pupils and reduces spasm of involuntary muscles. It is used mainly to relieve muscle rigidity and increase mobility in patients suffering from Parkinsonism. *Adverse effects:* Include dizziness, dryness of the mouth, nausea, vomiting and blurred vision. These symptoms are dose-related and disappear when the dose is reduced. *Precautions:* Benzhexol should not be used in patients suffering from closed-angle glaucoma. *Dose:* By mouth, 1 to 2 mg three times-daily, increasing to a maintenance dose of 20 mg daily in divided doses.

benzocaine (ethyl aminobenzoate) is a local anaesthetic much less toxic than cocaine. It is available in lozenges to relieve pain in the mouth and throat and also in an ointment for local application.

benzoic acid is used as an antiseptic, antifungal and preservative. Benzoic acid compound mixture contains benzoic acid and salicylic acid. Whitfield's ointment contains benzoic acid, salicylic acid and emulsifying ointment.

benzoin (Sumatra benzoin) is from a balsamic resin used in inhalations to treat catarrh and in skin applications as an antiseptic and protective agent.

benzoyl peroxide (AcetOxyl; Acnegel; Benoxyl; Benzagel; Nericur; Panoxyl; Theraderm) has a similar disinfectant action to hydrogen peroxide and is used in skin creams and ointments used to treat acne. **Benoxyl 5** contains benzoyl peroxide 5% and **Benoxyl 10** contains benzoyl peroxide 10%. **Benoxyl 20** is used to clean. cutaneous ulcers. It contains benozyl peroxide 20%.

benzphetamine is an amphetamine-like drug used for slimming. *Dose:* By mouth, 25 to 50 mg two or three times daily between meals.

benzthiazide is a diuretic with similar effects to chlorothiazide. *Dose:* 50 to 200 mg daily.

benztropine (Cogentin; benztropine mesylate) produces effects similar to those described under atropine. It also has some antihistamine properties. *Dose:* By mouth, 0·5 to 6 mg daily.

benzydamine (Difflam; benzydamine hydrochloride) is a topical pain killer and anti-inflammatory agent used both as a mouth rinse and a skin cream for the treatment of sprains and strains.

benzyl alcohol is used as an antiseptic, and as a weak local anaesthetic, in various skin applications.

benzyl benzoate is used to treat scabies.

benzyl cinnamate is used as a preservative in creams and ointments.

benzylpenicillin (Crystapen; benzyl penicillin potassium; benzyl penicillin sodium; crystalline penicillin G; penicillin; penicillin G) is a very effective antibiotic from which a group of semi-synthetic penicillins have been developed. It is usually given by injection. *Adverse effects:* All penicillins carry the risk of hypersensitivity (what most doctors and patients call allergy). This allergy is more likely to develop if the penicillin is applied to the skin. Allergic reactions include nettle-rash (urticaria), dermatitis, swelling of the throat (angioneurotic oedema), fever, and occasionally swollen joints. Very rarely death may occur in an allergic person. These allergic reactions are more likely to occur after injections but may occur if the penicillin is taken by mouth in a patient who has been made sensitive to penicillin. Patients allergic to one type of penicillin are allergic to *all* penicillins and some of them will also be allergic to cephalosporins. Penicillin skin rashes may occur in allergic patients after drinking milk from cows treated for mastitis with penicillin. Onset of allergic symptoms may occur immediately, within a few hours, after a few days, or not until the next course of penicillin treatment. Penicillin taken by mouth may cause nausea, diarrhoea and an itching anus (pruritus ani). If sucked, penicillin tablets can cause a sore tongue (glossitis), and sore gums and lips with small ulcers (angular and aphthous stomatitis). There is no suitable test for sensitivity to penicillin. *Precautions:* Penicillin ointment or lozenges should *never* be used. Caution is necessary when giving a large dose of potassium or sodium salts of penicillin to patients with impaired kidney function or congestive heart failure. *Dose:* By mouth, 125 to 500 mg every four hours; by intra-muscular injection, 150 to 600 mg every four hours or every twelve hours.

benzyl salicylate is used in skin applications as an antiseptic, keratolytic, and irritant.

bephenium (Alcopar) is used to treat infestation with hookworms and roundworms. *Adverse effects:* Nausea, diarrhoea and vomiting occasionally occur. *Dose:* By mouth, 5 g of granules to be taken on an empty stomach.

berberine is given by mouth as a bitter tonic.

bergamot oil is obtained from the fresh peel of fruit of *Citrus bergamia* (*Rutaceae*). It is used in perfumes and especially in hair preparations. It is also used in suntan applications where the active ingredient is considered to be a psoralen. There is doubt that concentrations below 1% have any tanning effect and there is evidence that psoralens produce skin cancer in mice.

Bergasol total block cream is a sunscreen containing annamic esters and zinc oxide.

Berkatens ◊ verapamil.

Berkmycen ◊ oxytetracycline.

Berkolol ◊ propranolol.

Berkozide ◊ bendrofluazide.

Berotec ◊ fenoterol.

Beta-Cardone ◊ sotalol.

Betadine ◊ povidone iodine.

Betadren tablets ◊ pindolol.

betahistine (Serc; betahistine hydrochloride) is used to treat dizziness and Ménière's disease. It produces effects similar to histamine. *Adverse effects:* Include flushing, tingling, chilliness, nausea, vomiting, diarrhoea, rapid beating of the heart and shivering. *Precautions:* It should be given with caution to patients with asthma or peptic ulcer. It should not be given to children and should not be given with antihistamines. *Dose:* By mouth, 8 to 48 mg daily, in divided doses.

betaine hydrochloride when dissolved in water forms hydrochloric acid. It is used for patients who no longer produce hydrochloric acid in their stomachs.

Betaloc ◊ metoprolol.

Betaloc-SA contains metroprolol 200 mg in a slow-release form ◊ metoprolol.

betamethasone (Betnelan) is a corticosteroid; it has effects and uses similar to those of prednisolone. *Dose:* By mouth, 0·5 to 4 mg daily.

betamethasone benzoate is used in a variety of topical preparations in the treatment of various skin disorders. It has effects and uses similar to prednisolone.

betamethasone dipropionate (Diprosone) has actions similar to betamethasone valerate.

betamethasone sodium phosphate (Betnesol) is available in eye drops, nose drops, tablets and injections. Betamethasone is a corticosteroid; it has effects and uses similar to those of prednisolone. *Dose:* Tablets, 0·5 to 4 mg daily in divided doses.

betamethasone valerate (Betnovate; Bextasol) is available in creams, ointments and aerosols. It has effects and uses similar to prednisolone.

betaxolol (Betoptic; Kerlone) is a beta-receptor blocker drug. It is used to treat raised blood pressure. *Adverse effects:* These include nausea, vomiting, diarrhoea, insomnia, lassitude and ataxia. *Precautions:* Dose should be reduced in patients suffering from impaired kidney function. *Dose:* 20 mg daily (elderly patients 10 mg).

bethanecol (Mechothane; Myotonine Chloride; bethanecol chloride) is given to relieve acute or chronic urinary retention. It is a parasympathomimetic drug (anticholinesterase). *Adverse effects:* Include sweating, slowing of the pulse rate and intestinal colic particularly in the elderly. *Dose:* By mouth, 30 to 120 mg daily in divided doses; by subcutaneous injection, 2·5 to 30 mg daily.

bethanidine (Bendogen; Esbatal; bethanidine sulphate) works on the endings of nerves which supply blood vessels. It is used to treat raised blood pressure. *Adverse effects:* Bethanidine reduces the blood pressure, particularly on standing (postural hypotension). This may produce faintness and dizziness. Other adverse effects are similar to those produced by guanethidine. It may interfere with sexual function in the male (failure to ejaculate) but produces less diarrhoea than similar drugs and it does not produce pain in the parotid salivary glands. Bethanidine rarely produces depression. *Precautions* ◊ guanethidine. *Dose:* By mouth, initially 10 mg three times daily; maintenance dose, up to 200 mg daily in divided doses.

Betim ◊ timolol.

Betnelan ◊ betamethasone.

Betnesol ◊ betamethasone sodium phosphate.

Betnesol N topical applications contain betamethasone sodium phosphate with added neomycin.

Betnovate ◊ betamethasone valerate.

Betnovate C (Betnovate with added clioquinol).

Betnovate N (Betnovate with added neomycin).

Betnovate RD is a 1 in 4 dilution of Betnovate.

Betoptic eyedrops contain a beta-blocker drug, betaxolol 0·5%. Used to treat glaucoma ◊ betaxolol.

Bextasol inhaler is an aerosol containing betamethasone. Each metered inhalation provides 0·001 mg of betamethasone valerate. ◊ betamethasone. *Adverse effects:* Hoarseness and thrush infections of the throat (*Candida albicans*) have occurred in a few patients. *Dose:* 2 puffs four times daily initially, taking several weeks to reduce to an effective minimum maintenance dose.

bezafibrate (Bezalip; Bezalip-Mono) is used to reduce high blood fat levels. *Adverse effects:* Include abdominal discomfort and hyper-sensitivity. *Precautions:* It should not be used in patients with severe liver or kidney impairment nor in pregnancy. *Dose:* 400 to 600 mg daily with or after food.

Bezalip ◊ bezafibrate.

Bezalip-mono tablets ◊ bezafibrate.

Biactol contains sodium lauryl ether sulphate 2·6% and propylene phenoxetol 2%.

Bicillin powder for injection. Each ml contains procaine penicillin 300 mg and benzylpenicillin 60 mg.

BiCNU ◊ carmustine.

Bilarcil ◊ metriphonate.

Bile Beans contain cascara dry extract 17·8 mg, jalap resin 3·09 mg, pepper-mint oil 890 micrograms, ginger oleoresin 1·57 mg, powdered ginger 12·59 mg, capsicum oleoresin 790 micrograms, simple aqueous extract of colocynth (1–4) 4·97 mg, powdered aloes 23·4 mg, cardamom fruit 1·82 mg, ipmoea resin 4·38 mg, sodium tauroglycocholate 11·24 mg, powdered gentian 5·11 mg, liquorice 14·81 mg, and aqueous extract of gentian (1–1) 10·37 mg.

Biltricide ◊ praziquantel.

BiNovum is a biphasic oral contraceptive.

Bio-Dyne is an alcohol soluble extract of live yeast cells.

Biogastrone ◊ carbenoxolone.

Biomin (sulphosuccinated undecyclenic monoalkylolamide) ◊ undecenoic acid.

Biophylline syrup: A sugar-free syrup containing theophylline hydrate 125 mg (as sodium glycinate) per 5 ml ◊ theophylline. Used to treat asthma.

Bioplex mouth wash granules contain 1% carbenoxolone sodium. Used to treat mouth ulcers ◊ carbenoxolone.

Bioral (carbenoxolone sodium gel and pellets for treating mouth ulcers) ◊ carbenoxolone.

Biorphen ◊ orphenadrine.

Bio-Strath Drops is a similar preparation to Bio-Strath Elixir (see below) but without malt, honey or orange juice.

Bio-Strath Elixir contains 84% candida, 7% extract of malt, 4·5% honey (natural), 4·5% orange juice.

biotin is also known as vitamin H. It is widely distributed in plants and animals. The daily human requirement is unknown but approximately 0·3 mg is considered adequate, which is provided by a normal diet. There is no evidence of biotin deficiency in adults.

Biovital Liquid: Each 20 ml contains vitamin B_1 hydrochloride 600 micrograms, riboflavine (as riboflavine 5′-phosphate sodium) 2·6 mg, vitamin B_6 hydrochloride 1 mg, nicotinamide 10 mg, cyanocobalamin 2 micrograms, vitamin C 20 mg, iron (as sodium ferric citrate) 12 mg, manganese (as manganese citrate) 60 micrograms, and alcohol 2·341 g.

Biovital Tablets: Each contains vitamin B_1 600 micrograms, vitamin B_2 600 micrograms, vitamin B_6 1 mg, nicotinamide 10 mg, vitamin B_{12} 2 micrograms, vitamin C 20 mg, iron 32·5 mg, and manganese 150 micrograms.

Birley's Antacid Powder contains dried aluminium hydroxide gel 1%, magnesium trisilicate 11·1%, and light magnesium carbonate 87·9%.

bisacodyl (Dulcolax) is a laxative. It may cause abdominal cramps and suppositories may produce local rectal irritation. *Dose:* 5 to 10 mg daily by mouth or by rectum.

Bisks are a range of slimming foods which contain hypromellose with added vitamins and iron.

Bisma-Calna Cream contains bismuth carbonate 82·5 mg, light magnesium carbonate 262·5 mg, chalk 250 mg, and sodium bicarbonate 187·5 mg.

Bismag Powder contains light magnesium carbonate 47·6%, heavy magnesium carbonate 3%, sodium bicarbonate 48·15%, and bismuth carbonate 1·25%.

Bismag Tablets: Each contains sodium bicarbonate 149 mg, heavy magnesium carbonate 130 mg, and light magnesium carbonate 26 mg.

Bisma-Rex Antacid Powder contains sodium bicarbonate 65%, calcium carbonate 15%, heavy magnesium carbonate 5%, light kaolin 4%, bismuth carbonate 1%, light magnesium carbonate 10%, peppermint oil 0·125%.

Bisma-Rex Antacid Tablets: Each contains bismuth carbonate 13 mg, magnesium trisilicate 90 mg, calcium carbonate 460 mg, magnesium carbonate 160 mg, and peppermint oil 2 mg.

Bismodyne ointment to treat haemorrhoids contains bismuth subgallate 2%, hexachlorophane 0·5%, lignocaine 0·5%, zinc oxide 7·5%. Suppositories contain 150 mg, 2·5 mg, 10 mg and 120 mg respectively.

bismuth aluminate is an antacid.

Bismuthated Magnesia Ovals Tablets contain bismuth carbonate 3·9 mg, sodium bicarbonate 15·6 mg, heavy kaolin 62·5 mg, heavy magnesium carbonate 220 mg, and calcium carbonate 220 mg with peppermint flavour.

bismuth carbonate ◊ bismuth salts.

bismuth oxide ◊ bismuth salts.

bismuth oxychloride ◊ bismuth salts.

bismuth oxyquinolinate is used in cosmetics and as a protective in skin applications.

bismuth salicylate has doubtful astringent, protective and antacid properties ◊ bismuth salts.

bismuth salts were once widely used to treat syphilis. They are used in some antacid mixtures and as protectives in some skin powders, pastes and in suppositories.

bismuth subgallate is used as a dusting powder in some skin disorders and in suppositories in the treatment of haemorrhoids. It has astringent properties. *Adverse effects:* These include stomach upset, anorexia, headache, malaise, skin reactions, discolouration of mucous membrane and mild jaundice.

bismuth subiodide ◊ bismuth salts.

bismuth subnitrate is used as an astringent.

bismuth subsalicylate ◊ bismuth salicylate.

BiSoDoL Powder contains light magnesium carbonate 37·58%, heavy magnesium carbonate 2%, sodium

bicarbonate 57·88%, and diastase 1·4%.

BiSoDoL Tablets contain calcium carbonate 518 mg, light magnesium carbonate 66·7 mg, sodium bicarbonate 63·3 mg, diastase 9·2 mg, and sucrose 538 mg.

bisoprolol (Emcor; Monocor) is a selective beta-blocker used to treat angina and raised blood pressure. *Adverse effects* and *precautions* ◊ propranolol. *Dose:* By mouth, 10 to 20 mg once daily.

bitoscanate is used to treat hookworms. *Adverse effects:* These include nausea, vomiting, anorexia, abdominal pain, diarrhoea, headache and dizziness. *Dose:* By mouth, a single dose of 150 mg or in 3 divided doses of 100 mg at 12-hourly intervals.

blackcurrant syrup contains vitamin C and is used as a flavouring agent.

Blake's Witch Hazel Cream contains olive oil 29%, distilled with hazel 40%, lanolin 5%, calamine 5%.

bleomycin is used as an anti-cancer drug. It interferes with DNA synthesis in cancer cells inhibiting growth and cell divisions. *Adverse effects:* These include fever, anorexia, tiredness, nausea and pain and inflammation at the injection site. Occasionally it may produce delayed effects on the lungs (interstitial pneumonia and fibrosis). Previous radiotherapy to the chest is an aggravating factor. The majority of patients may develop hard (indurated) red, tender swellings on their finger tips, ridging of the nails, lesions of the skin and mucous membranes, blisters (bullae) over pressure points and loss of hair. These usually disappear once the drug is stopped. *Precautions:* It should not be used in pregnant or breast-feeding women nor in patients with reduced lung function. Patients on treatment should have their chest X-rayed weekly. *Dose:* By injection in a dose which varies according to the disorder being treated.

Blisteze cream contains strong ammonia solution 0·2%, aromatic ammonia solution 6·04%, camphor 0·9%, and liquefied phenol 0·49%.

Blistik Medicated Lip Balm contains padimate O, camphor, and thymol.

Blocadren ◊ timolol.

BN Liniment contains turpentine oil 12%, ammonium carbonate 4%, ammonium chloride 2% and strong ammonia solution 2%.

Bocasan has similar effects to hydrogen peroxide. It contains sodium perborate monohydrate 68·635% and sodium hydrogen tartrate 29·415%. *Dose:* Contents of 1 sachet dissolved in 30 ml warm water and used as a mouth rinse three times daily after meals.

boldo is obtained from dried boldo leaves and acts as a diuretic.

Boldolaxine: Each tablet contains boldo 70 mg, phenolphthalein 75 mg, belladonna dry extract 3 mg, and Iceland moss 10 mg.

Bolvidon ◊ mianserin.

Bon Voyage: Each tablet contains cyclizine hydrochloride 50 mg.

Bonjela gel is used to treat ulcers of the tongue and mouth, contains choline salicylate 8·7%, cetalkonium chloride 0·01%, menthol 0·057%, alcohol 39% and glycerin 4·6%.

Bonomint Laxative Chewing Gum: Each tablet contains yellow phenolphthalein 97 mg, with sucrose, liquid glucose, starch, and peppermint oil in a chewing gum basis.

Boots Adrenaline Cream contains adrenaline acid tartrate equivalent to adrenaline 0·02%. It is used as a rubefacient.

Boots Antiseptic Cream contains dybenal (2,4-dichlorobenzyl alcohol) 0·5%, cetrimide 0·5%, and allantoin 0·2%.

Boots Antiseptic Lozenges: Each contains tyrothricin 1 mg and benzocaine 5 mg.

Boots Antiseptic Mouthwash & Gargle (Strepsol) contains dybenal (2,4-dichlorobenzyl alcohol) 0·5% and amylmetacresol 0·125%.

Boots Antiseptic Throat Drops each contain amylmetacresol 0·023% with menthol and eucalyptus, cherry menthol, or lemon flavour.

Boots Bronchial Cough Mixture contains in each 5 ml ammonium chloride 150 mg, ammonium carbonate 100 mg, and guaiphenesin 32·5 mg.

Boots Bronchial Lozenges contain balsam of tolu 0·75%, menthol 0·2%, anise oil 0·24%, alcoholic extract from 0·06% of capsicum, aqueous extracts from 0·1% of coltsfoot leaf and 0·15% of horehound, liquorice juice 6·3%, basis to 100%.

Boots Catarrh Cough Syrup: Each 10 ml contains codeine phosphate 3 mg, creosote 0·015 ml, and sucrose 7·8 g.

Boots Catarrh Pastilles contain menthol 1%, creosote 0·2%, and pine oil 0·45%.

Boots Chilblain Cream contains benzyl alcohol 7·5% and eucalyptus oil 1%.

Boots Chilblain Tablets each contain acetomenaphthone 7 mg, nicotinic acid 25 mg, and calcium hydrogen phosphate 320 mg.

Boots Children's Cough Linctus contains in each 5 ml ephedrine hydrochloride 3 mg, ipecacuanha liquid extract 0·00625 ml, tolu syrup 1·4 ml, citric acid 50 mg, sodium benzoate 10 mg, and sucrose 2·78 g.

Boots Children's Cough Pastilles contain honey 4·5%, glycerol 6·2%, ipecacuanha liquid extract 0·4%, and squill liquid extract 0·05%.

Boots Children's Soluble Aspirin*: Each tablet contains aspirin 75 mg, calcium carbonate 25 mg, and anhydrous citric acid 7·5 mg.

Boots Children's Vitamin Syrup contains in each 5 ml vitamin A 2500 units, thiamine hydrochloride 500 micrograms, riboflavine 600 micrograms, nicotinamide 5 mg, ascorbic acid 15 mg, and ergocalciferol 250 units.

Boots Cold and Influenza Mixture contains in each 10 ml camphor 0·015 g, ether spirit 0·062 ml, squill vinegar 0·35 ml, strong ammonium acetate solution 0·16 ml, benzoic acid 0·02 g, anise oil 0·003 ml, and rectified spirit 0·56 ml.

Boots Cold Relief: Each sachet contains paracetamol 650 mg, sodium citrate ·500 mg, and ascorbic acid 50 mg, in a blackcurrant-flavoured basis.

Boots Cold Sore Lotion contains camphor 3%, menthol 0·2%, dybenal (2,4-dichlorobenzyl alcohol) 0·25%, basis to 100%.

Boots Compound Laxative Syrup of Figs contains in each 5 ml: 45% alcoholic extract from 750 mg of senna fruit, aqueous extract from 550 mg of fig, malt extract 1·87 g, clove oil 0·001 ml, peppermint oil 0·00025 ml, and benzoic acid 10 mg.

Boots Corn Paint contains salicylic acid 14·3%, lactic acid 3%, ether solvent 10·4%, chlorophyll 0·3%, flexible collodion to 100%.

Boots Cough Relief for Adults: Each 10 ml contains pholcodine 7·5 mg, diphenhydramine hydrochloride 25 mg, and dehydrated alcohol 0·48 ml.

Boots Cough Relief for Children: Each 5 ml contains pholcodine 1·5 mg, diphenhydramine hydrochloride 12·5 mg, and dehydrated alcohol 0·24 ml.

Boots Cream of Magnesia Tablets each contain magnesium hydroxide 300 mg.

Boots Day Cold Comfort Linctus contains in each 30 ml pholcodine 10 mg, pseudoephedrine hydrochloride 40 mg, and paracetamol 600 mg.

Boots Decongestant Nasal Spray contains xylometazoline hydrochloride 0·1%.

Boots Deep Skin Cleanser contains dichlorobenzyl alcohol 0·2%, salicylic acid 0·25%, glycerol 0·5%, and industrial methylated spirit 44%.

Boots Diarrhoea Mixture: Each 20 ml contains activated attapulgite 3 g.

Boots Diarrhoea Tablets: Each white tablet contains codeine phosphate 10 mg and each brown tablet contains activated attapulgite 600 mg.

Boots Dusting Powder contains allantoin 0·5%.

Boots Dyspepsia Tablets each contain magnesium trisilicate 100 mg, ginger 5 mg, and sodium bicarbonate 150 mg.

Boots Effervescent Vitamin C Tablets each contain ascorbic acid 1 g.

Boots Embrocation contains acetic acid (80%) 6·27%, camphor 0·8%, and turpentine oil 40%.

Boots Eye Drops contain boric acid 2·5%, sodium borate 0·5%, hamamelis water 5%, and cetrimide 0·01%.

Boots Family Antiseptic contains chloroxylenol 3%, terpineol 5%, and aromatic pine oil 1%.

Boots Feeding Bottle Sterilizer Tablets contain sodium hypochlorite equivalent to 1% available chlorine.

Boots Foot Cream contains menthol 1%, cetrimide 0·5%, and distearyl-dimethylammonium chloride 3·75%.

Boots Foot Powder contains dichlorophen 0·2%, sodium polymetaphosphate 4%, light kaolin 20%, basis to 100%.

Boots Glycerin Honey and Lemon Linctus contains in each 5 ml glycerol 0·75 ml, honey 1·11 g, citric acid monohydrate 50 mg, lemon oil 0·006 ml, and sucrose 1·96 g. **Boots Glycerin Honey and Lemon Linctus with Ipecacuanha** contains, in addition, ipecacuanha liquid extract 0·015 ml.

Boots Glycerin of Thymol Pastilles with AMC contain sodium benzoate 0·49%, sodium salicylate 0·3%, sodium carbonate 1%, glycerol 3·8%, menthol 0·02%, thymol 0·03%, pumilio pine oil 0·03%, cineole 0·08%, methyl salicylate 0·02%, and amylmetacresol 0·036%.

Boots Gripe Mixture: Each 5 ml contains sodium bicarbonate 50 mg, weak ginger tincture 0·025 ml, concentrated caraway water 0·075 ml, concentrated spearmint water (*B.P.C. 1959*) 0·005 ml, concentrated peppermint water 0·0005 ml, and rectified spirit 0·15 ml.

Boots Indigestion Mixture contains in each 5 ml light magnesium carbonate 225 mg, sodium bicarbonate 225 mg, calcium carbonate 175 mg, peppermint oil 0·005 ml, and chloroform water to 5 ml.

Boots Indigestion Powder: Each teaspoonful (approximately 2·5 g) contains heavy magnesium carbonate 937·5 mg, sodium bicarbonate 312·5 mg, magnesium trisilicate 234·4 mg, light kaolin 78·1 mg, and prepared chalk 937·5 mg.

Boots Insect Repellent Gel contains diethyltoluamide; **Liquid** contains diethyltoluamide, dimethyl phthalate, and dibutyl phthalate; and **Spray** contains diethyltoluamide.

Boots Iodized Throat Tablets each contain iodophenol 0·4 mg, potassium iodide 0·4 mg, phenol 1·5 mg, and menthol 2 mg.

Boots Iron Tonic Tablets each contain ferrous fumarate 25 mg, dried yeast 300 mg, and thiamine hydrochloride 3 mg.

Boots Medicated Foot Spray contains chlorhexidine acetate 0·1% and dichlorophen 0·25%.

Boots Medicated Skin Treatment Gel contains glycerol 3%, allontoin 0·2%, industrial methylated spirit 50%, menthol 0·08%, and dichlorobenzyl alcohol 0·5%.

Boots Medicated Skin Wash: Active ingredients are cetrimide 0·5% and benzalkonium chloride solution 0·5%.

Boots Medicated Soap contains triclocarbon 2%.

Boots Menthol and Wintergreen Embrocation contains menthol 2·4%, cineole 2%, cajuput oil 0·5%, eucalyptus oil 1·5%, methyl salicylate 14·2%.

Boots Nappy Rash Cream contains dimethicone 10% and cetrimide 0·5%.

Boots Night Cold Comfort Linctus contains in each 30 ml pseudoephedrine hydrochloride 40 mg, pholcodine 10

Boots Ointment for Haemorrhoids contains boric acid 2·1%, zinc oxide 4·2%, methyl salicylate 0·05%, belladonna liquid extract 0·72%, tannic acid 0·6% and heavy kaolin 16·8%.

Boots Original Indigestion Tablets each contain calcium carbonate 200 mg, magnesium trisilicae 60 mg, heavy magnesium carbonate 60 mg, sodium bicarbonate 60 mg, and ginger 10 mg.

Boots Pain Relieving Balm contains glycol monosalicylate 7·5%, ethyl nicotinate 1%, and vanillylnonamide 0·015%.

Boots Pink Healing Ointment contains zinc oxide 8%, methyl salicylate 3·6%, liquefied phenol 2%, menthol 0·01%, basis to 100%.

Boots Senna Laxative Tablets each contain standardized senna equivalent to 7·5 mg of total sennosides.

Boots Sore Mouth Gel contains lignocaine 0·6% and cetylpyridinium chloride 0·02%.

Boots Sore Mouth Pastilles contain 2,4-dichlorobenzyl alcohol 0·1%, alcoholic (90%) extractive from 0·1% of myrrh, glycerol 4·5%, menthol 0·02%.

Boots Sparkling Health Salt contains sucrose 38·9%, sodium bicarbonate 22·5%, tartaric acid 6·9%, citric acid 13·8%, dried magnesium sulphate 17·3%, and sodium chloride 0·6%.

Boots Sting Relief contains zinc oxide 2%, benzyl alcohol 1·5%, chloroxylenol 1·5%, eucalyptus oil 1%, borax

mg, diphenhydramine hydrochloride 10 mg, paracetamol 600 mg, and alcohol 6 ml.
1%, menthol 0·5%, camphor 0·25%, basis to 100%.

Boots Suppositories for Haemorrhoids each contain zinc oxide 230 mg, glycol monosalicylate 104 mg, benzyl alcohol 52 mg, and methyl salicylate 10 mg.

Boots Tooth Tincture contains menthol 5%, camphor 3·5%, clove oil 0·1%, and rectified spirit 64%.

Boots Vapour Rub contains eucalyptus oil 1·5%, camphor 6%, turpentine oil 4%, menthol 1%, thymol 0·1%, and pumilio pine oil 0·4%.

Boots Vegetable Laxative Tablets: Each contains compound colocynth extract 60 mg, hyoscyamus dry extract 15 mg, jalap resin 15 mg, and peppermint oil 0·006 ml.

Boots Vitamin and Iron Tonic contains in each 10 ml ferrous gluconate 225 mg, calcium gluconate 200 mg, manganese glycerophosphate 6 mg, caffeine 32 mg, thiamine hydrochloride 700 micrograms, riboflavine 400 micrograms, and nicotinamide 6 mg.

Boots Vitamin E Tablets: Each contains vitamin E 100 mg.

Boots Vitamin Yeast Tablets each contain dried yeast 300 mg, thiamine 0·192 mg, riboflavine 0·215 mg, and nicotinic acid 2·144 mg.

boracic acid ◊ borax.

borax (sodium borate; sodium tetraborate) and boric acid (boracic acid) have feeble anti-bacterial and anti-fungal properties. They are used as solutions, dusting powders, mouthwashes and lotions. *Adverse effects:* Repeated use of boric acid (in any way) may lead to cumulation of the drug in the body. Poisoning can result in skin rashes, vomiting, diarrhoea, coma and death. Convulsions, kidney failure and alterations in body temperature may occur. Deaths of children have occurred after applying boric acid solution or powder to damaged skin surfaces. Deaths have also followed the washing out of internal organs (such as the bladder) with boric acid solution. Boric acid has been excluded from most reputable baby dusting powders for many years. Never use preparations which contain borax or boric acid (boracic acid).

boric acid ◊ borax.

bornyl acetate ◊ pumilio pine oil.

borotannic complex hydrolyzes to boric acid and tannic acid.

Box's Herbal Ointment contains slippery elm 10·5%, althaea 10·5%, and yellow soft paraffin to 100%.

Box's Indigestion Pills each contain myrrh 25 mg, gentian extract 7·5 mg, ginger 25 mg, capsicum 25 mg, aloes 27·5 mg, and cajuput oil 0·0045 ml.

Box's Multivitamin Capsules contain DL-Alpha tocopheryl acetate 2·2 mg, ergocalciferol 0·625 micrograms, vitamin A palmitate 5·5 mg, thiamine mononitrate 3·125 mg, riboflavine 2·75 mg, sodium ascorbate 19·52 mg, ascorbic acid 31·73 mg, nicotinamide 22 mg, pyridoxine 0·55 mg, calcium pantothenate 8·75 mg, cyanocobalamin 1·25 micrograms, and folic acid 0·55 mg.

Bradilan ◊ nicofuranose.

Bradosol ◊ domiphen.

Bragg's Charcoal Biscuits contain carbo ligni (*B.P.C. 1934*) 12·5%.

Bragg's Charcoal Tablets contain carbo ligni (*B.P.C. 1934*) 90%.

Brasivol contains aluminium oxide in large particles and is used as an abrasive together with a cleansing base to treat acne.

Bretylate ◊ bretylium.

bretylium (Bretylate; bretylium tosylate) is used to treat cardiac arrhythmias. *Adverse effects:* These include hypotension and nausea. *Precautions:* Do not give with adrenaline or related drugs. *Dose:* By intramuscular injection, 5 mg per kg body-weight.

Brevidil M ◊ suxamethonium.

Brevinor tablets contain ethinyloestradiol 0·035 mg and norethisterone 0·5 mg. It is an oral contraceptive.

Bricanyl ◊ terbutaline.

Bricanyl Compound tablets contain terbutaline sulphate 2·5 mg and guaiphenesin 100 mg. Used to treat bronchial asthma.

Bricanyl Expectorant: Each 5 ml contains terbutaline sulphate 1·5 mg and guaiphenesin 66·5 mg. Used to treat bronchial asthma.

Bricanyl ◊ terbutaline.

Brietal Sodium ◊ methohexitone.

brilliant green is used as an antiseptic. It may produce sensitivity of the skin.

Brinaldix-K is a diuretic with added potassium. Each effervescent tablet contains clopamide 20 mg and potassium 12 mmol.

Britcin ◊ ampicillin.

Britiazim tablets are used to treat angina ◊ diltiazem.

British Anti-Lewisite ◊ dimercaprol.

Brocadopa ◊ levodopa.

Broflex ◊ benzhexol.

Brolene eye drops ◊ dibromopropamidine isethionate. Contain antiseptic, benzalkonium. Not suitable for contact lenses.

bromazepam (Lexotan) is an antianxiety drug with similar effects and adverse effects to diazepam ◊ diazepam. *Dose:* 1·5 to 6 mg three times daily.

bromelains are enzymes derived from the pineapple plant. They are said to reduce pain and swelling arising from sprains, strains and other soft tissue injuries.

bromhexine (bromhexine hydrochloride) is used as a cough expectorant. It may cause nausea and occasionally give a false value on certain liver function tests (serum transaminase). It should be used with caution by patients with stomach ulcers. *Dose:* 24 to 32 mg daily in divided doses.

bromide ◊ potassium bromide.

bromocriptine (Parlodel; bromocriptine mesylate) stimulates dopaminergic receptors. It is used in the treatment of Parkinsonism. It stops production of the milk-producing hormone, prolactin, and it is used to prevent lactation after childbirth and to treat infertility. *Adverse effects:* These include nausea, vomiting, dizziness, fall in blood pressure, dryness of the mouth, leg cramps, headaches, nasal congestion, constipation, sedation, hallucinations, and dystonias in patients with Parkinsonism. *Dose:* Varies according to disorder being treated.

brompheniramine (Dimotane, also in Dimotapp) is an antihistamine drug. *Dose:* By mouth, 12 to 24 mg twelve-hourly.

Bronal Cough and Catarrh Elixir contains in each 5 ml dextromethorphan hydrobromide 10 mg, ephedrine hydrochloride 10 mg, tolu solution 156·25 mg, menthol 0·5 mg, glycerol 0·25 ml, and alcohol (90%) 1 ml. **Diabetic Bronal** contains the same active ingredients.

Bronalin: Each 5 ml contains ammonium chloride 135 mg, diphenhydramine hydrochloride 14 mg, and sodium citrate 57 mg.

Bronalin Paediatric: Each 5 ml contains diphenhydramine hydrochloride 7 mg and sodium citrate 28·5 mg.

Bronchilator is used to treat bronchial asthma. Each aerosol dose contains isoetharine mesylate 350 micrograms, phenylephrine hydrochloride 70 micrograms and thenyldiamine hydrochloride 28 micrograms. *Dose:* 1 or 2 puffs repeated after 30 minutes if necessary up to a maximum of 16 puffs in 24 hours.

Bronchipax: Extended-action tablets each containing ephedrine resinate equivalent to ephedrine hydrochloride 30 mg, theophylline 40 mg, and salicylamide 250 mg.

Bronchodil ◊ reproterol.

bronopol is an anti-infective drug used as a preservative in shampoos, cosmetics and suppositories.

Brontussin: Each 5 ml contains dextromethorphan hydrobromide 5·7 mg, ephedrine hydrochloride 14·25 mg, ammonium chloride 47·5 mg, ipecacuanha liquid extract 0·0052 ml, glycerol 0·75 ml, and menthol 1·1 mg, in a basis free from sugar.

Brooklax Chocolate Laxative tablets contain chocolate 90% and yellow phenolphthalein 10%.

Brovon inhaler contains adrenaline 0·5%, atropine 0·14%, papaverine 0·88% and chlorbutol 0·5%. *Dose:* 1 or 2 inhalations.

Broxil ◊ phenethicillin.

Brufen ◊ ibuprofen.

Brulidine ◊ dibromopropamidine isethionate.

Brush-off paint for cold sores contains Betadine ◊ povidone iodine.

Buccastem ◊ prochlorperazine. Each buccal tablet contains 3 mg of prochlorperazine which dissolves to a gel when sucked between the upper lip and the gums. It is used to treat nausea, vomiting, motion sickness, migraine and vertigo.

buchu is an alcoholic extract of buchu leaves. It is a weak diuretic and urinary antiseptic.

buclizine (buclizine hydrochloride) is an antihistamine drug. *Dose:* By mouth, 25 to 50 mg two or three times daily.

budesonide (Pulmicort) is a corticosteroid drug inhaled into the lungs to treat asthma. Fungal growth in the mouth (thrush) and throat can occur. *Dose:* 1 puff twice daily, up to 6 puffs daily if necessary. Also available as a nasal spray (Rhinocort).

Buf Acne Lotion contains benzoyl peroxide 5%.

bufexamac (Parfenac) is a synthetic non-corticosteroid drug used in skin applications to treat inflammatory skin disorders.

bufylline is a derivative of theophylline.

bumetanide (Burinex) is a fast-acting diuretic. *Adverse effects* and *Precautions* ◊ frusemide. It may produce skin rashes, swelling of the breasts, cramps and muscle pains. *Dose:* 0·5 to 1 mg by intravenous or intramuscular injection; by mouth, 1 to 4 mg.

bupivacaine (Marcain; bupivacaine hydrochloride) is a local anaesthetic with effects and uses similar to lignocaine, but it works for a longer duration. Overdose may cause a fall in blood pressure, muscle twitching, depression of respiration and convulsions. Its use in childbirth may cause the baby's heart to slow down.

buprenorphine (Temgesic) is a narcotic pain reliever. It is longer acting than morphine. ◊ morphine. *Dose:* 0·3 to 0·6 mg every six hours by intramuscular injection or 0·2 to 0·4 mg by mouth, dissolving the tablets under the tongue.

Burinex ◊ bumetanide.

Burinex K is a diuretic with added potassium. Each tablet contains bumetanide 0·5 mg, and potassium chloride 573 mg. *Dose:* 2 tablets daily, as a single dose.

Burn Aid Cream contains aminacrine hydrochloride 0·1% and antazoline hydrochloride 1%.

Burneze aerosol contains mepyramine maleate 0·5% and benzocaine 1%.

Buscopan ◊ hyoscine butylbromide.

Buserelin (Superfact) is a gonadotrophin releasing hormone analogue which is used to treat secondary cancers which are dependent on male sex hormones for their growth. It initially stimulates the pituitary to produce LH. This stimulates the testes to produce testosterone, thereby effecting a reduction in LH which causes the testes to stop producing testosterone. *Dose:* By injection (buserelin 1 mg/ml) under the skin, 500 micrograms every 8 hours for 7 days. Nasal spray contains 100 micrograms of buserelin acetate in a metered spray – apply 1 spray into each nostril 6 times daily for 7 days.

Buspar tablets ◊ buspirone.

buspirone (Buspar) is an anti-anxiety drug not related to the benzodiazepines. *Adverse effects:* Dizziness, headache, nervousness, lightheadedness, excitement, nausea. Rarely, rapid beating of the heart, chest pain, drowsiness, confusion, dry mouth, fatigue, sweating. *Precautions:* Do not use in patients with epilepsy or who suffer from severe kidney or liver impairment. Do not use in pregnancy or when breast-feeding. Use with caution in patients who have suffered from kidney or liver disease in the past. In order to avoid withdrawal symptoms reduce benzodiazepines slowly over several weeks before starting a patient on buspirone. *Dose:* By mouth, 10 to 45 mg daily in divided doses.

busulphan (Myleran) is an anti-cancer drug. *Adverse effects:* It may cause blood disorders producing haemorrhages and bone-marrow damage (this may be irreversible and come on several months after treatment is stopped). Loss of periods (amenorrhoea) may start up to six months after the drug is stopped. It may also produce an 'Addison's-like' disease of underworking of the adrenal glands. *Precautions:* It should not be used in pregnancy, by breast-feeding mothers and where there is a risk that bone-marrow function is not too good after radiotherapy. *Dose:* 2 to 4 mg daily

initially, reducing to a maintenance of 0·5 to 2 mg daily by mouth.

butacaine sulphate is a local anaesthetic drug.

Butacote ◊ phenylbutazone.

butamyrate citrate has been used as a cough mixture.

Butazolidin ◊ phenylbutazone.

Butazone ◊ phenylbutazone.

butethamate citrate relaxes the muscles in the bronchi, and is used to treat bronchial asthma.

butobarbital ◊ butobarbitone.

butobarbitone (Soneryl; butobarbital) is an intermediate-acting barbiturate. It is used as a hypnotic. *Dose:* By mouth, 100 to 200 mg at night.

butoxyethyl nicotinate is used as an irritant skin application in rheumatic liniments.

butriptyline (Evadyne; butriptyline hydrochloride) is a tricyclic antidepressant drug. *Adverse effects* and *Precautions* ◊ imipramine. *Dose:* By mouth, 75 to 150 mg daily.

Buttercup Baby Cough Linctus: Each 5 ml contains squill liquid extract 0·0015 ml, ipecacuanha liquid extract 0·01 ml, chloroform spirit 0·225 ml, tolu solution 0·04 ml, and glycerol 1 ml.

Buttercup Medicated Sweets each contain honey 1%, lemon oil 0·68%, menthol 0·15%, and eucalyptus 0·15%.

Buttercup Syrup: Each 5 ml contains squill liquid extract 0·0031 ml, stronger capsicum tincture 0·0025 ml, strong ginger tincture 0·005 ml, acetic acid 0·19 ml, and chloroform 0·025 ml.

butyl aminobenzoate is a local anaesthetic used in creams and ointments.

Buxton Rubbing Bottle contains capsicum oleoresin 2·19%, turpentine oil 12·69%, camphor 2·3%, methyl salicylate 2·3%, and soft paraffin to 100%.

Cabdrivers Adult Cough Linctus: Each 5 ml contains dextromethorphan hydrobromide 11·5 mg, terpin hydrate 11·5 mg, menthol 7 mg, pumilio pine oil 0·0015 ml, eucalyptus oil 0·0025 ml, glycerol 0·825 ml, glucose syrup 2·83 ml, and alcohol (90%) 0·79 ml.

Cabdrivers Decongestant Tablets are used to relieve nasal congestion. Each tablet contains paracetamol 250 mg, salicyclamide 150 mg, caffeine 30 mg, and phenylephrine hydrochloride 5 mg.

Cabdrivers Diabetic Cough Linctus contains in 5 ml ephedrine hydrochloride 6 mg and dextromethorphan hydrobromide 15 mg.

Cabdrivers Junior Glucose Linctus contains ephedrine hydrochloride 0·12%, vinegar of ipecacuanha 4·17%, red-poppy syrup 8·33%, anise syrup 4·17%, and glucose syrup 26%.

cade oil (juniper tar) has been used in skin applications, to treat eczema and psoriasis, and in medicated soaps.

Cafadol: Each tablet contains paracetamol 500 mg and caffeine 30 mg. *Dose:* By mouth, 2 tablets three to four hourly.

Cafergot Tablets contain ergotamine tartrate 1 mg and caffeine 100 mg; suppositories contain ergotamine tartrate 2 mg, caffeine 100 mg, belladonna alkaloids 0·25 mg and isobutyl-allyl-barbituric acid 100 mg. *Dose:* Tablets, 2 at onset, no more than 4 tablets in twenty-four hours and no more than 10 tablets in one week. Suppositories, 1 at onset, no more than 2 in twenty-four hours and no more than six per week.

caffeine has a stimulating effect upon the central nervous system and a weak diuretic effect. It is present in many over-the-counter pain relievers, tonics and pick-me-ups. Read section on stimulants – caffeine, tea, coffee, cocoa and cola.

caffeine citrate ◊ caffeine.

Caffexen contains caffeine 2·74%, sodium iodide 9%, liquorice liquid extract 8·33%, chloroform 0·21%, and ephedrine hydrochloride 0·3%.

cajuput is a mild rubefacient.

Caladryl cream and **lotion** contains calamine 8%, diphenhydramine hydrochloride 1% (an antihistamine) and camphor 0·1%.

calamine is a zinc salt (zinc carbonate) coloured with an iron salt (ferric oxide). It is a mild astringent and is used in various skin applications.

Calamine Mousse Aerosol contains calamine and aloe vera moisturiser in a non-greasy mousse to help prevent peeling of the skin.

Calamousse foam spray contains calamine 4% and witch hazel extract 5%.

Calavite is a multivitamin preparation. Each tablet contains vitamin A 4,000 units, thiamine hydrochloride 500 micrograms, riboflavine 100 micrograms, nicotinamide 20 mg, ascorbic acid 15 mg and ergocalciferol 12·5 micrograms.

Calcicard tablets ◊ diltiazem.

calciferol (vitamin D_2) has the same effects and uses as vitamin D. Deficiency of vitamin D causes rickets in children and osteomalacia (bone softening) in adults. *Adverse effects:* Excessive daily doses (150,000 units or more) may produce loss of appetite, nausea, vomiting, diarrhoea, loss of weight, headache, dizziness and thirst. The amount of calcium in the urine is raised and the patient may develop kidney stones and calcification of arteries. *Precautions:* If 4,000 units of calciferol a day cures rickets it does not follow that bigger doses will 'cure' any better. It may be dangerous and liquid doses given to children should be measured very carefully. *Dose:* Daily requirements for an adult: 100 units. To treat rickets, etc.: up to 4,000 units daily.

Calcimax vitamin syrup: Each 5 ml contains calcium 76 mg, calciferol 400 units, thiamine 0·5 mg, riboflavine 0·125 mg, pyridoxine 0·125 mg, cyanocobalamin 0·125 micrograms, ascorbic acid 5 mg, and calcium pantothenate 0·125 mg. *Dose:* By mouth, 20 ml two or three times a day.

Calciparine ◊ heparin.

Calcisorb ◊ sodium cellulose phosphate.

Calcitare ◊ calcitonin.

calcitonin (Calcitare) is a hormone which lowers the calcium content of blood and is used in the treatment of Paget's disease. *Adverse effects:* These include nausea, tingling of the hands, and an unpleasant taste. *Precautions:* It should be avoided during pregnancy and lactation. *Dose:* 40 to 160 units daily, by injection.

calcitriol (Rocaltrol) is a vitamin D derivative that is indicated in certain cases of bone disease complicating renal failure. *Dose:* 1 to 2 micrograms daily.

calcium: Various salts of calcium are used to supplement the diet, as antacids and in skin preparations.

calcium acetate is used as a source of calcium in solutions used for dialysing blood. The powder may be used in skin applications.

calcium alginate is a calcium salt of alginic acid. It is used in special dressings as an absorbable material to stop bleeding from wounds. Alginate dressings may be removed by applying 3% sodium citrate solution for a few minutes and washing out with sterile water.

calcium carbonate (chalk) is an antacid present in many antacid mixtures. *Adverse effects:* Calcium carbonate may cause constipation. *Precautions:* Avoid prolonged or excessive dosage along with an increased intake of milk or cream. *Dose:* By mouth, 1 to 5 g according to needs of the patient.

calcium gluconate is used as a source of calcium to treat and prevent calcium deficiency disorders.

calcium hydrogen phosphate is used as a source of calcium to treat and prevent calcium deficiency disorders. It is also used as a fine abrasive in toothpastes.

calcium hydroxide is a weak alkali used in skin applications. It has been used as an antacid and astringent.

calcium hypophosphite has been used as a tonic.

calcium lactate is used as a source of calcium to treat and prevent calcium deficiency disorders.

calcium lactophosphate is of little use as a dietary supplement of calcium or as a tonic.

Calcium Leucovorin ◊ folinic acid.

calcium pantothenate (pantothenic acid) is considered to be a member of the vitamin B group but its significance in human nutrition has not been shown. No specific signs of deficiency have been noted, but it is widely distributed in food.

calcium phosphate is used to make powders and tablets. It is also used as a fine abrasive in toothpastes.

calcium polystyrene sulphonate (Calcium Resonium) is an ion-exchange resin used to reduce abnormally high blood potassium levels. *Dose:* By mouth, 15 g three or four times daily.

Calcium Resonium ◊ calcium polystyrene sulphonate.

Calcium-Sandoz ◊ calcium.

calcium sulphaloxate has similar effects to phthalylsulphathiazole. *Dose:* By mouth, 1 g three times daily.

calcium tetrahydrogen phosphate is used as a source of calcium to treat and prevent calcium deficiency disorders.

calcium thioglycollate is used to remove hairs from the body.

California Syrup of Figs contains aqueous extract of senna leaf (1–1) 27·8%.

Callusolve ◊ benzalkonium.

Calmurid ◊ urea.

Calmurid HC cream contains hydrocortisone 1%, urea 10% in a water miscible base.

Calogen contains arachis oil in water and is low in electrolytes. Used to treat kidney failure where a high energy, low fluid and low electrolyte diet is needed.

Calpol Infant and Calpol Six-Plus ◊ paracetamol.

Calsalettes tablets contain aloin 38 mg, starch 16 mg, lactose 3 mg, and stearic acid 3 mg.

Calsynar ◊ Salcatonin.

Calthor ◊ ciclacillin.

CAM syrup is used to treat bronchial asthma. Each 5 ml contains ephedrine hydrochloride 4 mg and butethamate citrate 4 mg. *Dose:* By mouth, 20 ml three or four times daily.

Camcolit ◊ lithium.

camomile has a strong aromatic odour and is a constituent of Radox.

Camoquin is used to prevent and treat malaria. Each tablet contains amodiaquine 200 mg.

camphor is used in cough medicines and to treat flatulence. It is also used in liniments.

camphorated opium tincture is used in some cough mixtures.

Canada balsam has a pleasant smell and bitter taste. It is used in some solvents.

Candida ◊ yeast.

Canesten ◊ clotrimazole.

Canestan HC cream contains hydrocortisone 1% and clotrimazole 1% ◊ hydrocortisone ◊ clotrimazole.

canrenoate potassium (Spiroctan-M) is converted in the body to the major metabolite of spironolactone. *Use, Adverse effects* and *Precautions* ◊ spir-onolactone. *Dose:* Up to 800 mg daily by slow intravenous injection.

Cantab-17 consists of apricot kernel powder which contains laetrile.

Cantaba: Each tablet contains aminobenzoic acid 100 mg.

Cantapollen Naturtabs: Each tablet contains bee pollen 250 mg and dolomite 350 mg.

Cantarna: Each tablet contains ribonucleic acids 450 mg.

Cantassium Discs: Each contains ferrous fumarate 2 mg, potassium sulphate 4 mg, potassium iodide 2 mg, and potassium bicarbonate 296 mg.

canthaxanthin is a carotenoid used to colour foodstuffs an orange-red colour. It is also used to colour medicines and by mouth it was used to colour the skin to produce an artificial suntan but was withdrawn because it may damage the eyes.

Cantil ◊ mepenzolate.

Cantil with Phenobarbitone tablets contain mepenzolate bromide 25 mg and phenobarbitone 15 mg.

Capastat ◊ capreomycin.

Capitol gel ◊ benzalkonium.

Caplenal ◊ allopurinol.

Capoten ◊ captopril.

Capozide ◊ same as Acezide.

capreomycin (Capastat) is an antibiotic used to treat tuberculosis. It is a reserve drug and should only be used along with other anti-tuberculous drugs in order to reduce the development of resistant bacteria. It is not absorbed from the gut and has to be given by intramuscular injection. *Adverse effects:* It may produce vertigo, noises in the ears, and disturbances of salt and water balance in the body. The most serious adverse effect is irreversible deafness and also progressive kidney damage. Allergic skin rashes and fever and transient liver abnormalities have been reported. *Precautions:* It should be given with caution to patients with impaired kidney function and to those patients with a history of allergy and sensitivity reaction to drugs. *Dose:* 1 g daily by intramuscular injection.

Caprin: Each tablet contains aspirin 324 mg. The tablet is formulated to release the aspirin in the intestine rather than the stomach. *Dose:* By mouth, 1 to 4 tablets three or four times daily.

Capsicin ◊ capsicum.

capsicum is made from chillies. It is used in some indigestion mixtures, and in irritant skin applications.

captopril (Acepril; Capoten) is used to treat raised blood pressure. *Adverse effects:* Skin rashes, disturbances of taste, gastro-intestinal pain, pins and needles in the hands, cough and hypersensitivity, bronchospasm, enlarged lymph glands and serum sickness. It may cause blood disorders and protein to appear in the urine. *Precautions:* It should not be used in patients

with previous hypersensitivity to captopril. Blood tests and urine tests (for protein) should be carried out at two-weekly intervals. It should only be used in pregnancy and breast-feeding mothers with utmost caution. It may produce a marked fall in blood pressure in patients under anaesthesia for surgery and in patients who are receiving diuretic therapy. *Dose:* By mouth, 25 to 150 mg daily in three divided doses. Maximum daily dose is 450 mg.

caraway (caraway seed) is the dried fruits of *Carum carvi*. It is an aromatic carminative. Caraway water is used in mixtures for children to help them bring up wind.

caraway oil is obtained by distillation from caraway.

carbachol shares some of the actions of acetylcholine and is called a parasympathomimetic drug. It is given after an abdominal operation to patients whose bowels are inactive (atony), or who cannot empty their bladders. It is also used in eye drops to reduce the pressure inside the eye in patients with glaucoma. *Adverse effects:* Sweating, nausea and faintness may occur. *Precautions:* Carbachol should not be given to patients with acute heart failure, bronchial asthma or peptic ulcer. It should not be applied to the eye of a patient with corneal abrasions because it may be absorbed. *Dose:* 0·25 to 0·5 mg by subcutaneous injection. By mouth, 1 to 2 mg.

carbamazepine (Tegretol) is an anticonvulsant drug. It has been used to treat facial neuralgia (trigeminal neuralgia). *Adverse effects:* Dryness of the mouth, nausea, diarrhoea, dizziness and double vision may occur. Skin rashes, blood disorders and jaundice may rarely occur. *Precautions:* It should not be given to patients who are taking M.A.O. inhibitor antidepressant drugs. It should preferably not be given during the first three months of pregnancy. *Dose:* By mouth, 200 to 1,200 mg daily in divided doses.

carbamide ◊ urea.

carbaryl (Carylderm; Clinicide; Derbac with carbaryl; Suleo-C) is an insecticide used for treating head lice.

Carbellon tablets are used as an antispasmodic to treat indigestion and to relieve stomach and bowel pains. Each tablet contains belladonna dry extract 6 mg, magnesium hydroxide 100 mg, charcoal 100 mg and peppermint oil 0·003 ml.

carbenicillin (Pyopen; carbenicillin sodium) is a semi-synthetic penicillin. To prevent the development of resistant bacteria its use is restricted to treating serious generalized infections. *Adverse effects* and *Precautions* are similar to those described under benzylpenicillin. It should not be used in ointments and drops or for infections that would respond to other more active penicillins. *Dose:* By intravenous injection, 20 to 30 g daily in divided doses, usually by injection into a saline infusion apparatus.

carbenoxolone (Biogastrone; Bioplex; Bioral; Duogastrone; Pyrogastrone; carbenoxolone sodium) is used to treat peptic ulcers. It seems to work better in patients who are up and about. *Adverse effects:* Carbenoxolone may cause salt and water retention in the body, which leads to swelling (oedema) and an increase in weight and blood pressure. This may trigger off heart failure in patients who may have some underlying heart disorder. It also reduces the blood potassium level which may cause weakness and damage to muscles. It may affect enzyme actions in the liver. *Precautions:* Carbenoxolone should be used with caution in patients with heart disease or high blood pressure. Treatment should never be continued for more than four to six weeks. Potassium usually has to be added to the diet. *Dose:* By mouth, initially 50 mg three times daily, increasing to 100 mg three times daily for no more than six weeks. Bioral gel and Bioral pellets are used to treat mouth ulcers. *Dose:* Bioral pellets: 1 every four to six hours.

carbidopa blocks the breakdown of levodopa in the body. It is used levodopa to treat Parkinsonism.

carbimazole (Neo-Mercazole) is an anti-thyroid drug. It reduces the production of thyroid hormone and therefore reduces the rate at which the body burns up energy (metabolic rate). *Adverse effects:* These usually occur in the first few months of treatment and include nausea, headache, skin rashes, joint swelling and fever, blood disorders and loss of hair (alopecia). *Precautions:* Infants should not be breastfed by mothers taking carbimazole. Patients should report sore throats, skin rashes or fever immediately, since these may precede blood disorders by several days. Caution is necessary when using this drug during pregnancy and in patients with any evidence that the thyroid gland is pressing on the windpipe. The drug may produce enlargement of the thyroid gland in high doses. *Dose:* By mouth, 10 to 60 mg daily in divided doses, reducing to a maintenance dose of 5 to 20 mg daily for several months.

carbocisteine (Mucodyne) is used to liquefy sputum. *Adverse effects* and *Precautions* ◊ acetylcysteine. *Dose:* By mouth, initially 750 mg three times daily, reducing when a satisfactory response is obtained.

Carbo-Cort contains hydrocortisone 0·25% and coal tar solution 3%.

Carbo-Dome ◊ tar.

carbo ligni ◊ activated charcoal.

Carbomix is a preparation of activated charcoal used to treat acute poisoning by mouth and drug overdosage.

carboplatin (Paraplatin) is an anticancer drug similar to cisplatin but produces fewer and less severe adverse effects ◊ cisplatin.

carboxymethylcellulose is used in various drug preparations as a suspending agent, dispersal agent, and emulsifying agent. It is used as a bulk laxative, and is widely used in the food industry.

carboxypolymethylene is a synthetic polymer used as a suspending agent to make gels and ointments, etc. It is also used as a binder and an emulsifying agent in the preparation of emulsions and lotions.

Carbralax suppositories contain sodium acid phosphate 1·72 g in a fizzy base. It is a laxative. *Dose:* One suppository, inserted 30 minutes before evacuation of the bowel is required. Moisten with water before use.

Cardamom Fruit is used to prepare a volatile oil with a strong aromatic odour.

Cardene ◊ nicardipine.

Cardiacap: Each capsule contains pentaerythritol tetranitrate 30 mg in a sustained-release form ◊ pentaerythritol.

carfecillin (Uticillin; carfecillin sodium) is a semi-synthetic penicillin which reaches high concentrations in the urine. It is used to treat infections of the urinary system. *Dose:* By mouth, 500 to 1,000 mg three times daily.

Carisoma ◊ carisoprodol.

carisoprodol (Carisoma) is a centrally acting muscle relaxant.

carmellose is a suspending agent used to make medicines. It is used to make jellies, pastes and even a saliva substitute. It is widely used in the food industry.

Carmil: Each 5 ml contains pectin 40 mg, light kaolin 500 mg, morphine hydrochloride 350 micrograms, and atropine methonitrate 100 micrograms.

carmustine (BiCNU) is an alkylating agent used in the treatment of cancer. *Adverse effects:* These include nausea and vomiting, decreases in white blood cell count, burning at the site of injection and flushing of the skin. *Dose:* Varies according to the disorder being treated.

Carnation Callous. Caps contain an ointment of salicylic acid 40%.

Carnation Corn Caps contain an ointment of salicylic acid 40%.

carob bean flour (ceratonia) is a thickening agent used to treat vomiting and diarrhoea in infants.

carteolol is a beta-blocker used in Teoptic eyedrops to treat glaucoma ◊ Teoptic eyedrops.

Carters Infurno Embrocation contains methyl salicylate 17%, capsicin 1·25%, eucalpytus oil 4·25%, rectified camphor oil 4·25%, and menthol 0·8%.

Carters Little Pills each contain phenolphthalein 16 mg and aloin 8 mg.

Carylderm ◊ carbaryl.

caryophylli oil ◊ oil of cloves.

caryophyllum ◊ oil of cloves.

casanthranol is derived from cascara ◊ cascara.

cascara: The dried bark of *Rhamnus purshiana*. It is used to treat constipation.

cascarilla bark ◊ cascara.

casein is a protein obtained from milk.

cassia oil is similar to cinnamon oil and is used as a flavouring agent.

Castellan No. 10 Bronchial Pastilles contain liquorice extract 5·7%, menthol 0·5%, peppermint oil 0·025%, anise oil 0·3%, capsicin 0·001%, benzoin tincture 0·5%, and clove oil 0·05%.

Castellan No. 10 Cough Mixture contains morphine hydrochloride 0·025%, liquorice liquid extract 1%, squill liquid extract 1·5%, acetic acid 0·48%, ether 0·375%, chloroform 0·5%, anise oil 0·094%, and peppermint oil 0·094%.

Castellani's paint ◊ magenta paint.

castor oil is used as an irritant laxative. Large doses may produce nausea, vomiting, colic and severe loss of fluid with purgation. It is also used as a soothing application in eye drops and skin ointments.

Catapres ◊ clonidine.

catechu is an astringent and is given as an ingredient in some anti-diarrhoea mixtures. In a diluted dose it is used as a gargle.

Caved-S is used to treat indigestion and peptic ulcers. Each tablet contains powdered black liquorice 380 mg, bismuth subnitrate 100 mg, aluminium hydroxide gel 100 mg, light magnesium carbonate 200 mg, sodium bicarbonate 100 mg, and powdered frangula bark 30 mg. *Dose:* For gastric ulcer, 2 three times daily.

CCNU ◊ lomustine.

Ceanel Concentrate (shampoo for psoriasis) contains phenylethyl alcohol 7·5%, cetrimide 10% and undecenoic acid 1%.

Ce-Cobalin Syrup: Each ml contains cyanocobalamin 6 micrograms and ascorbic acid 2 mg. *Dose:* By mouth, 5 to 10 ml three times a day.

cedar wood oil (cedar oil) is used in perfumes.

Cedilanid ◊ deslanoside.

Cedocard ◊ isosorbide dinitrate.

Cedocard IV ◊ isosorbide dinitrate.

Cedocard Retard tablets contain isosorbide dinitrate 20 mg in sustained-release form ◊ isosorbide dinitrate.

cefaclor (Distaclor) is a cephalosporin antibiotic. *Adverse effects:* Nausea, vomiting, diarrhoea and allergic reactions, e.g., skin rashes. *Precautions:* Patients can be allergic to cephalosporin antibiotics. Its safety in pregnancy has not been shown. Patients allergic to penicillin may be allergic to cefaclor. It may produce a positive Coomb's test. *Dose:* By mouth, 250 mg every eight hours, maximum 2 g daily.

cefadroxil (Baxan) is a cephalosporin antibiotic with similar properties to cefaclor. *Adverse effects* and *Precautions* ◊ cefaclor. *Dose:* By mouth, 500 mg to 1 g twice daily.

cefamandole ◊ cephamandole.

Cefizox injection ◊ ceftizoxime.

cefotaxime (Claforan) is a cephalosporin antibiotic. *Adverse effects* and *Precautions* ◊ cefaclor. *Dose:* By intramuscular or intravenous injection, 1 g every twelve hours.

cefoxitin (Mefoxin) is a cephalosporin antibiotic. *Adverse effects* and *Precautions* ◊ cefaclor. Requires reduced dosage in patients with impaired kidney function. May give a false positive test for sugar in the urine. *Dose:* By intramuscular or intravenous injection, 1 to 2 g every eight hours.

cefsulodin (Monaspor) is a cephalosporin antibiotic with similar properties to cefaclor. *Adverse effects* and *Precautions* ◊ cefaclor. *Dose:* By injection, 1 to 4 g daily in divided doses.

ceftazidime (Fortum) is a cephalosporin antibiotic cefaclor. *Dose:* By injection, 1–6 g daily in divided doses.

Ceftizoxime (Cefizox) is a cephalosporin antibiotic available for injection. *Adverse effects:* Include swelling, pain and tenderness at the site of infection. Hypersensitivity reactions (rash, itching, fever), diarrhoea, nausea and vomiting, inflammation of the vagina (vaginitis) and blood disorders may occur. *Precautions:* It should be given with caution to patients sensitive to penicillin, and to patients with impaired function of their kidneys. It should be used with caution in pregnant and breast-feeding women and its benefits and potential risks carefully evaluated. *Dose:* Varies according to the disorder being treated, 0·5 to 3 g 8 to 12 hourly by intramuscular or intravenous injection. For gonorrhoea 1 g single dose by intramuscular injection.

cefuroxime (Zinacef, Zinnatt) is a cephalosporin antibiotic. *Adverse effects* and *Precautions* ◊ cefaclor. A reduced dosage is required in patients with impaired kidney function. *Dose:* By intramuscular or intravenous injection, 750 mg every eight hours.

Celaton CH3 Plus Tablets each contain riboflavine 0·6 mg, pyridoxine hydrochloride 0·7 mg, nicotinamide 6 mg, ascorbic acid 25 mg, vitamin E acetate 1·4 mg, rutin 1 mg, methionine 1 mg, calcium pantothenate 2·5 mg, thiamine hydrochloride 0·6 mg, cyanocobalamin 1 microgram, biotin 1 microgram, vitamin A acetate 2 mg, procaine hydrochloride 15 mg, ginseng powder 2 mg, and ergocalciferol 5 micrograms.

Celaton CH3 Strong and Calm Tablets each contain para-aminobenzoic acid 7·5 mg, biotin 1 microgram, vitamin A acetate 0·5 mg, vitamin B_1 0·6 mg, vitamin B_2 0·6 mg, vitamin B_6 0·7 mg, nicotinamide 6 mg, calcium pantothenate 2·5 mg, cyanocobalamin 1 microgram, ascorbic acid 25 mg, vitamin D_2 2·5 micrograms, vitamin E acetate 10·5 mg, sucrose 141 mg, acacia 3 mg, povidone 6·25 mg, methyl *p*-hydroxybenzoate 0·22 mg, and sodium propyl-*p*-hydroxybenzoate 0·11 mg.

Celaton CH3 Tri-Plus Tablets each contain vitamin A acetate 0·5 mg, vitamin B_2 0·6 mg, vitamin B_1 0·6 mg, vitamin B_2 0·7 mg, nicotinamide 6 mg, biotin 1 microgram, calcium pantothenate 2·5 mg, cyanocobalamin 2·5 micrograms, ascorbic acid 25 mg, vitamin D 2·5 micrograms, vitamin E 10·5 mg, para-aminobenzoic acid 7·5 mg, ginseng root 2 mg, heart powder 30 mg, brain powder 30 mg, and intrinsic factor 20 mg.

Celbenin ◊ methicillin.

Celerub is used to treat rheumatic pain, fibrositis and lumbago. It contains methyl salicylate 15%, celery seed oil 5%, clove oil 3·5%, thyme oil 3·5%, pumilo pine oil 3·5%, camphor liniment 20%, menthol 10% and salicylic acid 20%.

Celevac ◊ methylcellulose.

Cellucon ◊ methylcellulose.

Cendevax is a brand of rubella (German measles) vaccine.

Centurion pastilles are a vitamin supplement. Each pastille contains vitamin C 75 mg.

Centyl ◊ bendrofluazide.

Centyl-K is a diuretic with added potassium. Each tablet contains bendrofluazide 2·5 mg and potassium 7·7 mmol in sustained-release form.

cephalexin (Ceporex; Keflex; Keflex C) is a cephalosporin antibiotic. *Adverse effects* and *Precautions* ◊ cefaclor. Reduced dosage required in patients with impaired kidney function. May give a false positive for sugar in the urine. *Dose:* By mouth, 250 to 500 mg every six hours.

cephalosporin antibiotics. *Adverse effects:* These include nausea, vomiting, loss of appetite and diarrhoea. Skin rashes may occur particularly in patients who are allergic to penicillin. High doses may produce kidney damage, convulsions and a bleeding type of anaemia. They may interfere with certain blood tests used to cross-match blood for patients requiring a blood transfusion. *Precautions:* These drugs should be used with caution in patients who are allergic to penicillin. Some diuretics increase their toxicity. They should be given with caution to patients with impaired kidney function.

cephalothin (Keflin) is a cephalosporin antibiotic. *Adverse effects* and *Precautions* ◊ cefaclor. Reduced dosage is required in patients with impaired kidney function. Intramuscular injections are painful. *Drug interactions* may occur with ethacrynic acid, frusemide and gentamycin producing increased risk of kidney damage. *Dose:* By intravenous injection or infusion 1 g every four hours; maximum 12 g daily.

cephamandole (Kefadol) is a cephalosporin antibiotic. *Adverse effects* and *Precautions* ◊ cefaclor. Reduced dosage is required in patients with impaired kidney function. May give false positive test for glucose in the urine. *Dose:* By intramuscular or intravenous injection or infusion 0·5 to 2 g every four to eight hours.

cephamycins are related to cephalosporin. ◊ cephalosporin.

cephazolin (Kefzol) is a cephalosporin antibiotic. *Adverse effects* and *Precautions* ◊ cefaclor. Reduced dosage required in patients with impaired kidney function. May give false positive test for glucose in the urine. *Dose:* By intramuscular injection or intravenous injection or infusion, 0·5 to 1 g every six to twelve hours.

Cephos Powders each contain aspirin 570 mg, caffeine 20 mg, and salicylamide 40 mg.

Cephos Tablets: Each tablet contains aspirin 285 mg, salicylamide 20 mg, and caffeine 10 mg.

cephradine (Velosef) is a cephalosporin antibiotic. ◊ cefaclor. *Dose:* By mouth or by intravenous or intramuscular injection, 250 to 500 mg four times daily.

Ceporex (cephalexin) ◊ cephalosporin antibiotics.

Cepton Cleansing Milk contains chlorhexidine gluconate solution 2·5%.

Cepton Medicated Clear Gel contains chlorhexidine gluconate solution 2·5%.

Ceratonia ◊ carob bean flour.

Cerubidin ◊ daunorubicin.

Cerumol ear drops contain turpentine oil 10%, paradichlorobenzene 2% and chlorbutol 5% in arachis oil. Used to dissolve ear wax.

Cervagem pessaries ◊ gemeprost.

Cesamet ◊ nabilone.

cetalkonium is used as an antiseptic. It has effects like cetrimide.

Cetanorm is an antiseptic cream containing benzalkonium chloride 0·1%, chlorbutol 0·1%, cetrimide 0·4%, polyoxyethylenenony-phenol 2% and aluminium dihydroxyallantoinate 0·375%.

Cetavlex ◊ cetrimide.

Cetavlon ◊ cetrimide.

Cetavlon PC is a shampoo containing cetrimide 17·5% ◊ cetrimide.

cetomacrogol is used in the preparation of stable oil in water emulsions for skin creams and ear drops.

cetostearyl alcohol is used as a constituent in the preparation of ointments and creams, to increase the emollient properties.

Cetrimax Antiseptic Cream contains cetrimide 0·5%.

cetrimide (Cetavlon Cox antiseptic cream; Vesagex) is a surface active drug with antiseptic, emulsifying and detergent properties. It is used as a skin-cleansing agent in numerous preparations and also in shampoos. Some patients may develop sensitivity to cetrimide after repeated applications. It may cause the skin of the scalp to become very dry.

cetyl alcohol is used in the preparation of ointments and creams.

cetylpyridinium (cetylpyridinium chloride) is used as an antiseptic. It has effects and uses similar to those described under cetrimide. It is also used in cough medicines.

chalk (aromatic chalk powder) is an antacid.

chamomile (chamomile flowers) has a pleasant aromatic odour and appears in some cough medicines, indigestion remedies and hair preparations.

Chap Stick ointment contains wool fat 1%, padimate 0·4%, and camphor 1·6% in a wax basis.

charcoal is used to absorb gases in the treatment of flatulence and distension, as a deodorant for foul-smelling wounds and is given as a thick suspension in the first aid treatment of poisoning with some drugs to delay absorption into the body.

Chemocycline ◊ oxytetracycline.

Chemotrim ◊ co-trimoxazole.

Chendol ◊ chenodeoxycholic acid.

chenodeoxycholic acid (Chendol, Chenofalk) is used to dissolve cholesterol gallstones. Cholesterol stones, coated with calcium, or stones composed of bile pigments are not dissolved by chenodeoxycholic acid. It is a primary bile acid and reduces the output of cholesterol secreted into the bile. *Precautions:* It should not be used in

patients with radio-opaque calcified gallstones nor in patients with non-functioning gall-bladders. It should not be used in women of childbearing age, nor in patients with chronic liver disease or with inflammatory disorders of the gut. *Adverse effects:* Diarrhoea and pruritus (itching). *Dose:* By mouth, 10 to 15 mg per kg of body-weight daily in divided doses. Treatment may take up to two years.

Chenofalk ◊ chenodeoxycholic acid.

Cherrols are antiseptic lozenges used to treat sore throats. Each lozenge contains menthol 0·015% and eucalyptus oil 0·013%.

Chilblain Cream contains histamine acid phosphate 0·1% and methyl nicotinate 1%.

Child's Pain Elixir: Each 5 ml contains paracetamol 120 mg.

Chilvax Tablets: Each contain paracetamol 400 mg, thiamine hydrochloride 0·5 mg, caffeine 15 mg, and nicotinamide 5 mg.

Chloractil ◊ chlorpromazine.

chloral hydrate (Noctec) is a sleeping drug used mainly in children and the elderly. *Adverse effects:* Chloral hydrate may cause headache, nausea, dizziness, skin rashes and blood disorders. *Precautions:* It is a gastric irritant and must be taken well diluted. Chloral hydrate should not be used in patients with impaired liver, heart or kidney function or peptic ulcers. Some patients may develop drowsiness, disorientation and paranoid ideas. If the patient taking chloral hydrate regularly has a drink of alcohol he may experience flushing, rapid beating of the heart, and faintness due to a fall in blood pressure. *Drug dependence:* It produces drug dependence of the barbiturate/alcohol type and increases the effects of alcohol. *Dose:* By mouth, 300 mg to 2 g.

chlorambucil (Leukeran) is an anticancer drug. *Adverse effects:* Large doses can produce nausea and vomiting. Prolonged large doses can produce irreversible damage to the bone marrow, producing severe blood disorders. *Precautions:* It should not be used in pregnancy and not when there is a risk that bone-marrow function is decreased (e.g., within four weeks of radiotherapy or another anti-cancer drug). *Dose:* Varies according to the condition being treated.

chloramphenicol (Chloromycetin; Kemicetine) is an antibiotic which has a wide range of activity against infecting organisms. It is a drug of choice in treating typhoid and paratyphoid fever. Chloramphenicol eye drops and ear drops are used for superficial infections. *Adverse effects:* Serious effects include blood disorders which may be fatal, kidney damage, jaundice, inflammation of the main nerves of the eye (optic neuritis), and ulcers in the mouth with skin lesions (Stevens-Johnson syndrome). Ointments and drops may cause allergic skin rashes which may be serious in people sensitive to chloramphenicol. Dryness of the mouth, nausea, vomiting, diarrhoea and fungus infection (e.g., thrush – *Candida albicans*) of the gut may rarely occur; this causes a sore tongue and mouth, irritation and soreness in the anus and vagina and very rarely pneumonia. Blood disorders may occur with a relatively small dosage and develop up to several months after stopping treatment. *Precautions:* Chloramphenicol should not be used in bacterial infections except in typhoid and paratyphoid fever. *Dose:* By mouth, 1·5 to 3 g daily in divided doses.

chloramphenicol palmitate (Chloromycetin Palmitate) is used in mixtures, and chloramphenicol sodium succinate (Chloromycetin succinate) is used for injections. ◊ chloramphenicol.

Chlorasept ◊ chlorhexidine.

Chloraseptic ◊ phenol.

Chlorasol ◊ sodium hypochlorite.

chlorate of lime ◊ chlorinated lime.

chlorbutanol ◊ chlorbutol.

chlorbutol is a mild sedative with effects similar to chloral hydrate. It is also a local pain reliever, and has anti-bacterial and antifungal properties. It is used in nose sprays and ointments and also as a preservative in eye drops.

chlordiazepoxide (Librium; Tropium; chlordiazepoxide hydrochloride) is an anti-anxiety drug. *Adverse effects:* Chlordiazepoxide may produce drowsiness, dizziness, fatigue, apathy, irritability and unsteady walking (ataxia). It may also cause depression, indigestion and changes in sexual drive (libido). Large doses may cause faintness. Rarely it may produce skin rashes, headache, nausea, constipation, frequency of urination, and irregularities of menstruation. Blood and liver disorders have very occasionally been reported. Sometimes chlordiazepoxide may make some patients very excited and restless instead of sedated (what is called a paradoxical reaction). *Precautions:* Chlordiazepoxide should be given with caution to patients with impaired kidney or liver function and to the elderly or debilitated when 'normal' doses may make the patients unsteady on their feet, drowsy and confused. Its effects may be increased by alcohol, barbiturates, narcotics or any other drug that depresses brain function. It may rarely interfere with the effects of anticoagulant drugs. Chlordiazepox-

ide may interfere with ability to drive motor vehicles or operate moving machinery. *Drug dependence:* Chlordiazepoxide may rarely produce dependence of the barbiturate/alcohol type. *Dose:* By mouth, 30 to 100 mg daily in divided doses.

chlorhexidine (Acriflex; Chlorasept; Corsodyl; Eludril; Hibidil; Hibiscrub; Hibisol; Hibitane; Macroside; pHisoMed; Rotersept; Savloclens; Savlodil; Savlon; Travasept; chlorhexidine acetate; chlorhexidine hydrochloride; chlorhexidine gluconate) is used as an antiseptic and disinfectant. Occasionally it may cause skin sensitivity.

chlorinated lime is used as a disinfectant.

chlorinated soda (Dakin's solution) is prepared from chlorinated lime, sodium bicarbonate and boric acid. It is used as an antiseptic and disinfectant.

chlorine compounds are used as antiseptics and disinfectants.

chlormethiazole (Heminevrin) is used as a sleeping drug and sedative. *Adverse effects:* These include headache, nausea, vomiting, sneezing and dizziness. *Precautions:* It may increase the effects of alcohol and other depressant drugs. It may trigger off depression in someone who suffers from severe depressive illness (manic depressive psychosis). *Drug dependence* of the barbiturate/alcohol type may develop quickly in certain individuals, particularly those who are drug dependent. *Dose:* By mouth: for night sedation, 2 capsules, 2 tablets or

10 ml syrup; day-time sedation, 1 capsule, 1 tablet or 5 ml syrup three times daily; for alcohol or drug withdrawal, a nine-day course, starting with 3 capsules, 3 tablets or 15 ml syrup every six hours and gradually reducing.

chlormezanone (Trancopal) is an anti-anxiety drug. It has effects and uses similar to meprobamate. *Adverse effects:* It may cause drowsiness, nausea, dizziness, skin rash and dry mouth. Flushing of the skin and difficulty in passing water may rarely occur and, very occasionally, jaundice. *Precautions:* It may increase the effects of alcohol and it should not be given with other tranquillizers or monoamine oxidase inhibitor antidepressant drugs. It may interfere with ability to operate moving machinery or to drive motor vehicles. *Dose:* By mouth, 200 mg three times daily or 400 mg at night.

chlorocresol is used as an antiseptic, disinfectant, and preservative.

chloroform is now being gradually withdrawn as a preservative in medicines, because it may produce cancer in animals.

Chloromycetin ◊ chloramphenicol.

Chloromycetin Hydrocortisone eye ointment contains 1% chloromycetin and 0·5% hydrocortisone.

chlorophenothane (DDT) ◊ dicophane.

chlorophenoxyethanol has antibacterial and antifungal properties and is used in the treatment of skin infections.

chlorophyll is the green colouring matter from plants. It is used as a colouring agent in fats, oils and soaps. Copper complexes of chlorophyll are used to colour medicines and foods. It is used in dentifrices and in applications to treat wounds and ulcers, principally because of its deodorant properties. Its value in tablets and toothpaste to treat bad breath lacks evidence.

chloroquine (Avloclor; Malarivon; Nivaquine; chloroquine phosphate; chloroquine sulphate) is used to prevent and treat malaria, amoebiasis of the liver, and giardiasis. It is also used to treat rheumatoid arthritis and similar disorders. *Adverse effects:* Itching (pruritus), headache and visional disturbances may occur. Large doses over long periods may produce damage to the eyes (degeneration of the retina and opacities of the cornea). White patches on the skin due to loss of pigment may occur, and it may also cause whitening of the hair. Wasting of muscles and mental breakdown may rarely occur. These toxic effects were very rare with doses used to treat malaria. It was when doctors started using this drug to treat rheumatoid arthritis that most of the problems developed – they used it over prolonged periods. *Dose:* By mouth. Malaria: 1 g as first dose then 500 mg six hours later and 500 mg twice daily for 2 days. Amoebic hepatitis: 1 g daily for 2 days then 250 mg twice daily for 2 to 3 weeks. Rheumatoid arthritis: 250 mg daily at bedtime. Chloroquine sulphate (Nivaquine): malaria: prevention, 400 mg weekly by mouth; treatment, 800 mg daily, reducing to 400 mg daily by mouth; hepatic amoebiasis: 400 to 800 mg daily; giardiasis: 200 mg daily. Can also be given by injection.

chlorothiazide (Saluric) is a diuretic. It increases the excretion of sodium, potassium and chloride by the kidneys. These salts take water with them into the urine by a process of osmosis. Chlorothiazide works in about two hours and lasts from six to twelve hours. It does not lose its effect over time. It is used to treat an increase of body fluids (oedema). It is also used in the treatment of patients with a raised blood pressure. *Adverse effects:* Chlorothiazide occasionally causes allergies, skin rashes, nausea, dizziness, pains in the stomach, sensitivity of the skin to sunlight and weakness. It may rarely cause an acute disorder of the pancreas (acute pancreatitis) and blood disorders. Chlorothiazide and other thiazide diuretics may trigger off an attack of 'gout' or 'diabetes' in some patients. Prolonged use results in a fall in blood potassium which can sensitize the heart to digoxin. Ulcers in the gut have been caused by specially coated tablets of chlorothiazide containing a potassium chloride centre. *Precautions:* Chlorothiazide should be used with caution in patients with impaired kidney or liver function and in patients with diabetes. During prolonged treatment potassium supplements should be given. This needs to be taken at different times from the chlorothiazide because of the latter's effect upon potassium excretion by kidneys. *Dose:* By mouth, 1 to 2 g daily reducing to a maintenance dose of 500 mg to 1 g two or three times weekly. Potassium supplement, e.g., potassium chloride, 3 to 5 g daily in divided doses.

chlorothymol is used as an antiseptic in some skin applications.

chloroxylenol (in Dettol) is used as an antiseptic and disinfectant. It is less toxic than phenol. Wet dressings in contact with the skin may produce sensitivity reactions.

chlorphenesin (Mycil) is an antibacterial, antifungal drug used to treat fungus infections of the skin, e.g., athlete's foot.

chlorpheniramine (Alunex; Piriton; chlorpheniramine maleate; chlorprophenpyridamine maleate) is an antihistamine. *Dose:* By mouth, 2 to 4 mg three or four times daily. Also available as an elixir and injection.

chlorpromazine (Chloractil; Largactil; chlorpromazine hydrochloride) is a phenothiazine major tranquillizer (neuroleptic). It is also used to prevent nausea and vomiting. *Adverse effects:* Chlorpromazine may cause a fall in blood pressure, disorders of heart rate, drowsiness, depression, indifference, dry mouth, pallor, weakness, nightmares and insomnia. Agitation may occur and chlorpromazine may also cause disorders of the breasts in men and women (enlargement and production of milk – gynaecomastia and galactorrhoea), absence of menstrual periods (amenorrhoea), visional disturbances (opacities in the lens and cornea) and pigmentation of the skin and eyes. High doses may cause a fall in body temperature but sometimes an increase. It may also cause jaundice that mimics blockage of the bile ducts in the liver (cholestatic jaundice), blood disorders, skin rashes, sensitivity of the skin to sunlight and muscle tremblings and rigidity (Parkinsonism and dystonias). *Precautions:* It may cause severe dermatitis in sensitized people. Doctors, pharmacists, nurses and anyone who handles the drug frequently should wear masks and rubber gloves. Chlorpromazine should never be given to unconscious patients. It should be used with caution in the elderly and debilitated, in patients with impaired heart function, and in those with certain blood disorders. It should not be given to patients who have impaired liver function. It increases the effects of alcohol, barbiturates, narcotics, atropine-like drugs and other drugs which depress brain function. It also increases the effects of drugs used to treat high blood pressure and it should not be given along with drugs known to have a potential for producing blood disorders, e.g., phenylbutazone, thiouracil, amidopyrine. *Dose:* To prevent vomiting, 25 to 50 mg by mouth or injection into a muscle; in psychotic disorders, 75 to 300 mg daily in divided doses by mouth.

chlorpropamide (Diabinese; Glymese) is used to treat mild diabetes. It should not be used in obese diabetics to replace diet control. *Adverse effects:* Weakness, headache, skin rashes, blood disorders and jaundice may occur. A person on chlorpropamide may get intolerance to alcohol and develop flushing of his face after a drink. *Precautions:* Chlorpropamide should not be used in patients with impaired liver or kidney function or in patients with serious thyroid disorders. It should never be used in pregnancy. The blood sugar lowering effects may be increased by dicoumarol, M.A.O. inhibitor antidepressants, propranolol and other beta-blockers, and by aspirin. Its effects may be decreased by adrenaline, corticosteroids, oral contra-

ceptives and thiazide diuretics. *Dose:* 100 to 500 mg, daily by mouth.

chlorprothixene (Taractan) is a major tranquillizer. *Adverse effects:* It may cause dryness of the mouth, drowsiness, rapid beating of the heart, fall in blood pressure and vertigo. It may also cause skin rashes, fluid retention (oedema), nasal congestion, constipation, convulsions, insomnia, and fainting. Large doses may cause Parkinsonism effects and fits. Blood disorders, nerve damage and milk from the breasts have been reported as well as changes in liver function tests. *Precautions:* It should not be given to patients with heart failure, coronary artery disease or with disorders of the blood vessels supplying the brain. It should be given with caution to patients with epilepsy, and to those with impaired liver or kidney function. It may increase the effects of alcohol, barbiturates, narcotics and other depressant drugs and also drugs used to treat raised blood pressure. *Dose:* By mouth, 30 to 600 mg daily in divided doses.

chlorquinaldol has antibacterial and antifungal properties and is used in the treatment of skin infections.

chlortetracycline (Aureomycin; chlortetracycline hydrochloride) is a tetracycline antibiotic. *Dose:* By mouth, 1 g daily in divided doses.

chlorthalidone (Hygroton) is a thiazide diuretic ◊ chlorothiazide. It is effective for up to forty-eight hours. *Dose:* By mouth, for hypertension, 50 to 100 mg daily, for oedema, 100 to 200 mg on alternate days.

chlorthymol ◊ chlorothymol.

CHO/Vac is a cholera vaccine.

Chocovite tablets (contain calcium gluconate and calciferol 15 mg). *Dose:* By mouth, 1 to 3 tablets sucked three times daily.

cholecalciferol is vitamin D_3.

Choledyl ◊ choline theophyllinate.

cholesterol is a constituent of all animal cells and most foods. It is a 'fat' and raised blood levels in man have been associated with atherosclerosis leading to hypertension and coronary artery disease. In medicines it is used as an emulsifier and also in cosmetics and hair preparations.

cholestyramine (Cuemid; Questran) is used to lower blood fat levels. It may cause constipation, nausea, diarrhoea and large doses may interfere with the absorption of fat and vitamins A, D and K from the diet. *Dose:* By mouth, 8 to 16 g daily in divided doses.

choline is an essential factor in nutrition but it cannot be classified as a vitamin. It is the basic constituent of lecithin. Choline functions as a methyl donor in metabolism. The daily requirement has not been established and there are no valid reports of its effectiveness in any treatment. *Adverse effects:* Include nausea, vomiting, diarrhoea, depression, incontinence and a fishy odour.

choline dihydrogen citrate ◊ choline.

choline salicylate is used to relieve pain in local applications. It has effects similar to aspirin.

choline theophyllinate (Choledyl) is used to relax bronchial muscles in patients suffering from asthma and other respiratory disorders. *Adverse effects:* It produces irritation of the stomach and may cause nausea and vomiting, but less frequently than aminophylline. *Precautions:* It should be given with caution to young children. *Dose:* 400 to 1,600 mg daily in divided doses.

Choloxin ◊ dextrothyroxine sodium.

chondrus (Irish moss) from the dried seaweed *chondrus crispus* is used as an emulsifying agent for cod-liver and other oils and as a substitute for gelatin in the preparation of jellies for invalids. It is used in some cough medicines and extracts are used in the food industry.

chorionic gonadotrophin (Pregnyl; Profasi; Gonadotraphon LH) is a hormone secreted by pregnant women. It is given to stimulate ovulation in women who are infertile. *Adverse effects:* Tiredness, fluid retention and allergic reactions may occur. *Dose:* By injection, according to the patient's requirements.

cholinesterase is an enzyme which breaks down acetylcholine at parasympathetic nerve endings.

Christy's Skin Emulsion contains wool fat 4·8%, glyceryl monostearate 4·8%, white beeswax 0·7%, spermaceti 0·7%, propyl hydroxybenzoate

0·04%, methyl hydroxybenzoate 0·08%, glycerol 2·16%, industrial methylated spirit 7·5%, parachlorometaxylenol 0·05%, and aminacrine hydrochloride 0·00035%.

Chymar ◊ chymotrypsin.

Chymar-Zon ◊ chymotrypsin.

Chymocyclar: Each capsule contains tetracycline 250 mg and proteolytic enzymes in an enteric coated core. The enzymes are said to be useful where infections are associated with inflammation. *Dose:* By mouth, 1 to 2 capsules four times daily before meals.

Chymoral Forte: Each tablet contains trypsin and chymotrypsin equivalent to 100,000 units proteolytic activity. *Dose:* By mouth, 1 tablet four times daily 30 minutes before meals.

Chymoral tablets (enteric coated) contain trypsin and chymotrypsin providing 50,000 units proteolytic activity.

chymotrypsin (Chymar; Chymoral; Chymar-Zon; Zonulysin) is an enzyme secreted by the pancreas that breaks down protein. It is used to reduce inflammation from injuries to soft tissues, and to aid removal of cataracts from the eye.

Cicatrin cream and powder contains neomycin sulphate 3,300 units, bacitracin zinc 250 units, aminoacetic acid 10 mg, cysteine 2 mg, and threonine 1 mg in each 1 g. Also available as a spray.

ciclacillin (Calthor) is a semi-synthetic penicillin ◊ benzylpenicillin.

Cidal soap contains Irgasan 0·75%.

Cidomycin ◊ gentamicin.

cimetidine (Dyspamet; Tagamet) is an antihistamine drug which inhibits the production of acid in the stomach. It is used to treat peptic ulcers. *Adverse effects:* These include confusion, diarrhoea, muscle pains and dizziness. Skin rashes and breast enlargement have occasionally occurred. *Dose:* By mouth, 200 mg thrice daily and 400 mg at night for at least four weeks. It may be given by intravenous injection.

cinchocaine (Nupercainal; cinchocaine hydrochloride) is a local anaesthetic. Although it is much more toxic than procaine or cocaine it is relatively safer because its local anaesthetic effects are greater and it can therefore be used in lower concentration. It does not produce the idiosyncratic reactions that may occur with cocaine.

cinchona bark contains quinine. It has astringent properties.

cinchonidine sulphate ◊ cinchona bark.

cineole is an aromatic liquid found in eucalyptus oil. It is used as an inhalation in the treatment of catarrh and as an irritant skin application.

cinnamedrine is said to relieve painful spasms of the uterus. It is included in preparations used to treat painful periods (dysmenorrhoea).

cinnamic acid has a balsamic odour and is used with benzoic acid in cough medicines. It has antibacterial and antifungal properties.

cinnamon oil is used as a flavouring agent and in some indigestion mixtures. It has been used in inhalations and sprays and as a preservative. It can cause contact sensitivity to the skin.

cinnamon leaf oil is used as a flavouring agent and in some indigestion mixtures.

cinnarizine (Stugeron, Stugeron Forte) is used to treat nausea, dizziness and motion sickness. In high doses (75 mg three times a day) it is used to treat disorders of the peripheral circulation. *Adverse effects:* These include drowsiness, see cyclizine. *Dose:* By mouth, 30 mg three times daily.

Cinobac ◊ cinoxacin.

cinoxacin (Cinobac) is used to treat infections of the urinary system. *Adverse effects:* These include anorexia, nausea, vomiting, diarrhoea, rashes and swelling of the mouth (oral oedema), cramps, headache, noises in the ear (tinnitus), photophobia (discomfort on looking in bright light), and changes in liver function tests. *Precautions:* It should not be used in patients who have severe impairment of their kidney function. *Dose:* By mouth, 500 mg every twelve hours. Prophylaxis 500 mg at night.

cinoxate is a sunscreen agent. It may produce contact dermatitis on exposure to sunlight.

ciprofloxacin (Ciproxin) is a 4-quinoline antibiotic. *Adverse effects* include nausea, vomiting and diarrhoea, dizziness, headache and tiredness, and allergic reactions (skin rashes and itching). Injections may cause pain and inflammation at the site of injection. *Precautions:* The drug should be used with caution in patients who suffer from epilepsy. Patients should drink plenty of fluids and avoid their urine getting too alkaline. It should not be used in pregnancy or by breast-feeding mothers. It should not be used in patients who are allergic to it and preferably not in children. *Dose:* By intravenous infusion, 100 to 200 mg twice daily, given over 30 to 60 minutes. By mouth, 250 to 750 mg twice daily with fluids, but not within 1 to 2 hours of taking an indigestion mixture which will interfere with its absorption.

Ciproxin ◊ ciprofloxacin.

cisplatin (Platinex; Platosin) is an anticancer drug. It is of particular use in cancer of the testicles and cancer of the ovaries. *Adverse effects:* These include damage to the bone marrow producing blood disorders, damage to the kidneys, hearing, nervous system and gastrointestinal tract, a raised blood uric acid level and anaphylactic-like reactions characterized by swelling of the face, wheezing, rapid beating of the heart and falling blood pressure within a few minutes of drug administration. *Precautions:* It should not normally be used in patients with impaired function of their kidneys, bone marrow, nervous system or hearing. It should not be used in patients with a history of sensitivity to cisplatin or other platinum-containing compounds. It should not be used in pregnancy or in breast-feeding mothers. It may have an antifertility effect and because it is mutagenic to bacteria there is a possibility that it could be carcinogenic. Since anaphylactic-like reactions may occur in the first few minutes of administration, adrenaline, a corticosteroid and an antihistamine drug should always be at hand. Renal, neurological and hearing functions should be monitored throughout the period of treatment. *Dose:* By intravenous injection, varies according to the disorders being treated.

citric acid is obtained from lemons and other citrus fruits. It is used to give flavour to preparations.

citronella oil has a pleasant odour. It is obtained from *Cymtopogon nardus* or *C. Winterianus*. There are two types – Ceylon oil and Java oil. It is used as a perfume in soaps and brilliantines and as an insect repellent. Hypersensitivity has been reported.

Claforan ◊ cefotaxime.

Clairvan ◊ ethamivan.

Claradin: Each tablet contains aspirin 300 mg. *Dose:* By mouth, 2 to 3 tablets dissolved in water four hourly.

clavulanic acid has no antibacterial action of its own, but enhances the effects of penicillins. By inactivating penicillinase produced by bacteria, the resistance of these bacteria to penicillins is destroyed.

Clean & Care contains triclosan 0·5%, ethoxylated lauryl alcohol 40%, nonyl phenol ethylene oxide condensate 10%, with sodium salts of alkyl ether sulphate and sulphosuccinates.

Clearasil Clearguard Cleansing Lotion contains allantoin 0·1%, salicylic acid 0·25%, IMS 38·27%.

Clearasil Clearguard Cream contains sulphur 8% and triclosan 0·1%.

Clearasil Clearguard Soap contains colloidal sulphur 2%.

Clearine Eye Drops contain hamamelis water 12·5% and naphazoline hydrochloride 0·01%.

Clearsol is a disinfectant that contains xylenols and phenols.

clemastine (Aller-eze; Aller-eze Plus, Tavegil; clemastine hydrogen fumarate) is an antihistamine. *Dose:* By mouth, 1 mg night and morning.

clidinium (clidinium bromide) has actions and effects similar to atropine.

clindamycin (Dalacin C) is an antibiotic. It has similar effects and uses to those described under lincomycin. It may cause nausea, vomiting and severe diarrhoea. Skin rashes and blood disorders have been reported. *Dose:* By mouth, 150 to 450 mg six-hourly. Injections are also available.

Clinic Shampoo Cream Beauty contains 2,4,4'-trichloro-2-hydroxy diphenyl ether [triclosan] 0·03% and **Deep Health** contains 0·05%.

Clinicide lotion contains carbaryl 0·5% in a water base with 10% alcohol. Used to treat lice ◊ carbaryl.

Clinistix are reagent strips used for detecting glucose in the urine.

Clinitar cream contains coal tar extract 1%. Shampoo solution contains coal tar extract 2%.

Clinitest reagent tablets are used to check the urine for sugar.

Clinium ◊ lidoflazine.

Clinoril (sulindac) is an anti-rheumatic drug related to indomethacin ◊ indomethacin. *Dose:* By mouth, 100 to 300 mg daily.

clioquinol (Vioform; iodochlorhydroxyquinoline) is an antiseptic and amoebicide. It is used to treat amoebic and bacillary dysentery, and it was used to prevent travellers' diarrhoea (Entero-Vioform*). It is also used in lotions, creams and ointments. *Adverse effects:* It stains the skin yellow and may cause irritation. *Precautions:* It should not be taken by patients with impaired liver function or iodine sensitivity. It can affect iodine tests for thyroid function. It should not be used to prevent travellers' diarrhoea since it produces nerve damage. *Dose:* For amoebic dysentery: By mouth, 0·75 to 1·5 g in divided doses for ten days and repeat after one week.

clobazam (Frisium) is a benzodiazepine used to treat anxiety. It has effects and uses similar to those described under diazepam. *Dose:* By mouth, 20 to 60 mg daily in divided doses.

clobetasol (Dermovate; clobetasol propionate) is a corticosteroid used in skin applications.

clobetasone (Eumovate; clobetasone butyrate) is a corticosteroid used in skin applications.

clofazimine (Lamprene) is used in the treatment of leprosy and in skin problems resistant to other treatments. *Adverse effects:* The urine may be coloured red, and red pigmentation of the skin may occur. *Dose:* By mouth, depends on the needs of the individual patient.

clofibrate (Atromid-S) is used to reduce high blood fat levels. *Adverse effects:* Clofibrate may cause nausea, drowsiness, diarrhoea and gain in weight. Itching, skin rashes, loss of hair (alopecia), blood disorders and increased incidence of gallstones have been reported. *Precautions:* It should not be used by patients with impaired liver or kidney function. It should not be used in pregnancy. It may enhance the effects of anticoagulant drugs. *Dose:* By mouth, 20 to 30 mg per kg body-weight in divided doses after meals.

Clomid ◊ clomiphene.

clomiphene (Clomid, clomiphene citrate) is used to stimulate production of hormones in the treatment of infertility in women. *Adverse effects:* Related to dosage and include hot flushes, nausea, vomiting, depression, insomnia, breast tenderness, weight gain, abdominal discomfort and ovarian enlargement. *Precautions:* it is contraindicated in patients with liver disease, ovarian cysts, pregnancy, uterine cancer and bleeding. Patients should be warned of the possibility of multiple births. *Dose:* By mouth, 50 mg daily for 5 days starting on the fifth day of the cycle or at any time if cycles have stopped.

clomipramine (Anafranil; Anafranil SR, clomipramine hydrochloride) is a tricyclic antidepressant drug with effects, uses and adverse effects similar to those described under imipramine. *Adverse effects:* These include dryness of the mouth, blurred vision, and a fall in blood pressure on standing. *Dose:* By mouth, 50 to 150 mg daily in divided doses.

clomocycline (Megaclor; clomocycline sodium) is a tetracycline antibiotic ◊ tetracycline. *Dose:* By mouth, 170 mg to 340 mg four times daily.

clonazepam (Rivotril) is a benzodiazepine drug used in treating epilepsy. *Adverse effects:* Drowsiness, fatigue and difficulty in coordinating movements may occur in the first few weeks of treatment and can be avoided by starting with a low dose and slowly working up. It may produce drooling and an increase of sputum in young children who have some mental impairment. In some patients it may produce fits and aggressive behaviour (paradoxical reaction). *Precautions:* Patients should not drink alcohol when taking clonazepam and driving ability can be affected. Adverse effects may increase when given with hydantoins or phenobarbitone. It should be given with caution in pregnancy and the dose must be reduced slowly over several weeks if it is wished to stop the drug. *Dose:* By mouth, 4 to 8 mg daily in divided doses, varying according to the individual's needs.

clonidine (Catapres; Dixarit; clonidine hydrochloride) is used to treat raised blood pressure and also migraine. *Adverse effects:* These include dry mouth, drowsiness, and constipation. Slowing of the heart rate may occur in the first few weeks of treatment. It may produce impotence, itching, swelling of the throat and face (angioneurotic oedema), nausea and dizziness. *Precautions:* In patients on clonidine a general anaesthetic may cause a severe fall in blood pressure. It should be used with caution in pregnancy, in patients who are depressed and in patients with arterial disease (e.g., Raynaud's disease). The dosage should be reduced slowly if treatment is stopped. *Dose:* By mouth: for raised blood pressure, 0·05 to 0·15 mg daily in divided doses, increasing the daily dose slowly; for migraine, 0·05 to 0·075 mg twice daily.

clopamide (in Brinaldix-K) is a diuretic drug with effects and uses similar to those described under chlorothiazide. *Dose:* By mouth, 20 to 60 mg daily.

clopenthixol (Clopixol; clopenthixol hydrochloride, clopenthixol decanoate) is related to fluphenazine. *Dose:* By mouth 20 to 50 mg daily in divided doses. By intramuscular injection. 200 to 400 mg every 2 to 4 weeks.

Clopixol ◊ clopenthixol.

clorazepate potassium ◊ potassium clorazepate.

clotrimazole (Canesten) is an antifungal drug. *Dose:* Vaginal tablets (100 mg), 1 at night for six nights. Also available as a cream for skin infections.

clove oil ◊ oil of cloves.

cloves ◊ oil of cloves.

cloxacillin sodium (Orbenin) is a semi-synthetic penicillin which is mainly of use in treating infections produced by one particular group of bacteria which is resistant to penicillin (pencillinase-producing staphylococci). Otherwise it is not as potent as benzylpenicillin. _Adverse effects_ and _Precautions:_ These are similar to those described under benzylpenicillin. It should not be used on the skin. _Dose:_ By mouth, 500 mg before meals every six hours. By injection, 250 to 2,000 mg every six hours.

CMC ◊ carboxymethyl cellulose.

coal tar (Clinitar) ◊ tar.

Cobadex ◊ hydrocortisone.

Cobalin-H ◊ hydroxocobalamin.

cobalt sulphate has been used to treat cobalt deficiency in animals. Toxic effects on the heart were reported after its use to improve the 'head' on beer.

Co-Betaloc is used to treat raised blood pressure. Each tablet contains metoprolol 100 mg and hydrochlorothiazide 12·5 mg.

Co-Betaloc SA are sustained release tablets, containing metoprolol tartrate 200 mg ◊ metoprolol.

Cobutolin ◊ salbutamol.

cocaine is the oldest local anaesthetic, but because of adverse effects and risk of drug dependence it is hardly ever used except for local application to the eyes, ears or nose. Unlike all other local anaesthetics it constricts small blood vessels and need not be given with adrenaline. _Adverse effects:_ Some people have an idiosyncrasy to cocaine and may become seriously ill, even after a small dose. They develop headaches, faintness and may suddenly collapse and die. In other patients it may cause the general adverse effects of any local anaesthetic – excitation, restlessness, nausea, yawning and vomiting which may be followed by pallor, sweating, fall in blood pressure, twitching, convulsions and unconsciousness. _Precautions:_ It should not be given to patients with myasthenia gravis and it should be given with caution to patients with disordered heart rhythm or with impaired liver function. _Drug dependence:_ Cocaine causes stimulation and a lift in mood. Large doses cause restlessness, trembling and hallucinations. Its repeated use leads to drug dependence. Cocaine addicts inject it under the skin or use it in the form of snuff. The characteristics of cocaine dependence include a strong psychological dependence but no physical dependence. Persons dependent on cocaine develop an unbearable craving for the drug, loss of weight and memory and mental deterioration.

co-carboxylase is a form of thiamine found in the body.

cochineal is obtained by killing female insects (_Coccus cacti_) containing eggs and larvae by heating them. The wax melts and produces a purplish-black cochineal. It is used as a colouring agent in medicines and foods.

cocillana (liquid extract) is obtained from the bark of *Guarea rusbyi* and is used in expectorant cough medicines because it irritates the lining of the stomach which is said to produce a reflex cough. In large doses it causes vomiting.

coconut oil is used to form absorbable ointment bases for scalp applications. It is not precipitated by salt (sodium chloride) and is used in the manufacture of 'marine' soaps.

cod liver oil is a source of vitamins A and D. It also contains unsaturated fatty acids (of help in reducing cholesterol levels). It is included in some dressings and ointments without evidence of its effectiveness.

Coda-Med tablets contain paracetamol 450 mg, caffeine citrate 15 mg and codeine phosphate 8·1 mg ◊ paracetamol, caffeine and codeine.

Codanin tablets: Each contain paracetamol 500 mg and codeine phosphate 10 mg.

Co-danthrusate laxative capsules contain danthron with docusate sodium.

codeine (codeine sulphate; codeine phosphate) is a useful mild pain reliever. It is a weak cough suppressant and it is also of value in treating diarrhoea. *Adverse effects:* The commonest adverse effects are constipation, nausea, vomiting, dizziness and drowsiness. Very rarely skin rashes may occur in patients who are allergic to codeine. *Precautions:* Codeine should be given with caution to patients suffering from severe respiratory disorders (e.g., chronic bronchi-

tis). It may increase the effects of other drugs which depress brain function, e.g., sedatives, tranquillizers, hypnotics. *Drug dependence:* Prolonged use of high doses may rarely produce dependence of the morphine type. *Dose:* By mouth, 10 to 60 mg. Not more than 200 mg in twenty-four hours. Codeine, codeine phosphate or codeine sulphate appear in many pain-relieving mixtures, cough mixtures and anti-diarrhoeal mixtures.

Codella hand cream contains povidone-iodine 0·2%.

Codelsol ◊ prednisolone.

co-dergocrine mesylate ◊ Hydergine.

Codis: Each tablet contains soluble aspirin 500 mg and codeine phosphate 8 mg. *Dose:* 1 to 2 in water four-hourly.

Codural Period Pain Tablets each contain caffeine 50 mg, paracetamol 250 mg, and homatropine methylbromide 750 micrograms.

Cogentin ◊ benztropine.

Cojene: Each tablet contains aspirin 300 mg, caffeine citrate 105 mg, and codeine phosphate 8 mg.

colaspase (Crasnitin; 1-asparaginase) is an anti-cancer drug. *Adverse effects:* Include fever, nausea, vomiting, liver damage, nerve damage, allergic reactions, alterations in the levels of various chemicals in the blood and a fall in white blood cells. *Precautions:* It should not be used in pregnancy and it should be given with caution to patients with impaired liver function. *Dose:* Depends upon the disorder being treated.

colchicine is used for the relief of pain in acute gout. *Adverse effects:* Large doses quickly produce diarrhoea. Colchicine may also produce nausea, vomiting and abdominal pains. Kidney and liver damage, dehydration and loss of hair (after prolonged use) may rarely occur. *Precautions:* Colchicine should be given with caution to the elderly and debilitated and to patients who suffer from impaired heart, liver or kidney function. It should probably not be given to patients who suffer from disorders of the stomach or gut (e.g., colitis). *Dose:* Acute attack of gout: by mouth, 1 mg initially, followed by 0·5 mg every two hours until relief is obtained or until diarrhoea develops; the total amount in a course of treatment should not exceed 6 mg. Maintenance dose, 0·5 to 1 mg at night.

Cold and Influenza Capsules contain paracetamol 240 mg, ascorbic acid 66 mg, caffeine 10 mg, quinine sulphate 6 mg.

cold cream ◊ rosewater ointment.

Cold Discs tablets: Each contains ascorbic acid 50 mg, paracetamol 400 mg, phenylephrine hydrochloride 5 mg, terpin hydrate 25 mg, and noscapine 15 mg.

Coldrex Antiseptic Throat Lozenges contain menthol 3 mg and amylmetacresol 0·6 mg.

Coldrex Cold & Flu Treatment Tablets contain paracetamol 500 mg, phenylephrine hydrochloride 5 mg, caffeine 25 mg, terpin hydrate 20 mg, and ascorbic acid 30 mg.

Coldrex Nasal Spray contains phenylephrine hydrochloride 0·5%.

Coldrex Powders: Each sachet contains paracetamol 1 g, phenylephrine hydrochloride 10 mg, and ascorbic acid 60 mg.

Coldrex Tablets each contain paracetamol 500 mg, phenylephrine hydrochloride 5 mg, caffeine 25 mg, terpin hydrate 20 mg, and vitamin C 30 mg.

Colestid ◊ colestipol.

colestipol (Colestid; colestipol hydrochloride) is used to lower blood fat levels. *Adverse effects* ◊ cholestyramine. *Precautions:* The granules must be taken with a fluid. It may interfere with the absorption of drugs such as digoxin, penicillin and chlorothiazide. *Dose:* By mouth, 15 to 30 g daily in divided doses with plenty of fluid.

Colifoam ◊ hydrocortisone acetate.

colistin (Colomycin; colistin sulphate) is an antibiotic with a range of activity similar to polymyxin B. It is poorly absorbed from the gut and is therefore used for treating gastro-enteritis. *Adverse effects:* It may produce allergic skin rashes and, in high dose, it may cause kidney damage, dizziness and migraine. It may be used to treat blood poisoning (septicaemia), infections of the kidneys and bladder and meningitis. *Dose:* By mouth, 5 to 9 mega units daily in divided doses. Colistin sulphomethate sodium (a compound of colistin suitable for injection), by intramuscular injection, 5 to 9 mega units daily in divided doses.

Collins Elixir contains ethylmorphine hydrochloride 0·03%, chloroform 0·4%, tartaric acid 1·87%, and lemon oil 0·31%.

Collins Elixir Pastilles: Each contains chloroform 0·34%, citric acid 1·65%, lemon oil 0·6%, squill vinegar 0·42%, and glycerol 0·21%.

Collis Browne's (J.) Mixture: Each 5-ml dose contains: opium liquid extract equivalent to morphine 1 mg, peppermint oil 0·0015 ml, and capsicum tincture 0·0012 ml, in a vehicle containing chloroform water.

collodion ◊ pyroxylin.

colocynth (Bitter apple) is a drastic and obsolete purgative.

Colofac ◊ mebeverine.

Cologel ◊ methylcellulose.

Colomycin ◊ colistin.

colophony is obtained from volatile oils from various species of pine. It is an ingredient of some collodions and plaster-masses and was previously used in ointments for treating boils etc.

Colpermin ◊ peppermint oil.

Colsor Cream contains tannic acid 5%, camphor 5%, menthol 0·5%, phenol 1%, lanolin basis to 100%.

Colsor Lotion contains tannic acid 5%, camphor 5%, phenol 0·5%, and menthol 0·5%.

Coltex Cream contains diphenhydramine hydrochloride 2%.

coltsfoot (flower and liquid extract) is used as a demulcent in some cough medicines.

Colven sachets are used to treat irritable bowel syndrome. Each sachet contains mebeverine hydrochloride 135 mg and ispaghula husk 3·5 g.

Combantrin ◊ pyrantel.

Comox ◊ co-trimoxazole.

Complement Continus: Each tablet contains pyridoxine 100 mg in a sustained-release form. *Dose:* 1 daily by mouth.

compound chloroform mixtures ◊ chloroform.

Compound W contains salicylic acid 14·2%, glacial acetic acid 11%, menthol 1·9% and camphor 1·5%.

Comtrex tablets are used to treat cold symptoms. Each tablet contains paracetamol 325 mg, phenylpropanolamine hydrochloride 12·5 mg, dextromethorphan hydrobromide 10 mg and chlorpheniramine maleate 1 mg. **Comtrex Capsules** contain the same ingredients as the tablets in the same amount. **Comtrex liquid** contains the same ingredients as the tablets in each 15 ml.

Concavit is a multivitamin preparation. Each capsule contains vitamin A 5,000 units, thiamine hydrochloride 2·5 mg, nicotinamide 20 mg, riboflavine 2·5 mg, pyridoxine hydrochloride 1 mg, cyanocobalamin 5 micrograms, ascorbic acid 40 mg, ergocalciferol 500 units, calcium pantothenate 5 mg, vitamin E 2 units. Each 0·5 ml of drops and each 5 ml of syrup contain vitamin A 5,000 units, thiamine hydrochloride 2 mg, riboflavine 1 mg, nicotinamide 12·5 mg, pyridoxine hydrochloride 1 mg, cyanocobalamin 5 micrograms, ascorbic acid 50 mg, ergocalciferol 500 units, panthenol 2 mg.

Concordin ◊ probriptyline.

Congreve's Balsam Elixir contains aqueous extract of horehound 0·5%, coltsfoot leaf 0·5%, hyssop 0·25%, and rosemary 0·375%, alcoholic (48%) extracts of tolu balsam 2%, catechu 2%, guaiacum resin 1%, cochineal 0·2%, and squill 0·5%, turpentine oil 0·0625%, and alcohol 27·5%.

Conjuvac is used to treat allergy to pollens. It contains extracts of two grass pollens.

Conjuvac mite is used to treat allergy to house-dust mites. It contains a purified allergen extract.

Conotrane cream contains a silicone 20% and hydrargaphen 0·05%. ◊ mercury.

Conova 30 is an oral contraceptive drug containing ethinyloestradiol 0·03 mg and ethynodiol diacetate 2 mg.

Contac 400 are sustained-release capsules each containing phenylpropanolamine hydrochloride 50 mg and chlorpheniramine maleate 4 mg.

Controvlar: Each tablet contains norethisterone acetate 3 mg and ethinyloestradiol 0·05 mg. For control of menstrual irregularities.

Coparvax ◊ corynebacterium.

Copholco is used to treat coughs. Each 5 ml contains pholcodine 5·63 mg, menthol 1·41 mg, cineole 0·0026 ml, terpin hydrate 2·82 mg. *Dose:* By mouth, 10 ml four or five times daily.

Copholcoids is used to treat cough. Each pastille contains pholcodine 4 mg, menthol 2 mg, cineole 0·004 ml, terpin hydrate 16 mg. *Dose:* By mouth, 1 to 2 sucked three or four times daily.

copper acts as a contraceptive when present in the uterus. Copper is an essential trace element in the diet. There is no evidence that wearing a copper bracelet for the treatment of rheumatic disorders has any effect.

copper acetate is used as an astringent in skin applications.

copper carbonate is a copper salt said to aid absorption and use of iron in the body.

copper sulphate is used in very small amounts in people who are being fed entirely by the intravenous route, to make sure a deficiency does not occur. It is used to kill algae in ponds and swimming pools and as an astringent in skin applications. Crystals of copper sulphate are caustic.

Coppertone Supershade 15 ◊ dimethylaminobenzoate. Has an SPF of 15. **Coppertone Ultrashade 23** has an SPF of 23.

Cordarone X ◊ amiodarone.

Cordilox ◊ verapamil.

Corgard ◊ nadolol.

Corgaretic is used to treat raised blood pressure. Each tablet contains nadolol 40 mg and bendrofluazide 5 mg. *Dose:* By mouth, 1 or 2 daily.

coriander oil is aromatic and is used to treat wind.

Corlan ◊ hydrocortisone sodium succinate. For mouth ulcers – pellets (2·5 mg) dissolved in the mouth four times daily.

Coro-Nitro Spray ◊ glyceryl trinitrate.

Correctol Tablets contain docusate sodium 100 mg, yellow phenolphthalein 65 mg, sodium benzoate 18 mg, and calcium gluconate 59 mg.

Corsodyl gel and **mouthwash** ◊ chlorhexidine.

Cortelan ◊ cortisone.

Cortenema ◊ hydrocortisone.

corticotrophin (Acthar; ACTH; adrenocorticotrophic hormone) stimulates the cortex of the adrenal glands and produces an increased output of hormones. The effects produced are similar to, but not identical with, those produced by cortisone. *Adverse effects:* These are similar to those described under cortisone. Patients may sometimes become allergic to ACTH. *Precautions:* ACTH should not be given to patients with peptic ulcers, with active tuberculosis, with signs of mental instability or to patients with raised blood pressure. ACTH may

make diabetic patients worse and increase their insulin needs. It may also mask the signs and symptoms of underlying infections. *Withdrawal symptoms:* ACTH may depress the natural ACTH produced by the master gland – the pituitary. This leads to changes in the gland caused by its under-working so that if the ACTH drug is stopped, the pituitary gland cannot take over straight away. The patient may then experience severe symptoms. ACTH treatment should therefore be stopped very gradually in order to give the pituitary gland time to become active again. Corticotrophin is available for injection in two forms – corticotrophin gelatin injection (ACTH gel, Acthar gel) and corticotrophin injection (Acthar, ACTH). The gel is long acting and not suitable for injection into a vein.

cortisol ◊ hydrocortisone.

cortisone (Cortelan; Cortistab; Cortisyl) is a corticosteroid. It has the effects of the naturally occurring adrenocortical hormone, hydrocortisone. It is used in disorders of the adrenal glands which result in underproduction of hydrocortisone (Addison's disease) and it is used to treat inflammatory, allergic and rheumatic disorders. Its effects are transitory and relapse of the underlying condition soon occurs when the cortisone is stopped. With continued use of cortisone the master gland (the pituitary) stops producing the hormone which stimulates the adrenal glands to produce hydrocortisone. This results in disuse changes in the adrenal glands so that if the cortisone is stopped the adrenal glands are not in a position to produce even the body's normal requirements of hydrocortisone. This produces serious consequences. Prolonged use of cortisone also leads to changes in salt, sugar and protein used by the body. It reduces resistance to infection and also in the inflammatory response to infection; underlying infection may therefore go unnoticed. Cortisone should only be used for certain inflammatory disorders and when inflammation may be harmful, as in the eyes. It is better to use prednisolone to treat asthma, rheumatoid arthritis, certain blood disorders and other inflammatory or allergic disorders because it has less effect on body salts. *Adverse effects:* These are due to its effects upon salt, sugar and protein metabolism; to its effects upon healing and inflammation; and to its effects upon the pituitary and adrenal glands. These result in salt and water retention leading to oedema (a sign of which is ankle swelling), raised blood pressure and alterations in blood potassium which may cause heart failure. Calcium and phosphorus metabolism are affected which may result in bone softening and fractures. The blood sugar level increases. Cortisone may cause peptic ulcers with bleeding and perforation, delayed wound healing, and increased liability to infection. Prolonged application to the eyes may result in damage to the cornea and to the sight, and skin applications may cause wasting of skin tissues. Sudden collapse may occur if the drug is stopped (due to the adrenal glands not functioning) and growth may be slowed down in children. Large doses lead to development of moon face, hairiness (hirsutism), swelling of the tissues over the lower part of the back of the neck and shoulders (called a buffalo hump), flushing, increased bruising, acne and stripes (striae) on the skin, particularly around the lower abdomen and buttocks. Other adverse effects include disorders of the nervous system, mental disturbances, loss of periods (amenorrhoea) and muscle weakness. *Precautions:* Cortisone should not be given to patients with peptic ulcers, softening of bones (osteoporosis), or to patients with severe psychological disorders. It should be used with caution in patients with congestive heart failure, diabetes, infectious diseases, long-standing impairment of kidney function or kidney failure, or elderly patients. Patients with active or doubtfully active tuberculosis should not be given cortisone (unless it is part of the treatment and given along with antituberculous drugs). Normally the body produces more hydrocortisone in response to infection, anaesthetics, surgery, shock, and injury. Patients who are receiving cortisone or who have been on cortisone in the previous two years may not be able to produce sufficient hydrocortisone themselves during anaesthesia, surgery or injury. They will therefore need to be given a supplementary dose of cortisone. Cortisone may have its effects reduced by barbiturates and phenytoin. It may also affect the response to anticoagulant drugs. Applications to the skin, eyes or ears should not be used in the presence of infection. When applied to large areas of the body surface under plastic occlusive dressings, it is absorbed and may cause systemic adverse effects. In certain cases it may be used combined with an antibacterial drug for lesions of the eyes, ears or skin but such a mixture should never be used to treat viral inflammation of the eyes since there is a risk of causing blindness. *Dose:* By mouth or intramuscular injection, 25 to 400 mg daily in divided doses.

Cortistab ◊ cortisone.

Cortisyl ◊ cortisone.

Cortril (hydrocortisone spray, lotions, and ointments) ◊ hydrocortisone.

Cortucid eye drop cream contains sulphacetamide 10% and hydrocortisone acetate 0·5%.

corynebacterium parvum vaccine (Coparvax) used as a suspension of inactivated bacteria and administered into the chest or abdomen for the treatment of malignant pleural effusions and ascites. *Adverse effects:* These include fever, nausea, vomiting and abdominal discomfort.

Cosmegen ◊ actinomycin D.

Cosuric ◊ allopurinol.

Cosylan ◊ dextromethorphan.

Cotazym ◊ pancreatic enzymes.

Cotazym B is a pancreatin preparation containing cellulose, cholic acid 30 mg (ox bile extract), and pancreas powder.

Coterpin is a cough medicine containing in each 5 ml codeine phosphate 15 mg, terpin hydrochloride 30 mg, menthol 8 mg, ol. pini. pumil. 0·0025 ml, eucalyptol 0·004 ml and glycerin 1·7 ml.

Cotrimox ◊ co-trimoxazole.

co-trimoxazole (Bactrim; Chemotrim; Comox; Fectrim; Laratrim; Septrin) tablets contain sulphamethoxazole 400 mg and trimethoprim 80 mg. *Dose:* 1 or 2 twice daily. Range 1 to 3 twice daily. Double strength tablets, suspension and both I.M. and I.V. injections available.

Covermark is a masking cream for concealing scars, areas of discolouration and birthmarks.

Covonia Mentholated Bronchial Balsam contains dextromethorphan hydrobromide 0·075%, guaiphenesin 0·5%, menthol 0·05%, and eucalyptol 0·03%.

Cox antiseptic cream ◊ cetrimide.

Cox Antitussive Linctus is used to treat coughs. It contains in each 5 ml dextromethorphan hydrobromide 8 mg, ephedrine hydrochloride 10 mg, ammonium chloride 35 mg, ipecacuanha liquid extract 0·00375 ml, tolu solution 0·11 ml, glycerin 0·5325 ml, liquid glucose 2 g and sucrose 2·5 g.

Cox Bronchial Mixture contains in each 10 ml squill liquid extract 0·095 ml, senega liquid extract 0·0475 ml, ipecacuanha tincture 0·15 ml, tolu solution 0·12 ml, capsicum tincture 0·125 ml, camphor 2 mg, benzoic acid 12 mg, anise oil 0·002 ml, ammonium bicarbonate 235 mg, and glycerol 0·01 ml.

Cox Catarrh and Bronchial Syrup contains in each 10 ml codeine phosphate 2·125 mg, chloroform 0·006 ml, creosote 0·011 ml, alcoholic (68%) extract of aconite (0·05% aconitine) 0·0125 ml, calcium lactate 8 mg, calcium tetrahydrogen phosphate 10 mg, and cinnamon oil 0·00083 ml.

Cox Cetrimide Cream contains cetrimide 0·5%.

Cox Children Cherry Cough Syrup contains in each 5 ml tolu solution 0·067 ml, red-poppy syrup 0·535 ml, wild cherry syrup 0·535 ml, ipecacuanha tincture 0·1 ml, squill vinegar 0·33 ml, and glycerol 0·75 ml.

Cox Decongestant Tablets are used as a nasal decongestant. Each tablet contains methylephedrine hydrochloride 15 mg, menthol 1 mg, paracetamol 250 mg, guaiphenesin 50 mg and chlorpheniramine maleate 2 mg.

Cox Digestive Mints: Each contains dihydroxyaluminium sodium carbonate 300 mg.

Cox Extra Strong Bronchial Mixture is used to treat irritating coughs. Each 10 ml contains squill liquid extract 0·095 ml, senega liquid extract 0·0475 mg, ipecacuanha tincture 0·15 ml, tolu solution 0·12 ml, capsicum tincture 0·125 ml, camphor 2 mg, benzoic acid 12 mg, anise oil 0·002 ml, ammonium bicarbonate 235 mg, glycerol 0·01 ml and sucrose 3·25 g.

Cox Junior Multivitamins are a multivitamin supplement especially for children.

Cox Multivitamin and Cox Multivitamin with Iron are multivitamin preparations.

Cox Nasal Spray contains phenylephrine hydrochloride 0·5%.

Cox Pain Relief Tablets each contain paracetamol 450 mg, codeine phosphate 8·1 mg, caffeine citrate 15 mg, and nicotinamide 15 mg.

Cox Soothing Cream is used for bites, stings and minor skin irritations. It contains antazoline 1%, camphor 0·1%, calamine 8% and cetrimide 0·5%.

Cradocap is a shampoo containing cetrimide 10%, cetyl alcohol 15%, and lanolin 1%.

Crampex Tablets each contain guaiphenesin 60 mg, nicotinic acid 20 mg, calcium gluconate 200 mg, and ergocalciferol 20 micrograms.

Crasnitin ◊ colaspase.

cream of tartar is potassium acid tartrate and is used as a saline laxative. It has a mild diuretic action. It has been used as a dusting powder for surgical gloves and is used in some toothpastes.

Creds contain menthol 0·5%, peppermint oil 0·025%, aniseed oil 0·3%, benzoin tincture 0·5%, capsicin 0·001%, and clove oil 0·05%.

Cremaffin is a brand of liquid paraffin and magnesium hydroxide emulsion.

Cremalgin balm is a rubefacient. It contains methyl nicotinate 1%, histamine dihydrochloride 0·1%, capsicum 0·1% and glycol salicylate 10% in a base.

cremophor EL is an emulsifying agent.

Cremosan contains zinc oxide 5·3%, beeswax 10·7%, resin 10·7%, wool fat

22·2%, cresol 2·3%, formaldehyde solution 0·2%, thymol 0·2%, and paraffin basis to 100%.

Creon capsules are used as a replacement therapy in pancreatic insufficiency. Each capsule contains pancreatin 8,000 units and amylase 9,000 units and protease 210 units.

creosote is a disinfectant. It is used in small doses in some cough mixtures, but is an irritant.

Crescormon ◊ HGH.

cresol is used as an antiseptic and disinfectant. It has effects similar to phenol. It is also used as a rubefacient.

Crest Plus toothpaste contains sodium fluoride 0·24%.

Crookes Multivitamins: Each tablet contains vitamin A 5,000 units, vitamin B_1 2 mg, vitamin B_2 2 mg, vitamin B_6 1 mg, vitamin B_{12} 2 micrograms, vitamin C 50 mg, vitamin D 400 units, nicotinamide 20 mg, iron 15 mg, and copper 0·75 mg.

crotamiton (Eurax) is used as a skin application to relieve itching. *Precautions:* It should only be used on small areas of skin in babies and infants. It should not be used near the eyes or on areas of dermatitis.

Croupline Cough Syrup contains the water-soluble constituents of lobelia 3·62%, grindelia 0·36%, anise 0·9%, coltsfoot leaf 1·06%, and wild cherry bark (free from hydro-cyanic acid) 1·25%, together with guaiphenesin 0·25%, anise oil 0·1%, acetic acid 0·24%, and sucrose 75·93%.

Crown corn caps are used for removing corns. Each cap contains salicylic acid 40%.

crystal violet ◊ gentian violet.

crystalline penicillin G ◊ benzylpenicillin.

crystalline sodium penicillin ◊ benzylpenicillin.

Crystapen ◊ benzylpenicillin.

Crystapen V ◊ phenoxymethylpenicillin.

cubeb oil (fruit) from cubeb berries is used as a flavouring agent.

Cupal Burn Aid cream contains aminacrine hydrochloride 0·1% and antazoline hydrochloride 1%.

Cupal Child's Pain Elixir: Each 5 ml contains paracetamol 120 mg.

Cupal Cold Sore Lotion contains tannic acid 5%, salicylic acid 1%, and myrrh 10%.

Cupal Cold Sore Ointment contains allantoin 1%, diperodon hydrochloride 1%, camphor 1%, and zinc oxide 5%.

Cupal Insect Bite Cream contains antazoline hydrochloride 2%.

Cupal Nail Bite Lotion contains denatonium benzoate.

Cupal Verruca Ointment contains salicylic acid 50%.

Cupal Wart Solvent contains glacial acetic acid 86·25%.

Cupal Worm Elixir consists of Piperazine Citrate Elixir.

Cupal's oral rehydration glucolyte sachets contain sodium chloride and glucose powder for making up with 200 ml of drinking water. Used to treat dehydration caused by diarrhoea and vomiting.

Cuplex gel is used to treat warts. It contains salicylic acid 11%, lactic acid 4% and copper acetate 1%.

curare is an extract from bark of trees which grow in South America and is used to make poisoned arrows by the South American Indians. It paralyses muscles and was used in surgery. Tubocurarine has taken its place.

Cuticura Ointment contains mineral oil 28·5%, yellow soft paraffin 50·43%, beeswax 18·17%, pine oil 0·04%, rose geranium oil 0·17%, chlorophyll 0·04%, oxyquinoline 0·05%, sulphur praecip. 0·5%, and phenol 0·16%.

cyanocobalamin (Cytacon; Cytamen, Hepacon B_{12}) is a cobalt-containing substance used to treat anaemias caused by vitamin B_{12} deficiency. *Dose:* In pernicious anaemia, by intramuscular injection: initially, 0·25 mg to 1 mg on alternate days; maintenance 1 mg every four weeks.

cyclandelate (Cyclobral; Cyclospasmol) is a vasodilator drug. *Adverse effects:* In high dosage it may produce dizziness, flushing, headache, nausea and sweating. *Dose:* By mouth, 0·4 to 1·6 g daily in divided doses.

Cyclimorph 10 (each ml contains cyclizine tartrate 50 mg with morphine tartrate 10 mg); **Cyclimorph 15** (contains 15 mg of morphine tartrate and 50 mg of cyclizine tartrate). *Dose:* 1 ml ampoule by intramuscular injection when necessary for pain accompanied by nausea and vomiting.

cyclizine (Marzine; Valoid; cyclizine hydrochloride) is an antihistamine used to treat motion sickness, sickness of pregnancy and other disorders associated with nausea and vomiting. *Adverse effects:* Drowsiness and dizziness are the main adverse effects. *Dose:* By mouth, 50 mg, twenty minutes before a journey. Dose should *not* be repeated more than twice in twenty-four hours.

cyclobarbitone (Phanodorm; cyclobarbitone calcium) is an intermediate acting barbiturate. *Dose:* By mouth, 200 mg at night.

Cyclobral ◊ cyclandelate.

cyclofenil (Rehibin) is used in the treatment of female infertility. *Adverse effects:* These include hot flushes, abdominal discomfort, nausea and rarely cholestatic jaundice. *Precautions* ◊ clomiphene. *Dose:* 100 mg morning and evening for 10 days.

Cyclogest ◊ progesterone.

cyclopenthiazide (Navidrex) is a thiazide diuretic with effects and uses similar to those of chlorothiazide. It works in one to two hours and lasts about twelve hours. *Adverse effects* and *Precautions:* These are similar to those for chlorothiazide. *Dose:* By mouth, 0·25 to 0·5 mg once or twice daily.

cyclopentolate (cyclopentolate hydrochloride) has effects similar to those described under atropine. It is used in eye drops.

cyclophosphamide (Endoxana) is an anti-cancer drug. *Adverse effects:* It may cause nausea, vomiting and diarrhoea, and sometimes a bleeding colitis. A bleeding cystitis may be produced; this responds to high fluid intake. It may cause bone-marrow damage, producing blood disorders. Loss of hair (alopecia) is common at a dose of more than 35 mg per kg of body-weight in eight days. The hair regrows in two or three months even if the drug is continued. *Precautions:* It should not be given in pregnancy, to patients with any infection, nor to any patient whose bone-marrow function may be reduced. *Dose:* By mouth or injection – varies according to disorder.

Cyclo-Progynova 1 mg and 2 mg are hormone preparations containing oestradiol and norgestrel in varying proportions for the treatment of menopausal symptoms.

cyclopropane is a gas used as an anaesthetic.

cycloserine is an antibiotic drug active against many bacteria including tuberculosis. Its anti-bacterial activity is however lower than other antibiotics used to treat those infections; it is therefore only used as a reserve drug against bacteria resistant to other antibiotics or if the patient has become allergic to them. It is used principally to treat pulmonary tuberculosis and should be given in combination with other anti-tuberculous drugs in order to prevent resistance developing. *Adverse effects:* The incidence of adverse effects is high; these include headache, dizziness, drowsiness, twitching, speech difficulties, convulsions and even unconsciousness. Abdominal symptoms may occur. With daily doses of less than 500 mg, adverse effects are rare. Allergic skin rashes occasionally occur, blood sugar levels may be reduced and certain tests for liver function altered. *Precautions:* Cycloserine should not be given to patients with epilepsy, psychological disorders, or impaired liver function. It should be given with caution to alcoholics and patients with impaired kidney function. Blood levels of the drug should be checked frequently. *Dose:* By mouth, 250 to 750 mg daily in divided doses.

Cyclospasmol ◊ cyclandelate.

Cyclosporin is an immunosuppressant drug used to prevent patients rejecting bone marrow, kidney and heart transplants. *Adverse effects:* Impairment of kidney and liver function, tremor, gastro-intestinal disturbances and hirsutism. *Precautions:* Increased susceptibility to infections. Ketoconazole produces increased plasma concentrations of cyclosporin. *Dose:* By mouth or intravenous infusion. Dose varies according to disorder being treated.

Cyklokapron ◊ tranexamic acid.

Cymalon is used to relieve the symptoms of cystitis. Each sachet contains sodium citrate 4 g ◊ sodium citrate.

Cymex contains urea 1%, cetrimide 0·5%, dimethicone 9%, and chlorocresol 0·1%.

cyproheptadine (Periactin; cyproheptadine hydrochloride) is an antihistamine drug. It is effective in small doses but is short acting. It is also promoted as an appetite stimulant. *Dose:* By mouth, 4 to 20 mg daily in divided doses.

Cyprostat ◊ cyproterone.

cyproterone (Androcur; Cyprostat; cyproterone acetate) blocks the effects of male sex hormones (androgens) and has some progestogenic effects. The consequences of these effects is to reduce libido (sex drive) and cyproterone is used in 'patients' who are considered to have excessive or misdirected male libido. It is also used to treat cancer of the prostrate. *Adverse effects:* It stops sperm production and causes the testicles to shrink. These changes appear to be reversible but may take up to twenty months after stopping the drug. The consequences of long-term treatment are not known. It may produce swelling of the breasts, milk production and lumps in the breasts. Pain in the testicles may occur and there may be patchy loss of hair on the body with increased growth of hair on the scalp and lightening of hair colour. Increase in weight may occur with female distribution of fat – on the breasts and bottom. Stretch stripes (striae) may occur on the abdomen and the patient may complain of headache, flushing and sweating. *Precautions:* It should be used with caution in patients with liver disorders, diabetes or anaemia. Blood tests for these disorders should be carried out at monthly intervals. Alcohol reduces its effects and it is of no use in chronic alcoholics. A sperm count should be done before starting treatment to establish whether the patient is fertile or not. It should not be used in immature youths. It may affect the ability to drive motor vehicles because of the lassitude produced. *Dose:* By mouth, 100 to 300 mg daily in divided doses.

cysteine (l-cysteinc) is an amino acid which is an essential constituent of the diet to form body proteins.

Cystemime sachets contain sodium citrate and sodium bicarbonate. When dissolved in water the sachet contents form a fizzy lemon-flavoured drink. Used to reduce the acidity of the urine in the treatment of cystitis. *Adverse effects and precautions:* The preparation contains equivalent to 4 g of sodium citrate per sachet, and therefore it should be used with utmost caution in pregnancy and by any patient with raised blood pressure or heart disease. *Dose:* The contents of 1 sachet dissolved in a glass of water, 3 times daily for a maximum of 6 sachets over a 48-hour period.

Cystopurin is used to relieve the symptoms of cystitis. Each tablet contains hexamine 324 mg and sodium acetate 648 mg.

Cytacon ◊ cyanocobalamin.

Cytamen ◊ cyanocobalamin.

cytarabine (Alexan, Cytosar) is an anti-cancer drug used to treat leukaemia. *Adverse effects:* Include nausea, vomiting, diarrhoea, ulcers in the mouth, damage to the bone marrow, kidney disfunction, liver disfunction, skin rashes, joint pains, neuritis, skin and mucosal bleeding. *Precautions:* It suppresses bone-marrow function. It should not be given to patients who are pregnant or to breast-feeding mothers. Frequent tests of bone-marrow, liver and kidney function should be carried out. It should not be used in patients with impaired kidney or liver function. *Dose:* By injection – dose varies according to the disorder being treated.

Cyteal is an antiseptic skin cleanser containing chlorhexidine gluconate 0·5%, chlorocresol 0·3% and hexamidine isethionate 0·1%.

Cytosar ◊ cytarabine.

dacarbazine (DTIC) is an anti-cancer drug. *Adverse effects:* These include severe vomiting. *Precautions:* It is irritant to the skin and mucous membrane and should therefore be handled with great caution.

Dactil ◊ piperidolate.

Dakin's solution ◊ solution of chlorinated lime.

Daktacort cream and **ointment** contains miconazole 2% and hydrocortisone 1%.

Daktarin ◊ miconazole.

Dalacin C ◊ clindamycin.

Dalacin T solution contains clindamycin. ◊ clindamycin. Used to treat acne. May cause dry skin, dermatitis, boils, diarrhoea or colitis (stop immediately). Avoid contact with eyes and mouth.

Dalivit is a multivitamin preparation. Each capsule contains vitamin A 10,000 units, thiamine mononitrate 3 mg, riboflavine 3 mg, nicotinamide 25 mg, pyridoxine hydrochloride 1 mg, ascorbic acid 75 mg, vitamin D 1,000 units, calcium pantothenate 5 mg. Each 0·6 ml of oral drops contain vitamin A 5,000 units, thiamine hydrochloride 1 mg, riboflavine 400 micrograms, nicotinamide 5 mg, pyridoxine hydrochloride 500 micrograms, ascorbic acid 50 mg, vitamin D 400 units. Each 5 ml of syrup contains vitamin A 5,000 units, thiamine hydrochloride 2·5 mg, riboflavine 1 mg, nicotinamide 10 mg, pyridoxine hydrochloride 1 mg, ascorbic acid 25 mg, vitamin D 1,000 units, calcium pantothenate 5 mg.

Dalmane ◊ flurazepam.

danazol (Danol) is used to treat endometriosis, infertility associated with endometriosis, fibrocystic mastitis, virginal breast hypertrophy, gynaecomastia, precocious puberty and other endocrine disorders where control of the release of the pituitary gonadotrophic hormones LH and FSH would be therapeutic. *Adverse effects:* Acne, oily skin, fluid retention, mild hirsutism (hairiness), voice changes and rarely enlargement of clitoris, flushing, reduction of breast size, skin rashes, nausea, headache, dizziness, emotional upsets, nervousness, muscle spasms, loss of hair and increase in weight. *Precautions:* Should not be used in pregnancy. Use with caution in patients with impaired kidney, liver or heart function, epilepsy or migraine. It may potentiate the effects of anti-coagulant drugs. *Dose:* By mouth 200 to 800 mg daily in divided dose according to disorder being treated.

Daneral-SA (sustained-release tablets) ◊ pheniramine.

danthron is a stimulant laxative.

Danol ◊ danazol.

Dantrium ◊ dantrolene.

dantrolene (Dantrium; dantrolene sodium) is a muscle relaxant used to relieve spasm produced by conditions such as stroke, multiple sclerosis and spinal cord injury. *Adverse effects:* Transient drowsiness, dizziness, weakness, malaise, fatigue, diarrhoea, occasionally urinary or musculoskeletal disturbances, and, rarely, jaundice. *Precautions:* It should be given with caution to patients with impaired heart, lung and liver function; tests of liver function should be carried out six weeks after starting treatment. Desired effects may not develop for a few weeks but if the patient has not improved after about 45 days treatment should be stopped. Patients should not drive or operate machinery until therapy is stabilized. It should not be used in children or when spasticity serves a purpose e.g., in walking. It may enhance the effects of CNS depressant drugs. *Dose:* By mouth, initially 25 mg daily gradually increasing over 7 weeks to a maximum of 100 mg four times daily.

Daonil ◊ glibenclamide.

dapsone is used to treat leprosy and a skin condition known as dermatitis herpetiformis. *Adverse effects:* Neuropathy, allergic dermatitis, anorexia, nausea, vomiting, headache, insomnia, tachycardia, anaemia, hepatitis, blood disorders, lepra reactions (discontinue if eye or nerve trunks are affected). *Precautions:* Use with caution in patients with heart or lung disease and in breast-feeding mothers. Probenecid reduces the excretion of dapsone and will increase its adverse effects. It should not be used in pregnancy. *Dose:* By mouth, 25 to 50 mg twice weekly, gradually increased to 400 mg twice weekly or 100 mg daily.

Daranide ◊ dichlorphenamide.

Daraprim ◊ pyrimethamine.

daunorubicin (Cerubidin; daunorubicin hydrochloride) is an anti-cancer drug. *Adverse effects:* It may produce fever, nausea, vomiting, diarrhoea, abdominal pain, sore mouth, skin rash and loss of hair (alopecia). Damage to the bone marrow may produce severe blood disorders. It may also damage the heart. Injections may produce pain and irritation. *Precautions:* It should not be used in patients with heart disease and in patients with an infection. It should be used with utmost caution in pregnancy. *Dose:* Varies according to the disorder being treated.

Davenol: Each 5 ml of linctus contains carbinoxamine hydrochloride 2 mg, ephedrine hydrochloride 7 mg, pholcodine 4 mg. *Dose:* By mouth, 5 to 10 ml three or four times daily.

Day Nurse: Each 20 ml dose contains: paracetamol 500 mg, vitamin C 60 mg, phenylpropanolamine hydrochloride 25 mg, dextromethorphan hydrobromide 15 mg, and alcohol 3·08 ml.

DDAVP nose drops ◊ desmopressin.

DDD Lotion (Extra Strength) contains thymol 0·09%, methol 0·14%, salicylic acid 1·84%, resorcinol 0·74%, chlorbutol 1·1%, methyl salicylate 0·92%, glycerol 7·72%, liquefied phenol 0·98%, and alcohol 34·74%.

DDD Lotion (Ordinary Strength) contains thymol 0·09%, menthol 0·14%, salicylic acid 0·75%, resorcinol 0·75%, chlorbutol 1·13%, methyl salicylate 0·94%, glycerol 7·93%, liquefied phenol 0·98%, and alcohol 34·11%.

DDD Medicated Cream contains thymol 0·09%, menthol 0·15%, methyl salicylate 1·15%, chlorbutol 1·11%, resorcin 0·25%, liquefied phenol 0·98%, and titanium dioxide 0·5%.

DDT ◊ dicophane.

De Witt's Analgesic Pills: Each contains paracetamol 330 mg and caffeine 30 mg.

De Witt's Antacid Powder contains magnesium trisilicate 12%, light magnesium carbonate 10%, calcium carbonate 20%, sodium bicarbonate 48·5%, light kaolin 9% and peppermint oil 0·5%.

De Witt's Antacid Tablets: Each contains calcium carbonate 324 mg, heavy magnesium carbonate 194·4 mg, magnesium trisilicate 64·8 mg, peppermint oil 3·6 mg, and lactose 129·6 mg.

De Witt's Kidney and Bladder Pills: Each contains potassium nitrate 50 mg, juniper oil 2 mg, alcoholic (60%) extract of buchu (1–4) 10 mg, methylene blue 10 mg, aqueous extract of uva ursi (2–7) 20 mg, cascara dry extract 15 mg.

De Witt's Throat Lozenges: Each contains tyrothricin 1·25 mg, benzocaine 8 mg, and cetylpyridinium chloride 2 mg.

Deakin's Cough and Cold Healer contains camphor 0·05%, liquefied phenol 0·42%, anise oil 0·04%, benzoic acid 0·025%, glacial acetic acid 0·5%, aqueous extract (1 in 1) of coltsfoot flower 0·5%, senega liquid extract 0·25%, liquorice liquid extract 2·08%, squill liquid extract 0·25%, concentrated chloroform water 1·25%, and syrup 10%.

Deakin's Fever and Inflammation Remedy contains sodium salicylate 2·8%, sodium citrate 2·8%, concentrated quassia infusion 2%, alcoholic (25%) extract of bearberry (2 in 5) 2%, alcoholic (25%) extract of caryophyllum (1 in 5) 3%, taraxacum juice 5%, strong ginger tincture 0·5%, camphor 0·05%, peppermint oil 0·04%, liquefied phenol 0·41%, cinnamon oil 0·04%, and anise oil 0·04%.

Debrisan consists of beads of dextranomer which absorb exudate and tissue debris from wounds and ulcers. *Dose:* Replace with fresh beads one to five times daily.

debrisoquine (Declinax; debrisoquine sulphate) has effects and uses similar to those described under guanethidine. It is used to treat raised blood pressure. *Dose:* By mouth, 10 to 120 mg daily in divided doses or as a single dose.

Decadron ◊ dexamethasone.

Deca-Durabolin ◊ nandrolone.

Decaserpyl ◊ methoserpidine.

Decaserpyl Plus is used to treat raised blood pressure. Each tablet contains methoserpidine 10 mg and benzthiazide 20 mg. *Dose:* 2 to 3 daily.

Declinax ◊ debrisoquine.

Decortisyl ◊ prednisone.

Defencin ◊ isoxsuprine.

deglycyrrhinized liquorice is used to treat indigestion and peptic ulcers.

dehydrocholic acid increases the volume of bile fluid without increasing its total content of bile salts and pigments. It is given after surgery of the gall bag to flush out the ducts. It has also been used for the temporary relief of constipation.

Delax is an emulsion containing in each 5 ml liquid paraffin 2·5 ml, phenolphthalein 45 mg, and benzoic acid 5·5 mg.

Delfen ◊ nonoxynol.

Delial Factor 10 is a sunscreen preparation which contains 2-phenyl-1H-benzimidazole-5-sulphonic acid.

Delimon* is a pain reliever. Each tablet contains morazone 150 mg, paracetamol 50 mg and salicylamide 200 mg. *Dose:* By mouth, ½ to 1 tablet as required.

Delrosa Blackcurrant and Rose Hip Syrup is a sucrose-free syrup containing not less than 110 mg of ascorbic acid per fl oz.

Delrosa Real Orange Juice and Rose Hip Syrup is a sucrose-free syrup containing not less than 110 mg of ascorbic acid per fl oz.

Delrosa Rose Hip Syrup is a sucrose-free syrup containing ascorbic acid not less than 110 mg per fl oz.

Delta-Phoricol ◊ prednisolone.

Deltacortril Enteric ◊ prednisolone.

Deltalone ◊ prednisolone.

Deltastab ◊ prednisolone.

demecarium eye drops (Tosmilen; demecarium bromide) are used in the treatment of glaucoma. *Dose:* Apply 1 to 2 times daily.

demeclocycline (Ledermycin; demeclocycline hydrochloride; demethylchlortetracycline hydrochloride) is a tetracycline antibiotic. It is long acting. *Adverse effects* and *Precautions:* These are similar to those described under tetracycline but in addition demeclocycline may cause skin sensitivity to sunlight. Patients should therefore avoid exposure to sunlight when receiving treatment with this drug. Salts of aluminium, calcium, and magnesium (e.g., antacid mixtures) and iron may decrease the absorption of demeclocycline from the gut and should not be given to patients receiving treatment with this drug. Milk, which contains calcium, may also interfere with its absorption. *Dose:* By mouth, 300 to 900 mg daily in divided doses.

demethylchlortetracycline ◊ demeclocycline.

Demser ◊ metirosine.

De-Nol (tripotassium di-citrate bismuthate) is used to treat peptic ulcers. *Adverse effects:* Blackening of the stools usually occurs and darkening of the tongue has been reported. *Precautions:* It should not be used in pregnancy and in patients with severe kidney impairment. It may interfere with the absorption of tetracycline drugs. *Dose:* 5 ml of De-Nol diluted with 15 ml water or 1 tablet chewed and swallowed with water four times daily on an empty stomach.

De-Noltab (tripotassium dicitratobismuthate) ◊ De-Nol.

denatonium benzoate is used as a denaturant for alcohol in toilet preparations. It has a very bitter taste and is used on the nails to stop them being bitten.

Dentinox Colic Drops contain dimethicone 42 mg per ml and used to treat infant colic. They contain antifoam M (dimethicone plus silica) 4%.

Dentinox gel is used to treat infant teething. It has a local anaesthetic action. It contains lignocaine hydrochloride 0·03%, myrrh tincture 0·8%, chamomile extract 15% and cetylpyridinium chloride 0·1%.

Dentinox Teething Liquid contains lignocaine hydrochloride 0·33%, myrrh tincture 0·8%, alcoholic (60%) chamomile extract (1–5) 15%, honey 17%, cetylpyridinium chloride 0·1%, and alcohol 3%.

Dentosine mouthwash contains tannic acid 2·2%, phenol 2·2%, glycerol 11%, isopropyl alcohol 18%, tincture of krameria 7%, witch hazel (distilled extract) 10%.

deoxycortone (deoxycortone pivalate) is a corticosteroid ◊ cortisone. *Dose:* By intramuscular injection, 50 to 100 mg every 2 to 4 weeks.

deoxyephedrine ◊ methylamphetamine.

deoxyribonuclease (Deanase) is used to remove clots and exudates. It may be given by aerosol inhalation, intramuscular injection, local injection or as a bladder washout. *Adverse effects:* Local irritation and hypersensitivity, if given by inhalation may produce bronchospasm. *Dose:* Varies according to route of administration.

Depixol ◊ flupenthixol.

Depo-Medrone (methylprednisolone acetate – a long-acting injection) ◊ methylprednisolone. Available as 40 mg in 1, 2 and 5 ml suspensions for depot injections.

Depo-Provera (injection of 50 mg/ml of medroxyprogesterone) ◊ medroxyprogesterone.

Depocillin ◊ procaine penicillin.

Deponit 5 patch is designed to release glyceryl trinitrate from a plaster through the skin and into the blood stream ◊ glyceryl trinitrate.

Depostat ◊ gestronol.

Dequacaine lozenges are used to treat mouth and throat infections. Each lozenge contains dequalinium chloride 0·011% and benzocaine 0·45%.

Dequadin paint and **throat lozenges** ◊ dequalinium.

dequalinium (Dequadin; Labosept; dequalinium chloride) is used as an antibacterial drug and antifungal drug in throat lozenges and paints. *Precautions:* Its prolonged and repeated use should be avoided. It can cause the skin to ulcerate when applied under dressings and it should not be used around the anus and genitals.

Derbac-C ◊ carbaryl.

Derbac-M ◊ malathion.

Dermacolor is a masking cream for concealing scars, areas of discolouration and birthmarks.

Dermalex skin lotion is used to treat urinary rash and pressure sores. It contains squalane 3%, hexachlorophane 0·5% and allantoin 0·25%.

Dermidex Lotion is an antiseptic, anaesthetic creamy. It contains lignocaine 1·2%, aldioxa 0·25%, chlorbutol 1%, and cetrimide 0·5%.

Dermonistat cream ◊ miconazole.

Dermovate ◊ clobetasol.

Dermovate-NN cream contains clobetasol propionate 0·05% neomycin sulphate 0·5% and nystatin 100,000 units per g.

Deseril ◊ methysergide.

Desferal ◊ desferrioxamine.

desferrioxamine (Desferal) is used in the treatment of iron poisoning and in patients who store too much iron in their bodies. It joins with the iron, and the combination is excreted in the urine. *Adverse effects:* These include pain at the site of injection and hypotension if given too rapidly by IV injection. *Dose:* By injection, depending on the condition being treated.

desipramine (Pertofran; desipramine hydrochloride) is a tricyclic antidepressant drug. *Adverse effects* and *Precautions:* These are similar to those described under imipramine. *Dose:* By mouth, initially 25 to 150 mg daily in divided doses.

deslanoside (Cedilanid; lanatoside C) has similar actions to digoxin. *Dose:* By mouth, 0·25 to 1·5 mg per day. An injection is also available.

desmopressin (DDAVP nasal drops and injections, Desmospray nasal spray) is a synthetic relative of the natural antidiuretic hormone, arginine vasopressin (AVP) which is a hormone produced by the posterior pituitary gland. This hormone causes the kidneys to retain water from the urine. Desmopressin is used to treat diabetes insipidus – a condition in which the posterior lobe of the pituitary gland fails to produce the antidiuretic hormone with the result that the patient drinks excessive amounts of fluids and passes large volumes of weak urine. Desmopressin is also used to treat bed-wetting and to test kidney function. *Precautions:* It should be used with caution in patients with impaired kidney function or heart disease and in pregnancy. It should only be used to treat bed-wetting in patients who have a normal blood pressure. *Dose:* Up the nose, 10 to 20 micrograms once or twice daily. By intramuscular or intravenous injection, 1 to 4 micrograms daily. For bed-wetting, do not use nasal applications nightly for more than one month.

Desmospray ◊ desmopressin. It is a metered dose atomizer for administration up the nose.

desogestrel is a progestogen.

desonide (Tridesilon) is a potent corticosteroid used to treat severe skin disorders ◊ hydrocortisone.

desoxymethasone (Stiedex) is a topical corticosteroid used to treat skin disorders.

Destolit ◊ ursodeoxycholic acid.

Deteclo: Each antibiotic tablet contains chlortetracycline 115·4 mg, tetracycline hydrochloride 115·4 mg and demethylchlortetracycline hydrochloride 69·2 mg. *Dose:* 1 twice daily.

Dettol ◊ chloroxylenol.

Dexa-Rhinaspray is used to treat nasal allergy. Each aerosol dose contains tramazoline 0·12 mg, dexamethasone 0·02 mg and neomycin 0·1 mg.

dexamethasone (Decadron; Oradexon) has effects, uses and adverse effects similar to those of prednisolone but it is effective in lower doses. *Dose:* By mouth, 0·5 to 10 mg daily in divided doses.

dexamphetamine (Dexedrine; dexamphetamine sulphate; dextroamphetamine sulphate) produces similar effects to those described under amphetamine. *Dose:* By mouth, from 5 mg twice a day to 10 mg three times a day.

dexbrompheniramine (Halin) is an antihistamine drug.

Dexedrine ◊ dexamphetamine.

dexpanthenol is an alcohol analogue of pantothenic acid. It is present in some ointments, creams, solutions and cosmetics but for what reason is difficult to interpret.

dexpanthenol ethyl ether ◊ dexpanthenol.

dextran infusions are used to restore blood volume after accidents or operations.

Dextraven ◊ dextran.

dextrin is made from starch and is used in some infant foods, in surgical dressings and as a thickening agent.

dextroamphetamine ◊ dexamphetamine.

Dextrolyte is an oral solution of glucose, potassium chloride, sodium chloride and sodium lactate for rehydrating patients suffering from diarrhoea.

dextromethorphan (dextromethorphan hydrobromide) is a useful cough suppressant. *Adverse effects:* It may occasionally cause drowsiness and dizziness. No case of drug dependence has so far been reported. *Dose:* 15 to 30 mg by mouth once to four times daily.

dextromoramide (Palfium; dextromoramide tartrate) is used to relieve moderate to severe pain. It may be given by mouth, by rectum or by subcutaneous or intramuscular injection. It works for about four hours. *Adverse effects:* Dextromoramide may cause nausea, vomiting, dizziness, faintness (due to a fall in blood pressure) and insomnia. As with morphine these are more likely to occur if the patient is up and about. *Precautions:* It should be used with caution in patients with impaired liver function. It is a powerful respiratory depressant and should not be used in pregnant women or with drugs known to depress respiration, e.g. anaesthetics, sedatives, hypnotics and tranquillizers. After each of the first few doses the patient should lie down for half an hour because of the drug's effects. *Drug dependence:* Prolonged use of dextromoramide may lead to the development of tolerance, mood changes and drug dependence of the morphine type. *Dose:* By mouth or injection, 5 mg.

dextropropoxyphene (dextropropoxyphene hydrochloride; propoxyphene hydrochloride and also Doloxene; propoxyphene napsylate) is a mild pain reliever with probably similar potency to that of codeine, but it is less constipating. *Adverse effects:* Dextropropoxyphene may cause dizziness, headache, drowsiness, excitation, raised mood (euphoria), insomnia and skin rashes, nausea, vomiting, abdominal pains and constipation. Drug dependence may occur. *Precautions:* Dextropropoxyphene should be given with caution to patients with severe respiratory disorders. It may increase the effects of other respiratory depressant drugs (e.g., sedatives and hypnotics). *Dose:* Dextropropoxyphene hydrochloride: up to 400 mg daily in divided doses. Dextropropoxyphene napsylate: up to 260 mg daily in divided doses.

dextrose ◊ glucose.

Dextrostix is a reagent stick for the testing of glucose in the blood.

dextrothyroxine sodium (Choloxin) is used to lower blood fat levels. It lowers the concentration of cholesterol in the blood. *Adverse effects:* These include rapid heart beat, angina. *Dose:* By mouth, 1 to 2 mg daily increasing to a maximum of 8 mg daily.

DF 118 ◊ dihydrocodeine.

DHC Continus tablets contain 600 mg of dihydrocodeine in a controlled release form ◊ dihydrocodeine.

Diabinese ◊ chlorpropamide.

Diabur-Test 5000 is used to detect glucose in the urine.

Diamicron ◊ gliclazide.

Diamond Corn Treatment contains salicylic acid 13%, amyl acetate 2%, pyroxylin 1·625%, acetone to 100%.

Diamond Foot & Body Powder contains chlorphenesin 1·5%, zinc oxide 10%, and boric acid 10%.

diamorphine (heroin; diamorphine hydrochloride) has effects and uses similar to those described under morphine. It is more potent than morphine but is shorter acting – only about two hours. It has less tendency to produce vomiting and constipation. It is also a good cough suppressant. *Adverse effects* and *Precautions* ◊ morphine, *Drug dependence:* Diamorphine produces dependence of the morphine type. *Dose:* By mouth or injection, 5 to 10 mg, when necessary. To suppress coughs, 1·5 to 6 mg by mouth.

Diamox ◊ acetazolamide.

Dianette tablets contain the anti-male sex hormone cyproterone (2 mg) and the female oestrogen sex hormone ethinyloestradiol (35 micrograms). It is used to treat severe acne in females. The reason for using it is to try to block the effects of male sex hormones (androgens) which are considered to be a major factor in the development of acne. Dianette is also an effective oral contraceptive and women should *not* take any other oral contraceptive whilst on this treatment. It is not suitable for treating male acne. *Adverse effects:* Breast enlargement, bloated feeling, fluid retention, cramps, pains in the legs, depression, loss of libido, headaches, nausea, vaginal discharge, superficial ulcers on the neck of the womb, weight gain, breakthrough bleeding and brown patches on the skin of the face (chloasma). *Precautions:* Do not use in patients who suffer from or who have suffered from angina, coronary heart disease, thrombosis, valvular disease of the heart, sickle cell anaemia, jaundice, hepatitis, liver disease or any other disorder in which an oral contraceptive should not be taken. It should be used with caution in patients with hypertension, Raynaud's disease, diabetes, varicose veins, asthma or severe depression or in patients receiving kidney dialysis. For other precautions see oral contraceptives p. 235. *Dose:* By mouth, one tablet daily for 21 days starting on fifth day of menstrual cycle, then 7 free days.

Diarrest is used to treat diarrhoea. Each 5 ml contains codeine phosphate 5 mg, dicyclomine hydrochloride 2·5 mg, potassium chloride 40 mg, sodium chloride 50 mg and sodium citrate 50 mg. *Dose:* By mouth, 20 ml four times daily with water.

Diarrhoea & Sickness Mixture: Each 5 ml contains kaolin 1·83 g, pectin 50 mg, and belladonna tincture 0·1 ml.

diastase is a mixture of enzymes which break down starch to sugars.

Diastix reagent strip is used to test for glucose in the urine.

Diatensec ◊ spironolactone.

Dia-Tuss ◊ pholcodine.

Diazemuls ◊ diazepam.

diazepam (Alupram; Atensine; Diazemuls; Evacalm; Solis; Stesolid; Tensium; Valium) is a benzodiazepine anti-anxiety drug. It has effects and uses similar to those of chlordiazepoxide. It is used to relieve anxiety and tension. It also has muscle relaxant properties, produces sedation and is used to treat convulsions; read section on drugs used to treat epilepsy. *Adverse effects:* Drowsiness, fatigue and unsteady gait (ataxia), dryness of the mouth and fall in blood pressure may occur. In some patients it may produce excitement and aggression instead of sedation (paradoxical reaction). It may produce changes in libido, constipation, incontinence and trembling. Very rarely skin rashes and blood and liver disorders may occur. *Precautions:* Diazepam should be used with caution by patients with impaired kidney or liver function and by the elderly and debilitated. 'Normal' doses may make these patients unsteady on their feet, drowsy and confused. Its effects may be increased by alcohol, barbiturates, narcotics or any other drug which depresses brain function. Diazepam may interfere with ability to drive a motor vehicle or operate moving machinery. When given along with other anti-convulsant drugs, diazepam may increase the frequency and severity of major fits. This will require an increased dosage of the other anti-convulsant. Also, abrupt withdrawal may be associated with a temporary increase in frequency and severity of fits. *Drug dependence:* Diazepam may cause dependence of the barbiturate/alcohol type. *Dose:* By mouth, 5 to 30 mg daily in divided doses.

diazoxide (Eudemine) is used for disorders of low blood sugar levels and to treat raised blood pressure. *Adverse effects:* It causes water and salt retention and a diuretic may be given with it. If the blood sugar goes too high, insulin has to be given. *Precautions:* It can cause blood disorders and interfere with growth in children. *Dose:* By mouth – starting with 5 mg per kg of body-weight per day, the dose is increased until the required effect is achieved. Diazoxide given into a vein produces a rapid fall in blood pressure lasting up to twenty-four hours. It is used in emergencies to treat raised blood pressure in a dose of 300 mg.

dibenylamine (phenoxybenzamine hydrochloride) ◊ phenoxybenzamine.

Dibenyline ◊ phenoxybenzamine.

dibromopropamidine isethionate has antibacterial and antifungal properties and is used in skin applications.

dibutylphthalate is used as an insect repellent. It is not easily removed by washing and is used to impregnate clothing, giving protection for up to two weeks. It may produce hypersensitivity.

dichloralphenazone (Welldorm) has the effects of its constituents, chloral and phenazone. It is used as a hypnotic and sedative. *Adverse effects:* It may rarely produce nausea, headache, lassitude and skin rashes. *Precautions:* It may increase the effects of alcohol and other drugs that produce depression of brain function. It should not be given to patients who suffer from intermittent porphyria since it may trigger off an acute attack. It may also interfere with the actions of anticoagulant drugs. *Drug dependence:* Dichloralphenazone may produce dependence of the barbiturate/alcohol type. *Dose:* By mouth, to produce sleep, 0·65 to 1·3 g at night.

dichlorobenzyl alcohol is used as an antiseptic in throat lozenges and skin applications.

dichlorodifluoromethane is a propellent used in refrigerant sprays to relieve pain.

dichlorophen is used in the treatment of tapeworm infections. It is also used as a fungicide and as a germicide in soaps. Its use in cosmetics and toiletries is restricted. *Adverse effects:* In oral doses used to treat tapeworm it may produce nausea, vomiting, colic and diarrhoea. It may produce skin rash and jaundice. *Precautions:* It should not be used in patients with impaired kidney function and where purgation would be harmful – e.g. pregnancy, heart disease and acute fevers. *Dose:* By mouth, 6 g daily for 2 to 3 successive days. It is best taken in the mornings on an empty stomach.

dichloroxylenol is bactericidal and is used in antiseptic preparations.

dichlorphenamide (Daranide; Oratrol) is a diuretic, with effects and uses similar to those described under acetazolamide but it has a more prolonged action and it causes an increase in the excretion of chlorides. *Adverse effects* and *Precautions* are similar to those described under acetazolamide. It may rarely cause skin rash, and prolonged use causes the loss of salt and potassium which may require the addition of potassium to the treatment. No bone-marrow or kidney damage has been reported. *Dose:* By mouth, for glaucoma, 25 to 50 mg up to three times daily. It is also used as a diuretic to treat chronic chest disorders.

diclofenac (Voltarol) is an antirheumatic drug. *Adverse effects:* Transient symptoms may include epigastric pains, nausea, diarrhoea and headaches, skin rashes, oedema of the ankles and abnormal liver function tests may occur. Peptic ulceration with bleeding occurs rarely. *Precautions:* It should not be used in pregnancy and it should be used with the utmost caution in patients with a history of peptic ulcer, or in patients with impaired function of their liver or kidneys. It should not be used in patients who have a peptic ulcer or by patients who develop a reaction such as asthma, urticaria or rhinitis, to aspirin or other non-steroidal anti-rheumatic drugs: *Dose:* By mouth, 50 mg, two or three times daily with meals.

dicobalt edetate ◊ Kelocyanor.

Diconal is a moderate to severe pain reliever. Each tablet contains dipipanone hydrochloride 10 mg and cyclizine hydrochloride 30 mg. *Dose:* 1 tablet; repeat every six hours if necessary.

dicophane (DDT; chlorophenothane) is an insecticide. It is stored in the body fat and may cause chronic poisoning. It is used to treat lice.

dicyclomine (Merbentyl; dicyclomine hydrochloride) has weak atropine-like effects but it does not act upon the brain ◊ atropine. It is used to treat indigestion and peptic ulcer. *Dose:* By mouth, 30 to 60 mg daily in divided doses.

Dicynene ◊ ethamsylate.

Didronel ◊ etidronate.

dienoestrol ◊ has effects and uses similar to the female sex hormone stilboestrol but it is less potent. It is used as a vaginal cream (0·01%).

diethanolamine fusidate (Fucidin IV infusion) is an antibiotic. *Adverse* *effects:* These include nausea, vomiting, rashes and jaundice. *Dose:* It is given by slow intravenous infusion, 500 mg over 6 hours.

diethylamine salicylate has the actions of salicylates (◊ aspirin) and is used in rheumatic rubs.

diethylcarbamazine (Banocide; diethylcarbamazine citrate) is used in the treatment of parasitic worms. *Dose:* By mouth, depends on the type of worm.

diethyl phthalate is included in Three Flasks Cold Sore Lotion.

diethylpropion (in Apisate, Tenuate Dospan). Diethylpropion is used as a slimming drug. *Adverse effects:* Similar to those described under amphetamine, but diethylpropion produces less effect upon the heart and circulation. It may produce drug dependence of the amphetamine type. *Dose:* 25 mg three times daily before meals, 75 mg daily.

diethylstilboestrol ◊ stilboestrol.

diethyltoluamide is an insect repellent. It can occasionally cause hypersensitivity. *Adverse effects* and *Precautions*. It should not be applied near the eyes, to mucous membranes, to broken skin or near areas of skin flexion (e.g. elbows) – it can cause irritation and blistering.

Difflam ◊ benzydamine.

diflucortolone (Nerisone, Temetex; diflucortolone valerate) is a corticosteroid ◊ cortisone. It is used in skin applications.

diflunisal (Dolobid) is an aspirin derivative used to treat rheumatic disorders. *Adverse effects:* These include nausea, vertigo, somnolence, pruritis and skin rash. *Precautions:* It should not be used in pregnancy or nursing mothers. Care is necessary in patients on anticoagulants, patients with renal failure and those with a history of peptic ulcer. *Dose:* By mouth, 250 to 500 mg twice daily.

Digespirin Antacid Tablets each contain dihydroxyaluminium sodium carbonate 300 mg.

Digitaline Nativelle ◊ digitoxin.

digitalis: Read section on drugs used to treat heart failure.

digitoxin: (Digitaline Nativelle): Read section on drugs used to treat heart failure.

digoxin (Lanoxin): Read section on drugs used to treat heart failure.

Dihydergot ◊ dihydroergotamine.

dihydroallantoinate ◊ allantoin.

dihydrocodeine (DF 118; DHC Continus; dihydrocodeine tartrate; dihydrocodeine acid tartrate) is a mild to moderate pain reliever. It is also used as a cough suppressant. *Adverse effects:* These are similar to those described under morphine but less pronounced. *Precautions:* Dihydrocodeine should be given with caution to patients with impaired liver function and severe respiratory disorders (e.g., asthma). *Drug dependence:* It may produce dependence of the morphine type. *Dose:* By mouth, 30 to 60 mg when necessary, up to a maximum of 150 mg in twenty-four hours.

dihydroergotamine (Dihydergot, dihydroergotamine mesylate) is used to treat migraine. It has effects and uses similar to those described under ergotamine but it produces less vomiting and there is less risk of gangrene. *Dose:* By mouth, 1 to 2 mg repeated every half hour up to maximum of 10 mg; severe attacks, intramuscularly 1 to 2 mg.

dihydrostreptomycin ◊ streptomycin.

dihydrotachysterol (A. T. 10; Tachyrol) is vitamin D. *Dose:* By mouth, for hypercalcaemia, 0·2 mg daily.

dihydroxyacetone (Artificial Suntan Lotion) produces a slowly developing brown coloration of the skin. Its actions are unknown. It may occasionally produce skin rashes. It gives no protection against sunburn.

dihydroxyaluminium aminoacetate is used is antacid mixtures.

dihydroxyaluminium sodium carbonate (aluminium sodium carbonate hydroxide) is used as an antacid.

di-8-hydroxyquinoline p-aminosalicylate is used as an antiseptic in Valderma Antiseptic Cream.

di-iodohydroxyquinoline is used to treat amoebiasis of the gut. It has been used to treat *Trichomonas vaginalis* and fungal skin infections.

di-isobutylphenoxypolyethoxyethanol is used in contraceptive jellies and creams as spermicide.

di-isoephedrine ◊ aephedrine

Dijex Liquid is an antacid. Each 5 ml contains aluminium hydroxide gel 98% and magnesium hydroxide 1·7%. Dose 5 to 10 ml every two to four hours as required.

Dijex Tablets: Each contains aluminium hydroxide-magnesium carbonate co-dried gel 400 mg.

dill is obtained from the dried ripe fruit of *Anethum graveolens*. It is used as an aromatic carminative and the distilled water is used to relieve wind in babies.

dill oil ◊ dill.

dill water ◊ dill.

diloxanide (Entamizole; Furamide; dieoxanide furoate) is an amoebicide.

diltiazem (Britiazem; Calcicard; Tildiem) is used to treat and prevent angina. *Adverse effects:* These include slowing of the heart, ankle swelling, headache, nausea and rashes. *Precautions:* Do not use in pregnancy, in patients with severe heart block or slow pulse rate. Use with caution in patients with impaired kidney or liver function. *Dose:* By mouth, 60 mg to 120 mg three times daily.

Dimelor ◊ acetohexamide.

dimenhydrinate (Dramamine; Gravol; diphenhydramine theoclate) is an antihistamine drug. It is used to prevent and relieve motion sickness. One of its main adverse effects is drowsiness. *Dose:* By mouth, 25 to 50 mg (half an hour before a journey) and up to four times daily.

dimercaprol (British Anti-Lewisite) is used to treat poisoning with antimony, arsenic, bismuth, gold, mercury, and thallium.

dimethicone (silicone) is used as a water-repellent in skin applications, and as a dispersant in antacids.

dimethindene (Fenostil Retard; dimethindene maleate) is an antihistamine with similar effects to promethazine. *Dose:* 1 sustained-release tablet (2·5 mg) twice daily.

dimethylaminobenzoate (in Spectraban; in Coppertone supershade) is used as a sunscreen agent.

dimethylaminoethanol bitartrate and hydrogen tartrate has been used to relieve runny nose and as an antispasmodic.

dimethylphthalate (Sketofax) is used as an insect repellent.

dimethylpolysiloxane ◊ dimethicone.

dimethyl sulphoxide (Rimso-50) is used to relieve cystitis by instilling a solution into the bladder. It is also used as a penetrating basis for other drugs to be applied topically. *Adverse effects:* When applied to skin it may produce itching, burning and blisters. Nausea, vomiting, drowsiness and hypersensitivity reactions may occur. It produces a garlic odour in the breath. *Precautions:* It should not be applied to the eyes and it should not be used in pregnancy.

Dimotane ◊ brompheniramine.

Dimotane Plus: A cough liquid which is sugar-free. It contains brompheniramine maleate 4 mg and pseudoephedrine hydrochloride 30 mg in each 5 ml ◊ brompheniramine and pseudoephedrine. **Paediatric liquid** contains 2 mg and 15 mg in each 5 ml, respectively.

Dimotapp is used to treat upper respiratory symptoms and allergie. Each 5 ml contains brompheniramine maleate 4 mg, phenylephrine hydrochloride 5 mg and phenylpropanolamine hydrochloride 5 mg; Dimotapp L. A. as Dimotapp but each tablet contains 12 mg, 15 mg and 15 mg respectively. *Dose:* Dimotapp L. A. 1 or 2 tablets every twelve hours.

Dindevan ◊ phenindione.

Dinneford's Magnesia Gripe Mixture contains heavy magnesium carbonate 1·57%, citric acid monohydrate 3·54%, sodium bicarbonate 2·13%, sucrose 25%, and rectified spirit 5·28%.

dinoprost (Prostin F2 alpha) is a prostaglandin used to produce abortion and induce labour. *Adverse effects:* These include nausea, vomiting, headache, dizziness, temporary pyrexia and raised white blood count, and also redness at the site of injection. *Precautions:* Do not use in severe toxaemia, unrelated pelvic infection and where there may be a risk of uterine rupture. *Dose:* By intravenous infusion or intra-amniotic injection in a dose which varies according to the condition being treated.

dinoprostone (Prostin E2) is a prostaglandin used to produce abortion or induce labour. *Adverse effects, Precautions* and *Dose* ◊ dinoprost. It may be given by vaginal tablet.

Diocalm is used to treat diarrhoea. Each tablet contains morphine hydrochloride 0·36 mg and hydrated magnesium aluminium silicate (activated attapulgite) 280 mg.

Dioctyl ◊ docusate sodium.

dioctyl calcium sulphosuccinate lowers surface tension and has detergent properties. It is used to soften faeces in the treatment of constipation.

Dioctyl-medo ◊ docusate sodium.

Dioderm ◊ hydrocortisone.

Dioralyte sachets contain 0·2 g sodium chloride, 0·3 g potassium chloride, 0·3 g sodium bicarbonate and 8 g glucose. Used to treat fluid and salt loss, especially in babies with diarrhoea and vomiting. Each sachet to be added to 200 ml of water.

Dioralyte effervescent tablets contain sodium bicarbonate 300 mg, potassium bicarbonate 200 mg, citric acid 1·06 g, glucose 3·6 g. Plain or pineapple flavour. Note the tablets do not contain chlorides which are lost in diarrhoea and vomiting.

Diovol suspension is used to treat indigestion and peptic ulcer. Each 5 ml contains dimethicone 25 mg, aluminium hydroxide 200 mg, magnesium hydroxide 200 mg. *Dose:* By mouth, 10 to 20 ml three times daily and when necessary.

Diovol Fruit is used to treat indigestion and peptic ulcers. The contents are the same as Diovol Suspension but it is yellow and fruit flavoured.

dioxybenzone is a sunscreen agent.

Dip/Ser is a diphtheria antitoxin which is used to give protection after exposure (passive immunization) and in the treatment of diphtheria.

Dip/Vac/ads is a diphtheria vaccine.

dipentene ◊ terebene.

diperodon hydrochloride is a local anaesthetic.

diphenhydramine (Benadryl; diphenhydramine hydrochloride) is an antihistamine drug. It is one of the least effective antihistamines but produces more drowsiness. For this reason it is used to provide sleep, often in combination with a hypnotic drug. *Dose:* Diphenhydramine: by mouth, 50 to 200 mg daily in divided doses.

diphenoxylate (present in Lomotil) reduces the motility of the gut and is used to treat diarrhoea. *Adverse effects:* These include itching, skin rash, drowsiness, insomnia, dizziness, restlessness, changes in mood, abdominal distension and nausea. *Precautions:* It should not be used in patients with impaired liver function. It may increase the effects of barbiturates and other depressant drugs. Adverse effects may be exaggerated in infants and children and it should therefore not be used in children under two. *Drug dependence:* Diphenoxylate may produce drug dependence of the morphine type. *Dose:* By mouth, 5 to 40 mg daily in divided doses.

diphenylhydantoin ◊ phenytoin.

diphenylpyraline (Histryl; Lergoban; diphenylpyraline hydrochloride) is an antihistamine drug. *Dose:* 5 to 10 mg (slow-release preparations) every twelve hours.

dipipanone (piperidyl methadone hydrochloride) is a narcotic pain reliever which produces little sedation. After intramuscular injection it works in about fifteen minutes and lasts for about four to six hours. *Adverse effects:* Nausea, vomiting, dizziness, retention of urine and constipation may occur. *Precautions:* It should not be given intravenously because it may produce an alarming fall in blood pressure. It should be used with extreme caution in patients with impaired liver or kidney function. *Drug dependence:* Dipipanone may produce drug dependence of the morphine type. *Dose:* 25 to 50 mg subcutaneously or intramuscularly when necessary.

dipivefrin (Propine) is used in eye drops to treat open angle glaucoma.

Diprivan injection contains propofol 10 mg/ml. It is an intravenous anaesthetic.

Diprobase is a cream with a water miscible base. It contains liquid paraffin 6%, white soft paraffin 15%, ceto-macrogol 2·25% and cetostearyl alcohol 7·2%.

Diprosalic ointment and scalp lotion contain betamethasone and salicylic acid.

Diprosone ◊ betamethasone dipropionate.

dipyridamole (Persantin) is used to treat angina. It may cause headache, dizziness, faintness and gastric upsets. *Dose:* By mouth, 50 mg three times daily before meals. Also 100 mg three times daily to prevent thrombosis.

Dirythmin SA ◊ disopyramide.

Disadine DP is a dry powder spray of providone iodine.

Disalcid ◊ salsalate.

Disipal ◊ orphenadrine.

Di-Sipidin ◊ posterior pituitary extract.

disodium cromoglycate ◊ sodium cromoglycate.

disodium etidronate ◊ etidronate.

disodium phosphate ◊ sodium phosphate.

disopyramide (Dirythmin SA; Rythmodan; disopyramide phosphate) is used to treat disorders of heart rhythm. *Adverse effects:* Dry mouth, blurred vision, difficulty in passing water and adverse effects similar to those produced by quinidine. *Precautions:* It should be used with caution in patients with glaucoma or a tendency to retention of urine. *Dose:* By mouth, 300 to 800 mg daily in divided doses.

Disprin tablets each contain aspirin 300 mg, calcium carbonate 90 mg, and anhydrous citric acid 30 mg.

Disprin, Junior tablets each contain aspirin 75 mg, calcium carbonate 24 mg, and anhydrous citric acid 8 mg.

Distaclor ◊ cefaclor.

Distalgesic is a mild pain reliever. Each tablet contains dextropropoxyphene hydrochloride 32·5 mg and paracetamol 325 mg. *Dose:* 2 three or four times daily.

Distamine ◊ penicillamine.

Distaquaine V-K ◊ phenoxymethylpenicillin.

distearyldimethylammonium chloride is a skin irritant.

distigmine (Ubretid; distigmine bromide) acts on the parasympathetic division of the autonomic nervous system. Its effects are similar to those described under physostigmine. It is used in the treatment of urinary retention, myasthenia ‘gravis and paralysis of the bowel after surgical operations. *Dose:* By mouth, 5 mg daily or on alternate days. An injection is also available.

disulfiram (Antabuse) is used to treat alcoholism. It is not a cure and it is used because it produces unpleasant effects when alcohol is taken. These unpleasant effects are caused by an accumulation in the blood of a breakdown product of alcohol called acetaldehyde. Within fifteen minutes of taking alcohol, disulfiram may produce red eyes, flushed face, throbbing headache, fast beating heart, dizziness, nausea, sweating and vomiting. An irritation in the throat, deep breathing and a fall in blood pressure

may occur. The effects last from a half to one hour in mild cases and up to several hours in severe attacks. The intensity and duration vary greatly between individuals; initial treatment should therefore only be used in hospital. A careful dosage regimen needs to be worked out, starting with a high dose and slowly working down to a maintenance dose. *Adverse effects:* The use of disulfiram may cause indigestion, bad breath, body odour, drowsiness, headache, impotence, allergic skin rashes and nerve damage (peripheral neuritis). Even small quantities of alcohol may produce a severe reaction, which may result in heart failure, unconsciousness, convulsions and even death. *Precautions:* It should not be used in pregnancy, in patients with heart disease, with severe psychological disorders or with drug dependence. It should be used with the utmost caution in patients with impaired liver or kidney function, and in patients with epilepsy, chronic bronchitis or diabetes. It increases the effects of coumarin anticoagulants and phenytoin. Acute confusion may occur when given with metronidazole (Flagyl). *Dose:* By mouth, starting with 800 mg on first day and reducing the dose daily to a maintenance dose of about 100 mg to 200 mg daily.

dithranol (Anthranol; Antraderm; Dithrocream; Exolan) is used to treat psoriasis. Some patients are sensitive to it and a small area of skin should be tested first. It stains the skin, causes a burning sensation and irritates the eyes.

Dithrocream HP ◊ dithranol.

Dithrolan ◊ dithranol.

Diumide-K is a diuretic with added potassium. Each tablet contains frusemide 40 mg and potassium chloride 600 mg in sustained-release form. *Dose:* By mouth, 1 daily in the morning.

Diuresal ◊ frusemide.

Diurexan ◊ xipamide.

Dixarit ◊ clonidine.

Di-threonine ◊ threonine.

Doan's Backache Pills each contain paracetamol 97·2 mg, sodium salicylate 48·6 mg, and aloin 650 micrograms.

dobutamine (Dobutrex) is a sympathomimetic drug with effects similar to isoprenaline. It has less effect on heart rate than isoprenaline and is given by slow intravenous infusion (10 microgram per kg of body-weight) to treat shock.

Dobutrex ◊ dobutamine.

Doctor's Catarrh Pastilles (Sure Shield) contain menthol 0·36%, creosote 0·18%, and pine oil 0·36%.

docusate sodium (Audinorm, Dioctylmedo, Molcer, Soliwax, Waxsol) is a surface-active agent which lowers surface tension and has detergent properties. It is used as a laxative; to soften wax in the ears; as a tablet disintegrant and as a surface-active agent in industry. *Dose:* By mouth, 50 to 100 mg when necessary.

Do-Do tablets each contain ephedrine hydrochloride 22 mg, anhydrous caffeine 30 mg, and theophylline sodium glycinate 50 mg.

Dolmatil ◊ sulpiride.

Dolobid ◊ diflunisal.

Dolomite Tablets each provides calcium 90 mg and magnesium 55 mg.

Doloxene ◊ dextropropoxyphene.

Doloxene Compound is a mild pain-reliever. Each capsule contains dextropropoxyphene napsylate 100 mg, aspirin 375 mg and caffeine 30 mg. *Dose:* 1, three or four times daily.

Dols Rub Cream contains camphor 0·4%, methyl salicylate 9·5%, capsicum extract 0·075%, sodium iodide 0·45%, and chlorocresol 0·09%.

Dome-Acne cream contains sulphur 4% and resorcinol 3%.

Domestos is a disinfectant. It is a solution of sodium hypochlorite.

Domical ◊ amitriptyline.

domiphen (Bradosol; domiphen bromide; domiphen hydrochloride) is an antiseptic with properties similar to those described under cetrimide. It is used in throat lozenges and antiseptic skin applications. In higher concentration it may be used as a disinfectant.

domperidone (Evoxin; Motilium) is used for the prevention and relief of nausea and vomiting. It has similar effects to metaclopramide but is less likely to cause sedation and dystonia.

Dose: By mouth or injection, 10 to 20 mg every 4 to 8 hours.

Doom Insect Bite Repellent with Sunscreen contains diethyltoluamide 10% and cinoxate 2·5%.

Dopamet ◊ methyldopa.

dopamine (Intropin; dopamine hydrochloride) acts on nerve endings of the sympathetic nervous system. It is used in the treatment of shock which does not respond to replacement of fluid loss. *Adverse effects* ◊ adrenaline. *Dose:* By intravenous infusion, in a dose dependent upon the patient's condition.

Dopram ◊ doxapram.

Dorant Mouthwash: Each 100 mls contains parahydroxybenzoic acid esters: ethyl 250 mg, propyl 500 mg, and benzyl 250 mg; chloroform 4·9 ml.

Dormonoct ◊ loprazolam.

dothiepin (Prothiaden) is a tricyclic antidepressant drug with effects, uses and adverse effects similar to those described under imipramine. It may cause blurred vision, drowsiness, and a fall in blood pressure on standing. *Dose:* By mouth, 75 to 150 mg daily in single or divided doses.

Double Amplex is used to treat halitosis (bad breath).

Double Check ◊ nonoxynol.

doxapram (Dopram; doxapram hydrochloride) is used to stimulate breathing in patients with respiratory failure. *Adverse effects* ◊ nikethamide, also causes tachycardia, dizziness and perineal warmth. *Precautions* ◊ nikethamide. *Dose:* By intravenous infusion, 0·5 to 4 mg per minute according to patient's response.

doxepin (Sinequan; doxepin hydrochloride) is a tricyclic antidepressant drug. It has effects similar to imipramine but produces more drowsiness. *Dose:* By mouth, 30 to 300 mg daily in divided doses.

doxorubicin (Adriamycin) is an anticancer drug. *Adverse effects:* It colours the urine red. Doxorubicin produces damage to the bone marrow and ulcers of the mouth. It has toxic effects upon the heart, and produces alopecia, nausea, vomiting and diarrhoea. *Precautions:* Careful monitoring of the blood and heart should be carried out. It should be used with utmost caution in patients with impaired heart function. It should not be used in pregnancy or in breast-feeding mothers. Contact with the skin and eyes should be avoided. *Dose:* By injection in doses which vary according to the disorder being treated.

doxycycline (Nordox; Vibramycin; doxycycline hydrochloride). Doxycycline is an antibiotic and has effects, uses and adverse effects similar to those described under tetracycline. It is well absorbed, even when taken with food, and acts for a long time; its excretion is slow and it is possible to get high blood levels with a single daily dosage. *Dose:* By mouth, 100 to 200 mg daily.

doxylamine (doxylamine succinate) is an antihistamine drug.

Dozic ◊ haloperidol.

Dramamine ◊ dimenhydrinate.

Drapolene cream contains benzalkonium chloride 0·01% and cetrimide 0·2%. It is used as a protective skin application to prevent nappy rash etc.

Driclor ◊ aluminium chloride.

Dried Tub/Vac/BCG is Bacillus Calmette-Guérin vaccine. It is used in active immunization against tuberculosis.

dried yeast is used as a source of B vitamins.

Dristan Decongestant Tablets with Antihistamine each contain phenylephrine hydrochloride 5 mg, chlorpheniramine maleate 2 mg, aspirin 325 mg, and caffeine 16·2 mg.

Dristan Nasal Mist with Oxymetazoline contains oxymetazoline hydrochloride 0·05%.

Droleptan ◊ droperidol.

Dromoran ◊ levorphanol.

droperidol (Droleptan) is a major tranquillizer ◊ haloperidol. It is also used by injection with a narcotic analgesic to produce a specialized form of anaesthesia. *Dose:* By mouth, 5 to 20 mg every 4 to 8 hours.

drostanolone (Masteril; drostanolone propionate) is a male sex hormone. *Dose:* 100 mg three times weekly by intramuscular injection; 300 mg once weekly for breast cancer.

Droxalin: Each tablet contains polyhydroxyaluminium sodium carbonate 162 mg and magnesium trisilicate 162 mg. It is used to treat indigestion and peptic ulcers. *Dose:* 2 to 4 chewed every two to four hours.

Dry-Clear Acne Lotion contains benzoyl peroxide 5%.

Dryptal ◊ frusemide.

DT Per/Vac is diphtheria, tetanus and pertussis vaccine.

DT Per/Vac/ads is diphtheria, tetanus and pertussis vaccine adsorbed.

DT Vac/ads is diphtheria and tetanus vaccine adsorbed.

DTIC-Dome ◊ dacarbazine.

Dubam spray application is used as a rubefacient. It contains glycol salicylate 5%, methyl salicylate and methyl nicotinate 1·6%.

Dulcolax ◊ bisacodyl.

Duo-Autohaler is used to treat bronchial asthma. Each aerosol dose contains isoprenaline hydrochloride 0·16 mg, and phenylephrine bitartrate 0·24 mg. *Dose:* 1 to 3 puffs repeated after 30 minutes if necessary to a maximum of 24 puffs in 24 hours.

Duofilm paint contains salicylic acid 16·7%, lactic acid 16·7% in flexible collodion. It is used to treat warts. *Dose:* Apply daily.

Duogastrone ◊ carbenoxolone.

Duovent is used to treat bronchial asthma. Each aerosol dose contains fenoterol hydrobromide 0·1 mg and ipratropium bromide 0·04 mg. *Dose:* 1 to 2 puffs three or four times daily.

Duphalac ◊ lactulose.

Duphaston ◊ dydrogesterone.

Durabolin ◊ nandrolone.

Duracreme ◊ nonoxynol.

Duragel ◊ nonoxynol.

Duromine ◊ phentermine.

Duromorph ◊ morphine.

Dusk contains diethyltoluamide 20%.

Duttons Cough Mixture: Each 5 ml contains liquorice liquid extract 0·133 ml, acetic acid (80%) 0·133 ml, honey 0·267 ml, chloroform 0·025 ml, glycerol 0·2 ml, capsicum tincture 0·025 ml, treacle 2·275 ml.

Duvadilan ◊ isoxsuprine.

Duvadilan Retard capsules contain 40 mg of isoxsuprine hydrochloride in a slow-release form ◊ isoxsuprine.

Dyazide is a diuretic. Each tablet contains triamterene 50 mg and hydrochlorothiazide 25 mg. *Dose:* By mouth, 1 daily or 2 on alternate days.

dybenal ◊ dichlorobenzyl alcohol.

dydrogesterone (Duphaston) has effects similar to those described under progesterone. It is used to treat disorders of menstruation and to treat patients who have had repeated miscarriages. It is of no value as an oral contraceptive. *Adverse effects:* It may cause nausea, vomiting (which responds to a reduction in dose) and breakthrough bleeding (this usually responds to an increase in dose). *Dose:* By mouth. The dose varies according to the disorder being treated.

Dynese antacid suspension contains magaldrate 800 mg in each 5 ml.

Dyspamet chewable tablets of cimetidine ◊ cimetidine.

Dytac ◊ triamterene.

Dytide is a diuretic. Each capsule contains triamterene 50 mg and benzthiazide 25 mg. *Dose:* Initially, 2 at breakfast and 1 at lunchtime; maintenance, 1 or 2 on alternate days after food.

E45 cream contains light liquid paraffin 11·6%, white soft paraffin 14·5%, wool fat 1% with methyl hydroxybenzoate, self-emulsifying monostearin, stearic acid and triethanolamine. It is an emollient cream.

Earex eardrops contain arachis oil 33·3%, almond oil 33·3% and rectified camphor oil 33·3%.

Ebufac ◊ ibuprofen.

Ecdilyn Expectorant Syrup: Each 5 ml contains diphenhydramine hydrochloride 14 mg, ammonium chloride 135 mg, sodium citrate 57 mg, and menthol 1·1 mg.

Econacort cream contains 1% econazole nitrate and 1% hydrocortisone.

econazole (Ecostatin; Gyno-Pevaryl; Pevaryl) is a broad-spectrum antifungal drug. It is effective against thrush (*Candida albicans*). It is used to treat vaginal thrush as pessaries and cream (Ecostatin Pessaries and Twinpack). *Adverse effects:* It may produce local irritation. *Precautions:* Vaginal pessaries and cream should be used with utmost caution in the first three months of pregnancy. *Dose:* Insert vaginal pessaries at bedtime for three consecutive nights and apply cream around the anus and vagina twice daily for three days.

Econocil VK ◊ phenoxymethylpenicillin.

Economycin ◊ tetracycline.

Econosone ◊ prednisone.

Ecostatin ◊ econazole.

ecothiopate (Phospholine-iodine; ecothiopate iodide) is used in eye drops to constrict the pupil and reduce the pressure inside the eye in the treatment of glaucoma.

Ectodyne Worm Syrup contains piperazine citrate 12·6%.

Eczederm cream contains calamine 20·88% and starch 2·09%.

Edecrin ◊ ethacrynic acid.

edetic acid is used as a chelating agent in the preparation of pharmaceuticals.

edrophonium (Tensilon) has effects and uses similar to neostigmine. It is used to diagnose myasthenia gravis and has been used to treat disorders of heart rhythm.

Efavite tablets each contain ascorbic acid 125 mg, pyridoxine hydrochloride 25 mg, nicotinamide 7·5 mg, and zinc sulphate 2·5 mg.

Efcortelan (hydrocortisone in ointments and lotions; hydrocortisone acetate in creams; hydrocortisone semisuccinate sodium for injections) ◊ hydrocortisone.

Efcortelan P cream and ointment contains 1% hydrocortisone ◊ hydrocortisone.

Efcortesol ◊ hydrocortisone.

Effer-C: Effervescent tablets each containing ascorbic acid 1 g.

Effercitrate is used to relieve symptoms in infections of the urinary tract. Each tablet contains citric acid 1·14 g and potassium bicarbonate 1·39 g. *Dose:* By mouth, 2 tablets dissolved in water up to three times daily with meals.

Effico mixture contains two B vitamins (thiamine 0·18 mg and nicotinamide 2·1 mg), tincture of nux vomica 0·12 ml, caffeine 20·2 mg, compound infusion of gentian 2·1 ml, dilute hydrochloric acid 0·04 ml and orange and lemon syrup in each 5 ml. *Dose:* By mouth, 10 ml three times daily.

Eftab Effervescent Mouth Wash Tablets contain peppermint oil 0·56%, clove oil 0·33%, spearmint oil 0·03%, menthol 0·62%, thymol 0·23%, methyl salicylate 0·02%, effervescent basis to 100%.

Efudix ◊ fluorouracil.

Elantan (isosorbide mononitrate) ◊ isosorbide.

Elastoplast Antiseptic Cream contains chloroxylenol 0·3%, triclosan 0·3%, and edetic acid 0·2%.

Elastoplast Antiseptic Liquid contains cetrimide 3% and chlorhexidine gluconate solution 1·5%.

Elastoplast Antiseptic Wipes contain cetrimide 1%.

Elastoplast Insect Repel Wipes contains diethyltoluamide 20% and dimethylphthalate 10%.

Elavil ◊ amitriptyline.

Eldepryl ◊ selegiline.

Eldisine ◊ vindesine.

Electrolade sachets contain a powder for dissolving in cool drinking water for the treatment of fluid loss caused by, for example, diarrhoea and vomiting. The powder in each sachet contains sodium chloride 0·236 g, potassium chloride 0·3 g, sodium bicarbonate 0·5 g, glucose 4 g and saccharin sodium 0·01 g in each 5·1 g. *Precautions:* The made-up solution should be used with caution in patients with kidney failure and in patients with severe, acute abdominal pain. Diabetic patients should note the sugar content. *Dose:* The contents of each sachet should be dissolved in 200 ml of cool drinking water. The solution should be used immediately or refrigerated for no longer than 24 hours. It should not be boiled. Adults should take 1 to 2 sachets for every loose motion up to a maximum of 16 sachets in 24 hours. If vomiting is a problem, the solution should be frequently sipped. No solid food should be taken for 24 hours.

Electrosol: Effervescent tablets of sodium chloride 200 mg, potassium chloride 160 mg, and sodium bicarbonate 200 mg. 8 tablets dissolved in a litre of water provide electrolyte and water replacement for patients suffering from acute diarrhoea.

Elliman's Embrocation contains turpentine oil 35·41% and acetic acid 10·37%.

Eltroxin ◊ thyroxine.

Eludril is an antiseptic mouthwash and gargle. It contains chlorhexidine digluconate 0·1%, chlorbutol 0·1% and chloroform 0·5%. *Dose:* 10 ml in half a tumbler of warm water used as a mouthwash or gargle three or four times daily.

Elyzol ◊ metronidazole.

Emcor tablets ◊ bisoprolol.

Emeside ◊ ethosuximide.

emetine was used in the treatment of amoebic dysentery, amoebic hepatitis and liver abscess. It irritates the stomach lining. In small doses it increases bronchial secretion and causes sweating and vomiting. Prolonged use may cause damage to the liver, kidneys, muscles, nerves and heart muscle.

Emetrol oral solution for mild nausea.

Each 5 ml contains laevulose 1·87 g, dextrose 1·87 g and phosphoric acid 21·5 mg. *Dose:* By mouth, 15 to 30 ml as required.

Emko is a spermicidal contraceptive. It contains benzethonium chloride 0·2% and nonoxynol-9 8%. *Dose:* 1 applicatorful intravaginally not more than 1 hour before intercourse, together with a barrier contraceptive.

Emla cream is a local anaesthetic containing lignocaine and prilocaine.

Emlab Brewers' Yeast Tablets each contain dried yeast 300 mg.

Emlab Iron and Brewers' Yeast Tablets each contain dried yeast 300 mg and ferrous fumarate 15 mg.

empicol is used as an emulsifying agent in the preparation of medicated shampoos, etc. It is also used as a skin cleanser because it reduces surface tension and is a detergent and wetting agent.

Emtexate ◊ methotrexate.

Emulsiderm liquid emulsion is used as an emollient. It contains liquid paraffin 25%, isopropylmyristate 25% and benzalkonium chloride 0·5%. *Dose:* Add 2 to 3 capfuls to a warm bath or rub a small amount into areas of dry skin.

En-De-Kay ◊ fluoride.

enalapril (Innovace) is used to treat high blood pressure. *Adverse effects:* These include dizziness, headache, fatigue and weakness. *Dose:* By mouth, 5 mg to 40 mg daily.

Endet powder is used to treat infant teething. Each powder contains paracetamol 125 mg, promethazine hydrochloride 5 mg, heavy magnesium carbonate 100 mg and sucrose 30 mg.

Endoxana ◊ cyclophosphamide.

Enduron ◊ methyclothiazide.

Engerix B is a genetically engineered human vaccine against hepatitis B.

enflurane (Alyrane) is a volatile general anaesthetic with actions similar to halothane.

Eno: Each 5 g dose is prepared from sodium bicarbonate 2·99 g, tartaric acid 1·43 g, and citric acid 870 mg.

Entamizole: Each tablet contains diloxanide furoate 250 mg and metronidazole 200 mg ◊ diloxanide ◊ metronidazole.

Enteromide ◊ calcium sulphaloxate.

Enterosan: Each tablet contains kaolin 700 mg, morphine hydrochloride 275 micrograms, and belladonna dry extract 1·8 mg.

Entero-Vioform* ◊ clioquinol.

Entonox is a mixture of nitrous oxide 50% and oxygen 50% which is used to produce pain relief without loss of consciousness.

Entrotabs are used to treat diarrhoea. Each tablet contains light kaolin 700 mg, morphine hydrochloride 0·275 mg, belladonna dry extract 1·8 mg.

Dose: By mouth, initially 4 tablets, then 2 every three to four hours.

Envoy Pastilles contain benzalkonium chloride solution (50%) 0·00108 ml and hexylresorcinol 0·54 mg.

Epanutin ◊ phenytoin.

ephedrine (ephedrine hydrochloride, ephedrine sulphate) has stimulating effects which resemble adrenaline and amphetamines. When given by mouth it constricts small blood vessels and raises the blood pressure, it relaxes the muscles in the bronchi, slows down movements in the gut and contracts the uterus. It also has effects upon the bladder and the pupils, and it stimulates the central nervous system. It is used mainly to prevent attacks of asthma and in sprays for nasal congestion. *Adverse effects:* If given to patients sensitive to ephedrine or if given in large doses it may cause nausea, vomiting, giddiness, headache, sweating, thirst, palpitations, anxiety, restlessness, trembling, insomnia and muscular weakness. *Precautions:* It should not be used by patients with high blood pressure, coronary thrombosis or with overworking of their thyroid gland. It should be given with caution to patients with heart disease and it may cause retention of urine in patients with enlarged prostate glands (who may already have difficulty in passing urine). Ephedrine should not be used by patients being treated with monoamine oxidase inhibitor antidepressant drugs or within two weeks of stopping such drugs. *Dose:* By mouth, 30 mg three times daily, up to a maximum daily dose of 150 mg.

Ephynal ◊ alpha tocopheryl acetate.

Epifoam pressurized aerosol pack for treating perianal trauma including post-episiotomy pain and dermatitis disorders. It contains hydrocortisone acetate 1% and pramoxine hydrochloride 1%.

Epifrin eye drops contain 1% and 2% adrenaline.

Epilim ◊ sodium valproate.

epinephrine ◊ adrenaline.

epirubicin (Pharmorubicin) is an anticancer drug used to treat acute leukaemias and lymphomas. *Adverse effects:* These include nausea and vomiting, suppression of the bone marrow, loss of hair (alopecia) and inflammation of the tissues of the mouth, stomach and gut.

epithiazide (in Thiaver) is a thiazide diuretic. *Dose:* By mouth, 4 mg two to three times a day.

Epodyl ◊ ethoglucid.

epoprostenol (Flolan) is used to preserve platelet function during open heart surgery and as an alternative to heparin in kidney dialysis.

Eppy neutral adrenaline eye drops ◊ adrenaline.

Epsom salts ◊ magnesium sulphate.

EP Tablets each contain paracetamol 300 mg, caffeine 50 mg and codeine phosphate 8 mg. Used to relieve mild pain.

Equagesic: Each two-layer tablet contains aspirin 250 mg, calcium carbonate 75 mg, ethoheptazine citrate 75 mg and meprobamate 150 mg used to relieve mild pain with anxiety. *Dose:* 2 three or four times daily.

Equanil ◊ meprobamate.

Eradacin ◊ acrosoxacin.

Eraldin ◊ practolol.

ergocalciferol is vitamin D_2.

ergometrine (ergometrine maleate; ergonovine maleate) causes contractions of the uterus and is used to prevent bleeding from the uterus after childbirth. *Adverse effects:* These are rare if the drug is used properly. Nausea and vomiting may occur. Intravenous injection may cause the blood pressure to increase. *Precautions:* It should not be used during the first or second stages of labour since this may cause death of the foetus and rupture of the uterus. *Dose:* By mouth, 0·5 to 1 mg; by intravenous injection, 0·1 to 0·5 mg, when necessary.

ergotamine (Cafergot; Lingraine; ergotamine tartrate) stimulates and, in large doses, paralyses the endings of the sympathetic nerves. It constricts small blood vessels and also the uterus. Its main use is in the treatment of migraine. *Adverse effects:* It is isolated from ergot and is in fact a derivative of lysergic acid (LSD). The dose used to treat migraine may cause headache, nausea and vomiting and occasionally muscle weakness and pain. In large repeated doses it can produce all the symptoms of ergot poisoning – cold-

ness of the skin, severe muscle pains, gangrene of the hands and feet, thromboses, angina, alteration of heart rate and blood pressure, confusion, drowsiness, paralysis and convulsions. *Precautions:* It should not be used in pregnancy, in patients with diseases of the circulation or in patients with impaired kidney or liver function. Its effects are increased by adrenaline-like drugs. *Dose:* By mouth, 1 to 2 mg (maximum 4 mg in 24 hours and 10 mg in any one week); by subcutaneous and intramuscular injection, 0·25 to 0·5 mg.

Ermysin ◊ erythromycin.

Ervevax is a rubella (German measles) vaccine.

Erycen ◊ erythromycin.

Erymax capsules ◊ erythromycin.

Erytex ointment is used to treat eczema, it contains calamine 12·5%, zinc oxide 10% and salicylic acid 1·25%.

Erythrocin ◊ erythromycin stearate.

Erythrolar ◊ erythromycin.

Erythromid ◊ erythromycin.

erythromycin (Arpimycin; Ermysin; Erycen; Erymax; Erythrolar; Erythromid; Erythroped; Erythroped A; Ilosone; Ilotycin; Retcin) is an antibiotic. Bacteria may quickly become resistant to it. It is partly destroyed by acid in the stomach and has to be taken in specially coated tablets (enteric coated). *Adverse effects:* These are rare and usually mild. They include abdominal pains and skin rashes. *Dose:* By mouth, 1 to 2 g daily in divided doses.

erythromycin estolate (Ilosone): This preparation is rapidly absorbed, but can cause jaundice when treatment is repeated (see above).

erythromycin stearate (Erythrocin; erythromycin stearate) is more resistant to the acid in the stomach than erythromycin. It is given in the same dosages as erythromycin (see above).

Erythroped ◊ erythromycin.

Erythroped A ◊ erythromycin.

Esbatal ◊ bethanidine.

esculin is prepared from the horse chestnut, and is included in some suppositories for the treatment of haemorrhoids.

eserine ◊ physostigmine.

Esidrex ◊ hydrochlorothiazide.

Esidrex K is a diuretic with added potassium. Each tablet contains potassium chloride 600 mg in a slow-release core with 12·5 mg of hydrochlorothiazide in an outer coating. *Dose:* 2 to 4 tablets daily initially, maintenance 1 to 2 daily.

Eskamel is used to treat acne. It contains resorcinol 2% and sulphur 8%.

Eskornade is used to treat the common cold. Each capsule contains isopropamide 2·5 mg, phenylpropanolamine 50 mg, and diphenylpyraline 5 mg in sustained-release form. *Dose:* By mouth, 1 twelve hourly.

Eso-Dex Indigestion Tablets each contain dried aluminium hydroxide 130 mg, magnesium trisilicate 130 mg, magnesium carbonate 65 mg, and calcium carbonate 95 mg.

Eso-Pax Capsules each contain paracetamol 240 mg, ascorbic acid 60 mg, caffeine 10 mg, and quinine sulphate 6 mg.

Esopyn Inhalant Capsules contain camphor 8·15 mg, menthol 16·3 mg, eucalyptol 16·3 mg, pumilio pine oil 8·15 mg, thymol 3·26 mg.

Esotérica Facial and **Fortified** contain hydroquinone 2%, padimate O 3·3% and oxybenzone 2·5%; **Regular** contains hydroquinone 2%.

Estracyt ◊ estramustine.

Estraderm is a special application for applying to the skin to provide oestrogen replacement treatment for menopausal symptoms. Each transdermal patch contains 25, 50 or 100 micrograms of oestradiol, which is slowly released over a 24-hour period. *Adverse effects* include headache, nausea, breast tenderness and redness at the patch site. *Precautions:* Patients should have a full medical examination before starting treatment; this should include checking the blood pressure, examining the breasts and an internal examination to exclude any sign of cancer. Regular medical examination and cancer screening should be carried out during treatment. It should be used with caution in patients with a family history of breast cancer, gallstones or raised blood pressure. It should not be used in patients with a history of thrombosis or heart disease, severe kidney or liver disease, cancer of the breast or genital tract, endometriosis or any underdiagnosed vaginal bleeding. *Dose:* Apply patch to any clean, non-hairy area of skin below the waist and replace the patch every 3 to 4 days, using different sites. Start with a 50-microgram patch and adjust the dose in the following months; maximum dose 100 micrograms daily.

Estradurin ◊ polyoestradiol.

estramustine (Estracyt) is used as an anti-cancer drug to treat cancer of the prostate gland. *Adverse effects:* Nausea, vomiting, diarrhoea, transient impairment of the liver function tests and allergic skin rash and fever, rarely thrombocytopenia, enlarged breasts (gynaecomastia). *Precautions:* It should not be used in patients with peptic ulcers, severe liver disease or severe heart disease. It should be used with caution in patients with impaired bone-marrow function. *Dose:* By mouth, 140 mg capsules, 1 to 10 daily with meals.

estrogens ◊ oestrogens.

etafedrine is an ephedrine-like drug. ◊ ephedrine.

etamiphyllin (etamiphyllin camsylate) has similar effects to aminophylline but it is less likely to produce nausea and gastro-intestinal disturbances. *Dose:* By mouth, 100 to 300 mg three or four times daily after meals. An injection and suppositories are also available.

ethacrynic acid (Edecrin) is a rapidly acting diuretic drug. *Adverse effects:* It may cause loss of appetite, nausea, vomiting and diarrhoea in high doses. Single large doses or prolonged use may cause severe disturbances of the body's salt and water balance, resulting in weakness, muscle cramps, thirst, skin rashes, headaches, blurred vision, confusion and low blood sugar; increased blood uric acid levels may occur. Blood disorders and breast enlargement have been reported. *Precautions* ◊ frusemide. *Dose:* By mouth, 50 to 150 mg daily in divided doses.

ethambutol (Myambutol; ethambutol hydrochloride) is used to treat tuberculosis. *Adverse effects:* Its most serious adverse effect is progressive blindness associated with loss of copper and zinc from the body. It is reversible if the drug is stopped early enough. *Precautions:* It should be used with caution in patients with impaired kidney function. Blood levels must be checked. The eyes should be examined at frequent intervals. *Dose:* 25 mg per kg of body-weight daily for two months, followed by 15 mg per kg body-weight as a single daily dose.

ethamivan (Clairvan) is a respiratory stimulant. It increases the rate and depth of respiration. *Adverse effects:* These include restlessness, sneezing, twitching and itching. Overdose produces convulsions. *Precautions:* It should not be given to patients who suffer from epilepsy or other convulsive disorders. *Dose:* Varies according to disorder being treated.

ethamsylate (Dicynene) is used to reduce excess bleeding from small blood vessels e.g., in the treatment of menorrhagia. *Adverse effects:* These include nausea, headache and rashes. *Dose:* By mouth, 500 mg four times a day. By injection, dose depends on the condition being treated.

ethanol ◊ alcohol.

ethanolamine oleate is used in sclerosing therapy of varicose veins. *Adverse effects:* Leakage may lead to necrosis. *Precautions:* It should not be used in patients who cannot walk, who have acute phlebitis or who are taking oral contraceptive drugs or have obese legs. Allergic reactions may occur.

ether is occasionally used as a general anaesthetic.

ethinyloestradiol has the effects and uses of the oestrogens. It may cause headache, dizziness, nausea and vomiting. *Dose:* Varies according to disorder being treated.

ethisterone (Gestone Oral; ethinyltestosterone). Ethisterone has effects similar to progesterone. It is used to treat menorrhagia. *Dose:* By mouth 10 to 15 mg three times daily.

ethoglucid (Epodyl) is an anti-cancer drug. *Adverse effects:* These include nausea, vomiting, loss of hair (alopecia), fluid retention (oedema), pain and irritation at site of injection and bone-marrow damage leading to blood disorders. *Precautions:* It should be given with caution to patients whose bone-marrow function may be depressed. *Dose:* Varies according to the disorder being treated.

ethoheptazine (in Equagesic, Zactipar, Zactirin) is a mild pain reliever. It may produce stomach discomfort, nausea, dizziness, drowsiness and itching.

ethosuximide (Emeside; Zarontin) is an anti-convulsant drug used to treat epilepsy. *Adverse effects:* Mild transient effects include headache, nausea, drowsiness, apathy, mood changes, unsteadiness on the feet (ataxia) and loss of appetite. It may cause skin rashes, blood disorders, Parkinsonism, and difficulty in looking at bright light. If given to patients with temporal lobe epilepsy it may cause mental breakdown. *Precautions:* It should be given with extreme caution to patients with impaired liver or kidney function. *Dose:* By mouth, 500 to 2,000 mg daily in divided doses.

ethoxylated lauryl alcohol is a surfactant.

Ethrane ◊ enflurane.

ethyl acetate is used as a flavouring agent in medicines and as a solvent. It is also used in food.

ethyl alcohol ◊ alcohol.

ethyl aminobenzoate ◊ alcohol.

ethylenediamine (ethylenediamine hydrate) is used to prepare injections of aminophylline. It is irritant to the skin.

ethylene glycol is included in sunscreen lotions and protective creams. It should only be present in a very low concentration (less than 5%) and should *not* be applied extensively on the body. It can depress brain function and cause kidney damage.

ethylhexyl salicylate is included in some sunscreen preparations.

ethylmorphine hydrochloride is a salt of morphine.

ethyl nicotinate is used as an irritant in skin applications (rubefacient).

ethyl-paradimethylaminobenzoate is used in sunscreen preparations.

ethyl salicylate is used in rheumatic rubs as a rubefacient.

ethynodiol (ethynodiol diacetate) is a synthetic female sex hormone. Its effects and uses are similar to those described under norethisterone. It is used in conjunction with oestrogens as an oral contraceptive agent and in the treatment of disorders of menstruation. *Dose:* By mouth, 0·5 to 1 mg daily according to disorder being treated.

etidronate (Didronel; disodium etidronate) is used to treat Paget's disease of bone. *Adverse effects:* These include nausea, diarrhoea and increased bone pain. *Precautions:* Adequate intake of calcium and vitamin D must be maintained. Care is needed in renal failure. *Dose:* From 5 to 20 mg/kg body-weight per day for not more than 3 to 6 months. Available as tablets and injections.

etodolac (Lodine; Ramodar) is a non-steroidal anti-inflammatory drug. It is used in the treatment of rheumatoid arthritis. *Adverse effects:* These include nausea, stomach pain, diarrhoea, indigestion, heartburn, flatulence, abdominal pain, constipation, headaches, dizziness drowsiness, ringing in the ears (tinnitus), rash and fatigue. These are usually mild,

transient and reversible on stopping the drug. *Precautions:* It should be used with caution in patients with impaired kidney and liver function and in elderly patients. *Dose:* By mouth, 200 mg twice daily up to a maximum of 600 mg daily.

etomidate (Hypnomidate) is used as an intravenous anaesthetic.

etoposide (Vepesid) is used as an anticancer drug. *Adverse effects:* These include nausea, vomiting, loss of hair and blood disorders. *Dose:* By mouth or injection, according to disorder being treated.

etretinate (Tigason) is used to treat severe, resistant psoriasis and some congenital skin diseases. *Adverse effects:* These include cracked lips, loss of hair, generalized itching and nose bleeds. *Precautions:* This drug causes damage to the foetus and should be avoided in women who may become pregnant. *Dose:* By mouth, 0·25 to 0·5 mg/kg body-weight per day in divided doses for 6 to 9 months, followed by a rest period. *Contraceptive methods should be used during treatment and for two years after a course of the drug.*

Etsonal Stomach Treatment contains bismuth and ammonium citrate solution 14·4%, sodium citrate 1·16%, chloroform and morphine tincture 1·08%, chloroform emulsion 0·58%, and sodium bicarbonate 4·02%.

eucalyptol has the actions and uses of eucalpytus oil but it is less irritating. It is used in irritant skin applications, and it has some antiseptic properties. It is used in temporary dental fillings.

eucalyptus oil has a nice smell and is included in medicines used to treat symptoms of the upper respiratory tract. It is an irritant to the skin and mucous membranes and may be used in rheumatic liniments and to treat wind.

Eucarbon: Each tablet contains charcoal 180 mg, sublimed sulphur 50 mg, senna leaf 105 mg, rhubarb extract 25 mg, peppermint oil and fennel oil.

Eudemine ◊ diazoxide.

Euglucon ◊ glibenclamide.

Eugynon 30 tablets contain 0·25 mg levonorgestrel and 0·03 mg ethinyloestradiol. It is an oral contraceptive drug.

Eugynon 50 tablets contain 0·5 mg norgestrel and 0·05 mg ethinyloestradiol. It is an oral contraceptive drug.

Eumovate ◊ clobetasone.

Eumovate-N eye drops contain clobetasone butyrate 0·1% and neomycin sulphate 0·5%.

euphorbia is a drastic purgative and emetic that can cause kidney damage.

Eurax lotion and cream ◊ crotamiton.

Eurax-Hydrocortisone cream contains hydrocortisone 0·25% and crotamiton 10%.

eusol is chlorinated lime and boric acid solution used as an antiseptic ◊ chlorinated lime and boric acid.

Evacalm ◊ diazepam.

Evacort cream contains 1% hydrocortisone ◊ hydrocortisone.

Evadyne ◊ butriptyline.

Evening Primrose Oil contains linolenic acid which is used as a protective in skin applications. Claims for the other many uses need validating scientifically.

Evoxin tablets ◊ domperidone.

Exa-mol Antiseptic Ointment contains yellow soft paraffin 73·1%, wool fat 4·8%, phenol 3·5%, zinc oxide 6%, ammoniated mercury 1%, coal tar solution 2·4%, and starch 10%.

Exelderm cream is used for fungal infections. It contains sulconazole nitrate 1%.

Exirel ◊ pirbuterol.

Ex-Lax, Junior: Each tablet contains yellow phenolphthalein 48 mg in a chocolate basis.

Ex-Lax Pills: Each contains phenolphthalein 95 mg.

Ex-Lax Tablets each contain yellow phenolphthalein 98 mg in a chocolate basis.

Exolan ◊ dithranol.

Expulin linctus is used to treat coughs. Each 5 ml contains pholcodine 5 mg, ephedrine 8 mg, chlorpheniramine 2 mg, glycerin 190 mg, and menthol 1·1 mg. *Dose:* By mouth, 10 to 15 ml six hourly to a maximum of 45 ml in 24 hours.

Expurhin is a cough linctus for children containing chlorpheniramine maleate 1 mg, ephedrine hydrochloride 4 mg and menthol 1·1 mg in each 5 ml. *Precautions:* It may cause drowsiness.

Exterol ear drops contain urea hydrogen peroxide 5% in glycerine.

Extil Compound* is used to treat coughs. Each 10 ml contains noscapine 25 mg, pseudoephedrine 49·2 mg, and carbinoxamine 6 mg. *Dose:* By mouth, 10 ml three or four times daily.

Extra Energy Tablets each contain caffeine 50 mg, ascorbic acid 5 mg, thiamine hydrochloride 1 mg, riboflavine 1 mg, nicotinic acid 5 mg, dextrose 150 mg.

Extrapone No. 4 special is an ingredient of Spotaway Antiseptic cream.

Exyphen elixir* is a cough medicine. Each 5 ml contains brompheniramine maleate 2 mg, guaiphenesin 80 mg, phenylephrine hydrochloride 4·75 mg and phenylpropranolamine hydrochloride 5 mg. *Dose:* By mouth, 5 to 10 ml four times daily.

Eye dew eyedrops are used to treat eye irritation and bloodshot eyes, containing naphazoline hydrochloride 0·01% and distilled witch hazel 12·5%.

Fabahistin ◊ mebhydrolin.

Fabrol ◊ acetylcysteine.

Face-Savers Cream Medication contains colloidal sulphur 6·4% and resorcinol 1·5%.

Famel Catarrh & Throat Pastilles contain creosote 0·29%, cassia oil 0·21%, lemon oil 0·08%, and menthol 0·34%.

Famel Children's Cough Linctus contains pholcodine 0·039%, papaverine 0·0078%, glycerin 7·8% and syrup 81%.

Famel Expectorant Linctus contains guaiphenesin 50 mg in each 5 ml.

Famel Honey and Lemon Cough Linctus contains in each 5 ml guaiphenesin 50 mg, purified honey 250 mg, lemon juice 0·5 ml, and liquid glucose 4·68 g.

Famel Honey and Lemon Cough Pastilles: Each contain guaiphenesin 20 mg.

Famel Inhalant Capsules each contain pumilio pine oil 58·4 mg, chlorbutol 53·1 mg, menthol 47·8 mg, rectified camphor oil 21·3 mg, creosote 21·3 mg, and lavandin oil 10·6 mg.

Famel Linctus: Each 5 ml contains pholcodine 5 mg and papaverine hydrochloride 0·5 mg.

Famel Nasal Inhaler contains eucalyptol 10%, pumilio pine oil 10%, rectified camphor oil 7·5%, cinnamon oil 5%, menthol 50%, and creosote 17·5%.

Famel Original Cough Medicine: Each 5 ml contains creosote 16·75 mg and codeine 1·5 mg.

Famel Pastilles contain creosote 0·29%, cinnamon leaf oil 0·21%, lemon oil 0·08% and menthol 0·34%.

Famel Syrup (Original) contains creosote 0·335%, calcium lactate 0·051%, calcium hydrogen phosphate 0·01%, codeine 0·03%, and liquid glucose 94%.

Family Antiseptic Cream contains cetrimide 0·35% and benzalkonium chloride solution 0·3%.

Family Cherry Linctus: Each 5 ml contains dilute acetic acid 0·782 ml, ipecacuanha liquid extract 0·01 ml, glycerol 0·25 ml, and sucrose 2·1 g.

Fam-Lax Laxative Tablets each contain phenolphthalein 125 mg and powdered rhubarb 27·5 mg.

famotidine (Pepcid PM) is an H_2 blocker used to treat and prevent stomach ulcers and duodenal ulcers. *Adverse effects:* Headache, dizziness, constipation, diarrhoea. Less frequently, dry mouth, nausea, skin rash, stomach upsets, loss of appetite, fatigue. *Precautions:* Do not use if breastfeeding. Use with caution in patients with impaired kidney function or stomach cancer (may mask symptoms), and use with caution in pregnancy. *Dose:* By mouth, 40 mg at night for 4–8 weeks, prevention of relapse of duodenal ulcer, 20 mg at night.

Fansidar is an anti-malarial drug. Each tablet contains pyrimethamine 25 mg and sulfadoxine 500 mg.

Farlutal ◊ medroxyprogesterone.

Fasigyn ◊ tinidazole.

Faverin ◊ fluvoxamine.

Febrilix is a paediatric paracetamol elixir.

Febs Cold Relief Tablets with Vitamin C each contain paracetamol 400 mg, ascorbic acid 50 mg, caffeine 30 mg, and phenylephrine hydrochloride 5 mg.

Fectrim ◊ co-trimoxazole.

Feen-a-mint chewing gum tablets each contain phenolphthalein 97·2 mg.

Fefol: Each spansule contains ferrous sulphate 150 mg, and folic acid 0·5 mg. *Dose:* 1 daily.

Fefol-Vit: Each capsule contains ferrous sulphate 150 mg, folic acid 0·5 mg, thiamine 2 mg, riboflavine 2 mg, pyridoxine 1 mg, nicotinamide 10 mg, calcium pantothenate 2·17 mg, ascorbic acid 50 mg. *Dose:* By mouth, 1 daily.

Fefol Z spansules are sustained-release capsules containing dried ferrous sulphate 150 mg, folic acid 0·5 mg and zinc sulphate monohydrate (equivalent to 22·5 mg of zinc).

Feldene ◊ piroxicam.

felypressin (Octapressin) constricts small blood vessels and is mixed with injections of local anaesthetics to enable the anaesthetic effects to last longer at the site of injection. It is safe to use in patients who are taking antidepressants, unlike adrenaline.

Femafen ◊ ibuprofen.

Female Hormone Cream 1934 contains oestrone 330 units per g.

Femerital: Each tablet contains ambucetamide 100 mg and paracetamol 250 mg. *Dose:* By mouth, 1 to

2 tablets three times daily for period pains commencing two days before onset of menstruation.

Femfresh Intimate Deodorant Spray contains chlorhexidine hydrochloride 0·075%, talc, perfume, and propellants.

Femin-9 capsules are used to treat symptoms of pre-menstrual tension. They contain a range of vitamins.

Feminax tablets each contain paracetamol 250 mg, salicylamide 250 mg, codeine phosphate 8 mg, caffeine 50 mg, and hyoscine h drobromide 100 micrograms.

Femodene tablets contain gestodene 75 micrograms and ethinyloestradiol 30 micrograms. It is a combined oral contraceptive. Gestodene is a new progestogen related to norethisterone.

Femulen ◊ ethynodiol.

Fenbid sustained-release capsules contain 300 mg of ibuprofen ◊ ibuprofen.

fenbufen (Lederfen) is an anti-rheumatic drug. *Adverse effects:* These include nausea, vomiting, and stomach pains, skin rashes, dizziness, headache and drowsiness. Abnormal blood tests and liver function tests have been reported. *Precautions:* It should not be used in patients who are sensitive to aspirin or other similar anti-rheumatic drugs. It should be used with great caution in patients with a history of peptic or intestinal ulceration. Very careful consideration should be given before its possible use in pregnancy or in breast-feeding

mothers. Aspirin reduces its effective blood level. *Dose:* By mouth, 600 mg at night plus 300 mg in the morning if necessary.

fencamfamin is a weak central nervous stimulant, having a similar effect to caffeine ◊ caffeine. It is in the multi-vitamin preparation Reactivan.

fenfluramine (Ponderax) is a slimming drug. *Adverse effects:* It may cause drowsiness, dry mouth, dizziness, nausea, diarrhoea, fatigue and aching pains. It rarely causes itching of the skin and disturbed sleep. High doses may cause vivid and bad dreams. *Precautions:* Fenfluramine may increase the effects of certain drugs – bethanidine, guanethidine, methyldopa, and reserpine – used to treat blood pressure. It should not be given to patients on M.A.O. inhibitor antidepressant drugs and not to patients who are depressed or in the first three months of pregnancy. *Dose:* By mouth, 20 to 120 mg daily.

fennel oil is an aromatic carminative (for wind).

Fennings' Adult Cooling Powders: Each 300 mg powder contains anhydrous caffeine 30 mg, paracetamol 180 mg, heavy magnesium carbonate 30 mg, liquorice 24 mg, and light kaolin 26·67 mg.

Fennings' Children's Cooling Powders: Each 200 mg powder contains paracetamol 50 mg.

Fennings' Gripe Mixture: Each 5 ml contains sodium bicarbonate 50 mg, ginger tincture 0·025 ml, peppermint oil 0·000625 ml, dill oil 0·00125 ml, and caraway oil 0·00125 ml.

Fennings' Little Healers: Each tablet contains prepared ipecacuanha 20 mg.

Fennings' Mixture, Lemon Flavoured contains sodium salicylate 5%, sodium metabisulphite 0·1%, oil of lemon (terpeneless) 0·1%, spirit of chloroform 2·5%, and extract of quassia liq. (1–1) 0·5%.

Fennings' Original Mixture: Each 15 ml contains nitric acid 0·2 ml, peppermint oil 0·001 ml, and sanguis draconis 150 micrograms.

fenoprofen (Fenopron; Progesic) is used to treat rheumatic and arthritic disorders. *Adverse effects:* It may produce gastro-intestinal irritation and it may increase the effects of certain anticoagulant drugs. It may produce allergic reactions in patients allergic to aspirin. It should not be used in pregnancy and should only be used with caution in patients with a history of peptic ulcers or gastro-intestinal bleeding. *Dose:* By mouth, 300 to 600 mg three or four times daily.

Fenopron ◊ fenoprofen.

Fenostil Retard ◊ dimethindene.

fenoterol (Berotec; fenoterol hydrobromide) produces effects similar to those described under salbutamol. It is used to treat bronchial asthma. *Dose:* By inhalation, 200 to 400 micrograms twice daily.

Fenox (phenylephrine hydrochloride), available as **Nasal Drops** and as **Nasal Spray** each containing 0·5%.

fentanyl (Sublimaze) is a narcotic pain reliever that is also used in patients who need to be treated on ventilators. *Adverse effects:* Transient hypotension, bradycardia, nausea and vomiting. *Precautions:* Myasthenia gravis. *Dose:* By intravenous injection, 100 to 200 micrograms and then 50 micrograms every 20 to 30 minutes as required.

Fentazin ◊ perphenazine.

Feospan spansules are sustained-release (long-acting) capsules containing dried ferrous sulphate 150 mg (equivalent to 45 mg iron).

Feospan Z spansules are sustained-release capsules containing dried ferrous sulphate 150 mg and zinc sulphate monohydrate 61·8 mg (equivalent to 22·5 mg of zinc).

Feravol tablets contain dried ferrous sulphate 200 mg, thiamine hydrochloride 400 micrograms, riboflavine 1 mg and ascorbic acid 9 mg.

Feravol-F tablets contain ferrous gluconate 300 mg (35 mg iron) and folic acid 3 mg.

Feravol-G tablets contain ferrous gluconate 300 mg (35 mg iron), thiamine hydrochloride 400 micrograms, riboflavine 1 mg, ascorbic acid 9 mg, copper a trace.

Fergon ◊ ferrous gluconate.

ferric ammonium citrate is a form of iron. The mixture should be well diluted with water and sucked through a straw to prevent discoloration of the teeth. *Dose:* 6 g daily.

ferric hypophosphite is used in tonics.

Ferrocap: Each capsule contains ferrous fumarate 330 mg and thiamine 5 mg in slow-release form. *Dose:* By mouth, 1 daily. **Ferrocap-F 350** contains folic acid 350 micrograms in addition to ferrous fumarate 330 mg.

Ferrocontin Continus tablets contain ferrous glycine sulphate in slow-release form equivalent to 100 mg of ferrous iron.

Ferrocontin Folic Continus tablets contain ferrous glycine sulphate (equivalent to 100 mg ferrous iron) and 0·5 mg folic acid in slow-release form.

Ferrograd: Each timed-release tablet contains dried ferrous sulphate 325 mg. *Dose:* 1 daily before food. Not for children under seven years.

Ferrograd C: Each timed-release tablet contains ferrous sulphate 325 mg and ascorbic acid 500 mg. *Dose:* 1 daily.

Ferrograd Folic: Each timed-release tablet contains ferrous sulphate 325 mg and folic acid 0·35 mg. *Dose:* 1 daily before food during pregnancy.

Ferromyn elixir ◊ ferrous succinate.

ferrous carbonate is an iron salt.

ferrous fumarate (Fersaday; Fersamal; Galfer; Plancaps) An iron salt. *Dose:* By mouth, 400 to 500 mg daily, in divided doses.

ferrous gluconate (Fergon) is an iron salt. *Dose:* By mouth, 2·4 to 4·8 g daily, in divided doses for anaemia. Prevention, 600 mg daily.

ferrous glycine sulphate (Ferrocontin Continus, Kelferon, Plesmet) is an iron salt.

ferrous succinate (Ferromyn) is an iron salt. *Dose:* By mouth, 300 mg daily in divided doses.

ferrous sulphate (Feospan; Ferrograd; Ironorm; Slow-Fe) is an iron salt. *Dose:* By mouth, to treat anaemia, 0·9 to 1·8 g daily in divided doses. Prevention, 300 mg daily.

Fersaday ◊ ferrous fumarate.

Fersamal ◊ ferrous fumarate.

Fertiral injection is used to treat certain types of amenorrhoea (absence of periods) and infertility. It contains gonadorelin 500 mcg/1 ml ◊ gonadorelin.

Fesovit spansules are sustained release (long-acting) capsules containing dried ferrous sulphate 150 mg (equivalent to 47 mg iron), thiamine 2 mg, riboflavine 2 mg, nicotinamide 10 mg, pyridoxine 1 mg and ascorbic acid 50 mg.

Fesovit Z spansules are sustained-release capsules containing dried ferrous sulphate 150 mg, zinc sulphate monohydrate 61·8 mg (equivalent to 22·5 mg of zinc), ascorbic acid 50 mg, thiamine mononitrate 2 mg, riboflavine 2 mg, pyridoxine hydrochloride 1 mg and nicotinamide 10 mg.

fibrinogen is a factor in blood which helps it to clot.

Fibrosine Balm contains methyl nicotinate 1%, glycol salicylate 5%, histamine dihydrochloride 0·05%, and capsicum oleoresin 0·12%.

Fiery Jack Ointment contains iodine 0·28%, capsicum oleoresin 0·7%, arachis oil 0·72%, capsicum 20%, lard 8%, hard paraffin 8%, and yellow soft paraffin to 100%.

Fiery Jack Rubbing Cream contains capsicin 1·25%, histamine dihydrochloride 0·1%, methyl nicotinate 1%, glycol salicylate 5%, diethylamine salicylate 5%, water-miscible basis to 100%.

figs are a mild purgative and demulcent.

Finalgon is a rubefacient. It contains nonivamide 0·4% and butoxyethylnicotinate 2·5%.

Fisherman's Friend Aniseed Flavoured Cold and Flu Lozenges contain liquorice powder 7·6%, menthol 0·5%, and anise oil 0·17%.

Fisherman's Friend Extra Strong Throat & Chest Lozenges contain eucalyptus oil 0·153%, cubeb oil 0·305%, capsicum tincture 0·02%, liquorice extract 7·317%, and menthol 0·9%.

Fisherman's Friend Honey Cough Syrup contains honey 1·25 ml, squill vinegar 0·9 ml, citric acid 50 mg, saccharin solution 0·05 ml, anise oil 0·005 ml, benzoic acid 5 mg, peppermint oil 0·0025 ml, menthol 2·5 mg, and eucalyptol 0·001 ml.

Fisherman's Friend Rubbing Ointment contains capsicum oleoresin 2%, menthol 10%, chlorbutol 10%, and camphor 10%.

Flagyl ◊ metronidazole.

Flagyl compak contains 21 tablets of metronidazole 200 mg and 14 pessaries of nystatin 100,000 units. *Dose:* For mixed trichomonal and candida infection of the vagina – 1 tablet 3 times a day with water after food for seven days and 1 pessary inserted twice daily for seven days or one at night for 14 days.

Flamazine ◊ silver sulphadiazine.

flavoxate (Urispas) has similar effects to propantheline. It is used to relieve spasm and pain associated with the urinary tract. *Dose:* 200 mg three times a day.

Flaxedil ◊ gallamine.

flecainide (Tambocor; flecainide acetate) is used to treat disorders of heart rhythm. *Adverse effects:* Dizziness, visual disturbances and rarely nausea and vomiting. *Precautions:* It should be used with caution in patients with pacemakers, impaired kidney function and in pregnancy. It should not be used in heart failure or heart block. *Dose:* By mouth, 100 to 200 mg, twice daily (maximum 400 mg daily) reduce dose when possible and give a reduced dose to elderly patients (100 mg twice daily, reducing).

Fletchers' arachis oil retention enema is used to treat severe constipation. It lubricates and softens impacted faeces. *Precaution:* The enema should be warmed to body temperature before use.

Fletchers' enemette contains dioctyl sodium sulphosuccinate 90 mg, glycerol 3·78 g, macrogol 2·25 g and sorbic acid 5 mg, in each 5 ml. It lubricates and softens impacted faeces.

Fletchers' magnesium sulphate retention enema contains magnesium sulphate 50%.

Fletchers' phosphate enema contains sodium acid phosphate 12·8 g and sodium phosphate 10·24 g.

Flexin Continus is a controlled slow release tablet of indomethacin ◊ indomethacin. *Dose:* By mouth, one tablet (75 mg) once or twice daily with food, milk or an antacid.

Flolan ◊ epoprostenol.

Florinef ◊ fludrocortisone.

Floxapen ◊ flucloxacillin.

Flu-Amp capsules: Each antibiotic capsule contains ampicillin 250 mg (sodium salt) and cloxacillin 250 mg (sodium salt) ◊ ampicillin and cloxacillin.

Flu/Vac is an influenza vaccine, inactivated. It is used for active immunization against influenza.

Flu/Vac/SA is an influenza vaccine, inactivated (surface antigen). It is used for active immunization against influenza.

Fluanxol ◊ flupenthixol.

Flucaps Capsules each contain codeine phosphate 8 mg and paracetamol 500 mg.

fluclorolone (Topilar cream and ointment) is a cortico-steroid.

flucloxacillin (Floxapen; Ladropen; Stafoxil; Staphcil) is a semi-synthetic penicillin. ◊ benzylpenicillin. *Dose:* By mouth, 250 mg four times daily one hour before meals. Also available as an injection.

flucytosine (Alcobon) is an antifungal drug. It can cause changes in liver function. *Dose:* By mouth, 100 mg per kg of body-weight daily in four divided doses. Also available as an intravenous infusion.

fludrocortisone (Florinef; fludrocortisone acetate) is a corticosteroid. *Dose:* By mouth, 0·1 to 0·3 mg daily in the treatment of underworking of the adrenal glands.

flumazenil (Anexate) is the first benzodiazepine antagonist (antidote) to become available for use. It displaces benzodiazepines from their receptor sites and reverses their sedative and sleep-producing effects within 30 to 60 seconds of an intravenous injection. This could enable minor surgical procedures using benzodiazepines to be carried out in out-patients. *Adverse effects:* Nausea, vomiting, flushing, anxiety, agitation, transient rise in blood pressure, increase in heart rate and, rarely, seizures. *Precautions:* Do not use in patients allergic to benzodiazepines. Rapid or excessive amounts of injection may trigger off withdrawal symptoms in patients on long term treatment with benzodiazepines. Do not give to a patient under anaesthesia until the effects of any neuro muscular blocking drug has completely worn off. Flumazenil works for 2–3 hours so that any underlying sedation produced by a benzodiazepine may re-emerge. Use with caution in pregnancy and with breast-feeding mothers. *Dose:* Initially, 200 micrograms by slow intravenous injection over 15 seconds, repeat if necessary with 100 micrograms every 60 seconds up to a maximum of 1 mg (2 mg in an intensive care unit). Usual dose range 300–600 micrograms. Not recommended for children.

flumethasone (flumethasone pivalate). It is a corticosteroid used in skin applications.

flunisolide (Syntaris) is a corticosteroid used to treat nasal symptoms of hayfever. *Precautions:* It may mask some signs of infection. It should not be used in early pregnancy. *Dose:* 2 sprays into each nostril twice daily, reducing to the smallest amount necessary to control symptoms.

flunitrazepam (Rohypnol) is a benzodiazepine drug used as a sleeping drug. It has similar properties to diazepam. *Dose:* By mouth, 0·5 to 2 mg at night.

fluocinolone (Synalar; fluocinolone acetonide) is a corticosteroid used in skin applications.

fluocinonide (Metosyn) is a corticosteroid used in skin applications.

fluocortolone (Ultradil, Ultralanum; fluocortolone hexanoate) is a corticosteroid used in skin applications.

Fluor-a-day Lac ◊ fluoride.

fluoride (En-De-Kay, Fluor-a-day Lac, Fluorigard, Luride, Point-Two, Zymafluor; sodium fluoride). Forty years ago it seemed such a simple idea – put fluoride into drinking water to help reduce tooth decay. However, it is not that simple these days because people are taking in fluoride every day in different ways – in water, food, dental health products, medicines, pesticides, insecticides and in fertilizers. New evidence is emerging on the possible action of fluoride on human cells and tissues. It is now accepted that fluoride can be harmful but at what concentration does it become harmful to the body? The use of fluoride gels, toothpastes and tablets can raise the level of fluoride in the body and although some dentists claim that fluoride 'mottling' of the teeth is a sign of 'healthy' teeth it does nonetheless indicate that the person has had a toxic level of fluoride in his body when a child. The argument that if a little fluoride is good for you then more must be even better for you is dangerous. As yet we really do not know and we should be cautious about the indiscriminate use of fluoride-containing dental products.

Fluorigard ◊ fluoride.

fluorine is an essential trace element in the diet.

fluorometholone (FML) is a corticosteroid used to treat inflammation of the eye.

fluorouracil (Efudix) is an anti-cancer drug. *Adverse effects:* These include nausea, vomiting, loss of appetite, skin rash (dermatitis), loss of hair (alopecia), nail damage, and pigmentation of the skin. It may produce damage to the lining membrane of the mouth, stomach and gut, fever, haemorrhage and bone-marrow damage leading to blood disorders. *Precautions:* It should not be given to patients whose bone-marrow function may be depressed and it should be given with caution to patients whose liver function is impaired. *Dose:* Depends upon the condition being treated.

fluothane ◊ halothane.

flupenthixol (Depixol; Fluanxol; flupenthixol dihydrochloride) is related to fluphenazine. It is a major tranquillizer. *Dose:* By mouth, 0·5 to 9 mg daily. The last daily dose should be taken no later than 4 p.m. because it may occasionally cause insomnia. By oily, intramuscular injection, 20 to 40 mg every two to four weeks.

fluphenazine (Modecate, Moditen, Moditen Enanthate; fluphenazine decanoate, fluphenazine enanthate, fluphenazine hydrochloride) is a major tranquillizer. It also has anti-vomiting properties. *Adverse effects:* It may produce trembling, stiffness of the muscles and poor coordination of movement (Parkinsonism and dyskinesia). These effects are irreversible. Occasionally fluphenazine may cause milk to come from the breasts (galactorrhoea), abdominal pain and jaundice. For other adverse effects and precautions refer to chlorpromazine. *Dose:* By mouth; for anxiety states, 1 to 2 mg daily in divided doses; for schizophrenia, up to 15 mg daily in divided doses. Moditen (fluphenazine

enanthate) 25 mg every 10 to 28 days by intramuscular injection and Modecate (fluphenazine decanoate), 25 mg every 15 to 40 days by intramuscular injection. ˙

fluprednisolone is a corticosteroid. ◊ prednisolone.

flurandrenolide ◊ flurandrenolone.

flurandrenolone (Haelan; flurandrenolide) is a corticosteroid used in skin applications.

flurazepam (Dalmane; Paxane) is a benzodiazepine drug used to treat anxiety and insomnia. ◊ chlordiazepoxide. *Dose:* By mouth, 15 to 30 mg at night.

flurbiprofen (Froben) is an antirheumatic drug similar to ibuprofen. *Adverse effects:* These include anorexia, nausea, dyspepsia, diarrhoea, constipation and bleeding from the stomach. *Dose:* By mouth, 150 to 200 mg daily in divided doses.

Flu-rex: Each tablet contains paracetamol 400 mg, caffeine 30 mg, phenylephrine hydrochloride 5 mg, and noscapine 7.5 mg.

fluspirilene (Redeptin) is a major tranquillizer. It is available as a depot injection. *Adverse effects:* In the first 48 hours patients may develop Parkinsonism and dyskinesia (severe involuntary movements). They may also develop tremor and salivation (drooling from the mouth). These adverse effects can be controlled by reducing the next dose and by giving atropine-like drugs. It may also cause nausea, vomiting, drowsiness, insomnia, excitement, anxiety, headache and sweating. Blurred vision, dizziness, fall in blood pressure and skin rash may occur. Changes on the electrocardiograph (heart tracing) and electroencephalograph (brain tracing) have been reported. *Precautions:* Drowsiness may interfere with ability to drive or operate machinery. It should not be used in pregnancy and should be used with caution in patients with epilepsy. *Dose:* 2 to 8 mg weekly by intramuscular injection. Patients on depot injections like this should carry a warning card and be seen regularly by a psychiatrist.

Fluvirin is a brand of influenza vaccine.

Fluvoxamine (Faverin; fluvoxamine maleate) is an antidepressant drug. *Adverse effects* include sleepiness, agitation and trembling (tremor), nausea, loss of appetite, constipation, and slowing of the heart rate. *Precautions:* It should preferably not be used during pregnancy and breast feeding. Reduced dosage should be used in patients with impaired kidney and liver function. It may increase some of the harmful effects of alcohol. *Dose:* By mouth, 100 to 300 mg daily in two divided doses, morning and night. Daily doses of 100 mg or less should be taken as one dose at night.

FML eye drops contain fluorometholone.

FML-Neo eye drops contain fluorometholone 0·1% and neomycin sulphate 0·5%.

Folex-350: Each tablet contains ferrous fumarate 308 mg and folic acid 350 micrograms. *Dose:* By mouth, 1 daily.

folic acid (pteroylglutamic acid) is present in many foods; it is necessary for cell division and for the normal production of red blood cells. Symptoms of folic acid deficiency include sore tongue, anaemia, diarrhoea and loss of weight. Folic acid deficiency may occur in pregnancy, in patients with certain disorders of their stomach and bowels which interfere with absorption (e.g., coeliac disease, after gastrectomy), after prolonged use of large doses of pyrimethamine (used to prevent malaria) and in patients with epilepsy treated with anti-convulsant drugs (particularly primidone and phenytoin but also phenobarbitone). In this last disorder, folic acid deficiency can lead to mental deterioration, which can be prevented by giving folic acid and vitamin B_{12}. Folic acid is now often given as routine along with iron during the pre-natal period. *Adverse effects:* Large and continuous doses of folic acid may lower the blood level of vitamin B_{12} which is essential to the normal production of red blood cells. *Precautions:* Folic acid should not be used to treat pernicious anaemia since, unlike vitamin B_{12}, it does not prevent the spinal cord complications of pernicious anaemia. *Dose:* By mouth; initially: 5 to 20 mg daily; maintenance: 2·5 to 10 mg daily. 0·2 to 0·5 mg daily as a prophylaxis in pregnancy.

Folicin: Each tablet contains folic acid 2·5 mg, copper sulphate 2·5 mg, manganese sulphate 2·5 mg and ferrous sulphate 200 mg. *Dose:* By mouth, 1 to 2 daily.

folinic acid (Calcium Leucovorin; Refolinon; Rescufolin) is used in the treatment of megaloblastic anaemias and to lessen the side-effects of methotrexate which is a folic acid antagonist used to treat cancer. Folinic acid is closely related to folic acid.

fonazine ◊ dimethothiazine.

Forane ◊ isoflurane.

Forceval Capsules and Junior Capsules contain iron, minerals and vitamins.

formaldehyde solutions (formalin) are used in varying strengths as antiseptics, and disinfectants, to treat warts and verrucas, to treat sweaty feet and in throat lozenges.

formalin ◊ formaldehyde.

Fortagesic tablets contain pentazocine 15 mg and paracetamol 500 mg. It is a moderate pain-reliever. *Dose:* 2 three or four times daily.

Fortical is used to treat patients suffering from kidney and liver failure who require a high-energy, low-fluid, low-electrolyte diet. It contains glucose polymers providing carbohydrates.

Fortral ◊ pentazocine.

Fortum injection ◊ ceftazidime.

Fortunan ◊ haloperidol.

fosfestrol (Honvan; fosfestrol sodium) is broken down in the body to stilboestrol. It is used in the treatment of cancer of the prostate. *Adverse effects:* Injection may cause burning pain in the perineum. Nausea and vomiting may occur. *Dose:* By mouth, 100 to 600 mg daily, in divided doses. It is also available in injection.

Fosfor syrup is used as a tonic. It contains phosphorylcolamine 5%.

Frador contains menthol 0·1%, chlorbutol 1%; prep. storax 2%, and the alcohol-soluble matter of 15% of benzoin, in alcoholic solution.

framycetin (Framygen; Soframycin; framycetin sulphate) is an antibiotic of the neomycin group. It is too toxic to be used by mouth or by injection, and is used principally in skin applications and eye drops. *Adverse effects* and *Precautions:* These are similar to those described under neomycin.

Framycort preparations contain framycetin 0·5% and hydrocortisone acetate 0·5%.

Framygen ◊ framycetin.

frangula is used to treat constipation.

Franol is used to treat bronchial asthma. Each tablet contains ephedrine hydrochloride 11 mg, theophylline 120 mg and phenobarbitone 8 mg. *Dose:* 1 three times daily and 1 at bedtime.

Franol Plus: Each tablet contains ephedrine sulphate 15 mg, theophylline 120 mg, phenobarbitone 8 mg, and thenyldiamine hydrochloride 10 mg.

Franolyn Expect: Each 10 ml contains guaiphenesin 50 mg, ephedrine 9·5 mg, and theophylline 120 mg.

Franolyn Sed is used to treat dry coughs. Each 5 ml contains dextromethorphan hydrobromide 10 mg.

Freezone contains salicylic acid 14·41% and zinc chloride 2·36%.

Frisium ◊ clobazam.

Froben ◊ flurbiprofen.

fructose ◊ laevulose.

Frumil contains amiloride 5 mg, and frusemide 40 mg. It is used as a potassium sparing diuretic.

frusemide (Aluzine; Diuresal; Dryptal, Frusetic, Frusid, Lasix) is a diuretic. It works quickly when taken by mouth and lasts for about four to six hours. *Adverse effects:* It may produce nausea and diarrhoea. Continued use may cause salt and water loss resulting in weakness, muscle cramps, pins and needles, thirst and loss of appetite. It may trigger off an attack of gout in someone prone to gout. It may also produce blood disorders and cause the blood sugar to increase and sugar to appear in the urine. Prolonged use may cause a fall in blood sodium, calcium and potassium – the latter sensitizes heart muscle to digoxin. *Precautions:* Frusemide should be used with caution in patients with acute impairment of kidney function or when their blood potassium is low. It should be used with caution in patients with impaired liver function. *Dose:* By mouth, 20 to 80 mg daily in divided doses, reducing to a maintenance dose every other day or on three successive days each week.

Frusene ◊ triamterene.

Frusetic ◊ frusemide.

Frusid ◊ frusemide.

FSH ◊ gonadatrophon.

fuchsine ◊ magenta.

Fucibet cream contains betamethasone valerate 0·1% and fusidic acid 2%.

fucidic acid ◊ sodium fusidate.

Fucidin ◊ sodium fusidate.

Fucidin H ointment and **cream** contain hydrocortisone acetate 1% and sodium fusidate 2%.

Fucidin IV solution ◊ diethanolamine fusidate.

Fulcin ◊ griseofulvin.

Fungilin ◊ amphotericin.

Fungizone ◊ amphotericin.

Furadantin ◊ nitrofurantoin.

Furamide ◊ diloxanide.

fusafungine (Locabiotal) is an antibiotic with anti-inflammatory properties used for the treatment of infections of the upper respiratory tract. *Dose:* Three sprays into each nostril 5 times a day.

Fybogel ◊ ispaghula.

Fybranta is used to prevent and treat constipation. Each tablet contains bran 2 g. *Dose:* By mouth, 1 to 3 chewed and swallowed with a drink three or four times daily.

Fynnon Calcium Aspirin: Each tablet contains aspirin 500 mg, calcium carbonate 150 mg, and citric acid 50 mg.

Fynnon salts contain sodium sulphate 95·96%, sodium bicarbonate 1·95%, potassium sulphate 2·05%, lithium sulphate 0·033% and traces of iron and sodium chloride (common salt).

Fuller's earth consists mainly of native hydrated aluminium silicate. It is adsorbent and used in dusting powders.

Galcodine linctus and paediatric linctus are cough medicines containing codeine phosphate ◊ codeine.

Galenomycin ◊ oxytetracycline.

Galenphol linctus, strong linctus and paediatric linctus are cough medicines containing pholcodine ◊ pholcodine.

Galfer ◊ ferrous fumarate.

Galfer FA: Each capsule contains ferrous fumarate 290 mg and folic acid 350 micrograms.

Galfer-Vit: Each tablet contains ferrous fumarate 305 mg, sodium ascorbate 50 mg, riboflavine 2 mg, nicotinamide 10 mg, thiamine 2 mg and pyridoxine 4 mg. *Dose:* By mouth, 1 once or twice daily.

gall is obtained from growths on certain twigs caused by overgrowth of the tissues in response to the gall-moth. It is used as an astringent.

gallamine (Flaxedil; gallamine triethiodide) is a muscle relaxant which is used along with general anaesthetics in surgical operations. It may produce rapid beating of the heart. For precautions ◊ tubocurarine.

Galloways Baby Cough Linctus: Each 5 ml contains squill liquid extract 0·0015 ml, ipecacuanha liquid extract 0·01 ml, chloroform spirit 0·225 ml, tolu solution 0·04 ml, and glycerol 1 ml.

Galloways Bronchial Expectorant contains ether spirit 0·357%, ipecacuanha liquid extract 0·067%, squill vinegar 0·535%, acetic acid 4·2%, chloroform 0·2%, and syrup 78·6%.

Galloways Cough Syrup: Each 5 ml contains ipecacuanha liquid extract 0·0045 ml, chloroform 0·01 ml, acetic acid 0·21 ml, squill vinegar 0·0267 ml, and ether 0·0028 ml.

Galloways Honey and Lemon Cough Syrup contains ether spirit 0·00842 ml, acetic acid 0·21 ml, ipecacuanha tincture 0·045 ml, squill vinegar 0·0268 ml, honey 0·25 ml, syrup to 5 ml.

Galloways Junior Cough Linctus contains squill liquid extract 0·3%, ipecacuanha liquid extract 0·2%, chloroform spirit 4·5%, tolu solution 0·8%, glycerol 20%, and syrup.

Galpseud linctus and tablets contain pseudoephedrine hydrochloride ◊ pseudoephedrine.

Gamanil ◊ lofepramine.

Gamimune-N is a normal immunoglobulin injection.

gamma benzene hexachloride (Quellada) is used to treat scabies and lice.

Gamma Formula capsules contain evening primrose oil.

gammabulin is a normal immunoglobulin injection.

Ganda eye drops contain varying proportions of guanethidine sulphate and adrenaline for the treatment of glaucoma.

Gardenal ◊ phenobarbitone.

garlic has expectorant, disinfectant and diuretic properties. It should not be given to children for these purposes.

garlic oil ◊ garlic.

Garlisol ointment is used to treat bruises and minor skin irritations. It contains oil of garlic 0·625 mg, oil of aniseed 1·25 mg, thymol 1 mg, glycerin 200 mg and paraformaldehyde 50 mg.

Garlisol tablets are used to treat catarrh. Each tablet contains garlic oil 0·3 mg, thymol 0·4 mg, aniseed oil 0·5 mg and paraformaldehyde 7·5 mg.

Gastrils pastilles contain aluminium hydroxide and magnesium carbonate as a co-dried gel 500 mg. Used as an antacid.

Gastrobid continus tablets contain 15 mg of metoclopramide hydrochloride in a controlled release form ◊ metoclopromide.

Gastrocote is used to treat indigestion and peptic ulcer. Each tablet contains alginic acid 200 mg, aluminium hydroxide 80 mg, magnesium trisilicate 40 mg, and sodium bicarbonate 70 mg. *Dose:* By mouth, 1 to 3 chewed four times daily after meals and at bedtime.

Gastromax is a controlled slow release capsule of metoclopramide ◊ metoclopramide. *Dose:* One daily before meals.

Gastron tablets are used to treat heartburn and acid reflux. Each tablet contains alginic acid 600 mg, dried aluminium hydroxide 240 mg, sodium bicarbonate 210 mg and magnesium trisilicate 60 mg. See entry on each drug.

Gastrozepin ◊ pirenzepine.

Gaviscon is used to treat indigestion, peptic ulcer, oesophagitis, hiatus hernia and heartburn. Each tablet contains alginic acid 250 mg, sodium alginate 250 mg, magnesium trisilicate 25 mg, dried aluminium hydroxide gel 100 mg and sodium bicarbonate 170 mg. **Gaviscon Liquid** contains sodium alginate 500 mg, sodium bicarbonate 267 mg, calcium carbonate 160 mg per 10 ml. *Dose:* By mouth, 1 or 2 tablets or 10–20 ml after meals and at bedtime.

Gee's Linctus ◊ opiate squill linctus.

Gee's Pastilles ◊ opiate squill linctus.

gelatin (Gelofusine) is a protein extracted from animal tissues. It is used in the preparation of capsules and suppositories, in the preparation of pastes, pastilles and pessaries, in preparing lubricating eye drops and to make a solution used to restore blood volume after haemorrhage. It is taken by mouth to treat brittle nails.

Gelcosal gel contains strong coal-tar solution 5%, tar 5%, and salicylic acid 2%. Used to treat psoriasis and chronic dermatitis ◊ tar and salicylic acid.

Gelcotar gel contains strong coal tar solution 5%, and tar 5%.

Gelofusine is an injection used to increase the volume of the blood. It contains gelatin 4% and sodium chloride 0·9%.

Gelusil is an antacid. Each tablet contains magnesium trisilicate 250 mg and dried aluminium hydroxide 500 mg. Also available as a suspension. *Dose:* 1 to 2 tablets or 5 to 20 ml of suspension after meals and when required.

gemeprost (Cervagem) is a synthetic prostaglandin. It has been used for the termination of pregnancy.

gemfibrozil (Lopid) is used to lower blood fat levels. *Adverse effects* include nausea, diarrhoea, vomiting and wind, headache, dizziness, blurred vision, impotence, pains in the hands and feet, painful muscles and itching. *Precautions:* Before starting treatment patients should have at least two tests for anaemia, liver function and blood fat levels. It should be used with caution in patients with impaired kidney function and patients should have a specialist examination of their eyes every 12 months. Their blood fat levels should be measured at regular intervals. If there is no response or the blood fats go up (a paradoxical response), the drug should be stopped. The latter can happen in alcoholic liver

disease. Tests for anaemia should be carried out every two months during the first 12 months of treatment. It should not be used in patients with alcoholic liver disease, gall stones or impaired liver function. It should not be used in pregnancy. *Dose:* By mouth, 1,200 to 1,500 mg daily in two divided doses.

Genexol ◊ nonoxynol.

Genisol is a shampoo containing tar used for psoriasis of the scalp.

gentamicin (Cidomycin; Genticin; gentamicin sulphate) is an antibiotic. It is not absorbed by mouth and has to be given by injections; it is also used in ointments. *Adverse effects:* Gentamicin by injection may produce deafness and disorders of balance – these may be permanent. It may also produce kidney damage, skin rashes and fevers. *Precautions:* Gentamicin should only be used in pregnancy or infancy if no safer treatment is available. *Dose:* By intramuscular injections, 80 mg every 8 hrs.

gentian compound infusion is used as a bitter tonic. See tonics.

gentian violet (crystal violet) is used in antiseptic skin applications against bacteria, worms and fungi.

Genticin ◊ gentamicin.

Genticin HC cream and ointment contains hydrocortisone 1% and gentamicin 0·3%.

Gentran ◊ dextran.

George's American Marvel Liniment contains alcoholic (45%) extract of arnica flower (10–1) 3·7%, alcoholic (60%) capsicum extract (5–1) 3·7%, turpentine oil 5%, water 6%, camphor 2%, eucalyptus oil 2%, rosemary oil 0·3%, soft soap 8%, and industrial methylated spirit to 100%.

geranium oil is used for perfuming tooth powders, ointment, talcum powders, and various cosmetics.

Germ Ointment contains zinc oxide 8%, starch 5%, phenol 0·5%, methyl salicylate 3%, chloroxylenol 0·25%, basis to 100%.

Germolene Footspray contains triclosan 0·03% and dichlorophen 0·1%.

Germolene Medicated Plasters are adhesive plasters with a medicated pad containing domiphen bromide 0·15%.

Germolene New-Skin contains ethyl acetate 57·3%, alcohol 25·1%, pyroxylin 6·9%, butyl alcohol 5%, castor oil 3%, amyl acetate 2%, and camphor 0·6%.

Germolene Ointment contains anhydrous lanolin 35%, yellow soft paraffin 36%, liquid paraffin 7·9%, starch 10%, phenol 1·19%, zinc oxide 6·55%, methyl salicylate 3%, octaphonium chloride 0·3%, and menthol 0·01%.

Germolene 2 Antiseptic Cream contains phenol 1·2% w/w and chlorhexidine gluconate 0·25% w/w.

Germoloids Moist Toilet Tissues contain benzalkonium chloride 0·133%, chlorhexidine gluconate 0·2%, and menthol 0·04%.

Germoloids Ointment contains yellow soft paraffin 84·5%, zinc oxide 6·6%, wool fat 3·5%, methyl salicylate 3·05%, bismuth oxychloride 1·1%, phenol 1%, menthol 0·2%, and chloroxylenol 0·05%. **Suppositories** each contain lignocaine hydrochloride 13·2 mg and zinc oxide 284 mg.

Gerovital H3 Face Cream contains procaine hydrochloride 100 mg in each 27-g pack.

Gerovital H3 Tablets each contain procaine hydrochloride 100 mg, benzoic acid 6 mg, potassium metabisulphite 5 mg, and disodium phosphate 500 micrograms.

Gestanin ◊ allylostrenol.

Gestodene is a progestogen related to norethisterone (see p. 232).

Gestone Oral ◊ ethisterone.

gestronol (Depostat; gestronol hexanoate) is a long-acting progestogen. It is used to treat cancer of the endometrium (lining of the womb) and benign enlargement of the prostate. *Dose:* By intramuscular injection 200 to 400 mg once every 5 to 7 days.

Gevral is a compound iron preparation. Each capsule contains ferrous fumarate 30·8 mg, vitamin A 5,000 units, thiamine mononitrate 5 mg, riboflavine 5 mg, nicotinamide 15 mg, pyridoxine hydrochloride 500 micrograms, cyanocobalamin 1 microgram, ascorbic acid 50 mg, vitamin D 500 units, d-alpha-tocopheryl acetate 10 units, calcium pantothenate 5 mg, choline bitartrate 50 mg, copper 1 mg, iodine 100 micrograms, inositol 50 mg, lysine hydrochloride 25 mg, magnesium 1 mg, calcium 145 mg, phosphorus 110 mg, potassium 5 mg, zinc 500 micrograms.

Gibbs SR toothpaste contains sodium monofluorophosphate 0·8% and zinc citrate trihydrate 0·5%.

Gill's Medicated Dandruff Remover Shampoo: Active ingredients are methyl salicylate 1·5% and rosemary oil 0·5%.

ginger is obtained from the scraped and dried rhizome of *Zingiber officinale*, known in commerce as unbleached Jamaica ginger. It is used as a flavouring agent and carminative.

gingerin ◊ ginger.

ginger linctus ◊ ginger.

ginseng: Various parts of the ginseng plant are used to make medicines. The leaves are used to make tea and said to help digestion, the roots are used in tonic remedies. There are as many uses as there are preparations available. The most popular types come from China, Manchuria and Korea. If you think it will do you good it probably will but we need documented scientific evidence if we are to assess its value. *Adverse effects:* Raised blood pressure, nervousness, sleeplessness, skin rashes and diarrhoea in the mornings, the *ginseng abuse syndrome*.

Givitol is a compound iron preparation. Each capsule contains ferrous fumarate 305 mg, folic acid 500 micrograms, thiamine mononitrate 2 mg, riboflavine 2 mg, nicotinamide 10 mg, pyridoxine hydrochloride 4 mg, sodium ascorbate 56 mg.

Glacier Cream. Green tube: a nongreasy cream containing ethylparadimethylaminobenzoate 1% and titanium dioxide 1%. **Red tube:** a greasy cream containing ethylparadimethylaminobenzoate 1%, titanium dioxide 1%, and zinc oxide 1%. **Lip Salve** contains ethylparadimethylaminobenzoate 1%.

Glandosane spray is used to treat a dry mouth. It contains carboxymethylcellulose sodium 0·5 g, sorbital 1·5 g, potassium chloride 60 mg, sodium chloride 42·2 mg, magnesium chloride 2·6 mg, calcium chloride 7·3 mg, dipotassium hydrogen phosphate 17·1 mg per 50 ml.

Glauber's salts ◊ sodium sulphate.

Glauline eye drops contain the beta-blocker metipranolol in concentrations of 0·1%, 0·3%, 0·6%. *Adverse effects:* Stinging of the eyes, transient headache. See propranolol for adverse effects of beta-blockers taken by mouth. *Precautions:* Do not use in patients who suffer from asthma or other chronic wheezing disorders, or from heart failure. Do not use in pregnancy or if you wear soft contact lenses. Use with caution in patients with a slow pulse rate or heart block. *Dose:* Apply 1 drop twice daily.

Glempec contains glycerol 5%, citric acid 0·6%, acetic acid 1·2%, ipecacuanha liquid extract 0·13%, camphor 0·04%, liquid glucose 3·7%, and lemon juice 5%.

glibenclamide (Daonil; Euglucon; Libanil; Malix; Semi-Daonil) is an oral anti-diabetic drug. It may cause headache, indigestion, diarrhoea, skin rashes and affect tests for liver function. *Dose:* Initially, 2·5 to 5 mg daily at breakfast increasing by 0·5 mg daily at weekly intervals. Maximum daily dosage is 15 mg.

Glibenese ◊ glipizide.

glibornuride (Glutril) is an oral anti-diabetic drug. *Adverse effects* and *Precautions:* ◊ chlorpropamide. *Dose:* By mouth, 12·5 to 50 mg daily.

gliclazide (Diamicron) is an oral anti-diabetic drug. *Adverse effects:* Nausea, headache, rashes and gastro-intestinal upsets. *Precautions:* Should not be used in juvenile-onset diabetes, diabetes complicated by ketosis and acidosis, pregnancy, in diabetics undergoing surgery or in patients known to be sensitive to other sulphonylureas. It should be used with caution in patients suffering from impaired renal or hepatic function. It should be given with caution with other drugs such as sulphonamides, salicylates, phenylbutazone, beta-blocking drugs, MAOIs, thiazide diuretics and corticosteroids. *Dose:* By mouth, 40 to 320 mg daily in divided doses.

Glinteel Lotion contains tannic acid 5·25%, Peru balsam 6·25%, cinnamon oil 0·5%, water 8·6%, and industrial methylated spirit to 100%.

glipizide (Glibenese; Minodiab) is an oral anti-diabetic drug. *Adverse effects* and *Precautions* ◊ chlorpropamide. *Dose:* By mouth, 2·5 to 30 mg daily.

gliquidone (Glurenorm) is an oral anti-diabetic drug. *Adverse effects* and *Precautions* ◊ chlorpropamide. *Dose:* By mouth, 45 to 60 mg daily in divided doses. Maximum 180 mg daily.

glucagon is a peptide hormone produced by the body. It increases the blood level of glucose by activating glycogen stored in the liver to produce glucose. It can be given by injection as an alternative to glucose in hypoglycaemia (low blood-sugar level).

Glucodin ◊ glucose.

Glucophage ◊ metformin.

glucose (Gleucodin) is a readily absorbable carbohydrate which acts as a source of energy. It may be given by mouth or injection.

Glucotard ◊ guar gum.

Glurenorm ◊ gliquidone.

glutamic acid hydrochloride releases hydrochloric acid when dissolved in water and is used in patients who are not producing acid in their stomach.

glutaraldehyde (Glutarol; Verucasep) is a disinfectant. It is also used as a paint in the treatment of warts.

Glutarol ◊ glutaraldehyde.

Glutril ◊ glibornuride.

glycerides are surfactants.

glycerin (glycol) is a sweet-tasting, syrupy liquid used in some cough medicines and in some skin preparations.

glycerine ◊ glycerol.

glycerol is used as a sweetening agent in mixtures and pastilles. Externally, it is used in creams for its water-retaining and emollient properties. It is used in some ear drops to soften wax. It has been given orally to reduce high pressure in the brain. It is included as a demulcent in some cough medicines.

glycerophosphates and **hypophosphites.** These have been used as *tonics* for decades in the belief they would be easily assimilated into the brain and help convalescence. There is no evidence of this at all and their effects are placebo.

glyceryl aminobenzoate is used as a sunscreen.

glyceryl mono-oleate is an emulsifying agent.

glyceryl monostearate is used as a stabilizer in the preparation of emulsions. It has emollient properties.

glyceryl trinitrate (Coro-Nitro; Deponit; GTN 300 mcg; Nitrocontin; Nitrocine; Nitronal; Percutol; Sustac; Suscard Buccal; Transiderm-Nitro; Tridil; nitroglycerin; trinitrin) is principally used to treat angina. It may also be used to relieve pain from kidney stones or gallstones. *Adverse effects:* Large doses cause flushing of the face, severe throbbing headache and faintness. In severe cases restlessness, blueness, vomiting and fainting may occur

but these only last for a short time. *Precautions:* Glyceryl trinitrate should be used with caution in patients with marked anaemia, head injury, or acute coronary thrombosis. *Dose:* Tablets to be dissolved in the mouth: 0·5 to 1 mg as required. **Sustac** is in the form of sustained-release tablets, taken two or three times daily. **Percutol** ointment contains 2% glyceryl trinitrate.

glycine ◊ aminoacetic acid.

glycocol ◊ aminoacetic acid.

glycol ◊ glycerin.

glycol monosalicylate is used in rheumatic rubs as a skin irritant.

glycol salicylate is related to aspirin and is used in rheumatic rubs.

Glyconon ◊ tolbutamide.

glycopyrronium (Robinul; glycopyrronium bromide) is used to treat symptoms of peptic ulcer and spasm of the gastro-intestinal tract. *Adverse effects* and *Precautions* ◊ atropine. *Dose:* By mouth, 1 to 4 mg two to three times daily. Intravenous or intramuscular injection (200–400 micrograms) as a pre-medication before a general anaesthetic.

Glykola is a compound iron preparation. Each 5 ml of syrup contains ferric chloride solution 0·01 ml, caffeine 20 mg, calcium glycerophosphate 30 mg, kola liquid extract 0·12 ml.

Glymese ◊ chlorpropamide.

glymidine (Gondafon) is an oral anti-diabetic drug. *Adverse effects:* Stomach upsets and skin rashes may occasionally occur and rarely blood disorders. In some patients anti-histamines may make these allergic skin rashes worse. *Precautions:* It should probably not be given in pregnancy and it should not be given to patients with severe impairment of kidney function. *Dose:* Initially 1·5 g with breakfast; maintenance 0·5 to 1 g with breakfast.

Glypressin ◊ terlipressin.

Goddard's White Oil Embrocation contains turpentine oil 22%, dilute acetic acid 30%, and dilute ammonia solution 14%.

gold (Myocrisin; sodium aurothioma-late; sodium aurothiosuccinate) is a compound of gold used to treat rheumatoid arthritis. It is given in a water solution by deep intramuscular injection. It is slowly absorbed, stored in the body and slowly excreted in the urine. It is not known how it works. *Adverse effects:* Skin rashes, itching, blood disorders, liver damage, kidney damage, colitis, stomatitis, sensitivity of the skin to sunlight and occasionally neuritis and encephalitis may occur. An injection may set off an attack of acute rheumatoid arthritis. *Precautions:* Gold should not be given to patients with impaired kidney or liver function, to patients with blood disorders or to patients with dermatitis or other skin disorders. It should be given with caution in pregnancy and to patients with high blood pressure. Before each injection patients should be carefully examined particularly for stomatitis, fever, debility, bleeding disorders, sore throats, and skin rashes. The urine should be examined and repeated blood tests should be carried out. Any sign of intolerance to gold is an indication for immediately stopping the drug and starting an anti-dote – dimercaprol or penicillamine. Patients should report any untoward symptoms such as fever, debility, sore throat, sore mouth, skin rash or di-arrhoea as soon as they occur. *Dose:* By deep intramuscular injection, 10 to 50 mg weekly. No more than 1 g in one course.

Gold Label tablets: Each contain Korean ginseng 200 mg.

Gon tablets: Each contain ace-tomenaphthone 10 mg and nicotina-mide 50 mg.

gonadorelin (Fertiral) is gonadot-rophin-releasing hormone. When in-jected intravenously it leads to a rapid rise in plasma-luteinizing hormone (LH) and follicle-stimulating hor-mone (FSH) concentrations. It is used to assess pituitary function. *Adverse effects:* These include nausea, headaches, abdominal pain and in-creased menstrual bleeding rarely occur.

Gonadotraphon LH ◊ chorionic gona-dotrophin.

Gondafon ◊ glymidine.

goserelin (Zoladex) mimics the action of the gonadotrophin-releasing hor-mone which stimulates the pituitary gland to release luteinizing hormone (LH) which stimulates the testes to produce the male sex hormone, tes-tosterone. It is 100 times more potent than the natural hormone and its effects last longer. After initial stimulation it leads to a reduction in testosterone production by the testes equivalent to castration. It is used to treat cancers of the prostate gland which are dependent on testosterone for growth. *Adverse effects:* Hot flushes, decreased libido, breast swelling and tenderness, skin rashes, mild bruising at injection site. Initial increase in testosterone level in the blood may cause an increase in bone pain from secondary prostatic cancer deposits. *Precautions:* monitor patient carefully in first four weeks because of risk of secondaries getting worse. *Dose:* One 3 to 6 mg depot injection under the skin in the abdominal wall every 28 days.

gramicidin is an antibiotic used in skin applications.

Graneodin applications contain neomycin sulphate 0·25% and gramicidin 0·025%.

Grapefruit Health Salts contain tartaric acid 40%, sodium bicarbonate 42·04%, dried magnesium sulphate 17·66%, saccharin sodium 0·05%, and grapefruit oil 0·25%.

grapefruit oil is used as a flavouring agent. It has an irritant effect on the skin and lining of the gut.

Grasshopper Ear Drops contain docusate sodium 5%.

Grasshopper Ointment contains colophony 31·68%, yellow beeswax 7·94%, larch oleoresin 23·74%, arachis oil 15·84%, white soft paraffin 19·81%, and copper acetate 0·99%.

Gregoderm applications contain neomycin sulphate 0·4%, nystatin 100,000 units/g, and polymyxin B 7250 units/g and hydrocortisone 1%.

grindelia (gum plant) has expectorant properties and is included in some cough medicines. Large doses can affect kidney function.

griseofulvin (Fulcin; Grisovin) is an antibiotic used to treat fungus infections of the nails, hair, and skin. *Adverse effects:* It may cause headaches, stomach upsets and skin rashes which are usually mild and short-lasting. Rarely severe allergic reactions to griseofulvin may produce dermatitis, swelling of the throat, blood disorders, skin sensitivity to sunlight and bad headaches. Swelling of the breast and brown coloration of the area round the nipples have occurred in children. *Precautions:* Griseofulvin should not be used in patients suffering from porphyria. It may increase the effects of alcohol and decrease the effects of anticoagulant drugs. Barbiturates can reduce the effectiveness of griseofulvin. *Dose:* By mouth, 0·5 to 1 g daily in single or divided doses.

Grisovin ◊ griseofulvin.

GTN 300 mcg ◊ glyceryl trinitrate.

guaiacum resin has mild laxative and diuretic actions. It has an aromatic odour and has been included in rheumatic treatments. It is used to detect blood in the faeces and as an antioxidant in food.

guaiphenesin (in Robitussin and various cough mixtures) reduces the stickiness of sputum and is used as a cough expectorant. *Dose:* 100 to 200 mg every two or four hours.

guanethidine (Ismelin; guanethidine sulphate) lowers the blood pressure. *Adverse effects:* The commonest adverse effects at the start of treatment with guanethidine are diarrhoea and a drop in blood pressure on exertion, producing dizziness, faintness, weakness and lassitude (particularly in the mornings). These decrease in severity as treatment is continued. Other frequent adverse effects are slowing of the heart rate, breathlessness and oedema (often recognized because the ankles swell). Nausea, vomiting, pain in the cheeks (parotid glands), stuffy nose, blurred vision, muscle pains, trembling, dermatitis, failure to ejaculate, frequency in passing urine and depression of mood may occur. *Precautions:* Guanethidine should be used with caution in patients with defective blood supply to the brain, kidneys or heart. The blood pressure lowering effects are decreased by antidepressant drugs. Patients may become sensitive to the effects of amphetamines and other similar drugs. *Dose:* By mouth, 20 to 100 mg daily in divided doses until the desired reduction in blood pressure is obtained.

Guanor Expectorant is used to treat coughs. Each 5 ml of syrup contains ammonium chloride 135 mg, diphenhydramine hydrochloride 14 mg, menthol 1·1 mg and sodium citrate 57 mg. *Dose:* 5 to 10 ml every 2 to 3 hours.

guar gum (Glucotard; Guarem; Guarina, Lejguar) is used as a thickening agent in medicines. Also as an additional treatment in patients with diabetes.

Guarem ◊ guar gum.

Guarina sachets ◊ guar gum.

gum arabic is the dried gummy exudation from the stems and branches of *Acacia senegal*. It is used to make mixtures, linctuses and powders. It is also used as a soothing agent in skin applications.

Gum-eze contains myrrh tincture 10%, krameria tincture 2·5%, thymol 0·1%, oil of cloves 0·1%, propylene glycol 50%, glycerol 37·0875%, sodium benzoate 0·1%, cetylpyridinium chloride 0·1%, and saccharin 0·0125%.

Gynatren is a vaccine prepared from inactivated lactobacillus acidophilus. It is used to treat recurrent trichomoniasis infections of the neck of the womb and vagina.

Gyno-Daktarin vaginal cream and pessaries ◊ miconazole.

Gyno-Pevaryl ◊ econazole.

Gynol 11 ◊ nonoxynol.

Gynovlar 21: Each tablet contains norethisterone acetate 3 mg and ethinyloestradiol 0·05 mg. It is an oral contraceptive drug.

H11 injection* contains a protein extract from male urine and is said to be useful in palliating the effects of advanced cancer.

Hacks contain menthol 0·1%, eucalyptus oil 0·06%, anise oil 0·11%, tolu liquid 0·02%, coltsfoot extract equivalent to coltsfoot 0·008%, horehound extract equivalent to horehound 0·03%, compound benzoin tincture 0·02%, sucrose 63·7%, and liquid glucose 31·9%.

Hactos Chest & Cough Mixture contains chloroform 0·5%, capsicum extract 0·01%, peppermint oil 0·01%, anise oil 0·01%, clove oil 0·01%, and sucrose 10%.

Haelan cream and **ointment** contain flurandrenolone 0·0125%.

Haelan-C cream contains flurandrenolone 0·0125% and 3% clioquinol in a diluent aqueous cream. The ointment is in a base of diluent white soft paraffin.

Haelan-X cream and **ointment** contains flurandrenolone 0·05%.

Haemaccel infusion contains gelatin and is used to restore blood volume after haemorrhage.

haematoporphyrin is a red pigment free from iron obtained from haematin (which is an iron complex from haemoglobin in red blood cells). It is used as a tonic ◊ tonics in Part Two.

Haemorex ointment contains zinc oxide 7·5%, diperodon hydrochloride 1%, allantoin 1%, and basis to 100%.

Haemorrhoidal Spray contains lignocaine 0·08% and chlorhexidine hydrochloride 0·1%.

Haemostatic Dressing Strip contains sodium alginate, calcium alginate, domiphen bromide 0·15%.

Halaurant liquid is a multivitamin supplement.

halazone has a strong smell of chlorine. It is used to disinfect drinking water.

Halciderm ◊ halcinonide.

halcinonide (Halciderm Topical) is a corticosteroid used to treat skin disorders. ◊ corticosteroids in Part Two.

Halcion ◊ triazolam.

Haldol ◊ haloperidol.

Half-inderal LA: Each capsule contains propranolol hydrochloride 80 mg in sustained-release form ◊ propranolol.

Haliborange Tablets: Each contain vitamin A 2,500 units, cholecalciferol 200 units, and ascorbic acid 25 mg.

halibut liver oil is a rich source of vitamin A and vitamin D.

Hall's Cherry Flavour Cough Drops contain menthol 1·5 mg and eucalyptus oil 1 mg.

Hall's Mentho Lyptus pastilles contain menthol, eucalyptus, citric acid and sugar and glucose.

haloperidol (Dozic; Fortunan, Haldol, Serenace) is a major tranquillizer. It also has anti-vomiting effects. *Adverse effects:* Dose-related adverse effects commonly include muscle rigidity, trembling and incoordination, depression, blood disorders, and loss of weight with high doses. *Precautions:* Haloperidol should not be given to patients with Parkinsonism. It may reduce the effects of anticoagulant drugs. *Dose:* By mouth, 1 mg to 200 mg daily according to condition being treated. Haldol Decanoate (haloperidol decanoate) is a depot intramuscular injection – 100 to 400 mg every four weeks.

halothane is a general anaesthetic which may cause liver damage.

halquinol is used in the treatment of infected skin conditions.

Halycitrol emulsion contains vitamin A 4,600 units and vitamin D 460 units in each 5 ml.

hamamelis ◊ witch hazel.

Hamarin tablets ◊ allopurinol.

hard soap was used as an excipient to make pills and plasters.

Harmogen ◊ oestrone.

Haymine tablets contain chlorpheniramine maleate 10 mg and ephedrine hydrochloride 15 mg. Used to treat hay-fever symptoms. *Dose:* By mouth, one tablet morning and evening.

Hayphryn is a nasal decongestant. It contains phenylephrine hydrochloride 0·5% and thenyldiamine hydrochloride 0·1%. *Dose:* 2 sprays in each nostril three or four hourly.

H-B-Vax is a brand of hepatitis B vaccine.

HC4 cream contains 1% hydrocortisone ◊ hydrocortisone.

HCG ◊ chorionic gonadotrophin.

Head & Shoulders shampoo contains zinc pyrithione 1%.

Healthy Feet Cream contains glycerol 5%, menthol 1·5%, undecylenic acid 2·5%, and dibromopropamidine isethionate 0·15%.

heavy kaolin is a purified native hydrated aluminium silicate of variable composition. It is used to prepare kaolin poultices.

heavy magnesium carbonate ◊ magnesium carbonate.

Hedamol ◊ ibuprofen.

Hedex tablets: Each contain paracetamol 500 mg.

Hedex Plus is used to relieve mild pain. Each capsule contains paracetamol 500 mg, codeine phosphate 8 mg and caffeine 30 mg.

Hedex Seltzer sachets each contain paracetamol 1 g, caffeine 60 mg, sodium bicarbonate 1·54 g, and anhydrous citric acid 1·25 g.

Heminevrin ◊ chlormethiazole.

Hemocane cream contains lignocaine hydrochloride 0·65%, zinc oxide 10%, bismuth oxide 2%, benzoic acid 0·4%, and cinnamic acid 0·45%. **Suppositories** contain 11 mg, 300 mg, 25 mg, 8 mg, and 9 mg respectively. See entry on each drug. Used to relieve symptoms produced by haemorrhoids.

Hep-flush ◊ heparin.

Hepacon-B₁₂* ◊ cyanocobalamin.

Hepacon-B Forte* contains folic acid 2·5 mg, liver extract equivalent to vitamin B₁₂ 15 micrograms and cocarboxylase 50 mg.

Hepacon-Plex* is a vitamin B complex preparation containing thiamine hydrochloride 50 mg, riboflavine 1 mg, nicotinamide 75 mg, pyridoxine hydrochloride 2·5 mg, cyanocobalamin 4 micrograms, calcium pantothenate 5 mg/ml. *Dose:* By injection.

heparin (see preparations, p. 176) prevents the blood from clotting. Its main use is in the treatment of patients suffering from thrombosis in a vein or artery. It is ineffective by mouth and must be given by injection every four or six hours because it is short acting. *Adverse effects:* The main adverse effect is bleeding – from any site. Rarely fever and allergic reactions may occur. Nosebleeds, red blood cells in the urine, and bruising are the signs of overdosage. Transient loss of hair and diarrhoea may occur. *Precautions:* It should not be used in patients with jaundice or in those with bleeding disorders (e.g., haemophilia), or in patients with peptic ulcers, or with impairment of kidney or liver function. *Dose:* 5,000 to 15,000 units by intramuscular or intravenous injection. Heparin is also given subcutaneously for prophylactic use – 5,000 units two or three times daily.

heparinoid (Hirudoid) has anti-inflammatory, anti-clotting and anti-exudative actions. It inhibits hyaluronidase and is used as an anti-spreading agent in applications to relieve rheumatic pains and other painful conditions of muscles and joints.

Hepsal ◊ heparin.

heroin ◊ diamorphine.

Herpid solution contains 5% idoxuridine in dimethyl sulphoxide. It is used to treat shingles (herpes zoster).

Hespan ◊ hetastarch.

hetastarch (Hespan) is used to produce an expansion of the blood volume in injury or shock. *Adverse effects:* include vomiting, fever, chills, itching and urticaria.

Hewlett's Antiseptic Cream contains zinc oxide 80 mg, boric acid 25 mg, lanolin 40 mg, in each g of cream.

hexachlorophane (Ster-Zac DC) is used as an antiseptic. By mouth it may produce diarrhoea, drowsiness and dizziness. Repeated skin application may rarely make the skin sensitive to sunlight. When applied repeatedly to the skin in premature babies it may produce brain damage.

hexachlorophene ◊ hexachlorophane.

hexalated metacresol is used as an antiseptic.

hexamethonium (hexamethonium bromide) was previously used to treat raised blood pressure. Its prolonged use may produce bromism (◊ potassium bromide).

hexamidine is used topically as a wound antiseptic, and also as a mouthwash.

hexamine (Hiprex; methenamine; methenamine mandelate; hexamine mandelate) is used to treat chronic and recurrent infections of the urinary system. It only works if the urine is made acid by taking a preparation such as ammonium chloride. *Adverse effects:* If taken in large doses it may cause painful and frequent micturition, cystitis and blood in the urine due to its conversion into formaldehyde. Skin rashes may occasionally occur. *Precautions:* It should not be given with sulphonamides since crystals may develop in the urine. It should not be given to patients with impaired kidney function. *Dose:* 250 to 1,000 mg up to four times daily by mouth.

hexamine hippurate (Hiprex) ◊ hexamine. It makes the urine acid. *Dose:* By mouth 1 g twice daily.

hexetidine (Oraldene) has an antiseptic action and is used in a 0·1% solution as a mouthwash.

hexobarbitone is a barbiturate sleeping drug. *Dose:* By mouth, 250 to 500 mg at bedtime.

Hexopal ◊ inositol.

hexyl nicotinate is used as a rubefacient.

hexylresorcinol is an antiseptic included in throat lozenges for the treatment of sore throat.

HGH is a growth hormone.

Hibidil solution ◊ chlorhexidine.

Hibiscrub cleansing solution ◊ chlorhexidine.

Hibisol solution ◊ chlorhexidine.

Hibitane cream and **liquid** ◊ chlorhexidine.

Hill's Bronchial Balsam: Each 5 ml contains morphine hydrochloride 900 micrograms, ammonium acetate 180 mg, capsicum tincture 0·0105 ml, compound benzoin tincture 0·3125 ml, ipecacuanha liquid extract 0·025 ml, acetic acid 0·11 ml, and simple lobelia tincture 0·125 ml.

Hill's Bronchial Balsam Pastilles contain compound benzoin tincture 0·793%, capsicum oleoresin 0·001%, peppermint oil 0·04%, ipecacuanha liquid extract 0·5%, simple lobelia tincture 2·5%, and menthol 0·11%.

Hill's Junior Balsam contains compound benzoin tincture 3·125%, ipecacuanha liquid extract 0·2%, simple lobelia tincture 1·25%, acetic acid (80%) 1·13%, capsicum tincture 0·1%, ammonium acetate 1·8%, and squill vinegar 3·12%.

Hioxyl cream ◊ hydrogen peroxide.

Hip-C rose hip syrup contains vitamin C not less than 3 mg per ml.

Hiprex ◊ hexamine hippurate.

Hirudoid cream ◊ heparinoid.

Hismanal ◊ astemizole.

Histalix syrup is used to treat coughs. Each 5 ml contains diphenhydramine 14 mg, ammonium chloride 135 mg, sodium citrate 57 mg, menthol 1·1 mg. *Dose:* 5 to 10 ml every 3 hours.

histamine ◊ see antihistamines, Part Two.

histamine acid phosphate is used to diagnose and to test acid secretion function of the stomach. It is also used to test patients with Ménière's disease to see if they are sensitive to histamine. *Adverse effects:* These include headache, wheezing, rapid beating of the heart, flushing, blurred vision, vomiting and diarrhoea. *Precautions:* It should not be given to patients with asthma or allergy. Applied to the skin it will cause redness and flushing.

histamine dihydrochloride ◊ histamine acid phosphate.

histamine hydrochloride ◊ histamine acid phosphate.

Histergan cream is used to treat insect bites and stings. It contains diphenhydramine 2%.

Histergan syrup is used to treat hay fever, allergic rhinitis and skin allergies. It contains diphenhydramine hydrochloride 10 mg in each 5 ml. **Histergan tablets** contain diphenhydramine hydrochloride 25 mg.

Histofax cream contains 2% chlorcyclizine hydrochloride and 8% calamine. It is an antihistamine skin application.

Histryl ◊ diphenylpyraline.

HNIG (Normal immunoglobulin injection) is an immunoglobin prepared from pools of at least 1000 donations of human plasma. It is used to provide protection against hepatitis A virus, measles and to a lesser extent rubella.

homatropine has uses and effects similar to those described under atropine.

homatropine methylbromide is an atropine-like drug. It is a mild antispasmodic and is included in some over-the-counter remedies for the treatment of period pains.

Homocea Ointment contains coconut oil 20%, lard 2%, white beeswax 7·5%, hard paraffin 20%, soft white paraffin 30%, camphor 2%, eucalyptus oil 0·5%, rosemary oil 0·5%, cajuput oil 2·5%, turpentine oil 10%, strong ammonia solution 3%, and water 2%.

honey is used as a demulcent and sweetening agent especially in cough mixtures and in linctuses.

Honey Kof Syrup contains honey 13·5%, glycerol 8%, lemon tincture 0·2%, chloroform 0·1%, benzoic acid 0·025%, lemon juice 7%, ipecacuanha liquid extract 0·25%, dilute sulphuric acid 0·56%, acetic acid 1·5%, and sucrose 52%.

Honvan ◊ fosfestrol.

hop (*Lupulus*) **extracts** are used as flavouring agents and in perfumes.

They are used to give the characteristic flavour to beer.

horehound aqueous extract is an expectorant and in large dose a laxative.

Hormofemin ◊ dienoestrol.

Hormonin tablets contain oestradiol 600 micrograms, oestriol 270 micrograms and oestrone 1·4 mg. Used to treat menopausal symptoms. *Dose:* By mouth, ½ to 1 tablet daily.

horse-chestnut (*aesculus*) has been used to reduce traumatic swelling but its use is of doubtful value.

Hot Measure (Solution): Each liquid dose contains paracetamol 600 mg, dextromethorphan hydrobromide 15 mg, chlorpheniramine maleate 4 mg, phenylpropanolamine hydrochloride 25 mg, and alcohol 5·7 ml.

H₃ Plus: Each capsule contains vitamin A 2,850 units, vitamin D 250 units, vitamin B_{12} 0·5 micrograms, vitamin C 40 mg, aminobenzoic acid 25 mg, thiamine hydrochloride 5 mg, riboflavine 5 mg, nicotinamide 12 mg, pyridoxine hydrochloride 500 micrograms, calcium pantothenate 3 mg, inositol 30 mg, choline dihydrogen citrate 42 mg, tocopherol acid succinate 10 units, biotin 0·5 micrograms, folic acid 25 micrograms, L-lysine monohydrochloride 24 mg, iron 10 mg, iodine 150 micrograms, calcium 46·5 mg, phosphorus 37 mg, copper 1 mg, manganese 1 mg, potassium 5 mg, zinc 500 micrograms, and magnesium 1 mg.

HRF ◊ gonadorelin.

human insulin ◊ insulin.

Human Protaphane: Read section on insulins.

Humiderm emollient cream contains sodium pyrrolidine carboxylate 5%. It is used to treat dry, thickened skin (e.g. eczema). It acts as a moisturizer.

Humotet injection is used to give passive immunization against tetanus.

Hyalase ◊ hyaluronidase.

hyaluronidase is an enzyme from mammals' semen which makes tissues more permeable. It is used to increase the spread and absorption of drugs from injections and applications.

Hydergine tablets contain a mixture of ergot alkaloids. They are used to improve the blood circulation in disorders which affect the blood vessels supplying the brain. *Adverse effects:* It may produce nausea, flushing, skin rashes, stuffiness of the nose, abdominal pains, and a fall in blood pressure on standing in patients with a raised blood pressure. *Dose:* By mouth, 1 tablet three times daily.

hydralazine (Apresoline; hydralazine hydrochloride) is used to treat raised blood pressure. *Adverse effects:* These include nausea, vomiting, headache, a fall in blood pressure on standing, rapid beating of the heart, flushing, sweating, pins and needles, and numbness in the hands and feet, trembling, breathlessness, skin rashes, difficulty in passing water and depressed mood. These usually occur in the first few weeks of treatment. Prolonged use may produce signs and symptoms of rheumatoid arthritis or acute lupus erythematosus. *Precautions:* It should be used with caution in patients with coronary artery disease or in patients with rapid beating of the heart. As with most of these drugs a severe fall in blood pressure may occur in patients given a general anaesthetic. *Dose:* By mouth, 25 mg three times daily rising to a maximum of 50 mg four times daily. Also available as an injection.

hydrargaphen is used as an antifungal and antibacterial drug in skin applications and vaginal pessaries. ◊ mercury.

Hydrea ◊ hydroxyurea.

Hydrenox ◊ hydroflumethiazide.

hydrochloric acid (dilute) is used in disorders where the stomach is not producing acid e.g., pernicious anaemia, chronic gastritis. *Dose:* Not more than 20 ml of dilute hydrochloric acid (10%) must be given in 24 hours.

hydrochlorothiazide (Direma; Esidrex; HydroSaluric) is a diuretic. It has effects and uses similar to those described under chlorothiazide but it is effective in smaller doses. It works in about two hours, reaches a maximum in four and lasts for about six to twelve hours. *Adverse effects* and *Precautions* ◊ chlorothiazide. *Dose:* By mouth, 25 to 200 mg daily or on alternate days.

hydrocodone has similar properties to codeine. It is included in cough medicines.

hydrocortisone (Cortisol; Cortril; Dioderm, Hydrocortone) in many skin preparations. It occurs naturally in the body and is produced by the adrenal glands. It has similar effects and uses to those described under cortisone.

It is given by mouth, injections, and enemas, and it is applied externally in ointments, creams and lotions. ◊ corticosteroids. *Adverse effects* and *Precautions:* These are discussed in the section on corticosteroids, and under cortisone. *Dose:* By mouth, 10 to 300 mg daily in divided doses.

hydrocortisone acetate (cortisol acetate) has effects and uses similar to those described under cortisone. It is used in eye drops, creams and ointments. It may also be injected into painful joints, ligaments and muscles. Read section on corticosteroids. *Dose:* 5 to 50 mg by injection into a joint or painful lesion.

hydrocortisone butyrate is a more potent form of hydrocortisone used in skin preparations.

hydrocortisone hydrogen succinate is used in hydrocortisone preparations for injection, as also is hydrocortisone sodium phosphate (Efcortesol). ◊ hydrocortisone.

hydrocortisone sodium succinate (Corlan; Efcortelan soluble; Solu-Cortef) is used in hydrocortisone preparations for injection and in lozenges in the treatment of aphthous ulcers in the mouth. ◊ hydrocortisone.

Hydrocortistab ◊ hydrocortisone.

Hydrocortisyl ◊ hydrocortisone.

Hydrocortone ◊ hydrocortisone.

Hydroderm applications contain hydrocortisone 1%, neomycin sulphate 0·5% and zinc bacitracin 1,000 units/g.

hydroflumethiazide (Hydrenox) is a diuretic. It has effects and adverse effects similar to those described under chlorothiazide. *Dose:* By mouth, 25 to 100 mg daily.

hydrogen peroxide is used as a disinfectant and deodorant, to clean wounds and as a mouthwash.

Hydromet is used to treat raised blood pressure. Each tablet contains methyldopa 250 mg and hydrochlorothiazide 15 mg. *Dose:* By mouth, 1 twice daily increasing gradually to a maximum of 12 daily.

Hydromol is a bath emollient containing light liquid paraffin 37·8% and isopropyl myristate 13%. It is used to treat dry and thickened skin conditions (e.g. eczema). It acts as a moisturizer.

hydroquinone is used in cosmetics and toiletries as an anti-oxidant. It is also used as a depigmenting agent for the skin in the form of 2–5% ointment.

Hydrosaluric ◊ hydrochlorothiazide.

hydrotalcite (Altacaps; Altacite) is a magnesium and aluminium compound used as an antacid. It rarely produces diarrhoea and vomiting. *Adverse effects;* It may reduce the absorption of tetracyclines from the gut. *Dose:* By mouth, 500 mg tablets or 5 ml of suspension between meals and at bedtime.

hydrous lanolin ◊ hydrous wool fat.

hydrous ointment (oily cream) is used to treat dry skin and as a vehicle for drugs which need to be applied to the skin. It contains dried magnesium sulphate 0·5%, phenoxyethanol 1%, water 48·5% in wool alcohols ointment.

hydrous wool fat (hydrous lanolin; lanolin) is a yellowish-white base for ointments prepared from seven parts wool fat and three parts water.

hydroxocobalamin (Cobalin-H, Neo-Cytamen, vitamin B_{12}) is used to treat pernicious anaemia. *Dose:* By intramuscular injection, 1 to 2 mg in first week. Maintenance, 0·25 mg every three to four weeks.

hydroxyapatite (Ossopan) contains calcium, phosphorus and trace elements and is used in the treatment of osteoporosis and related conditions. *Dose:* By mouth 10 g powder or up to 16 tablets daily, in divided doses, before meals.

hydroxychloroquine (Plaquenil; hydroxychloroquine sulphate) is an antimalarial drug. It has effects and uses similar to those described under chloroquine. Its main use however has been in the treatment of rheumatoid arthritis and lupus erythematosus. *Adverse effects* and *Precautions:* These are similar to those listed under chloroquine. Prolonged use of hydroxychloroquine may cause nausea, diarrhoea and cramps in the abdomen. Its use for long periods exceeding one to two years may irreversibly damage the eyes (retinopathy). *Dose:* By mouth; anti-malarial suppression, 400 mg weekly; malarial treatment, 400 to 1,200 mg daily in divided doses. Giardiasis: 200 to 400 mg three times daily for five days.

Rheumatoid arthritis, etc.: 200 to 1,200 mg daily in divided doses.

hydroxycholecalciferol ◊ alfacalcidol.

hydroxyethylcellulose has similar properties to methylcellulose.

hydroxyethylrutosides reduce the fragility and permeability of capillary blood vessels and are used to treat haemorrhoids and venous disorders of the lower limbs.

hydroxyprogesterone (Proluton Depot; hydroxyprogesterone hexanoate; hydroxyprogesterone caproate) has effects and uses similar to progesterone. It is used in threatened and habitual miscarriage, and to treat disorders of menstruation. *Dose:* 250 to 500 mg once or twice weekly by intramuscular injection.

hydroxyquinoline is used as an antibacterial and antifungal in skin applications. It is also used as a keratolytic and as a deodorant.

hydroxyurea (Hydrea) is an anticancer drug. *Adverse effects:* These include nausea, vomiting, confusion, skin rashes, loss of hair (alopecia), abdominal pain, diarrhoea, blood in the motions and convulsions. A common effect is reversible damage to the bone marrow, producing blood disorders. *Precautions:* It should not be used in pregnancy and because it may cause kidney damage it shuld be used with caution in patients with impaired kidney function. *Dose:* 20 to 30 mg per kg of body-weight daily as a single dose, or 80 mg per kg every third day by mouth.

hydroxyzine (Atarax; hydroxyzine embonate; hydroxyzine hydrochloride) is used to treat nausea and vomiting. It is also used as an anti-anxiety drug and it has antihistamine properties. *Adverse effects:* These include drowsiness, headache, dry mouth and itching. High doses may produce trembling and convulsions. *Precautions:* It increases the effects of alcohol and other depressant drugs. It should not be given during pregnancy and it must be used with caution by those who drive motor vehicles or operate moving machinery. It increases the effects of coumarin anticoagulant drugs. *Dose:* By mouth, 25 to 100 mg three times daily.

Hygroton ◊ chlorthalidone.

Hygroton K is a diuretic with added potassium. Each tablet contains chlorthalidone 25 mg and potassium chloride 500 mg in sustained-release form. *Dose:* By mouth, 1 twice daily or 2 at breakfast.

hyoscine (Buscopan; Kwells; Serene hyoscine hydrobromide; scopolamine) has effects and uses similar to those described under atropine. It depresses the brain and produces drowsiness and is therefore used to treat patients who are excited. It is used along with morphine as a medication before surgical operations. It is also used to prevent motion sickness and in the treatment of Parkinsonism. *Adverse effects* and *Precautions:* These are similar to those listed under atropine. *Dose:* Preoperative medication: 0·6 mg of hyoscine (scopolamine) with 10 to 15 mg morphine by subcutaneous or intramuscular injection. Motion sickness: 0·6 mg by mouth. Parkinsonism: 0·3 to 0·6 mg three times daily by mouth.

hyoscine butylbromide (Buscopan) is used to relax involuntary muscles to relieve spasmodic colic. *Adverse effects* and *Precautions* are similar to those described under atropine. *Dose:* By mouth, 20 mg four times daily or 20 mg by intramuscular or intravenous injections as required.

hyoscine hydrobromide is used to relieve spasm in abdominal and pelvic organs. *Adverse effects* and *Precautions:* As for atropine. *Dose:* By mouth, 20 mg four times a day. Injection is also available.

hyoscine methonitrate ◊ hyoscine.

hyoscyamine (hyoscyamine hydrobromide and hyoscyamine sulphate) has effects similar to those described under atropine.

hyoscyamus contains hyoscyamine. It has actions and effects similar to those described under atropine.

Hypercal ◊ rauwolfia.

Hypercal-B tablets, contain rauwolfia alkaloids 2 mg and amylobarbitone 15 mg.

Hyperdrol cream or roll-on gel contains aluminium chlorohydrate (19%). It is a drying agent (astringent) used to prevent excessive sweating.

Hypertane tablets, contain hydrochlorothiazide 50 mg and amiloride 5 mg ◊ hydrochlorothiazide and amiloride.

Hypnomidate ◊ etomidate.

Hypnovel ◊ midazolam.

Hypon is a mild pain-reliever. Each tablet contains codeine phosphate 5 mg, aspirin 325 mg, caffeine 10 mg and phenolphthalein 5 mg. *Dose:* By mouth, 1 to 2 four-hourly.

hypophosphorus acid ◊ glycerophosphates and hypophosphites.

Hypotears drops contain polyethylene glycol 2% and polyvinyl alcohol 1%. They are used to lubricate dry eyes.

Hypovase ◊ prazosin.

hypromellose has effects and uses similar to those produced by methylcellulose. It is mainly used as eye drops, for artificial tears.

hyssop is a constituent of Congreve's Balsamic Elixir.

Hytrin ◊ terazosin.

Ibu-Slo ◊ ibuprofen.

Ibular ◊ ibuprofen.

Ibumetin tablets ◊ ibuprofen.

ibuprofen (For preparations see p. 196) is an anti-rheumatic drug. *Adverse effects* and *Precautions:* See p. 197. Like all anti-rheumatic drugs it may produce irritation of the stomach and it should be taken with or after meals. It may cause nausea, indigestion and skin rash. It should probably not be used in patients with impaired liver function and it should be used with caution in the first three months of pregnancy. *Dose:* By mouth, 600 to 1,600 mg in divided doses daily after meals.

Iceland moss has demulcent properties.

ichthammol is slightly antibacterial and it irritates the skin. It has been used in skin applications.

idoxene ◊ idoxuridine.

Idoxuridine (Dendrid; Herpid; Idoxene; Ophthalmadine; Kerecid) is an antiviral agent. It is used as drops to treat virus ulcers on the eye and also cold sores (herpes simplex) and shingles (herpes zoster). It should not be used during pregnancy.

Iduridin solution contains 5% or 40% idoxuridine in dimethyl sulphoxide. It is used to treat shingles (herpes zoster).

ifosfamide (Mitoxana) is an alkylating agent given by direct intravenous injection after dilution or by intravenous infusion. It is used to treat cancer ◊ cyclophosphamide. *Dose:* Depends upon the disorder being treated.

Iglodine is an antiseptic solution containing the equivalent of phenol 0·089% and combined iodine 0·04%.

Iglodine Ointment contains combined iodine 0·14%, zinc oxide 1·43%, phenol 0·32%, bismuth oxychloride 2·86%.

Iloderm contains zinc oxide 19·8%, talc 3·3%, kaolin 2·5%, wool fat 2·5%, and cod-liver oil 1·5%.

Ilonium ointment contains colophony 15·6%, larch turpentine 8·1%, turpentine oil 8%, phenol 0·1%, and thymol 0·03%.

Ilosone ◊ erythromycin estolate.

Ilotycin ◊ erythromycin.

Ilube eye drops contain acetylcysteine and pseudophendrine.

Imbrilon ◊ indomethacin.

Imdur sustained-release tablets contain isosorbide mononitrate 60 mg ◊ isosorbide mononitrate.

Imferon ◊ iron dextran solution.

imipramine (Praminil, Tofranil; imipramine hydrochloride) is a tricyclic antidepressant drug. The relief of symptoms is slow and it may be up to two or three weeks before the patient feels any improvement. It has also been used to treat bed-wetting in children. *Adverse effects:* During the first few weeks of treatment dose-related adverse effects occur. These usually disappear; they include dryness of the mouth, blurred vision, constipation, retention of urine, rapid beating of the heart, fall in blood pressure and sweating. Nausea, vomiting, fatigue, trembling, unsteadiness when walking, excessive energy and milk from the breasts (galactorrhoea) may occur. *Precautions*: Imipramine should be given with caution to patients with heart disease, glaucoma, epilepsy, enlarged prostate gland or pyloric stenosis (a narrowing of the outlet from the stomach). Local anaesthetic solutions containing adrenaline should be used with care in patients taking imipramine or any other tricyclic antidepressant drug. Caution is also necessary when giving imipramine to patients taking alcohol, barbiturates and atropine-like drugs. It should not be given to patients who are taking M.A.O. inhibitor antidepressants and preferably not within two weeks of stopping such drugs. Imipramine may decrease the effectiveness of the blood pressure lowering drugs guanethidine and methyldopa. *Dose:* By mouth, 75 to 225 mg daily in divided doses, using smaller doses (e.g., 10 to 30 mg daily) in the elderly.

Imodium ◊ loperamide.

Imperacin ◊ oxytetracycline.

Imunovir tablets ◊ inosine pranobex.

Imuran ◊ azathoprine.

Inabrin ◊ ibuprofen.

indapamide (Natrilix; indapamide hemihydrate) is used to treat high blood pressure. It is related to thiazide diuretics but is claimed to produce fewer metabolic effects. *Precautions:* It may cause low blood potassium if given with other diuretics. *Dose:* By mouth, 2·5 mg each morning.

Inderal ◊ propranolol.

Inderal-LA: Each capsule contains propranolol hydrochloride 160 mg in sustained-release form ◊ propranolol.

Inderetic: Each capsule contains propranolol 80 mg and bendrofluazide 2·5 mg.

Inderex is used to treat raised blood pressure. Each capsule contains propranolol 160 mg and bendrofluazide 5 mg in sustained-release form. *Dose:* By mouth, 1 daily.

Indocid PDA powder for injection ◊ indomethacin. Used to treat patent ductus arteriosus in premature babies.

Indocid ◊ indomethacin.

Indocid-R capsules contain indomethacin 75 mg in slow-release form. ◊ indomethacin. *Dose:* By mouth, one or two daily.

Indoflex ◊ indomethacin.

Indolar SR are sustained-release capsules of indomethacin 200 mg ◊ indomethacin.

indomethacin (Artracin; Flexin Continus; Imbrilon; Indocid; Indocid PDA; Indoflex; Indolar; Indomod) relieves inflammation, reduces high temperature and relieves pain. It is used to treat gout, rheumatoid arthritis and other rheumatic disorders. *Adverse effects:* The most common adverse effects are headache and dizziness. These are dose-related and disappear if the dose is reduced. Loss of appetite, nausea, vomiting, dyspepsia and diarrhoea may occur and are not dose related. Ulceration of the stomach with bleeding may occur sometimes without the warning symptoms of dyspepsia. Blood disorders, skin rashes and oedema may also occur. Drowsiness, confusion and depression, sensitivity reactions (asthma, rashes and swelling of the throat), hearing disturbances, blurred vision, corneal deposits, nerve damage and fainting may occur. *Precautions:* Indomethacin should be given with caution to patients with impaired liver or kidney function. It should not be given to patients with a history of peptic ulcer and probably not to pregnant women. It should be used with caution in patients with epilepsy, Parkinsonism, psychiatric disturbances and in elderly patients. Regular eye and blood tests should be carried out. It may impair ability to drive and operate moving machinery. *Dose:* By mouth after food, 50 to 150 mg daily in divided doses; by suppository, 100 mg once or twice daily.

Indomod capsules ◊ indomethacin.

indoramin (Baratol) is used to treat raised blood pressure. *Adverse effects:* Sedation, dry mouth, nasal congestion, weight gain, dizziness, depression and failure to ejaculate. *Precautions:* Drowsiness may occur in the first few days of treatment and patients should be warned not to drive motor vehicles or operate moving machinery. It should be used with caution in patients with heart failure, impaired kidney or liver function or in patients with Parkinsonism. It should only be used with the utmost caution in pregnancy. *Dose:* By mouth, 25 mg twice daily.

Infacol liquid contains activated dimethicone ◊ activated dimethicone. It is used to treat griping pain and infant colic.

Infant Gaviscon powder in sachets contain sodium bicarbonate 340 mg, magnesium trisilicate 50 mg and dried aluminium hydroxide 200 mg per 2 g sachet. In addition to these antacids the sachets contain alginic acid 924 mg/2 g. *Note:* Each sachet contains 4 mmol of sodium. *Dose:* ½ to 1 sachet with feeds when required.

Influvac Sub-unit ◊ influenza virus.

Innovace tablets ◊ enalapril.

inosine pranobex (Imunovir) is used as an antiviral drug to treat herpes simplex (cold sores). *Precautions:* It should be used with caution in patients with renal impairment, gout or hyperuricaemia. *Dose:* Usually 4 g daily for seven to fourteen days.

inositol is a member of the B group of vitamins. Inositol nicotinate (Hexopal) is a drug used to improve the circulation. In high doses it may cause a slight fall in blood pressure and slowing of the pulse. *Dose:* By mouth, 500 to 1,000 mg three times daily.

insulins: See general discussion on insulins under the section on drugs used to treat diabetes.

Intal ◊ sodium cromoglycate.

Intal Compound is used to treat allergic asthma. Each capsule contains sodium cromoglycate 20 mg and isoprenaline sulphate 0·1 mg. *Dose:* 4 daily at regular intervals.

Integrin ◊ oxypertine.

Interlene is a medicated shampoo containing undecylenic monoalkylolamide sodium sulphosuccinate 2%.

Intraglobin is an immunoglobulin preparation.

Intralgin gel and liquid contains salicylamide 5%, benzocaine 2% and isopropyl alcohol 60%. It is a rubefacient.

Intraval sodium ◊ thiopentone sodium.

Intron A (interferon alfa-2b) is a water-soluble human protein produced by recombinant DNA techniques. It is used to treat hairy cell leukaemia. *Adverse effects:* Raised liver function tests, reduced white blood and platelet counts, flu-like symptoms, lethargy, confusion, depression, changes in blood pressure and disorders of heart rhythm. *Precautions:* Do not use in patients who are allergic to it or related drugs. Safety below the age of 18 years not established nor in pregnancy or breast-feeding. Patients on treatment should practise contraception. *Dose:* 2 million iu/m^2 subcutaneously every other day.

Intropin ◊ dopamine.

iodine is used by the thyroid gland to make thyroid hormone. It has been used to prepare a patient for surgical removal of an overworking thyroid gland. Iodine is also used as an antiseptic. *Adverse effects:* Those due to allergy to iodine include skin rashes, runny eyes, runny nose, bronchitis and sore throat. It can produce goitre when taken by mouth and also depression, nervousness, sexual inpotence and insomnia.

iodochlorhydroxyquin ◊ clioquinol.

iodoform has an anaesthetic action when applied to mucous membranes.

It slowly releases iodine and has a mild disinfectant action. It is not very effective as a wound dressing.

iodophenol has antiseptic properties.

Iodosorb powder contains an iodine compound in modified starch gel microbeads. It is used in the treatment of leg ulcers.

Ionamin ◊ phentermine.

Ionax Scrub is a skin cleaner for acne containing benzalkonium chloride.

Ionil T shampoo application contains salicylic acid 2%, benzalkonium chloride 0·2% and tar solution 4·25% in an alcoholic base.

ipecacuanha (the dried roots of *Cephaelis ipecacuanha*) in small doses is used as a cough expectorant. *Adverse effects:* Ipecacuanha has an irritant effect upon the stomach and gut. Large doses produce vomiting and diarrhoea. It may also produce irregular heart beats and cause protein to appear in the urine (albuminuria). It is used to produce vomiting after swallowing certain poisons.

ipecacuanha liquid extract is obtained from ipecacuanha.

ipomoea resin has a drastic purgative action.

Ipral ◊ trimethoprim.

ipratropium (Atrovent; ipratropium bromide) is an anticholinergic drug used to treat bronchial asthma. *Dose:* By inhalation, 20 to 40 micrograms three or four times daily.

iprindole (Prondol) is a tricyclic antidepressant drug with effects, uses and adverse effects similar to those described under imipramine. *Adverse effects* ◊ imipramine. Jaundice may occur in the first two weeks of treatment. *Precautions* ◊ imipramine. It should not be given to patients with impaired liver function or with a history of liver disease. *Dose:* By mouth, 45 to 180 mg daily in divided doses.

iproniazid (Marsilid; iproniazid phosphate) is an M.A.O. inhibitor antidepressant drug. ◊ phenelzine. *Dose:* By mouth as a single dose, 100 to 150 mg daily reducing to maintenance dose of 25 to 50 mg daily.

Irgasan ◊ triclosan.

Irofol C: Each tablet contains ferrous sulphate 325 mg in sustained-release form, folic acid 350 micrograms and ascorbic acid 500 mg. *Dose:* By mouth, 1 daily before food.

iron: Read section on iron.

Iron Blood Tonic Number 20 contains concentrated compound sarsaparilla decoction 0·08%, potassium iodide 0·5%, ferric ammonium citrate 2·5%, sassafras oil 0·05%.

iron dextran solution (Imferon) is given by injection to treat iron-deficiency anaemia. *Adverse effects:* It may produce pain and brown staining at the site of injection. Fever, allergic reactions and rapid beating of the heart may occur. After intravenous injection an allergic reaction causing death may very rarely occur and thrombosis may occur at the site of injection. Repeated use of deep injec-

tions in rats has produced a cancer but no such change has been shown in man. *Precautions:* It should be given with caution to anyone who has suffered from a previous adverse drug reaction. The patient should be kept under close observation for at least one hour after an intravenous injection. It should not be given to patients with severe impairment of liver function or with depression of blood cell production in the bone marrow. *Dose:* According to level of anaemia.

Iron Jelloids: Each contains dried ferrous sulphate 65 mg, copper carbonate 170 micrograms, dried yeast 138 mg, thiamine hydrochloride 170 micrograms, riboflavine 290 micrograms, nicotinamide 1·67 mg, and ascorbic acid 4·17 mg.

Ironorm ◊ iron dextran.

iron phosphate is used to treat iron-deficiency anaemia. *Dose:* By mouth. 0·3 to 2 g daily in divided doses.

Ironplan sustained-release capsules each contain exsiccated ferrous sulphate 150 mg and vitamin B_1 3 mg.

iron sorbitol (Jectofer) is used to treat iron-deficiency anaemia. *Adverse effects:* These include flushing, nausea, vomiting, metallic taste in the mouth, loss of taste, dizziness, disorientation, blurred vision, headache, and painful muscles. It turns the urine black in some patients and may produce pain and staining at the site of injection. *Precautions:* It should not be given to patients with kidney disease and not within 24 hours of taking iron by mouth. *Dose:* According to level of anaemia; 1·5 mg per kg body-weight intramuscularly as a single dose.

isoniazid 473

Ismelin ◊ guanethidine.

Ismo ◊ isosorbide mononitrate.

isoaminile (Dymiril, isoaminile citrate) is a cough suppressant. It may occasionally cause nausea, dizziness and diarrhoea or constipation. *Dose:* 40 mg three to five times daily.

Iso-Autohaler ◊ isoprenaline.

isocarboxazid (Marplan) is an M.A.O. inhibitor antidepressant drug. *Adverse effects* and *Precautions:* These are similar to those discussed under phenelzine. *Dose:* By mouth, 10 to 30 mg daily in divided doses.

isoconazole (Travogyn; isoconazole nitrate) is an antifungal and antibacterial drug used in topical applications. *Dose:* 2 vaginal tablets at night, the cream is applied twice daily.

isoetharine (Numotac; isoetharine hydrochloride) has effects and uses similar to those described under isoprenaline. *Dose:* By mouth, 10 to 20 mg three to four times daily. The tablets are in a sustained-release form and should be swallowed whole.

isoflurane (Aerrane; Forane) is a volatile general anaesthetic with actions similar to halothane.

Isogel is a preparation of ispaghula which is used to treat constipation.

Isoket 0·1% ◊ isosorbide dinitrate.

Isoket tablets ◊ isosorbide dinitrate.

Isoket Retard tablets contain isosorbide dinitrate 20 mg in sustained release form ◊ isosorbide dinitrate.

isometheptene mucate (Midrid) is used to treat migraine. *Adverse effects:* These include dizziness and disturbances of the circulation. *Precautions:* It should be used with caution in patients suffering from disorders of the heart and circulation. It should *not* be used in patients with glaucoma. *Dose:* By mouth, two capsules at start of migraine attack and then one every hour if necessary to a maximum of five capsules in twelve hours. For *headache* 1 to 2 capsules every 4 hours to a maximum of 8 daily.

isoniazid (in Rifater; Rimifon; isonicotinic acid hydrazine) is an anti-bacterial drug used to treat tuberculosis. It is used principally in the treatment of tuberculosis of the lungs, but it may also be used to treat tuberculous meningitis and tuberculosis of the kidneys and bladder. Bacterial resistance develops within a few weeks of use so it should always be given with other antituberculous drugs. This greatly reduces the risk of resistance developing. *Adverse effects:* Isoniazid may cause constipation, difficulty in starting urination, dryness of the mouth and vertigo. In doses above 10 mg per kg of body-weight per day patients may develop inflammation of nerves (peripheral neuritis) producing numbness, pins and needles and weakness. This may be prevented by giving vitamin B_6 (pyridoxine) 100 mg daily. Isoniazid usually lifts the mood but it may also cause mental disturbances which are usually reversed on withdrawal of the drug. Allergic reactions include fever, skin rashes, swollen glands (lymphadenopathy) and, rarely, blood disorders and jaundice.

Raised blood sugar and swollen breasts (gynaecomastia) have been associated with isoniazid treatment. Withdrawal symptoms may occur on stopping the drug; these include headache, irritability, nervousness, insomnia and excessive dreaming. *Precautions:* Isoniazid should be given with caution to patients suffering from convulsive disorders, chronic alcoholism or with impaired kidney or liver function. It should preferably not be used in pregnant women. Some patients inactivate it slowly and therefore they may develop adverse effects on smaller doses. Tuberculosis bacteria rapidly become resistant to isoniazid and therefore it should not be used alone. *Dose:* By mouth, 300 to 600 mg daily in divided doses.

isoprenaline (Aleudrine; Isuprel; Medihaler-Iso; Saventrine; isoprenaline hydrochloride; isoprenaline sulphate; isoproterenol hydrochloride; isoproterenol sulphate) acts like adrenaline on special nerve endings. It relaxes bronchial muscles, dilates peripheral blood vessels, causes a fall in blood pressure, increases the heart rate and stimulates the heart muscle. It is used to treat bronchial asthma. It is also used to treat heart block and severe slowing of the heart (bradycardia). *Adverse effects:* Isoprenaline may cause rapid beating of the heart, chest pain, faintness, dizziness, headache, nervousness, trembling and weakness. Irregularities of the heart may occur. *Precautions:* Isoprenaline should not be used in patients with acute coronary heart disease or in patients with asthma due to heart disease. It should be used with caution in patients with overworking thyroid glands (hyperthyroidism). It should never be given at the same time as adrenaline but may be used simultaneously with phenylephrine. Tolerance may develop to isoprenaline taken in an aerosol: in such cases the dose should not be increased but the drug should be stopped and an alternative drug used. There were reports of increasing deaths amongst asthmatics below twenty years of age, which were thought to be related to the use of aerosols containing high doses of isoprenaline and similar drugs. It has been suggested that the use of these aerosols should not be repeated within the hour and if relief is not obtained then an alternative drug should be used. *Doses:* When necessary. By mouth 30 mg eight hourly; by aerosol, 0·1 to 0·25 mg; by subcutaneous or intramuscular injection, 0·2 mg; by intravenous injection, 0·01 to 0·02 mg.

isopropamide has similar effects to atropine. ◊ atropine.

isopropamide iodide has atropine-like effects ◊ atropine.

isopropyl alcohol is used in skin applications as a cleansing agent, degreaser, and antiseptic. It is used as a solvent in cosmetics and perfumes.

isopropyl linoleate has similar properties to those described under isopropyl myristate.

isopropyl myristate is resistant to oxidation and hydrolysis and does not become rancid. It is used in ointments, etc., to make them relatively free from greasiness. It is also used as a solvent and is absorbed readily by the skin. It is also used as a food additive.

Isopto Alkaline eye drops contain hypromellose 1%.

Isopto Atropine eye drops contain atropine sulphate 1% and hypromellose 0·5%.

Isopto Carbachol eye drops contain carbachol 3% and hypromellose 1%.

Isopto Carpine eye drops contain pilocarpine hydrochloride 0·5, 1, 2, and 3% all with hypromellose 0·5%.

Isopto Epinal eye drops contain adrenaline 0·5 and 1% with hypromellose 0·5%.

Isopto Frin eye drops contain phenylephrine hydrochloride 0·12% and hypromellose 0·5%.

Isopto Plain eye drops contain hypromellose 0·5%.

Isordil ◊ isosorbide dinitrate.

Isordil Tembids: Each capsule contains isosorbide dinitrate 40 mg in sustained-release form ◊ isosorbide dinitrate.

isosorbide dinitrate (Cedocard; Isoket; Sorbichew; Sorbid; Isordil; Sorbitrate; Vascardin; sorbide dinitrate) has effects and uses similar to those described under glyceryl trinitrate. It is used to treat angina. *Dose:* Sublingually when required 5 to 10 mg; by mouth 30 to 120 mg daily in divided doses; by intravenous infusion 2 to 10 mg/hour.

isosorbide mononitrate (Elantan, Imdur, Ismo) is used to treat angina. It has very similar effects to isosorbide dinitrate, but has a longer action and is more reliably absorbed ◊ isosorbide dinitrate. *Dose:* 40 to 120 mg daily in divided doses; the tablets should be swallowed whole without chewing.

isotretinoin (Roaccutane) is used to treat severe acne. *Adverse effects:* These include dry lips, sore eyes, nose bleeds, mild transient, loss of hair and joint pains. *Precautions:* It should not be used by women who are or may become pregnant (unless concomitant effective contraception is used). Contraception should continue for one month after stopping isotretinoin. *Dose:* By mouth, 500 mg per kg per day for three to four months. The acne may flare up after two to four weeks of starting treatment but then subsides after a few weeks.

isoxsuprine (Defensin; Duvadilan; isoxsuprine hydrochloride) is a vasodilator drug used to treat disorders of the circulation. It may cause transient dizziness, nausea and vomiting. It should be used with caution in patients with rapid heart beat and those with disorders of blood pressure. *Dose:* By mouth, 10 to 20 mg three or four times daily; 5 to 10 mg by intramuscular injection. Also given by I.V. infusion to treat premature labour.

ispaghula (Fybogel) is the dried ripe seeds of *Plantago ovata*. It is used as a bulk laxative, because the seeds take up a large amount of water in the gut to form a mucilaginous mass. *Dose:* By mouth, 3 to 10 g in one dose when necessary.

Isuprel ◊ isoprenaline.

Ivy Leaf Corn Plaster contains salicylic acid 40% and chlorbutol 2%.

Izal antiseptic liquid contains dichloroxylenol 1·25%, chlorophene 1·25% and terpenes 4·5%.

Jaap's health salt contains sodium potassium tartrate 0·94%, tartaric acid 20·8%, sucrose 56%, dextrose monohydrate 0·94% and sodium bicarbonate 21·32%.

Jackson's All Fours Cough Mixture contains in each 5 ml anise oil 0·00325 ml, peppermint oil 0·0006 ml, chloroform spirit 0·0125 ml, chloroform 0·01185 ml, anaesthetic ether 0·003 ml, capsicum extract 0·02375 ml, and liquorice extract 0·125 ml.

Jackson's Antiseptic Throat Pastilles contain liquorice extract 5·7%, acetic acid 0·9%, menthol 0·12%, camphor 0·03%, terebene 0·49%, benzoic acid 0·01%, thymol 0·003%, methyl salicylate 0·005%, cineole 0·005%, capsicum oleoresin 0·00001%, and pumilio pine oil 0·2%.

Jackson's Bronchial Catarrh Pastilles contain creosote 0·15%, chloroform 1·5%, menthol 0·6%, anise oil 0·02%, peppermint oil 0·02%, capsicin 0·001%, and benzoin tincture 0·5%.

Jackson's Catarrh Pastilles contain menthol 0·6%, sylvestris pine oil 0·3%, Siberian fir oil 0·3%, and creosote 0·2%.

Jackson's Children's Cough Pastilles contain honey 12%, ipecacuanha liquid extract 0·36%, squill liquid extract 0·73%, and citric acid 0·9%.

Jackson's Eucalyptus & Menthol Pastilles contain eucalyptus oil 0·6% and menthol 0·8%.

Jackson's Febrifuge contains sucrose 4·19%, sodium sulphate 4·19%, potassium nitrate 0·76%, chloroform 0·13%, ammonium chloride 0·76%, liquorice liquid extract 2%, rhubarb liquid extract 0·19%, taraxacum extract 0·66%, burnt sugar 0·66%, strong ginger tincture 0·47%, potassium iodide 0·04%, iodine 0·04%, capsicum tincture 0·1%, camphor 0·02%, alcohol 1·4%, anise oil 0·02%, and clove oil 0·04%.

Jackson's Glycerin Thymol Pastilles contain sodium benzoate 0·3%, thymol 0·04%, menthol 0·03%, cineole 0·06%, Siberian fir oil 0·02%, methyl salicylate 0·01%, and glycerol 3%.

Jackson's Iodised Throat Lozenges contain citric acid 10·27 mg, phenol 6·5 mg, menthol 2·86 mg, aqueous iodine solution 0·0039 ml, and methyl salicylate 0·920 mg.

Jackson's Night-Cough Pastilles contain cinnamic acid 0·009%, benzoic acid 0·002%, aqueous extract of wild cherry bark (1–1) 3·2%, and codeine phosphate 0·178%.

Jackson's Pholcodine Pastilles each contain pholcodine 2·2 mg, menthol 1·1 mg, aniseed oil 540 micrograms, peppermint oil 120 micrograms, and eucalyptus oil 120 micrograms.

jalap resin is a drastic purgative.

Jectofer ◊ iron sorbitol.

Jexin injection ◊ tubocurarine.

Johnson's Celebrated Liniment contains eucalyptus oil 27% and dipentene 73%.

Johnson's XX Oils contains castor oil 88%, dipentene 9%, and eucalyptus oil 3%.

Jojoba oil has largely replaced spermaceti (a waxy substance obtained from the head of the sperm whale) as a base for cold creams etc.

Joy-rides: Each tablet contains hyoscine hydrobromide 150 micrograms.

Junior disprol tablets ◊ paracetamol.

juniper berry oil and juniper oil have carminative effects and diuretic effects. They should *not* be taken in pregnancy or by patients with impaired kidney function.

juniper tar ◊ cade oil.

Juno Junipah Salts contain anhydrous sodium sulphate 88%, anhydrous sodium phosphate 0·8%, sodium bicarbonate 11%, saccharin 0·04%, and juniper oil 0·1%.

Juno Junipah Tablets contain anhydrous sodium sulphate 450 mg, anhydrous sodium phosphate 60 mg, phenolphthalein 25 mg, and juniper oil 0·00025 ml, with sodium chloride and terpeneless lime oil.

Juvel is a multivitamin preparation. Each tablet contains vitamin A 5,000 units, thiamine hydrochloride 2·5 mg, riboflavine 2·5 mg, nicotinamide 50 mg, pyridoxine hydrochloride 2·5 mg, ascorbic acid 50 mg, vitamin D 500 units. Each 5 ml of syrup contains

vitamin A 4,000 units, thiamine hydrochloride 2 mg, riboflavine 2 mg, nicotinamide 40 mg, pyridoxine hydrochloride 2 mg, ascorbic acid 40 mg, vitamin D 400 units.

JW Glycerin Lemon and Honey contains in each 5 ml glycerin 0·5 ml, honey 1·5 ml and syrup of lemon 3 ml.

JW Indian Brandee is used to treat stomach upsets, it contains in each 5 ml cardamom compound tincture 0·187 ml, capsicum tincture 0·125 ml and concentrated ethyl nitrate solution 0·031 ml.

Kabiglobulin is a normal immune human serum globulin injection. *Adverse effects:* allergic reactions may occur.

Kabikinase ◊ streptokinase.

Kalms are used as a nerve tonic. Each tablet contains hops 45 mg, asafetida 30 mg, aqueous ext. gentian 90 mg and aqueous extract of valerian 35 mg.

Kalspare is a diuretic. Each tablet contains chlorthalidone 50 mg and triamterene 50 mg. *Dose:* By mouth, 1 to 2 daily.

Kalten capsules contain atenolol 50 mg, amiloride hydrochloride 2·5 mg and hydrochlorothiazide 25 mg ◊ atenolol ◊ amiloride ◊ hydrochlorothiazide.

Kamillosan contains extracts from the chamomile herb and hexylresorcinol and is used as a soothing skin application.

kanamycin (Kannasyn; kanamycin sulphate) is an antibiotic. It is used to treat serious infections caused by organisms resistant to the more commonly used antibiotics, in the treatment of certain infections of the urinary tract and in the treatment of tuberculosis. *Adverse effects:* Adverse effects occur with sufficient frequency to make kanamycin only of use in treating infections resistant to other antibiotics. Skin rashes, nausea and vomiting may occur. Reversible kidney damage is relatively common. The most serious adverse reaction is deafness. This is irreversible and may follow intramuscular injections, particularly if the patient has impaired kidney function or if the drug is used for a prolonged period as in the treatment of tuberculosis. Some organisms develop resistance to kanamycin. *Precautions:* Kanamycin should only be given by intramuscular injection when there is no safer alternative. If the patient develops noises in the ears (tinnitus) or dizziness the drug should be stopped immediately. It should be used with caution in patients with impaired kidney function. Adverse reactions may be greatly reduced by keeping the blood level at no more than 30 mg per ml. The total dose in acute infections should not exceed 15 g over fourteen days – provided the patient is not allowed to become dehydrated. *Dose:* By mouth, 1 to 2 g per day in divided doses; by intramuscular injection or intravenous infusion, 15 mg per kg body-weight given 12 hourly.

Kannasyn ◊ kanamycin.

Kao-C Adults' Diarrhoea Mixture contains light kaolin 10% and calcium carbonate 5%.

Kao-C Junior Diarrhoea Mixture contains light kaolin 10% and calcium carbonate 5%.

Kaodene is used to treat diarrhoea. Each 10 ml contains codeine phosphate 10 mg and kaolin 3 g. *Dose:* By mouth, 20 ml three or four times daily. **kaolin** is purified native hydrated aluminium sylicate; it is used to treat diarrhoea. *Dose:* Light kaolin 15 to 75 g by mouth; or kaolin and morphine mixture (light kaolin 2 g, sodium bicarbonate 500 mg and tincture of morphine 0·4 ml in each 10 ml) 10 ml three or four times daily until diarrhoea stops.

Kaopectate* ◊ kaolin.

Kap-ind ◊ indomethacin.

Karvol inhalant capsules contain menthol, chlorbutol, cinnamon oil, pine oil, terpineol, and chlorothymol. They are inhaled to relieve nasal congestion.

Kay-Cee-L syrup: Each ml contains potassium chloride 75 mg. *Dose:* By mouth, 10 to 50 ml daily in divided doses after food.

K-Contin Continus: Each tablet contains potassium chloride 600 mg in sustained-release form. *Dose:* By mouth, 2 to 5 daily or on alternate days.

Kefadol ◊ cephamandole.

Keflex ◊ cephalexin.

Keflex-C ◊ cephalexin.

Keflin ◊ cephalothin sodium.

Kefzol ◊ cephazolin.

Kelfizine W ◊ sulfametopyrazine.

Kelocyanor injection contains dicobalt edetate and is used as an antidote for cyanide poisoning.

Kemadrin ◊ procyclidine.

Kemazoid Throat Lozenges each contain benzalkonium chloride 1 mg.

Kemazoid Throat Lozenges with Benzocaine each contain cetrimide 1 mg and benzocaine 5 mg.

Kemicetine ◊ chloramphenicol.

Kenalog ◊ triamcinolone.

Keralyt ◊ salicylic acid.

Kerecid ◊ idoxuridine.

Kerfoot cream contains 1% hydrocortisone ◊ hydrocortisone.

Keri Lotion ◊ paraffin.

Kerlone ◊ betaxolol.

Keroderm: An ointment containing titanium dioxide 2%, zinc oxide 10%, bismuth oxyquinolinate 0·25%, in a water-in-oil emulsion basis.

Keromask masking cream is used for concealing scars, areas of discolouration and birthmarks.

Kest is used to treat constipation. Each tablet contains magnesium sulphate 300 mg and phenolphthalein 50 mg. *Dose:* By mouth, 1 at night, 2 in the morning.

Ketalar injection ◊ ketamine.

ketamine (Ketalar) is an injectable anaesthetic, mainly used for children. *Adverse effects:* These include increased arterial pressure, tachycardia (rapid beating of the heart), hallucinations.

ketazolam (Anxon) is a benzodiazepine anti-anxiety drug. *Adverse effects* and *Precautions* ◊ diazepam. *Dose:* By mouth, 15 to 60 mg daily, preferably at bedtime.

ketoconazole (Nizoral) is a broad-spectrum antifungal drug. *Adverse effects:* Nausea, stomach upsets and pruritus (itching). *Precautions:* Its absorption from the stomach depends upon the presence of acid; it is therefore better absorbed when taken with a meal and poorly absorbed if taken along with any drug that reduces acid production e.g., anticholinergics, cimetidine, antacids. Such drugs should be taken not less than two hours after a dose of ketoconazole. It should not be used in pregnancy. *Dose:* By mouth, 200 to 400 mg daily.

ketoprofen (Alrheumat; Orudis; Oruvail) is an anti-rheumatic drug. *Adverse effects:* Like all anti-rheumatic drugs it may produce irritation of the stomach and it should be taken with meals. *Precautions:* It should be used with caution by patients with peptic ulcers, in the first three months of pregnancy, or with impaired liver function. It may increase the effects of other drugs such as anticoagulants, phenytoin and certain sulphonamides. *Dose:* By mouth with food, 50 mg two to four times daily.

Ketostix is used to detect ketones in the urine.

480   *ketotifen*

ketotifen (Zaditen; ketotifen hydrogen fumarate) is an antihistamine drug which also has some effect in preventing attacks of asthma. *Adverse effects:* May enhance the effects of sedatives, hypnotics, alcohol and other antihistamine drugs. *Precautions:* It should be used with caution by those who drive motor vehicles or operate moving machinery, particularly at the start of therapy. *Dose:* By mouth, 1 mg (capsule in the evening, increasing to 1 mg twice daily.

Ketovite is a multivitamin preparation available in both tablet and liquid form.

Keybells glycerin, lemon and ipecac family cough mixture contains in each 5 ml ipecacuanha liquid extract 0·0119 ml, chloroform 0·01125 ml, squill vinegar 0·1124 ml and capsicum oleoresin 0·175 mg.

KH3 Geriatricum Capsules each contain procaine hydrochloride 50 mg and haematoporphyrin base 200 micrograms.

Kiditard ◊ quinidine.

Kilpain Menthol & Wintergreen Cream with Mustard contains eucalyptus oil 1·3%, menthol 0·23%, methyl salicylate 11·22%, thymol 0·75%, phenol 0·38%, camphor 0·38% and volatile mustard oil 0·07%.

Kinidin Durules ◊ quinidine.

KLN anti-diarrhoea mixture contains kaolin 1·15 g, pectin 57·5 mg and sodium citrate 17·25 mg in each 5 ml. *Dose:* By mouth, 20 mls every 4 hours.

Kloref effervescent tablets of potassium chloride (500 mg) in solution.

Kloref-S effervescent granules. Each sachet contains betaine hydrochloride 2·07 g, potassium bicarbonate 1·35 g and potassium chloride 500 mg. *Dose:* By mouth, 1 or 2 sachets in water daily, after food.

Klyx enema ◊ dioctyl sodium sulphosuccinate.

kola: The therapeutic use of kola derives from its caffeine content. It is used in cola drinks which may contain up to 20 mg of caffeine/100 ml ◊ caffeine.

Koladex Tablets each contain caffeine 21 mg, stabilized kola extract 4·5 mg (equivalent to 80 mg dry kola nuts), and glucose 700 mg.

Kolanticon: Each 10 ml of gel contains light magnesium oxide 200 mg, dried aluminium hydroxide gel 400 mg, dicyclomine hydrochloride 5 mg and dimethicone 40 mg. It is used to treat indigestion and peptic ulcers. *Dose:* 10 to 20 ml three- to four-hourly.

Kolantyl: Each 5 ml of gel contains dried aluminium hydroxide gel 200 mg, magnesium oxide 100 mg and dicyclomine hydrochloride 2·5 mg. It is used to break indigestion and peptic-ulcers. *Dose:* 10 to 20 ml every four hours.

Kompbo contains black catechu 6%, clove oil 0·065%, cassia oil 0·09%, and capsicum oleoresin 0·019%.

Konakion ◊ phytomenadione.

krameria (krameria root) is used as an astringent in throat lozenges and gargles. The dried root is used in preparations to treat haemorrhoids.

Kruschen Salts contain sodium chloride 10%, anhydrous sodium sulphate 2%, potassium chloride 1%, potassium sulphate 5·5%, citric acid 1·5%, potassium iodide 0·001%, magnesium sulphate, exsiccated (MgSO₄, $MgSO_4$, 2·75H_2O) to 100%.

Kwells ◊ hyoscine and read section on drugs used to treat nausea, vomiting and motion sickness.

labetalol (Labrocol; Trandate; labetolol hydrochloride) is a beta-receptor blocking drug with additional vasodilator effects on peripheral blood vessels. It is used to treat raised blood pressure. *Adverse effects:* Postural hypotension, headache, tiredness, weakness, nausea, vomiting, rashes, tingling of the scalp, difficulty in passing water, pains in the stomach and skin rash. *Precautions:* It should be used with utmost caution in patients suffering from heart block, heart failure and asthma; and particularly in late pregnancy and breast-feeding mothers. The dose should be reduced in liver disease and abrupt withdrawal of the drug should be avoided. It can interfere with laboratory tests for adrenaline-like substances. *Dose:* By mouth, 200 to 400 mg daily in divided doses with food and with an increase in dose at 14-day intervals. By intravenous injection 50 mg over 1 minute, repeated after 5 minutes if necessary to a maximum of 200 mg. By intravenous infusion, 2 mg/minute to a maximum of 200 mg.

Labiton is a tonic containing alcohol and caffeine together with other ingredients. *Dose:* 10 to 20 ml twice daily.

Labophylline injections contain theophylline 200 mg and lysine 122 mg/ml ◊ theophylline. Lysine is an amino acid.

Laboprin: Each tablet contains aspirin 300 mg and lysine 245 mg. *Dose:* By mouth, 1 to 2 four hourly.

Labosept ◊ dequalinium.

Labrocol tablets ◊ labetalol.

lachesine chloride (Lachesine eye drops) is used to dilate the pupil in the treatment of eye disorders. ◊ atropine.

Lacri-Lube eye ointment contains liquid paraffin and lanolin.

lactic acid is used to prepare compound sodium lactate injections which are given for acidosis (when the blood acid/base balance becomes disturbed). It may be used in vaginal douches for the treatment of vaginal discharge and as a paint to treat warts.

Lacticare lotion contains lactic acid 5%, sodium pyrrolidone-carboxylate 2·5% in an emulsion basis.

Lactocalamine is used to treat sunburn. It contains calamine 4%, hamamelis water 5% and phenol 0·2%.

lactulose (Duphalac) is used as a laxative. *Dose:* By mouth, 7·5 to 20 g at breakfast.

Ladropen ◊ flucloxacillin.

Ladycare No. 1, No. 2 and No. 3 are multivitamin and mineral supplements.

laetrile is a substance obtained from apricot kernels. Evidence of its effects in treating cancer is confused and emotive. Orthodox cancer specialists regard it as ineffective.

laevo-amphetamine ◊ amphetamine.

laevulose (fructose) is a sugar, used medicinally in the same way as glucose.

Lamprene ◊ clofazimine.

Lanacane is a cream containing benzocaine 3%, resorcinol 2%, and chlorothymol 0·0325%.

Lanacort cream contains 1% hydrocortisone ◊ hydrocortisone.

lanatoside C (Cedilanid): See general discussion in section on drugs used to treat heart failure. *Dose:* By mouth for digitalization, 1 to 1·5 mg; maintenance 0·23 mg six-hourly reducing according to desired results.

Lance B + C is a multivitamin preparation. Each tablet contains thiamine hydrochloride 50 mg, riboflavine 5 mg, nicotinamide 200 mg, pyridoxine hydrochloride 5 mg, ascorbic acid 100 mg.

Langdale's Cinnamon Essence contains cinnamon oil 2·72%, alcohol (60%) 54·35%, ipecacuanha tincture 0·85%, squill tincture 0·85%, and senega tincture 0·47%.

Langdale's Tablets contain cinnamon oil 1%, squill liquid extract 0·006%, senega liquid extract 0·001%, and ipecacuanha liquid extract 0·001%.

lanolin ◊ hydrous wool fat.

lanosterol is obtained from wool fat of sheep.

Lanoxin ◊ digoxin.

Lantex Moist Tissues contain methylbenzethonium chloride 0·25%.

Lanvis ◊ thioguanine.

Laractone ◊ spironolactone.

Laraflex ◊ naproxen.

Laratrim ◊ co-trimoxazole.

larch (larch oleoresin and larch turpentine) is a rubefacient.

Largactil ◊ chlorpromazine.

Larodopa ◊ levodopa.

Lasikal is a diuretic with added potassium. Each tablet contains 20 mg frusemide and 750 mg slow-release potassium chloride. *Dose:* By mouth, two each morning.

Lasilactone is a diuretic. Each capsule contains frusemide 20 mg and spironolactone 50 mg. *Dose:* By mouth, 1 to 4 daily.

Lasipressin is used to treat raised blood pressure. Each tablet contains frusemide 20 mg and penbutolol 40 mg. *Dose:* By mouth, 1 daily or twice daily.

Lasix ◊ frusemide.

Lasix + K is a diuretic with added potassium. Each tablet contains frusemide 40 mg and potassium chloride (Potassium 10 mmol).

Lasma sustained-release tablets ◊ theophylline.

Lasonil ointment contains heparinoid 5,000 units and hyaluronidase 15,000 units per 100 g. Used to treat sprains and bruises. Also used in suppositories to treat haemorrhoids.

Lasoride tablets contain frusemide 40 mg and amiloride 5 mg ◊ frusemide and amiloride.

l-asparaginase ◊ colaspase.

Lassar's Paste ◊ zinc and salicylic acid paste.

latamoxef (Moxalactam; latamoxef sodium) is a cephalosporin antibiotic which has similar effects to cefaclor. *Dose:* By injection, 0·25 to 3 g every 12 hours.

Lauromacrogol 400 ◊ lauromacrogol.

lauromacrogols are used as lubricants, surfactants and as spermicidal agents in some contraceptive preparations.

lavandin oil is a substitute for lavender oil and is more fragrant ◊ lavender oil.

lavender oil (lavandin oil) is used as a carminative, colouring agent and as a flavouring agent. It is used as an insect repellent and in ointments and perfumes for its pleasant smell.

Laxoberal ◊ sodium picosulphate.

L-cystene ◊ cystine.

L-dopa ◊ levodopa.

Lecigran consists of vegetable (soya) lecithin.

lecithins consist of groups of fatty acids obtained from animal and vegetable sources, e.g., egg lecithins, vegetable lecithins, soya lecithins. Vegetable lecithin differs from egg lecithin in so far as it does not contain cholesterol and contains a lower percentage of phosphorus. They are used in skin applications. **Lecithins** have no therapeutic effects. They occur in all animal and vegetable cells – e.g., egg lecithins and vegetable lecithin.

Ledclair ◊ sodium calciumedetate.

Ledercort ◊ triamcinolone.

Lederfen ◊ fenbufen.

Lederfen-F are effervescent tablets of fenbufen ◊ fenbufen.

Ledermycin ◊ demeclocycline.

Lederspan ◊ triamcinolone.

Lejfibre biscuits contain 4·04 g of oat bran meal.

Lemeze Cough Syrup contains in each 5 ml cetylpyridinium chloride 2 mg, ipecacuanha liquid extract 0·003 ml, lemon oil 0·006 ml, purified honey

500 mg, ammonium chloride 30 mg, glycerol 500 mg, and citric acid monohydrate 125 mg.

Lemon Flu Cold Syrup contains in each 5 ml codeine phosphate 5 mg, ephedrine hydrochloride 7·5 mg, and diphenhydramine hydrochloride 5 mg, in a basis containing terpeneless lemon oil 0·01 ml.

lemon oil (juice) is used as a flavouring agent and as a carminative.

Lemonexa syrup is used to relieve cold symptoms. Each 5 ml contains codeine phosphate 5 mg, diphenhydramine hydrochloride 5 mg and ephedrine hydrochloride 7·5 mg.

Lem-Plus Cough Linctus with Honey and Lemon: Each 5 ml contains ipecacuanha liquid extract 0·015 ml, honey 1·12 g, glycerol 0·75 ml, citric acid 50 mg, terpeneless lemon oil 0·00006 ml, lemon oil 0·006 ml, lime oil 0·00125 ml, and sucrose 1·96 g.

Lem-Plus Instant Hot Lemon Drink Granules for solution contain paracetamol 650 mg, sodium citrate 500 mg, and ascorbic acid 50 mg.

LemSip: Each sachet contains paracetamol 650 mg, phenylephrine hydrochloride 5 mg, ascorbic acid 10 mg, and sodium citrate 500 mg, in a flavoured basis.

LemSip, Junior: Each sachet contains paracetamol 217 mg, phenylephrine hydrochloride 1·7 mg, ascorbic acid 3·3 mg, and sodium citrate 167 mg, in a blackcurrant-flavoured basis.

Lenium ◊ selenium.

Lentizol capsules contain amitriptyline hydrochloride 25 mg and 50 mg in slow-release form.

Leo K: Each tablet contains potassium chloride 600 mg in a sustained-release form.

Lergoban ◊ diphenylpyraline.

Leukeran ◊ chlorambucil.

Levius: Each tablet contains aspirin 500 mg in a sustained-release form.

levodopa (Broçadopa; Larodopa; L-dopa) is used to treat Parkinsonism. *Adverse effects:* Levodopa may produce loss of appetite, nausea, vomiting, dizziness and faintness (due to a fall in blood pressure on standing), and irregularities of heart rate. It may also produce involuntary movements of the tongue, jaw and neck. These are dose-related. It may also produce mental disturbances and depression; psychosis and mania have been reported. *Precautions:* Levodopa should not be used in patients with disorders of the heart or circulation. It should be used with caution in patients with mental disorders. Its effects may be reduced by phenothiazine major tranquillizers, pyridoxine, methyldopa and reserpine. Its effects may be increased by atropine-like drugs and by M.A.O. inhibitors. It should not be used whilst taking, or within two weeks of stopping, M.A.O. inhibitor drugs. *Dose:* By mouth, 125 mg to 8 g daily in divided doses.

levonorgestrel ◊ norgestrel.

Levophed ◊ noradrenaline.

levorphanol (Dromoran; levorphanol tartrate) has effects and uses similar to those described under morphine, but it differs from morphine by being almost as effective by mouth as by injection. For *Adverse effects, Precautions* and *Drug dependence* ◊ morphine. *Dose:* By mouth, 1·5 to 4·5 mg; by subcutaneous or intramuscular injection, 2 to 4 mg; and by intravenous injection in doses of 1 to 1·5 mg.

Lexotan ◊ bromazepam.

Lexpec ◊ folic acid.

Lexpec syrup with iron contains ferric ammonium citrate equivalent to 80 mg iron and folic acid 2·5 mg in each 5 ml.

Lexpec syrup with iron-M contains ferric ammonium citrate equivalent to 80 mg iron and folic acid 0·5 mg in each 5 ml.

L H–R H ◊ gonadorelin.

Libanil ◊ glibenclamide.

Librium ◊ chlordiazepoxide.

Librofem ◊ ibuprofen.

lidocaine ◊ lignocaine.

lidoflazine (Clinium) is an anti-angina drug. It is a long-acting coronary vasodilator with calcium antagonist effects. *Adverse effects:* Dizziness, tinnitus, headache, stomach upsets. *Precautions:* It may precipitate ventricular tachycardia. *Dose:* By mouth, first week, 120 mg once daily; second week, 120 mg twice daily; third and subsequent weeks, 120 mg three times daily.

light magnesium carbonate ◊ magnesium carbonate.

lignocaine (Xylocaine; Xylotox; Xylocard; lignocaine hydrochloride; lidocaine hydrochloride) is a local anaesthetic. It is used to treat disorders of heart rhythm.

Limbitrol 5 is a combined anti-anxiety and antidepressant drug. Each capsule contains amitriptyline hydrochloride 12·5 mg and chlordiazepoxide 5 mg). **Limbitrol 10** (contains 25 mg of amitriptyline and 10 mg of chlordiazepoxide). *Dose:* 1 to 3 times daily of Limbitrol 5 or 10 according to patient's needs.

Limclair ◊ trisodium edetate.

lime juice is used as a flavouring agent.

lime oil is used as a flavouring agent. It is irritant to the skin and mucous membranes.

lime water ◊ calcium hydroxide.

Limmits are a range of slimming foods that contain sodium carboxymethylcellulose with added vitamins, calcium and iron. ◊ methylcellulose.

linalyl acetate ◊ lavender oil.

Lincocin ◊ lincomycin.

lincomycin (Lincocin; Mycivin; lincomycin hydrochloride) is an antibiotic. It is active against a narrow range of bacteria. As it penetrates bone it is used for the treatment of bone infections (osteomyelitis). Bacterial resistance is induced easily, but cross-resistance is rare except with erythromycin. *Adverse effects:* Lincomycin may produce severe diarrhoea and colitis, nausea and abdominal cramps, an itching anus (pruritus ani) and sore gums (stomatitis) occasionally. Allergic reactions may produce skin rashes. Sensitivity of the skin to sunlight and supra-added infection with yeasts may occur. Rarely blood disorders and liver damage may occur. *Precautions:* It should not be given in pregnancy or to women who are breast feeding. It should be given with caution to patients with impaired kidney function. *Dose:* By mouth, 1·5 g daily in divided doses, half an hour before food; by intramuscular injection, 0·6 to 1·2 g daily in divided doses (twelve-hourly).

Linctoid C contains oxymel 6%, chloroform spirit 3%, tolu syrup 30%, horehound syrup 12%, ipecacuanha tincture 2%, and blackcurrant syrup 20%.

Lindane ◊ gamma benzene hexachloride.

Lingraine ◊ ergotamine.

Linituss is a cough medicine. Each 5 ml contains chloroform and morphine tincture 0·4 ml, camphorate opium tincture 0·2 ml, liquorice liquid extract 0·35 ml, ipecacuanha liquid extract 0·02 ml, capsicum tincture 0·002 ml, tolu syrup 0·125 ml, linseed 40 mg and vinegar of squill 0·4 ml.

Linoleic acid and **linolenic acids** are unsaturated fatty acids from oils of certain seeds such as sunflower and maize. They have been used to lower saturated blood fat levels and as a food in the treatment of multiple sclerosis.

linseed preparations are used as demulcents in cough medicines.

Linus Brand Vitamin C Powder consists of ascorbic acid.

Lion ointment contains rosin 5% and methylated spirit 5%.

Lioresal ◊ baclofen.

liothyronine (Tertroxin; liothyronine sodium; 1-tri-iodothyronine sodium) is a hormone produced by the thyroid gland, it has the effects and uses of thyroxine. It is effective in smaller doses, it works quicker but its effects do not last as long. It is used to treat thyroid disorders. *Dose:* Starting with 0·01 to 0·02 mg daily, and gradually increasing by 0·01 mg daily every week up to a total of 0·08 to 0·1 mg daily.

Lipoflavonoid is a vitamin B complex preparation. Each capsule contains thiamine hydrochloride 330 micrograms, riboflavine 330 micrograms, nicotinamide 3·33 mg, pyridoxine hydrochloride 330 micrograms, hydroxocobalamin 1·66 micrograms, ascorbic acid 100 mg, choline bitartrate 233 mg, inositol 111 mg, lemon bioflavonoid complex 100 mg, methionine 28 mg, dexpanthenol 330 micrograms.

Lipotriad is a vitamin B complex preparation. Each capsule contains thiamine hydrochloride 330 micrograms, riboflavine 330 micrograms, nicotinamide 3·33 mg, pyridoxine hydrochloride 330 micrograms, hydroxocobalamin 1·66 micrograms, choline bitartrate 233 mg, inositol 111 mg, methionine 28 mg, dexpanthenol 330 micrograms. Each 5 ml of elixir contains thiamine hydrochloride 1 mg, riboflavine 1 mg, nicotinamide 10 mg, pyridoxine hydrochloride 1 mg, cyanocobalamin 5 micrograms, inositol 334 mg, methionine 84 mg, panthenol 1 mg, tricholine citrate 460 mg (≡ choline 334 mg).

Lipsavers contain 2-ethylhexyl salicylate 4%, sorbic acid 0·5%, and allantoin 0·25%.

Liptrex contains lanolin, modified wheat-germ oil, and nipastat in a vegetable-oil basis.

Liqfruta Honey: Each 5 ml contains chondrus 20 mg, liquorice extract 37 mg, linseed 33 mg, chamomile 6·25 mg, peppermint oil 0·005 ml, anise oil 0·002 ml, ipecacuanha liquid extract 0·008 ml, and honey 840 mg.

Liqfruta Lemon contains the water-soluble constituents of linseed 0·66%, and chamomile 0·125%, with noscapine 0·08%, ipecacuanha liquid extract 0·15%, tolu solution 2%, and lemon basis to 100%.

Liqfruta Medica contains the water-soluble constituents of linseed 0·66%, chondrus 0·4%, and chamomile 0·125%, together with garlic oil 0·0195%, peppermint oil 0·104%, anise oil 0·052%, ipecacuanha liquid extract 0·165%, liquorice juice 0·75%, burnt sugar 1·25%, and sucrose 1·25%.

Liqfruta Standard contains the water-soluble constituents of linseed 0·66%, chondrus 0·4%, and chamo-mile 0·125%, together with garlic oil 0·013%, peppermint oil 0·104%, anise oil 0·052%, ipecacuanha liquid extract 0·165%, liquorice juice 0·75%, burnt sugar 1·25%, and sucrose 1·25%.

liquid paraffin ◊ paraffin.

Liquifilm Tears ◊ polyvinyl alcohol.

liquorice is used as a demulcent and expectorant in cough medicines. Liquorice extracts are also used to treat peptic ulcer.

Liskonum ◊ lithium.

Listerine Antiseptic contains alcohol (95%) 28·4%, benzoic acid 0·12%, eucalyptol 0·09%, menthol 0·04%, methyl salicylate 0·05%, thymol 0·06%, water to 100%.

Listermint mouthwash is used to treat halitosis (bad breath). It contains alcohol (96%) 12·8%, cetylpyridinium chloride 0·1%, glycerol 7·5% and zinc chloride 0·05%.

Litarex ◊ lithium citrate.

lithium (Camcolit; Liskonum; Phasal; Priadel; Lithium carbonate; lithium sulphate) is used to treat mania and manic-depressive illness. *Adverse effects:* These develop slowly as the drug accumulates in the body; they are related to dosage. They include transient nausea, trembling, weakness and drinking and passing a lot of water (polydipsia and polyuria). Higher dosage results in higher blood levels which produce more serious adverse effects – confusion, slurred speech, diarrhoea, drowsiness, trembling, and ataxia. It may also precipitate goitre. Changes on electrocardiograms have been reported. *Precautions:* Lithium should not be given to patients with impaired heart or kidney function and preferably not during pregnancy. Blood levels should be monitored regularly. *Dose:* By mouth, 0·25 to 1·5 g daily in divided doses.

lithium citrate (Litarex) has similar properties to lithium carbonate ◊ lithium.

Lloyd's Cream contains diethylamine salicylate 10%.

L-lysine monohydrochloride ◊ lysine.

LoAsid tablets contain dried aluminium hydroxide 230 mg, magnesium hydroxide 230 mg and activated dimethicone 12 mg. It is used to treat indigestion and peptic ulcer.

Lobak is used to treat muscle pain and spasm. Each tablet contains paracetamol 450 mg and chlormezanone 100 mg. *Dose:* 2 three times daily.

lobelia: The action of lobelia is due principally to one of its constituents – lobeline. Lobelia is contained in some asthma powders which are burned and the fumes inhaled.

lobeline (lobeline hydrochloride) is included in anti-smoking remedies. It produces effects in the body similar to nicotine. It may cause nausea, vomiting and coughing, headache, dizziness, trembling and rapid beating of the heart. Its use in helping patients to reduce the amount they smoke has not been proved.

Locabiotal ◊ fusafungine.

Locan cream contains local anaesthetics – amethocaine 0·8%, amylocaine 1%, and cinchocaine 0·4%.

Lockets Lozenges contain eucalyptol 0·25%, menthol 0·27%, honey 14·7%, and glycerol 2·4%.

Locoid ◊ hydrocortisone butyrate.

Locoid C cream contains hydrocortisone butyrate 0·1% and chlorquinaldol 3%.

Locobase cream is a base used for Locoid cream.

Locorten-Vioform ear drops contain clioquinol 1% and flumethasone 0·02%.

Lodine capsules ◊ etodolac.

Loestrin 20 tablets contain ethinyloestradiol 0·02 mg and norethisterone acetate 1 mg. It is an oral contraceptive drug.

Loestrin 30 tablets contain ethinyloestradiol 0·03 mg and norethisterone acetate 1·5 mg. It is an oral contraceptive drug.

lofepramine (Gamanil, lofepramine hydrochloride) is a tetracyclic antidepressant and has similar effects to mianserin. *Dose:* by mouth, 70 mg morning and evening.

Logynon is a triphasic oral contraceptive.

Logynon ED is an oral contraceptive drug.

Lomodex ◊ dextran.

Lomotil (each tablet and each 5 ml of liquid contain diphenoxylate hydrochloride 2·5 mg and atropine sulphate 0·025 mg). It is used to treat diarrhoea. *Dose:* 4 tablets or 20 ml liquid initially and then 2 (or 10 ml) every six hours until condition is controlled.

lomustine (CCNU, Cee NU) is an anticancer drug. *Adverse effects:* These include anorexia, nausea and vomiting. Blood disorders, mouth ulcers, loss of hair and liver toxicity have been reported. *Dose:* By mouth, up to 130 mg per square metre of body surface every six weeks.

Loniten ◊ minoxidil.

loperamide (Arret; Imodium; loperamide hydrochloride) acts on the muscles of the gut wall and slows down its movements. It is used to treat diarrhoea. *Dose:* By mouth, 6 to 8 mg daily in divided doses; maximum daily dose is 16 mg.

Lopid ◊ gemfibrozil.

loprazolam (Dormonoct) is a benzodiazepine drug used to produce sleep. *Adverse effects* and *precautions* are similar to those described under diazepam. *Dose:* 1 to 2 mg at night.

Lopresor ◊ metoprolol.

Lopresor SR: Each tablet contains metoprolol tartrate 200 mg in sustained-release form.

Lopresoretic is used to treat raised blood pressure. Each tablet contains metoprolol 100 mg and chlorthalidone 12·5 mg.

Loramet ◊ lormetazepam.

lorazepam (Almazine, Ativan) is a benzodiazepine drug used to treat anxiety and insomnia. *Adverse effects:* and *Precautions* ◊ diazepam. *Dose:* 1 to 10 mg daily in divided doses for anxiety. For sleep, 1 to 4 mg at bedtime.

Lorexane Cream contains lindane 1% and it is used to treat scabies and pediculosis (lice).

Lorexane No. 3 shampoo contains lindane 2% in a detergent base and is used to treat pediculosis (lice).

lormetazepam (Loramet) is a benzodiazepine drug used as a hypnotic. *Adverse effects* and *Precautions* ◊ diazepam. Its use during pregnancy is not recommended. *Dose:* By mouth, 1 mg at bedtime.

Lotil contains wool alcohols 6%, self-emulsifying glyceryl monostearate 10%, glycerol 6%, benzyl alcohol 5%, cetostearyl alcohol 3%, chlorocresol 0·2%.

Lotio Rubra ◊ zinc sulphate lotion.

Lotriderm cream contains the corticosteroid betamethasone (0·05%) and the antifungal drug clotrimazole 1% ◊ betamethasone and clotrimazole. Used to treat fungal infections of the skin associated with inflammation.

Lotussin linctus is used to treat coughs. Each 5 ml contains diphenhydramine hydrochloride 5 mg, dextromethorphan hydrobromide 6·25 mg, ephedrine hydrochloride 7·5 mg and guaiphenesin 50 mg. *Dose:* By mouth, 10 ml three times daily.

Loveridge Adults' Cough Mixture contains euphorbia extract 0·21 ml, cocillana liquid extract 0·021 ml, squill liquid extract 0·021 ml, senega liquid extract 0·021 ml, menthol 1·1 mg, anise oil 0·0105 ml, in each 5 ml.

Loveridge Children's Cherry Bark Cough Syrup contains wild cherry syrup 0·175 ml, acetic acid 0·075 ml, ipecacuanha liquid extract 0·0025 ml, camphor 2·5 mg, anise oil 0·0004 ml, in each 5 ml.

Loveridge Children's Cough Mixture contains cocillana extract 0·008 ml, squill liquid extract 0·02 ml, vinegar of ipecacuanha 0·16 ml, in each 5 ml.

Lucozade contains glucose syrup 22·4%, lactic acid 0·11%, caffeine 0·018%, and vitamin C 0·0082%, with flavouring and preservative.

Ludiomil ◊ maprotiline.

Lugacin ◊ gentamicin.

Lugol's Solution ◊ aqueous iodine solution.

Luma Bath Salts contain methyl salicylate, capsicum oleoresin, potassium iodide, and sodium carbonate.

Luminal ◊ phenobarbitone.

Luride ◊ fluoride.

Lurselle ◊ probucol.

lymecycline (Tetralysal) is an antibiotic having effects and uses described under tetracycline. It is rapidly absorbed from the gut. *Adverse effects* and *Precautions:* These are similar to those discussed under tetracycline. *Dose:* By mouth, 408 mg twice daily.

lynoestrenol is a synthetic progestogen. It is used principally with oestrogens as an oral contraceptive agent but may be used to treat disorders of menstruation. *Adverse effects:* It may cause headache, tension, fullness of the breasts, fluid retention, weight gain, breakthrough bleeding, acne and deepening of the voice, and it may make premenstrual tension worse. *Precautions:* It should not be used by patients with impaired liver function. *Dose:* 5 to 15 mg daily in divided doses.

lypressin (Syntopressin) is a nasal spray for the treatment of diabetes insipidus. It has similar effects to vasopressin.

lysine is an amino-acid – an essential part of the diet which goes to form body proteins.

Maalox and **Maalox TC** preparations contain aluminium hydroxide and magnesium hydroxide in varying proportions. **Maalox plus** preparations also contain dimethicone. They are used to treat indigestion and peptic ulcers.

Mac Blackcurrant Lozenges each contain amylmetacresol 600 micrograms, with sucrose and glucose syrup solids.

Mac Lozenges Honey-Lem: Each lozenge contains amylmetacresol 600 micrograms, sucrose and glucose syrup solids 2·4 g.

Mac Lozenges Medicated: Each lozenge contains amylmetacresol 600 micrograms, menthol 4 mg, glucose syrup solids 2·7 g.

Mackenzie Decongestant Tablets: Each contains paracetamol 250 mg, guaiphenesin 50 mg, methylephedrine hydrochloride 15 mg, chlorpheniramine maleate 2 mg, and menthol 1 mg.

Mackenzies Smelling Salts contain ammonia 15% and eucalyptus oil 3%.

Macleans Indigestion Powder contains heavy magnesium carbonate 15·5%, calcium carbonate 37·2%, and stabilized aluminium hydroxide equivalent to 17·4% of dried aluminium hydroxide.

Macleans Indigestion Tablets: Each contain light magnesium carbonate 150 mg, calcium carbonate 400 mg, and stabilized aluminium hydroxide equivalent to 183 mg of dried aluminium hydroxide.

Macrocide skin cleanser ◊ chlorhexidine.

Macrodantin ◊ nitrofurantoin.

Macrodex ◊ dextran.

macrogol ◊ cetomacrogol.

Madopar 125 capsules contain 100 mg of levodopa and 25 mg of benserazide hydrochloride. It is used to treat Parkinsonism. *Dose:* By mouth. The initial dose will depend upon the patient's needs and previous treatments; maintenance dose is 4 to 6 capsules daily of the 125 strength. Madopar 250 is double the strength of Madopar 125.

Madribon ◊ sulphadimethoxine.

mafenide (Sulfamylon; Sulfomyl) is a sulponamide cream used to prevent infections of burns. *Adverse effects:* Allergic reactions include rashes, metabolic acidosis. *Precautions:* It should be used with caution in patients with pulmonary dysfunction. It is also available as eye drops (Sulfomyl).

magaldrate (Dynese; hydrated magnesium aluminate) is used as an antacid. *Dose:* By mouth 400 to 800 mg as required.

magenta (fuchsine; basic fuchsine; triphenylmethane) is used as a skin antiseptic.

magenta paint (magenta and resorcinol paint; Castellani's paint a mixture of magenta, boric acid, phenol, resorcinol, and industrial methylated spirit). It is used as a skin antiseptic.

Magnapen preparations contain ampicillin and flucloxacillin in equal parts.

magnesium is an essential body electrolyte.

magnesium aluminate is used as an antacid. *Dose:* By mouth, 400 to 800 mg as requred.

magnesium aluminium trisilicate is used as an antacid.

magnesium carbonate: Heavy magnesium carbonate and light magnesium carbonate have antacid and laxative properties. Magnesium carbonate is less effective than magnesium hydroxide in neutralizing gastric acid and it liberates carbon dioxide. *Adverse effects:* It releases carbon dioxide in the stomach which may produce belching. It acts as a laxative. It is absorbed into the blood-stream and is rapidly excreted by the kidneys, but if kidney function is impaired the blood level of magnesium may rise resulting in magnesium intoxication (fall in blood pressure and paralysis of respiration). *Precautions:* Magnesium salts should be used with caution in patients with impaired kidney function. *Dose:* By mouth; antacid, 250 to 500 mg; laxative, 2 to 5 g.

magnesium hydroxide is used as an antacid (500 to 750 mg) and as a laxative (2 to 4 g).

magnesium oxide is used as an antacid (250 to 500 mg) and as a laxative (2 to 5 g).

magnesium phosphate is used as an antacid and mild laxative.

magnesium silicate ◊ magnesium trisilicate.

magnesium stearate is used in dusting powders, barrier creams, cosmetics and tablet making.

magnesium sulphate (Epsom salts) is used as a laxative. The usual dose is 5 to 15 g.

magnesium trisilicate is used as an antacid. It is absorbent and slow acting. The dose is 0·5 to 2 g.

malachite green is a brilliant dye used as an antiseptic in skin applications.

Malarivon ◊ chloroquine.

Malatex cream is a desloughing agent. It is used to remove dead tissue from around pressure sores. It contains propylene glycol 40%, malic acid 2·25%, benzoic acid 0·15% and salicyclic acid 0·0375%.

malathion (Derbac with Malathion liquid; Prioderm shampoo and liquid; Suleo-M) is an insecticide used for treating head lice.

malic acid is present in apples, pears and many other fruits. It is used as a food additive.

Malinal chewable tablets and suspension contain almasilate 500 mg in each tablet or 5 ml of suspension ◊ almasilate.

Malix ◊ glibenclamide.

Maloprim: Each tablet contains dapsone 100 mg and pyrimethamine 12·5 mg. *Dose:* By mouth, 1 tablet once a week to protect against malaria.

Malt extract has nutritional properties and is used also as a flavouring agent.

manganese is an essential trace element (an element needed by the body in very small amounts). It is concerned in several chemical reactions in the body.

manganese glycerophosphate is used as a tonic. See general comment under

glycerophosphates and **hypophosphites**.

manganese hypophosphite is used as a tonic. See general comment under **glycerophosphates** and **hypophosphites**.

manganese sulphate is an ingredient of compound ferrous sulphate tablets BP. Manganese salts are supposed to increase the effects of iron salts.

mannitol is an osmotic diuretic. *Adverse effects:* It may produce diarrhoea when given by mouth. Rapid injection into a vein may cause headache and chest pains and depress the respiration. *Precautions:* It should be used with caution in patients with heart failure or in those with impaired kidney function. *Dose:* Varies according to the disorder being treated.

mannomustine (mannomustine hydrochloride) is an anti-cancer drug. *Adverse effects* and *Precautions* are similar to those described under mustine. *Dose:* Varies according to disorder being treated.

Mansil ◊ oxamniquine.

Manusept ◊ triclosan.

maprotiline (Ludiomil; maprotiline hydrochloride) is a tetracyclic antidepressant drug. *Adverse effects* ◊ imipramine. Maprotiline produces sedation which may be useful in treating patients who are anxious. *Precautions* ◊ imipramine. *Dose:* By mouth, 25 to 150 mg daily in divided doses or in a single dose.

Marcain ◊ bupivacaine.

Marevan ◊ warfarin.

Marplan ◊ isocarboxazid.

Marvelon tablets contain desogestrel 0·15 mg, and ethinyloestradiol 0·03 mg. It is an oral contraceptive.

Marzine ◊ cinnarazine.

Massé Breast Cream contains arachis oil, cetyl alcohol, glycerol, glyceryl monostearate, wool fat, polysorbate 60, potassium hydroxide, sorbitan monostearate and stearic acid. It is used in pre- and post-natal nipple care.

Masteril ◊ drostanolone.

Matthews' Fullers Earth Cream contains Matthews' fullers earth 5·3%, zinc oxide 2·9%, calcium carbonate 2·9%, and lanolin 3·4% in an emollient basis.

Maw's Baby Lotion contains chlorhexidine gluconate 0·01%.

Maw's Cold Sore Ointment contains tannic acid 5%.

Maw's Orange Halibut Tablets each contain vitamin A 2,500 units, ergocalciferol 250 units, and ascorbic acid 25 mg.

Maxagesic ◊ ibuprofen.

Maxamaid XP contains essential and non-essential amino acids, carbohydrate, vitamins, minerals and trace elements in a phenylalanine-free powder.

Maxepa capsules and liquids contain fish oil made up of fatty acids, 18%

eicosapentaenoid acid and 12% docosahexaenoic acid. The products contain less than 100iu/g of vitamin A and less than 10 iu/g of vitamin D. Used to treat certain raised blood fats (triglycerides). *Adverse effects* include nausea and belching. Patients with bleeding disorders and patients taking anti-blood-clotting drugs should be carefully monitored. *Dose:* By mouth, 5 capsules with food twice daily or 5 ml of liquid twice daily with food.

Maxidex eye drops contain dexamethasone 0·1% and hypromellose 0·5%.

Maxipro HBV is supplemented whey protein powder 88%.

Maxitrol eye drops contain dexamethasone 0·1%, neomycin sulphate 0·35%, hypromellose 0·5% and polymyxin B sulphate 6,000 units per ml.

Maxolon ◊ metoclopramide.

Maxtrex tablets ◊ methotrexate.

mazindol (Teronac) is used to suppress the appetite. *Adverse effects:* These include constipation, dry mouth, insomnia, nervousness, headache, dizziness and chills. High doses may occasionally produce rapid beating of the heart. *Precautions:* It should not be used in pregnancy, in patients with a peptic ulcer or glaucoma. It should not be given in conjunction with M.A.O. inhibitor drugs and drugs such as guanethidine and debrisoquine, which are used to lower the blood pressure. These drugs should not be taken within one month of stopping mazindol. No cough medicines or cold remedies containing sympathomimetic drugs should be taken while taking mazindol or within one month of stopping it. Also, patients taking mazindol should seek medical advice before having a dental anaesthetic and for one month after stopping the drug. It should be used with caution in patients with coronary heart disease or severe anxiety states, and patients taking thyroid drugs or stimulants. *Dose:* By mouth, 1 tablet (2 mg) after breakfast for up to three months.

Meas/Vac is measles vaccine live. It is used for active immunization against measles.

mebendazole (Vermox) is used to treat infestation with threadworms, hookworms, whipworms and roundworms. *Dose:* By mouth, 100 mg as a single dose, or twice daily for two days, depending on the type of worms.

mebeverine (Colofac; mebeverine hydrochloride) is used to treat gut colic. It has atropine-like effects ◊ atropine.

mebhydrolin (Fabahistin; mebhydrolin napadisylate) is an antihistamine drug. *Dose:* By mouth, 100 to 300 mg daily in divided doses.

mechlorethamine ◊ mustine.

Mechothane ◊ bethanechol.

mecillinam (Selexidin) is a penicillin antibiotic active against gram-negative enteric bacteria. *Adverse effects* and *Precautions:* Benzylpenicillin. In long-term use kidney and liver function tests should be carried out. *Dose:* 5 to 15 mg/kg every 6 to 8 hours by intramuscular or slow intravenous injection or infusion.

meclozine (Sealegs; meclozine hydrochloride) is an antihistamine drug. It is used mainly to treat motion sickness, nausea and vomiting, nausea and vertigo due to disorders of the organ of balance and pregnancy sickness. *Adverse effects* and *Precautions:* These are similar to those discussed under promethazine. It is suggested that meclozine should not be used during the first three months of pregnancy – similar caution is recommended in the use of chlorcyclizine and cyclizine. *Dose:* By mouth, 25 to 50 mg daily in divided doses. The effect of a single dose lasts up to 24 hours. For motion sickness the dose is taken one hour before travelling.

Medacalm Tablets contain activated magnesium aluminium trisilicate 225 mg and pectin 50 mg.

medazepam (Nobrium) is a benzodiazepine drug used to treat anxiety. It has effects, uses and adverse effects similar to those described under chlordiazepoxide. *Dose:* By mouth, 10 to 30 mg daily.

Medex Elixir: Each 5 ml contains diphenhydramine hydrochloride 14 mg, ammonium chloride 100 mg, and sodium citrate 44 mg.

Medicaid cream contains cetrimide 0·5% in a hydrophilic basis.

Medicalm: Each 5 ml contains light kaolin 1·83 g and belladonna tincture 0·1 ml, in an aqueous pectin suspending vehicle.

Medicoal effervescent granules contain activated charcoal and are used as an absorbent by mouth in drug poisoning.

Medicol Liquid Antiseptic contains dichloroxylenol 2·5%, terpineol 5%, and isopropyl alcohol 13·5%.

Medicort cream contains 1% hydrocortisone ◊ hydrocortisone.

medigoxin (Lanitop) has similar properties to digoxin. *Dose:* By mouth, 0·1 mg two or three times daily.

Medihaler-Duo: Each aerosol dose contains isoprenaline hydrochloride 0·16 mg and phenylephrine bitartrate 0·24 mg. It is used to treat asthma. *Dose:* 1 to 3 puffs repeated after 30 minutes if necessary, up to a maximum of 24 puffs in 24 hours.

Medihaler-Epi is a pressurized spray containing adrenaline, 0·28 mg per dose. It is used in allergic emergencies to relieve wheezing. *Dose:* 1 to 3 doses. May be repeated in half an hour. Maximum twenty-four doses in 24 hours.

Medihaler-Ergotamine ◊ ergotamine.

Medihaler-Iso is a pressurized spray containing isoprenaline 0·08 mg per dose. It is used to treat bronchial asthma. *Dose:* 1 to 3 doses, repeated in half an hour. Maximum twenty-four doses in 24 hours.

Medihaler-Iso Forte is a pressurized spray inhaler used for treating bronchial asthma. It contains five times as much isoprenaline as Medihaler-Iso. ◊ isoprenaline.

Medijel anaesthetic gel contains glycerol 5%, lignocaine hydrochloride 0·66%, and aminacrine hydrochloride 0·05%.

Medijel Soft Pastilles contain lignocaine hydrochloride 0·25% and aminacrine hydrochloride 0·025%.

Medilave solution contains cetylpyridinium chloride 0·025%. It is used as a mouthwash or gargle.

Medipain Tablets: Each contain paracetamol 500 mg, codeine phosphate 8 mg, and casein 30 mg.

Medised: Each tablet contains paracetamol 500 mg and promethazine hydrochloride 10 mg. *Dose:* By mouth, 2 at night, or at four-hourly intervals to a maximum of 8 tablets in 24 hours. Also available as a suspension. Each 5 ml contains paracetamol 120 mg and promethazine hydrochloride 2·5 mg.

Meditar ◊ tar.

Medocodene: Each tablet contains paracetamol 500 mg and codeine phosphate 8 mg. *Dose:* By mouth, 1 to 2 hourly up to a maximum of 8 tablets in 24 hours.

Medomet ◊ methyldopa.

Medrone ◊ methylprednisolone.

medroxyprogesterone (Depo-Provera; Farlutal; Provera, medroxyprogesterone acetate) is a progestogen used to treat uterine disorders, secondary amenorrhoea, as a contraceptive and to treat cancer of the breast, uterus, prostate, kidney and testis. *Adverse effects* and *Precautions* ◊ progesterone. Disturbances of normal menstrual cycle and irregular bleeding may occur. *Dose:* By mouth, 2·5 to 10 mg daily for 5 to 10 days from 16th to 21st day of cycle. By deep intramuscular injections for endometriosis, 50 mg weekly or 100 mg every two weeks. For use as a contraceptive ◊ progestogen only contraceptives in Part Two.

mefenamic acid (Ponstan) relieves pain and brings down a high temperature. It has a weak anti-inflammatory action. It is used to relieve symptoms of rheumatic disorders and as a mild pain reliever. *Adverse effects:* Mefenamic acid may cause indigestion, constipation, diarrhoea, and irritation of the stomach with bleeding. It may also cause drowsiness, skin rashes and blood disorders. *Precautions:* Mefenamic acid should be taken with caution by patients with a history of peptic ulcer or impaired kidney function. It should not be taken during pregnancy or when breast feeding. It may increase the effects of certain anticoagulant drugs. *Dose:* By mouth, 1·5 g daily in divided doses.

Mefoxin ◊ cefoxitin.

mefruside (Baycaron) is a diuretic with similar properties to chlorothiazide. *Dose:* 25 mg daily or on alternate days.

Megace ◊ megestrol.

Megaclor ◊ clomocycline.

megestrol (Megase) is a progestogen ◊ progesterone.

Meggezones Pastilles each contain menthol 15 mg, benzoin 5·5 mg, peppermint oil 3·1 mg, liquorice liquid extract 17·5 mg and myrrh 0·09 mg.

melaleuca oil contains products which resemble terpineol. It is added to disinfectant preparations.

melissa is a lemon-scented herb containing a small amount of volatile oil which acts as an irritant to the skin and mucous membranes. It is included in some cough medicines.

Melissin contains in each 5 ml guaiphenesin 100 mg, menthol 1 mg, glycerol 1·66 ml, melissa, dried 125 mg, benzoic acid 5 mg, citric acid 50 mg, and aromatic oils.

Melleril ◊ thioridazine.

Melo glycerin, lemon and honey with ipecacuanha is a cough medicine containing in each 5 ml honey 1·82 ml, citric acid 75 mg, sodium benzoate 5 mg, glycerin 0·5 ml, lemon essence 0·001 ml and ipecacuanha 0·0025 ml.

Meloids lozenges: Each containing liquorice juice 93·3%, menthol 1·5%, cinnamon oil 0·37%, and stronger capsicum tincture 0·12%.

melphalan (Alkeran) is an anti-cancer drug. *Adverse effects:* These include nausea, vomiting, diarrhoea, mouth ulcers, bleeding from the gut, and loss of hair (alopecia). It damages the bone marrow, producing blood disorders. *Precautions:* It should not be used in pregnancy and in the presence of an infection. It should be used with caution in patients with blood disorders and evidence of impaired

bone-marrow function. *Dose:* Varies according to the condition being treated.

Melrose contains hard paraffin 27·9%, yellow soft paraffin 67·3%, wool fat 1·9%, isopropyl linoleate 1·5%, and chloroxylenol 0·1%.

Meltus Adult Cough & Catarrh Linctus contains in each 5 ml guaiphenesin 25 mg, cetylpyridinium chloride 2·5 mg, sucrose 1·75 g, and purified honey 500 mg.

Meltus Junior Cough & Catarrh Linctus contains in each 5 ml guaiphenesin 12·5 mg, cetylpyridinium chloride 2·5 mg, sucrose 2 g, and purified honey 500 mg.

menadiol (Synkavit tablets and injections; menadiol sodium diphosphate) is a water-soluble preparation of vitamin K used to prevent vitamin K deficiencies in malabsorption syndromes. It is also used as an antidote to oral anticoagulant drugs. *Precautions:* It should be given with caution in pregnancy. *Dose:* Varies according to the disorder being treated.

Menophase is used to treat the symptoms of the menopause. It is supplied in a calendar pack containing 5 pink tablets, mestranol 12·5 micrograms; 8 orange tablets, mestranol 25 micrograms; 2 yellow tablets, mestranol 50 micrograms; 3 green tablets, mestranol 25 micrograms and norethisterone 1 mg; 6 blue tablets, mestranol 30 micrograms and norethisterone 1·5 mg; 4 lavender tablets, mestranol 20 micrograms and norethisterone 750 micrograms. *Dose:* 1 tablet daily, starting with a pink tablet on

Sunday then in sequence (without interruption).

menotrophin (Pergonal) is a gonadotrophic hormone used in the treatment of female infertility. *Adverse effects:* Sensitivity reactions, ovarian hyperstimulation and enlargement, multiple pregnancy. *Dose:* By injection, according to the patient's response.

menthol is used in numerous preparations for treating cough and common cold symptoms. It also relieves itching and is used in skin applications.

Menthol and Wintergreen Cream contains eucalyptus oil 1·25%, methyl salicylate 11·2%, menthol 0·22%, camphor 0·34%, and volatile mustard oil 0·1%.

Mentholated Balsam contains ipecacuanha tincture 2%, chloroform and morphine tincture 5%, liquorice liquid extract 5%, squill oxymel 25%, menthol 0·05%, camphor spirit 2%.

Mentholatum Antiseptic Lozenges each contain menthol 16 mg, eucalyptus oil 12 mg, and amylmetacresol 600 micrograms.

Mentholatum Balm contains menthol 1·66%, camphor 10%, eucalyptus oil 0·66%, pumilio pine oil 0·66%, and methyl salicylate 0·66%.

Mentholatum Deep Heat Lotion contains menthol 1·58%, methyl salicylate 18·94%, and liquid lanolin 1·9%.

Mentholatum Deep Heat Rub contains menthol 5·91%, eucalyptus oil 1·97%, methyl salicylate 12·8% and turpentine oil 1·47%.

Mentholatum Deep Heat Spray is a non-metered aerosol containing glycol salicylate 5%, methyl salicylate 1%, methyl nicotinate 1·6%, and ethyl salicylate 5%.

Mentholatum Nasal Inhaler contains menthol 40%, camphor 40%, methyl salicylate 11%, eucalyptus oil 5%, and pine oil 4%.

Mentho Lyptus Extra Strong contains menthol 0·39% and eucalyptus oil 0·14%.

Mentho Lyptus Original contains menthol 0·1% and eucalyptus oil 0·08%.

Mentho Lyptus Spearmint Lozenges contain menthol 0·04% and eucalyptus oil 0·1%.

menthyl salicylate is used as a sunscreen agent.

menthyl valerianate is a menthol compound used in anti-smoking.

Mepacrine was used for the suppression and treatment of malaria but it has now been replaced by newer drugs. *Adverse effects:* These include dizziness, headache and mild stomach upset. *Dose:* 100 mg to 900 mg per day.

meparfynol ◊ methylpentynol.

mepenzolate (Cantil; mepenzolate bromide) has similar properties to atropine. It is used to relieve pain and spasm of the gastro-intestinal tract.

Dose: 25 to 50 mg three or four times daily.

meperidine ◊ pethidine.

mepivacaine (mepivacaine hydrochloride) is a local anaesthetic.

Meprate ◊ meprobamate.

meprobamate (Equanil; Meprate) is an anti-anxiety drug. *Adverse effects:* Meprobamate may produce loss of appetite, nausea, vomiting, diarrhoea and headache. Blood disorders have been reported and some patients become excited instead of calm. *Precautions:* Meprobamate may trigger off convulsions in someone with a history of epilepsy. It may also increase the effects of alcohol. *Dose:* By mouth, 400 to 1,200 mg daily in divided doses.

meptazinol (Meptid; meptazinol hydrochloride) is a narcotic analgesic with similar properties to morphine but it is less likely to depress breathing. *Adverse effects* and *Precautions* ◊ morphine. *Dose:* By injection, 50 to 100 mg, repeated 2 to 4 hourly as necessary.

Meptid ◊ meptazinol.

mepyramine (Anthisan; mepyramine maleate) is an antihistamine drug. It has similar effects and uses to those described under promethazine but it is less potent and shorter acting. *Dose:* By mouth, 200 to 1,000 mg daily in divided doses.

mequitazine (Primalan) is an antihistamine with similar effects to promethazine. *Dose:* By mouth, 5 mg twice daily.

Merbentyl ◊ dicyclomine.

mercaptopurine (Puri-Nethol) is an anti-cancer drug. *Adverse effects:* These include nausea, vomiting, diarrhoea, and occasionally ulceration of the lining of the gut and liver damage. It causes bone-marrow damage, which produces blood disorders. *Precautions:* It should not be given in early pregnancy. *Dose:* By mouth, varies according to disorder being treated.

Mercilon is an oral contraceptive tablet containing the oestrogen ethinyloestradiol 20 micrograms and the progestogen desogestrel 150 micrograms.

mercury salts have been widely used in the past as antibacterial and antifungal agents in applications to be applied to skin, eyes, ears, nose and wounds, to clean the skin for surgery, to wash out the bladder, in the treatment of syphilis, as purgatives, in contraceptive creams (to kill sperms), and as teething powders. *Adverse effects:* Mercury and its salts can damage the lining of the mouth, stomach and gut, damage the kidneys and produce bleeding from the gut. In children it can produce pink disease (acrodynia) which produces hot red skin and nerve damage. The use of mercury and its salts is seldom, if ever, necessary.

Merieux Tetavex contains tetanus formol toxoid. It is used as a tetanus vaccine.

Merocaine antiseptic lozenges contain cetylpyridinium chloride 1·4 mg and benzocaine 10 mg. *Dose:* 1 lozenge dissolved in the mouth 2 hourly to a maximum of 8 in 24 hours.

Merocet lozenges ◊ cetylpyridinium.

Merothol lozenges contain cetylpyridinium chloride 1·4 mg with menthol and eucalyptus. Used to treat sore throats ◊ cetylpyridinium, menthol, and eucalyptus.

mersalyl is a diuretic. It is rarely used now. *Adverse effects:* It may cause stomatitis, gastric upset, vertigo, fever, skin irritation and rarely blood disorders. *Precautions:* It must be given by intramuscular injection.

Meruvax II is a brand of rubella (German measles) vaccine.

mesalazine (Asacol) is used to treat ulcerative colitis in patients intolerant to sulphasalazine. *Dose:* 3 g to 6 g daily.

mesna (Uromitexan) is used in patients who are receiving ifosfamide or cyclophosphamide therapy to prevent damage to the bladder. *Adverse effects:* Stomach upsets, headaches and fatigue if given above maximum recommended dose. *Dose:* Varies according to the disorder being treated.

mesterolone (Pro-Viron) is a male sex hormone. ◊ testosterone. *Dose:* 25 mg two to four times daily.

mestranol is a synthetic oestrogen used in oral contraceptive drugs ◊ oestradiol.

metacresol (hexalated metacresol) is used as an antiseptic.

Metamucil contains psyllium mixed with dextrose. It is used to treat constipation.

Metanium dusting powder ◊ titanium.

metaraminol (Aramine) is a sympathomimetic drug which has been used to maintain blood pressure in shock.

Metatone mixture contains calcium, potassium, sodium and manganese glycerophosphates and thiamine 0·5 mg in each 5 ml. It is used as a tonic. *Dose:* 5 to 10 ml two or three times daily.

Metenix ◊ metolazone.

Meterfer ◊ ferrous fumarate.

Meterfolic tablets contain ferrous fumarate (equivalent to 100 mg of iron) and folic acid 350 micrograms.

metformin (Glucophage; metformin hydrochloride) is an oral anti-diabetic drug. *Adverse effects:* Anorexia, nausea and vomiting may occur and are usually related to the dose. Skin rashes, loss of weight and weakness may rarely occur. *Precautions:* Metformin should be used with caution by patients with impaired liver or kidney function. It should not be used during pregnancy. It should not be used by patients with infections or after operations or injury – such patients will require insulin. *Dose:* By mouth, initially 1,500 to 1,700 mg daily in divided doses with meals.

methadone (Physeptone; amiodarone hydrochloride) is a narcotic pain reliever. It has effects and uses similar to those described under morphine. It is used as a cough suppressant and also in treating heroin addicts. It blocks the withdrawal effects of heroin and is used as a substitute, because it is said to be easier to withdraw methadone subsequently. Methadone produces less sedation than morphine and it is therefore not used as a pre-operative medication. *Adverse effects:* Minor adverse effects particularly in ambulant patients include nausea, vomiting, dizziness, faintness, dry mouth and constriction of the pupils. Methadone may cause a fall in blood pressure and depress respiration. Children tolerate only very small doses. *Precautions:* Methadone depresses respiration; it is therefore undesirable as a pain reliever in childbirth. *Drug dependence:* Methadone produces drug dependence of the morphine type. *Dose:* For pain, 5 to 10 mg by mouth or subcutaneously every four hours; to suppress cough, 1 to 2 mg as a linctus.

methenamine ◊ hexamine.

methenamine mandelate ◊ hexamine.

methicillin (Celbenin; methicillin sodium) is a semi-synthetic penicillin. It is given by injection because it is not well absorbed by mouth. It is used to treat infections by bacteria which produce a substance which destroys natural penicillin (penicillinase). *Adverse effects* and *Precautions:* These are similar to those described under benzylpenicillin. *Dose:* Intramuscular injections, 1 g every four to six hours.

methionine is an antidote used for paracetamol overdosage. It protects the liver if given within 10 to 12 hours of ingestion of paracetamol. Liver damage is the cause of death in paracetamol overdose.

methixene (Tremonil; methixene hydrochloride) produces mild atropine-like effects and antihistamine effects. It also relieves spasm and is used to treat Parkinsonism. *Adverse effects* and *Precautions* ◊ atropine. *Dose:* By mouth, 2·5 to 60 mg in divided doses. Maintenance, 15 to 30 mg daily.

methocarbamol (Robaxin) is a muscle relaxant. *Adverse effects:* Light headedness, dizziness, drowsiness, nausea, allergic reactions (e.g. skin rash, itching, conjunctivitis, blocked nose, headache and fever). May cause blurred vision. *Precautions:* Do not use in patients allergic to it. Do not use if breast-feeding or in first three months of pregnancy, and use with utmost caution in last six months of pregnancy. May increase effects of alcohol, sleeping drugs, sedatives and anti-anxiety drugs. *Dose:* by mouth, 1·5 to 2 g four times daily, maintenance 1 g four times daily.

methohexitone (Brietal sodium; methohexitone sodium) is a barbiturate drug used to produce anaesthesia for surgical operations.

methoserpidine (Decaserpyl) is used to treat high blood pressure. It has effects and uses similar to those described under reserpine – its onset of effect is slow and may take up to two or three weeks. *Adverse effects:* These are similar to those described under reserpine. It may cause congestion of the nose, mild sedation, diarrhoea and other disturbances of the bowel. *Precautions:* Methoserpidine should not be taken by patients with certain types of depressive disorders. *Dose:* By mouth, 15 to 60 mg daily in divided doses, starting with 15 to 30 mg daily and slowly increasing.

methotrexate (Emtexate; Maxtrex) is an anti-cancer drug and is used to treat psoriasis. *Adverse effects:* These include nausea, vomiting, diarrhoea, abdominal pain, skin rashes and loss of hair (alopecia). Ulceration of the mouth and gut may occur with high doses. Severe allergic reactions may occur (sometimes fatal). It may cause sensitivity of the skin to sunlight and bone-marrow damage leading to serious blood disorders. *Precautions:* It should not be given in early pregnancy and it should be used with caution in patients with impaired kidney, liver or bone-marrow function. Its effects may be increased by aminobenzoic acid, aspirin, sulphonamides and thiazide diuretics. *Dose:* Varies according to the condition being treated.

methotrimeprazine (Nozinan; Veractil; methotrimeprazine hydrochloride; methotrimeprazine maleate) is a major tranquillizer. *Adverse effects* and *Precautions* ◊ chlorpromazine. It is more sedating and produces more hypotension and should be used with caution in patients over 50 years. *Dose:* By mouth, 25 to 1,000 mg daily. By intramuscular or intravenous injection in terminal care 12·5 to 50 mg 6 to 8 hourly.

methoxamine (Vasoxine) is an adrenaline-related drug which constricts blood vessels and raises the blood pressure. It is used to treat a fall in blood pressure that can occur under a general anaesthetic. *Adverse effects* include raised blood pressure, headaches, and slowing of the heart rate. *Precautions:* It should not be used in patients with serious heart disease. *Dose:* By intramuscular injection 5 to 10 mg. By slow intravenous injection 5 to 10 mg at a rate of 1 mg per minute.

methoxyphenamine (Orthoxine hydrochloride; methoxyphenamine hydrochloride) is a sympathomimetic drug used to treat bronchial asthma. *Adverse effects:* It may cause nausea, dizziness and dry mouth. *Precautions:* It should not be given to patients who are receiving, or who have received in the preceding two weeks, M.A.O. inhibitor drugs. *Dose:* By mouth, 50 to 100 mg every four hours.

methyclothiazide (Enduron) is a diuretic drug with effects and uses similar to those described under chlorothiazide. *Dose:* By mouth, 2·5 to 5 mg daily; to a maximum of 10 mg daily.

methyl benzethonium chloride is a surfactant like cetrimide. It is used as an antiseptic.

methylcellulose (Celevac; Cellucon; Cologel) is an emulsifying agent which swells in water and is used to treat constipation as a bulk laxative. It also absorbs water in the stomach and is said to relieve hunger because it swells and makes the stomach feel full. It is used as a slimming drug.

methyl cysteine (Visclair; methyl cysteine hydrochloride) is used to liquefy sputum production to treat coughs. *Dose:* By mouth, 200 mg three or four times daily before meals.

methyldopa (Aldomet; Dopamet, Medomet) is used to treat raised blood pressure. *Adverse effects:* Drowsiness may occur in the first few days of treatment; this usually disappears on its own or on reduction of the dose. Other adverse effects include diarrhoea, dryness of the mouth, nausea, depression, mental disturbances, nightmares, oedema, stuffiness of the nose, fever, dizziness and failure to ejaculate. Rarely, joint and muscle pains, impotence, skin rashes and weakness may occur. Blood disorders have been reported and liver function may be impaired in the first few weeks of treatment. Methyldopa may occasionally make the urine dark. *Precautions:* Methyldopa should be used with caution by patients with impaired kidney or liver function or with a history of liver disease or mental depression. A severe fall in blood pressure may occur during anaesthesia in patients on methyldopa. Amphetamines and antidepressant drugs decrease the effects of methyldopa. *Dose:* By mouth, 500 mg to 2 g daily in divided doses.

methyldopate ◊ methyldopa.

methylene blue is used in the treatment of drug-induced methaemoglobinaemia. A weak solution has been used to treat infections of the urinary tract.

methylephedrine (methylephedrine hydrochloride) has effects and uses similar to those described under ephedrine. It is used to treat bronchial asthma. *Dose:* By mouth, 40 mg three times daily and at bedtime.

methyl hydroxybenzoate is used as a preservative in creams and ointments and also in foods.

methyl nicotinate is used as a rubefacient skin application.

methylphenobarbitone (Prominal) is a long-acting barbiturate used in the treatment of epilepsy ◊ phenobarbitone. *Dose:* 100 to 600 mg daily.

methylprednisolone (Depo-Medrone; Medrone, Solu-Medrone) is a corticosteroid. ◊ prednisolone. *Dose:* By mouth, 8 to 80 mg daily in divided doses. By intramuscular or slow intravenous injection or infusion, up to 120 mg daily for up to 3 days. Shock: by intravenous infusion 30 mg/kg.

methylpolysiloxane ◊ dimethicone.

methyl salicylate (oil of wintergreen) has the actions of salicylates ◊ aspirin. It is used in rheumatic rubs and liniments.

methyltestosterone (Viroromone-Oral) is a male sex hormone. It has similar effects and uses to those described under testosterone. It has the advantage that it is absorbed when taken by mouth or sucked under the tongue. *Adverse effects:* Jaundice may occur after prolonged use. In women excessive libido may develop and with larger doses masculinization may occur – deep voice, acne, facial hair, male-type baldness and body hair. *Precautions:* Methyltestosterone should not be used by patients with impaired liver function or in pregnancy. For other precautions ◊ testosterone. *Dose:* By mouth: men, 25 to 50 mg daily: women, 5 to 20 mg daily.

methyprylone (Noludar) is used as a sleeping drug. *Adverse effects:* Minor side-effects may occasionally occur and include drowsiness, dizziness,

headache, excitation, skin rashes, nausea and vomiting. *Precautions:* Methyprylone may interfere with the ability to drive motor vehicles and operate machinery. It increases the effects of alcohol. *Drug dependence:* Methyprylone may produce drug dependence of the barbiturate/alcohol type. *Dose:* By mouth, 200 to 400 mg at night. For sedation: 50 to 100 mg three times daily.

methysergide (Deseril; methysergide maleate) is used to treat migraine. *Adverse effects:* It may produce nausea, stomach pains, drowsiness, dizziness, restlessness, cramps in the legs and mood changes. It may also cause vomiting, diarrhoea or constipation, ataxia, weakness, weight gain, disorders of circulation in the arms and legs, confusion, insomnia, skin rashes, loss of hair, painful joints and muscles, fall in blood pressure on standing, rapid beating of the heart, and blood disorders. Prolonged use may produce fibrosis (scar tissue) of tissues at the back of the abdomen (retroperitoneal). *Precautions:* It should not be taken during pregnancy, and should not be taken by patients with heart or circulatory disorders, with high blood pressure, impaired kidney or liver function or oedema, or with peptic

ulcers. *Dose:* By mouth, 2 to 6 mg daily in divided doses with food.

metirosine (Demser) is used to treat phaechromocytoma, a disease where the adrenal glands produce too much of the hormone adrenaline. *Adverse effects:* Sedation, severe diarrhoea and involuntary movements may occur. *Precautions:* A high fluid intake must be maintained; the ability to drive or operate machinery may be impaired.

Dose: 250 mg 4 times daily to a maximum of 4 g daily.

metoclopramide (Gastrobid; Gastromax; Maxolon; Metox; Metramid; Mygdalon; Parmid; Primperan; metoclopramide hydrochloride) is used to treat nausea and vomiting. It is also used to hurry emptying of the stomach during X-rays of the stomach and duodenum. *Adverse effects:* It may cause constipation. In large doses especially in children and young adults it may cause drowsiness and affect movements of muscles (dystonia). *Precautions:* It should be used with caution in patients with psychological disorders. It should be used with care during pregnancy and in patients receiving phenothiazine major tranquillizers. Its effects are decreased by atropine-like drugs. *Dose:* 10 mg by mouth, intramuscular or intravenous injection.

metolazone (Metenix) is an oral diuretic drug. *Adverse effects* ◊ chlorothiazide. It may cause headache, nausea, vomiting, loss of appetite, dizziness, abdominal pains, skin rashes, blood disorders and flare-up of gout. *Precautions* ◊ chlorothiazide. It should not be used in patients with impaired kidney or liver function. It may trigger off gout by increasing the blood uric acid level and it may affect the dose of insulin or oral anti-diabetic drugs required in diabetic patients. *Dose:* By mouth, 5 to 10 mg once daily according to the disorder being treated.

Metopirone ◊ metyrapone.

metoprolol (Betaloc; Co-Betaloc; Lopresor) is a beta-receptor blocker used to treat angina and raised blood pressure. *Adverse effects* ◊ propranolol and read the section in Part Two on drugs used to treat angina. Metoprolol has less effect upon the beta-receptors in the bronchi but even so it should be given with caution to patients with chronic obstructive lung disorders. It may change the insulin requirements of diabetic patients and it should not be given during pregnancy. *Dose:* Angina: by mouth, 50 to 100 mg two or three times daily. Raised blood pressure: 100 to 400 mg daily in divided doses.

Metosyn cream contains fluocinonide.

Metox ◊ metoclopramide.

Metramid ◊ metoclopramide.

metriphonate (Bilarcil) is an organo-phosphorus compound which is effective against schitosoma haematobium worms which live in the genito-urinary veins.

Metrodin injection contains human follicle stimulating hormone (FSH) 75 i.u.

Metrolyl ◊ metronidazole.

metronidazole (Elyzol; Entamizole; Flagyl; Metrolyl; Vaginyl; Zadstat) is used to treat inflammation of the vagina and penis (*Trichomonas* vaginitis and urethritis). It is also effective against amoebic infections, infections of the mouth (Vincent's angina) and giardiasis of the gut. It has no effect on thrush (*Candida*). Many relapses of vaginitis may be due to re-infection by the male partner and therefore both should be treated. Gonorrhoea should be tested for and excluded. It is widely used in hospitals to treat and to prevent anaerobic infections. *Adverse effects:* Metronidazole may cause loss of appetite, nausea, headache, malaise, coated tongue, dryness of the mouth and skin rashes. Less often it may cause drowsiness, vertigo, depression, peripheral neuropathy and insomnia. It may cause the urine to be stained brown. *Precautions:* When taken with alcohol the patient may experience flushing of the face, headache, dizziness and nausea. *Dose:* By mouth; 200 to 400 mg three times daily. It may also be given by injection and as suppositories.

metyrapone (Metopirone) is used to treat Cushing's syndrome. It is also used to assess the function of the pituitary gland in hypopituitarism and after prolonged treatment with corticosteroids which can depress the function of the adrenal and pituitary glands. *Adverse effects:* Nausea and vomiting. *Dose:* By mouth, 750 mg every four hours with food for six doses.

Mevilin-L is a brand of measles vaccine.

mexenone (in Uvistat) is a sunscreen agent.

mexiletine (Mexitil; mexiletine hydro-chloride) is used to treat disorders of heart rhythm. *Adverse effects:* These include nausea, vomiting, dizziness, drowsiness, confusion, pins and needles, double vision, alterations of heart rate, fall in blood pressure, tremor, difficulty in speaking and ataxia. *Precautions:* Tremor may be increased in patients with Parkinsonism. *Dose:* By intravenous infusion, 100 to 250 mg slowly over five to ten minutes, then slowly reducing to 1 mg per minute. By mouth, 400 to 600 mg, then 200 to 250 mg after two hours, repeated six to eight hourly.

Mexitil ◊ mexiletine.

Mexitil PL is a slow-release capsule of mexiletine 360 mg.

mezlocillin (Baypen) is a broad-spectrum penicillin antibiotic. *Adverse effects* and *Precautions:* See benzyl-penicillin. It should not be used during the first three months of pregnancy. *Dose:* By intramuscular injection, 1 to 2 g every six to eight hours, or by intravenous infusion or injection.

MFV-Ject is a brand of influenza vaccine.

mianserin (Bolvidon; Norval; mianserin hydrochloride) is a tetracyclic antidepressant. *Adverse effects:* Drowsiness, dry mouth, blurred vision, constipation. *Precautions* ◊ imipramine. *Dose:* By mouth, 30 to 90 mg daily in divided doses or as a single dose at night.

Micolette Micro-enema contains sodium citrate 450 mg, sodium lauryl-sulphoacetate 45 mg and glycerol 625 mg in each 5 ml single disposable pack with nozzle.

miconazole (Daktarin; Dermonistat; Monistat; miconazole nitrate) is an antifungal and antibacterial drug used in skin applications and as an oral gel for mouth infections. Gyno-Daktarin and Monistat are vaginal preparations. It is also used to treat systemic fungal infections by mouth and by intravenous infusion. *Adverse effects:* Nausea, vomiting, pruritus and rash. *Dose:* By mouth, 250 mg 6 hourly, by intravenous infusion 600 mg 8 hourly.

Micralax Micro-enema contains sodium citrate 450 mg, sodium alkyl-sulphoacetate 45 mg, sorbic acid 5 mg in each 5 ml single-dose disposable pack with nozzle.

Micro-K ◊ potassium.

Microgynon 30 tablets contain 0·15 mg levonorgestrel and 0·03 mg ethinyloestradiol. It is an oral contraceptive drug.

Micronor ◊ norethisterone.

Microval tablets contain levonor-gestrel 0·03 mg – a progestogen-only oral contraceptive.

Mictral effervescent granules are used to treat urinary infections. Each sachet contains nalidix acid 660 mg, sodium citrate 3·75 g, citric acid 250 mg, sodium bicarbonate 250 mg. *Dose:* Contents of 1 sachet dissolved in water and taken by mouth three times daily for 3 days.

Midamor ◊ amiloride.

midazolam (Hypnovel) is a benzodiazepine drug used before surgical procedures to produce sedation with amnesia. *Adverse effects* and *Precautions* ◊ diazepam. *Dose:* By slow intravenous injection 70 micrograms/kg until patient becomes drowsy – range 2·5 to 7·5 mg.

Midrid ◊ isometheptene mucate.

Migen is used to treat allergy to house dust mites.

Migraleve (pink tablets each contain buclizine hydrochloride 6·25 mg, paracetamol 500 mg, codeine phosphate 8 mg and dioctyl sodium sulphosuccinate 10 mg; yellow tablets each contain paracetamol 500 mg, codeine phosphate 8 mg and dioctyl sodium sulphosuccinate 20 mg). It is used to treat migraine. *Dose:* Two pink tablets at the start of an attack, then two yellow tablets every three to four hours if required. Maximum daily dose, 2 pink tablets and 6 yellow tablets.

Migralift tablets contain the same drugs as Migraleve ◊ Migraleve. Used to treat migraine.

Migravess tablets are used to treat acute attacks of migraine. Each effervescent tablet contains metoclopramide 5 mg and aspirin 325 mg. *Dose:* By mouth, two tablets dissolved in water at start of attack then every four hours if necessary. Maximum of 6 tablets in 24 hours.

Migril: Each tablet contains ergotamine tartrate 2 mg, cyclizine hydrochloride 50 mg and caffeine hydrate 100 mg. It is used to treat migraine.

Dose: 1 to 2 at onset of attack, then ½ to 1 half-hourly. Maximum for one attack is 4 tablets. Maximum for a week is six tablets.

Mijex contains diethyltoluamide and citronella oil.

mild silver protein has antibacterial properties and is included in some eye drops and nose drops used to treat infections.

Milk of Magnesia: Each 5 ml contains magnesium hydroxide 415 mg.

Milk of Magnesia Tablets: Each contains magnesium hydroxide 300 mg.

Mill-Par contains approx. 6% magnesium hydroxide and 25% liquid paraffin.

Milton ◊ sodium hypochlorite.

Milton crystals ◊ potassium monopersulphate.

Minadex is an orange-flavoured syrup containing in each 5 ml vitamin A 650 units, vitamin D 65 units, ferric ammonium citrate 150 mg, calcium glycerophosphate 22·5 mg, potassium glycerophosphate 2·25 mg, manganese sulphate 0·5 mg and copper sulphate 0·5 mg. *Dose:* 10 ml three times a day after meals.

Minalka: Each tablet contains calcium gluconate 243 mg, potassium citrate 132 mg, disodium phosphate 19 mg, magnesium phosphate 4 mg, ferrous gluconate 540 micrograms, manganese sulphate 540 micrograms, copper sulphate 270 micrograms, zinc sulphate

270 micrograms, cobalt sulphate 270 micrograms, potassium iodide 3 micrograms, and vitamin D_3 1·25 micrograms, with excipients.

Minamino is a multivitamin preparation. Each 5 ml of syrup contains thiamine hydrochloride 15 mg, riboflavine 2 mg, pyridoxine hydrochloride 1·75 mg, nicotinamide 20 mg, cyanocobalamin 5 micrograms, with amino acids, extracts of liver, spleen, and gastric mucosa, iron citrate, manganese sulphate, and copper sulphate.

Minihep ◊ heparin.

Minihep Calcium ◊ heparin.

Minilyn: Each tablet contains lynoestrenol 2·5 mg and ethinyloestradiol 0·05 mg. It is an oral contraceptive drug.

Minims amethocaine single dose eyedrops contain amethocaine 0·5% or 1%. It is used to anaesthetize the eye.

Minims atropine single dose eyedrops contain atropine 1% ◊ atropine.

Minims benoxinate single dose eyedrops contain oxybuprocaine hydrochloride 0·4% ◊ oxybuprocaine.

Minims chloramphenicol single dose eyedrops contain chloramphenicol 0·5% ◊ chloramphenicol.

Minims cyclopentolate single dose eyedrops contain cyclopentolate hydrochloride 0·5%. It is used to dilate the pupil to help examination of the eye.

Minims fluorescein single dose eyedrops contain fluorescein sodium 1% or 2%. It is used as a stain to diagnose damage to the cornea of the eye.

Minims gentamicin single dose eyedrops contain gentamicin sulphate 0·3% ◊ gentamicin.

Minims homatropine single dose eyedrops contain homatropine hydrobromide 2% ◊ homatropine.

Minims lignocaine & fluorescein single dose eyedrops contain lignocaine hydrochloride 4% and florescein sodium 0·25%. It is used as a stain to diagnose damage to the cornea of the eye.

Minims metipranolol single dose eye drops contain the beta-blocker metipranolol in concentrations of 0·1%, 0·3% and 0·6% *Adverse effects:* Stinging of the eyes, transient headache. See propranolol for adverse effects of beta-blockers taken by mouth. *Precautions:* Do not use in patients who suffer from asthma or other chronic wheezing disorder, or from heart failure. Do not use in pregnancy or if you wear soft contact lenses. Use with caution in patients with a slow pulse rate or heart block. *Dose:* Apply 1 drop twice daily.

Minims phenylephrine single dose eyedrops contain phenylephrine hydrochloride 10% ◊ phenylephrine.

Minims pilocarpine single dose eyedrops contain pilocarpine nitrate 1%, 2% or 4% ◊ pilocarpine.

Minims prednisolone single dose eyedrops contain prednisolone sodium phosphate 0·5% ◊ prednisolone.

Minims rose bengal single dose eye-drops contain rose bengal 1% and is used as a stain to diagnose damage to the cornea of the eye.

Minims saline single dose eyedrops contain sodium chloride 0·9% and is used to irrigate the eye.

Minims sulphacetamide single dose eyedrops contain sulphacetamide sodium 10% ◊ sulphacetamide.

Minims thymoxamine single dose eye-drops contain thymoxamine hydro-chloride 0·5% ◊ thymoxamine. Used to reverse effects of sympathomimetic drugs that cause constriction of the pupil.

Minims tropicamide single dose eye-drops contain tropicamide 0·5% or 1% ◊ tropicamide.

Min-i-Jet ◊ adrenaline.

Minocin ◊ minocycline.

minocycline (Minocin; minocycline hydrochloride) is a tetracycline anti-biotic. *Dose:* By mouth, 200 mg initially and then 100 mg every twelve hours.

Minodiab ◊ glipizide.

Minodiab tablets ◊ glipizide.

Minovlar: Each tablet contains norethisterone acetate 1 mg and ethinyloestradiol 0·05 mg. It is an oral contraceptive drug.

Minovlar ED is an oral contraceptive. Each tablet contains ethinyloestradiol

0·05 mg and norethisterone acetate 1 mg. The ED pack contains seven in-active tablets so that one tablet has to be taken each day for 28 days and the next pack started without a break.

minoxidil (Loniten) is a vasodilator drug used to treat severe hypertension. *Adverse effects:* Increase in oede-ma and heart rate. Increased growth of hair which is reversible, skin rashes, weight gain, gastro-intestinal discom-fort and breast tenderness may occur. *Precautions:* It should not be given to patients with oedema and it should always be given along with a diuretic or reduced salt intake. It may aggravate heart failure and angina. Lower doses are needed in patients on renal dialysis. Its combination with guane-thidine-like drugs may produce a sev-ere reduction in blood pressure. *Dose:* By mouth, 5 to 50 mg daily in divided doses.

Mintec capsules ◊ peppermint oil.

Mintezol ◊ thiabendazole.

Minulet is an oral contraceptive tablet containing the oestrogen ethinyloes-tradiol 30 micrograms and the prog-estogen gestodene 75 micrograms.

Miochol ◊ acetylcholine.

Miol antiseptic cream contains sodium chloride 2·1%, calcium chloride 0·2%, magnesium chloride 1·5%, alu-minium chlorhydroxyallantoinate 1%, chlorphenesin 0·1%, camphor 4%.

Miol antiseptic lotion contains sodium chloride 1·98%, calcium chloride 0·17%, magnesium chloride 1·42%, aluminium chlorhydroxyallantoinate 1% in a saturated aqueous solution of camphor.

Miraxid tablets contains pivmpicillin 125 mg and pivmecillinam 100 mg ◊ pivampicillin ◊ pivmecillinam. *Dose:* 2 twice daily.

Mist Nerve Sedative contains potassium bromide mixture 100%.

mithracin ◊ plicamycin.

mitobronitol (Myelobromol) is an anti-cancer drug. *Adverse effects:* It may produce nausea, vomiting and diarrhoea, loss of hair (alopecia), skin rashes, irregular periods and bone-marrow damage leading to severe blood disorders. *Precautions:* It should be given with utmost caution to patients suspected of having impaired bone-marrow function. *Dose:* Varies according to disorder being treated.

mitomycin (Mitomycin C K yowa) is an anti-cancer antibiotic. It interferes with cell multiplication. *Adverse effects:* These include blood disorders, loss of hair, impairment of kidney and liver function, fever, nausea and vomiting. *Dose:* By intravenous injection, depends upon the condition being treated.

Mitoxana ◊ ifosfamide.

mitozantrone (Novantrone) is an anti-cancer drug. *Adverse effects:* These include loss of hair (alopecia), blood disorders, anaemia, loss of appetite, diarrhoea, fatigue, weakness, fever, bleeding from the gut, changes in liver function and heart failure. *Precau-*

tions: It should not be used in women who are pregnant or breast feeding. *Dose:* 14 mg/m^2 as a single intravenous dose every three weeks, dose should be adjusted according to blood count results.

Mobilan ◊ indomethacin.

Modantis cream contains antazoline hydrochloride 1%, cetrimide 0·5%, titanium dioxide 2%, and allantoin 0·5%, with cetostearyl alcohol, liquid paraffin, and water.

Modecate ◊ fluphenazine.

Moditen ◊ fluphenazine.

Moditen Enanthate ◊ fluphenazine.

Modrasone cream and ointment ◊ alclometasone.

Modrenal ◊ trilostane.

Moducren is used to treat raised blood pressure. Each tablet contains hydrochlorothiazide 25 mg, amiloride 2·5 mg and timolol 10 mg.

Moduret 25 is a diuretic. Each tablet contains amiloride hydrochloride 2·5 mg and hydrochlorothiazide 25 mg.

Moduretic is a diuretic. Each tablet contains hydrochlorothiazide 50 mg and amiloride hydrochloride 5 mg. *Dose:* 1 to 2 daily, maximum 4 daily.

Mogadon ◊ nitrazepam.

Molcer ◊ docusate sodium.

Molipaxin ◊ trazodone.

molybdenum is a trace element essential to life. It is a component of several enzymes.

Monaspor ◊ cefsulodin.

Moncler Derma Gel contains *N*-ethyl-9-(4-methoxy-2,3,6-trimethylphenyl)-3, 7-dimethyl-2, 4, 5, 8-nonatetraenamide (Vibenoid) and D-panthenol.

Moncler Derma Lotion: Active ingredients are allantoin, salicylic acid, phenoxyethanol, and D-panthenol ethyl ether.

Monistat ◊ miconazole.

Monit (isosorbide mononitrate) ◊ isosorbide.

monocalcium phosphate ◊ calcium tetrahydrogen phosphate.

Mono-Cedocard (isosorbide mononitrate) ◊ isosorbide.

Monocor tablets ◊ bisoprolol.

Monoparin ◊ heparin.

Monoparin CA ◊ heparin calcium.

Monophane: Read section on insulins.

monosulfiram (Tetmosol) is used to treat scabies. *Adverse effects:* Rarely it can produce a rash. *Precautions:* It contains 25 per cent industrial methylated spirit and is *highly inflammable*. It should not be stored in a cold place because it crystallizes. The drinking of alcohol should be avoided for 48 hours before and 48 hours after the application of monosulfiram to the skin. (It is related to disulfiram.) *Application:* Apply diluted two to three parts with water to the entire body after a good wash in soap and water. Can be repeated daily for two to three days in difficult cases.

Monotrim ◊ trimethoprim.

Monovent ◊ terbutaline.

Monovent LA are sustained release tablets of terbutaline ◊ terbutaline.

Monphytol paint for athlete's foot. Contains boric acid 2%, chlorbutol 3%, methyl undecenoate 5%, salicylic acid 31% and propyl undecenoate 1%.

Moorland Indigestion Tablets: Each contain bismuth aluminate 5·4 mg, magnesium trisilicate 29 mg, dried aluminium hydroxide 11·6 mg, heavy magnesium carbonate 94 mg, light kaolin 27 mg, and calcium carbonate 464 mg.

MOPP contains four anti-cancer drugs: mustine, vincristine (Oncovin), procarbazine and prednisolone. Read entries on each individual drug.

morazone is a mild pain-relieving drug, which has been used in combination with other pain-relieving drugs.

Morhulin ointment contains cod-liver oil 11.4% and zinc oxide 38%.

morphine (Duromorph; MST Continus; Oramorph solution, morphine hydrochloride and morphine sulphate; Nepenthe) is a narcotic pain reliever. It is more effective when injected than by mouth. Morphine is also used as a pre-operative medication combined with hyoscine or atropine. *Adverse effects:* Nausea, loss of appetite, constipation, vomiting and confusion may occur. It may also produce difficulty in passing urine, vertigo, drowsiness, restlessness, and change in mood. These effects occur more often if the patient is up and about rather than in bed. Sneezing and skin rashes may occur. *Precautions:* Babies and young children are very sensitive to the effects of morphine and it is not usually given to children under one year of age. Alarming and unusual reactions may occur in the elderly and the debilitated. It should not be used in patients with severe respiratory disorders and after operations on the gall-bladder. It should not be used in acute alcoholism and convulsive disorders. Its effects may be increased by M.A.O. inhibitor anti-depressant drugs and depressant drugs such as anaesthetics, sleeping drugs, sedatives and phenothiazine major tranquillizers. Tolerance quickly develops. *Drug dependence:* Drug dependence of the morphine type is a state arising from repeated use of morphine or a morphine-like drug. It is characterized by an overwhelming desire to go on taking the drug, by a tendency to increase the dose, and by psychic and physical dependence. Withdrawal symptoms include running eyes and nose, sneezing, trembling, headache, weakness, sweating, anxiety, insomnia, restlessness, nausea, loss of appetite, vomiting, diarrhoea, muscle cramps and a rise in temperature. *Dose:* By subutaneous or intramuscalar injection 10–15 mg every 4 hours for acute pain and 5–20 mg for chronic pain (or by mouth).

Morsep cream contains cetrimide 0·5%, vitamin A 70 units/g and calciferol 10 units/g.

Mothereze Tablets each contain dry extracts of raspberry leaf 27·7% and of senna leaf 11·1%.

Motilium ◊ domperidone.

Motipress is used to treat depression. Each tablet contains fluphenazine hydrochloride 1·5 mg and nortriptyline 30 mg. *Dose:* By mouth, daily, preferably at bedtime, for a maximum of 3 months.

Motival is used to treat depression. Each tablet contains nortriptyline 10 mg and fluphenazine hydrochloride 0·5 mg. *Dose:* 1 tablet two to four times daily.

Motretinide is used in a similar way to tretinoin to treat acne.

Motrin ◊ ibuprofen.

Movelat cream is a rubefacient. It contains corticosteroid extract 1%, heparinoid 0·2% and salicylic acid 2%.

Moxalactam ◊ latamoxef.

Mrs Cullen's Cuts 'n' Grazes Antiseptic Cream contains chlorhexidine gluconate solution 0·5%.

Mrs Cullen's Lem-Clear: Each single-dose sachet contains aspirin 585 mg, salicylamide 95 mg, caffeine 60 mg, and ascorbic acid 80 mg.

Mrs Cullen's Powders contain aspirin 600 mg, caffeine 62 mg, calcium phosphate 34.08 mg, saccharin sodium 3·84 mg, and sodium lauryl sulphate 80 micrograms.

MST Continus ◊ morphine.

Mucaine: Each 5 ml contains oxethazine 10 mg, aluminium hydroxide gel 4·75 ml and magnesium hydroxide 100 mg. It is an antacid mixture containing a topical anaesthetic. It is used to treat oesophagitis. *Dose:* 5 to 10 ml four times daily before meals and at bedtime.

Mucodyne ◊ carbocisteine.

Mucogel suspension is an antacid mixture containing dried aluminium hydroxide gel 220 mg and magnesium hydroxide 195 mg in each 5 ml.

Mucogel tablets contain 400 mg of dried aluminium hydroxide gel and 400 mg of magnesium hydroxide ◊ aluminium hydroxide and magnesium hydroxide. Used as antacids to treat indigestion and peptic ulcers.

Mu-Cron liquid contains phenylpropanolamine 0·2% and guaiphenesin 0·5%. It is used to treat coughs.

Mu-Cron Liquid for Children contains phenylpropanolamine hydrochloride 0·2% and guaiphenesin 0·5%.

Mu-Cron Tablets each contain guaiphenesin 32 mg, phenylpropanolamine hydrochloride 25 mg, prepared ipecacuanha 11 mg, and paracetamol 250 mg. It is used to treat coughs and the common cold.

Muflin syrup is used to treat coughs. Each 5 ml contains dextromethorphan hydrobromide 10 mg, sodium citrate 130 mg, pheniramine maleate 7·5 mg and citric acid 20 mg. *Dose:* By mouth, 5 to 10 ml three or four times daily.

Mulcets Mouth Ulcer Tablets each contain ascorbic acid 25 mg and cetylpyridinium chloride 1 mg.

Multibionta injection is a vitamin supplement.

Multilind ◊ nystatin.

Multiparin ◊ heparin.

Multivite pellets contain 2,500 units of vitamin A, thiamine 0·5 mg, vitamin C 12·5 mg, and calciferol 0·0625 mg. *Dose:* 2 pellets daily by mouth.

Multone Iron Vitamin Tonic Tablets each contain ferrous gluconate 150 mg, ascorbic acid 5 mg, nicotinamide 3 mg, thiamine hydrochloride 0·5 mg, and riboflavine 0·3 mg.

Mumpsvax is a brand of mumps vaccine.

mupirocin (Bactroban) is used to treat bacterial skin infections.

Murine eye-drops contain naphazoline hydrochloride 0·012%.

Muripsin: Each tablet contains glutamic acid hydrochloride 500 mg and pepsin 35 mg. It is used to treat patients who are not producing enough acid and pepsin in their stomachs. *Dose:* 1 to 2 tablets with meals.

muscarine ◊ acetylcholine.

mustard oil is very irritant to the skin

and can produce blistering. In very dilute concentrations it is used as a rubefacient.

mustine (mustine hydrochloride; mechlorethamine) is an anti-cancer drug. *Adverse effects:* These include nausea, vomiting, diarrhoea, peptic ulceration, drowsiness, psychosis, loss of hair (alopecia), deafness and noises in the ears (tinnitus), several months without a period (amenorrhoea), reduced sperm count and skin rashes. Damage to the bone marrow may occur, leading to severe blood disorders. Injections may produce pain, irritation and thrombophlebitis at the site. *Precautions:* It should not be used in pregnancy, or in the presence of any infection or blood disorder. Evidence of impaired bone-marrow function should give rise to utmost caution in its use. *Dose:* Varies according to the disorder being treated.

MVPP contains four anti-cancer drugs: mustine, vinblastine, procarbazine and prednisolone. Read entries on each individual drug.

Myambutol ◊ ethambutol.

Mycardol ◊ pentaerythritol.

Mycifradin ◊ neomycin.

Myciguent ◊ neomycin.

Mycil ◊ chlorphenesin.

Mycota ◊ undecenoic acid.

Mydriacyl ◊ tropicamide.

Mydrilate ◊ cyclopentolate.

Myelobromol ◊ mitobronitol.

Mygdalon ◊ metoclopramide.

Myleran ◊ busulphan.

Mynah is used to treat tuberculosis. The tablets contain ethambutol and isoniazid in various strengths. *Dose:* Varies according to the severity of the disorder.

Myocrisin ◊ gold.

Myolgin pain-relievers: Each tablet contains paracetamol 200 mg, aspirin 200 mg, codeine phosphate 5 mg and caffeine citrate 15 mg. *Dose:* By mouth, 1 or 2 tablets in water three or four times daily.

Myotonine ◊ bethanecol.

myrrh is a gum-resin obtained from the stem of *Commiphora molmol*. It acts as an astringent to mucous membranes and is used in mouth washes and gargles. It has a carminative effect when taken by mouth.

Mysoline ◊ primidone.

Mysteclin tablets contain tetracycline hydrochloride 250 mg and nystatin 250,000 units. *Dose:* 1 four times daily.

Mysteclin syrup contains tetracycline 125 mg and amphotericin 25 mg per 5 ml.

N Tonic: Each 5 ml contains calcium hypophosphite 7·5 mg, potassium hypophosphite 7·5 mg, manganese hypophosphite 2·5 mg, ferric hypophosphite 1·25 mg, thiamine hydrochloride 0·53 mg, potassium citrate 2·2 mg, phosphoric acid 0·0009 ml, and quassia extract 2·5 mg.

nabilone (Cesamet) is chemically related to one of the constituents of cannabis. It is used to control nausea and vomiting in patients taking anti-cancer drugs. *Adverse effects:* These include drowsiness, confusion, depression, tremors and blurred vision. *Precautions:* It should be used with care in patients taking depressant drugs such as narcotic analgesics. *Dose:* By mouth, 1 to 2 mg twice daily.

nabumetone (Relifex) is a non-steroidal anti-inflammatory pain reliever used to treat rheumatoid arthritis and related disorders. *Adverse effects* include nausea, indigestion, diarrhoea, constipation, stomach pain and wind, headache, drowsiness, skin rash and itching. *Precautions:* Patients allergic to aspirin should not take this drug. It should be used with caution in patients with impaired kidney function and in patients with a history of peptic ulcers. *Dose:* By mouth, two 500 mg tablets at night and a third one in the morning if the pain is severe. Elderly people should not take more than two tablets in 24 hours (i.e. not more than 1 g).

Nacton ◊ poldine.

nadolol (Corgard) is a beta-receptor blocker used to treat angina, and hypertension. *Adverse effects* and *Precautions* ◊ propranolol. *Dose:* By mouth, for raised blood pressure 80 mg daily; angina 40 mg daily. Increase dose at weekly intervals to a maximum of 240 mg daily.

naftidrofuryl (Praxilene; naftidrofuryl oxalate) dilates blood vessels and is used in the treatment of disorders of the circulation. *Adverse effects:* Nausea and epigastric pain. *Dose:* By mouth, 100 to 200 mg three times daily. By injection, 200 mg over at least 90 minutes, twice daily.

nalbuphine (Nubain) is a moderate to severe pain reliever used preoperatively. *Adverse effects* and *Precautions* ◊ morphine. It may produce sedation and the dose should be reduced in patients with impaired kidney function. *Dose:* By subcutaneous, intramuscular or intravenous injection, 10 to 20 mg every three to six hours, as required.

Nalcrom is an oral preparation of sodium cromoglycate used to treat ulcerative colitis and other ulcerative disorders of the bowel. ◊ sodium cromoglycate. *Dose:* By mouth, 200 mg four times daily.

nalidixic acid (Negram; Uriben) is an anti-bacterial drug. It is used in the treatment of infections of the bladder and kidneys and gut. *Adverse effects:* Nausea, vomiting, diarrhoea, dizziness, drowsiness, weakness, itching skin and rashes may occur. Muscle weakness and pains, bleeding from the gut, fever and sunlight sensitivity of the skin have been reported. Occasionally, headache, blurred vision, depression, confusion, hallucinations and excitement may occur. These are transient and reversible. Blood disorders and convulsions have occurred very rarely. *Precautions:* Nalidixic acid should be given with caution to patients with impaired kidney or liver function or with disorders of the nervous system. It should also be given with caution to patients subject to convulsions or with severe respiratory disorders. It should not be given during the first three months of pregnancy or to babies under one month of age. Exposure to strong sunlight should be avoided during treatment. *Dose:* By mouth, 1 g four times daily. Half this dosage for prolonged treatment.

nalorphine (nalorphine hydrobromide) reduces or abolishes most of the effects produced by morphine and related substances. It is used to treat acute poisoning by these drugs. Read section on morphine and narcotic pain relievers. *Adverse effects:* Nalorphine may cause drowsiness, irritability, sweating, restlessness, nausea, slowing of the heart rate, and a fall in blood pressure. Given alone it may produce severe mental disturbance and when given to narcotic addicts it may trigger off withdrawal symptoms. *Dose:* 5 to 10 mg intravenously up to a maximum of 40 mg.

naloxone (Narcan; naloxone hydrochloride) has similar uses to those described under nalorphine, but it is more potent and it is a specific antagonist of pentazocine. *Adverse effects:* In patients dependent upon narcotic drugs naloxone will produce typical withdrawal symptoms. It may produce nausea and vomiting. *Dose:* 0·1 to 0·2 mg by intravenous, intramuscular or subcutaneous injection – repeated every two to three minutes according to needs of the patient.

nandrolone (Deca-Durabolin; nandrolone decanoate) is an anabolic (body-building) steroid. *Adverse effects* and *Precautions:* These are similar to

those discussed under testosterone. Jaundice has not been reported after its use. *Dose:* By intramuscular injection, 50 to 100 mg every three or four weeks. Durabolin (nandrolone-phenylpropionate): by intramuscular injection, 25 to 50 mg weekly.

naphazoline (naphazoline nitrate, naphazoline hydrochloride) constricts small blood vessels and is used in nose drops to reduce stuffiness and running noses. It is also used in eye drops to relieve inflammation of the eyes. *Adverse effects:* overdose or accidental swallowing may produce drowsiness or coma. *Precautions:* Frequent or prolonged use of naphazoline nose drops may produce congestion in the nose; therefore use the smallest dose at not less than four- or six-hour intervals.

Napisan is a preparation for cleansing and disinfecting babies' napkins, based on potassium monopersulphate and sodium chloride.

Naprosyn ◊ naproxen.

naproxen (Laraflex; Naprosyn; Synflex) is an anti-rheumatic drug. *Adverse effects:* Skin rashes, and angio-oedema (swelling of the lips and mouth) have been reported in patients who are hypersensitive to aspirin. Naproxen may precipitate bronchial asthma in a patient with a history of bronchial asthma or allergic disorders. Caution should be used in patients who have developed similar sensitivities to other related anti-theumatic drugs. Patients may experience abdominal discomfort, headache, insomnia, inability to concentrate, tinnitus and vertigo. Blood disorders, peptic ulceration and kidney damage may occur rarely. *Precautions:* It should be used with caution in patients with a history of peptic ulcers, allergic disorders (particularly asthma, and hypersensitivity to aspirin, other salicylates and related anti-rheumatic drugs) and renal or hepatic impairment. Its use in suppositories must be with caution in patients with proctitis and haemorrhoids. Patients receiving hydantoins and anticoagulants should be carefully observed for signs of overdose. *Dose:* By mouth, 500 to 1,000 mg per day in two divided doses (e.g., twelve-hourly) with meals. Also available as suppositories, one at night.

Narcan ◊ naloxone.

narcotine ◊ noscapine.

Nardil ◊ phenelzine.

Narphen ◊ phenazocine.

Nasciodine contains iodine 1·26%, menthol 0·59%, methyl salicylate 3·87%, essential oil of camphor 3·87%, and turpentine oil 3·87%.

Naseptin cream contains chlorhexidine hydrochloride 0·1% and neomycin sulphate 0·5%. It is applied to the inside of the nostrils to eradicate staphylococcal bacteria (which cause boils) from the nose.

natamycin (Pimafucin; Tymasil) is an antifungal drug. *Adverse effects:* These include nausea and diarrhoea. It may irritate the skin. *Dose:* Varies according to disorder being treated. Used in suspensions, creams and vaginal tablets.

Natirose is an anti-anginal drug containing glyceryl trinitrate 750 micrograms, ethylmorphine hydrochloride 3 mg and hyoscyamine hydrobromide 50 micrograms in each tablet.

Natrilix ◊ indapamide.

Natuderm is an emollient cream containing lipids and glycerol.

Natulan ◊ procarbazine.

Natusan Baby Cream contains boric acid 2·85%, borax 0·15%, and glycerol in an emollient basis.

Natusan Baby Lotion contains polyoxyethylene alcohol 0·55%, polyoxyethylene derivative of wool fat 0·87%, carboxypolymethylene 0·78%, and glycerol 2·73%, in an emollient basis.

Navidrex ◊ cyclopenthiazide.

Navidrex-K is a combined diuretic and potassium supplement containing cyclopenthiazide 0·25 mg and potassium 8·1 mmol for sustained release ◊ cyclopenthiazide ◊ potassium.

Naxogin-500 ◊ nimorazole.

Nazex Nasal Spray contains phenylephrine hydrochloride 0·5% in an iso-osmotic basis.

Nebcin ◊ tobramycin.

Necol paint is used for removing warts. It contains salicylic acid 25%.

nedocromil sodium (Tilade aerosol) is used to prevent attacks of asthma. It stops the inflammation that follows an allergic reaction. *Adverse effects* include a bitter taste in the mouth, nausea and headache. *Precautions:* It should be used with caution in pregnancy and breast-feeding mothers, particularly during the first three months of pregnancy. *Dose:* Two doses, twice daily from a metered dose, pressurized aerosol.

nefopam (Acupan) is a non-narcotic pain reliever which is rapidly acting. *Adverse effects:* Nausea, vomiting, dry mouth, lightheadedness, blurred vision, drowsiness, insomnia, sweating, headache and rapid beating of the heart. *Precautions:* It should not be used in the treatment of myocardial infarction. It should be used with caution in patients with impaired kidney or liver function. It should not be used in patients with a history of convulsions. Its effects may be additive to the effects produced by anti-cholinergic drugs and sympathomimetic drugs. *Dose:* By mouth, 30 to 90 mg three times daily. Intramuscular or intravenous injections 20 mg every six hours. Intravenous injections should be given slowly with the patient lying down for 20 minutes afterwards.

Negram ◊ nalidixic acid.

Nella Red oil is a rub for muscular pain, rheumatism and lumbago. It contains methyl nicotinate 1 g, ol. sinapis 25 ml, ol. caryoph. 1·5 ml, ol. red tax 0·01 g and ol. arachis to 100 ml.

Neo Baby Cream contains cetrimide 0·2%, benzalkonium chloride solution 0·1%, in a silicone/lanolin basis.

Neo Baby Mixture: Each 5 ml contains sodium bicarbonate 50 mg, ginger tinc-ture, strong 0·01 ml, and dill oil 0·005 ml.

Neocon 1/35 tablets contain ethinyloestradiol 35 micrograms and norethisterone 1 mg. It is an oral contraceptive.

Neo-Cytamen ◊ hydroxocobalamin.

Neogest tablets contain norgestrel 0·075 mg. It is a progestogen-only oral contraceptive.

Neolate ◊ neomycin.

Neo-Medrone cream contains methylprednisolone acetate 2·5 mg, neomycin sulphate 2·5 mg, aluminium chlorhydroxide complex 100 mg and sulphur 50 mg. It is used to treat acne.

Neo-Mercazole ◊ carbimazole.

neomycin (Mycifradin, Myciguent; Nivemycin; neomycin sulphate) is an antibiotic. Its use is restricted to treating infections of the skin, ears and eyes, and also bowel infections. *Adverse effects:* Neomycin should not be given by injection because it causes kidney damage, deafness, and disorders of balance after a few days of treatment. The deafness is permanent. Allergy may occur, producing skin rashes and itching after local application to the eye, ears or skin. Neomycin increases the effects of drugs used to treat blood pressure, thiazide diuretics and certain neuromuscular blocking agents used in surgical anaesthesia. *Precautions:* It should not be given by injection, applied to raw areas or wounds, or given by mouth for prolonged periods. Prolonged use in creams, ointments and drops should be avoided as it leads to allergy which may be obscured but not prevented by the use of preparations of neomycin containing corticosteroids. *Dose:* As an intestinal antiseptic, 2 to 8 g by mouth daily in divided doses.

Neo-Naclex ◊ bendrofluazide.

Neo-Naclex-K is a diuretic with added potassium. Each tablet contains 2·5 mg of bendrofluazide and 630 mg of potassium chloride in a two-layer tablet, the potassium chloride having a special coating. *Dose:* 1 to 4 tablets daily as a single dose.

Neophryn nasal spray ◊ phenylephrine.

Neosporin eye drops contain polymyxin B sulphate 0·25% and gramicidin 25 units in each ml.

neostigmine (Prostigmin; neostigmine; bromide; neostigmine methylsulphate) acts upon the parasympathetic division of the autonomic nervous system. It is an anticholinesterase drug which prevents the destruction of acetylcholine by cholinesterase thus allowing the concentration of acetylcholine to build-up. It is used in the treatment and diagnosis of myasthenia gravis, to reverse the effects of muscle relaxant drugs such as tubocurarine used in surgery and to prolong the action of muscle relaxant drugs such as suxamethonium. *Adverse effects:* Nausea, vomiting, increased salivation, diarrhoea, abdominal cramps. Signs of overdose are increased gastrointestinal discomfort, bronchial secretions, and sweating, involuntary defaecation and micturition, miosis, nystagmus, bradycardia, hypotension, agitation, excessive dreaming, and weakness eventually leading to fasciculation and paralysis. *Precautions:* It should be used with caution in patients suffering from asthma, bradycardia, recent myocardial infarction, epilepsy, hypotension, Parkinsonism, vagotonia, pregnancy. Atropine or other antidote to muscarinic effects may be necessary (particularly when neostigmine is given by injection) but it should not be given routinely as it may mask signs of overdosage. It should not be used in patients with intestinal or urinary obstruction. *Dose:* By mouth, neostigmine bromide 75 to 300 mg or more, daily in divided doses at suitable intervals. For a child, neonate 1 to 5 mg every 4 hours, for older children 15 to 60 mg daily in divided doses. By subcutaneous, intramuscular, or intravenous injection, neostigmine methylsulphate 1 to 2·5 mg daily in divided doses at suitable intervals. For a child, neonate 50 to 250 micrograms every 4 hours, for older children 200 to 500 micrograms daily in divided doses.

Neovita Capsules each contain vitamin A 2,400 units, vitamin B_1 2·5 mg, vitamin B_2 2·5 mg, vitamin B_6 1 mg, vitamin B_{12} 4·9 micrograms, vitamin C 40 mg, vitamin D 240 units, vitamin E 2 mg, nicotinamide 20 mg, calcium phosphate 100 mg, ginseng 100 mg, magnesium oxide 10 mg, copper sulphate 2 mg, zinc oxide 5 mg, manganese sulphate 2 mg, dried ferrous sulphate 33 mg, calcium pantothenate 10 mg, and lecithin 9·5 mg.

Nepenthe ◊ morphine.

Nephril ◊ polythiazide.

Nericur gel is used in the treatment of acne. It contains benzoyl peroxide ◊ benzoyl peroxide.

Nerisone ◊ diflucortolone.

Nestargel is used for habitual vomiting in infants. It consists of carob seed flour 96·5% and calcium lactate 3·5%.

Nethaprin expectorant contains in each 10 ml etafedrine hydrochloride 40 mg, bufylline 120 mg, doxylamine succinate 12 mg and guaiphenesin 200 mg. It is used to treat coughs. *Dose:* 5 to 10 ml three- to four-hourly.

Netillin ◊ netilmicin.

netilmicin (Netillin; netilmicin sulphate) is an antibiotic with similar effects and adverse effects to gentamicin. *Dose:* By injection, 4 to 6 mg per kg body-weight daily, in divided doses every 8 to 12 hours.

Neulactil ◊ pericyazine.

Neurodyne is a mild pain-reliever. Each tablet contains paracetamol 500 mg and codeine phosphate 8 mg. *Dose:* 1 to 2 three- to four-hourly.

Neutradonna powder and tablets contain aluminium sodium silicate 650 mg with belladonna alkaloids 0·048 mg (powder contains 0·075 mg). It is used to treat indigestion and peptic ulcers. *Dose:* Powder: 1 to 2 level teaspoonfuls in milk or water up to four times daily after meals. Tablets: 2 to 3 chewed three times daily and at bedtime.

niacin ◊ nicotinic acid.

niacinamide (nicotinamide) is a member of the vitamin B group. For effects see nicotinic acid.

nicardipine (Cardene; nicardipine hydrochloride) is a calcium anatagonist used to treat angina and raised blood pressure. *Adverse effects* include dizziness, headache, nausea, swelling of the ankles and palpitations. It may also cause abdominal pain, diarrhoea, constipation, vomiting, loss of appetite, heartburn, lassitude, drowsiness, itching, skin rash, backache, frequency of passing urine and insomnia. It may make angina worse, cause disorders of heart rhythm and impair the functioning of the kidneys and liver. *Precautions:* A change from a beta-blocker to nicardipine should be carried out with caution. The dose of beta-blocker should be reduced slowly over ten days. Some patients can get angina within half an hour of starting the drug; if this happens the treatment should be stopped. It should be used with caution in patients with impaired kidney or liver function. Infrequently, it can cause a fall in blood pressure upon standing up from a sitting or lying position (orthostatic or postural hypotension). *Dose:* By mouth, 60 mg to 120 mg per day in three divided doses.

niclosamide (Yomesan) is used to treat infestation with tapeworms. *Dose:* 2 g as a single dose. The tablets should be chewed.

Nicrobrevin Anti-Smoking Capsules each contain menthyl valerianate 100 mg, quinine 15 mg, camphor 10 mg, and eucalyptus oil 10 mg.

nicofuranose (Bradilan) dilates blood vessels and is used in the treatment of Raynaud's disease and similar disorders of the circulation. It is also used to lower high blood fat levels. *Adverse effects* and *Precautions* ◊ nicotinic acid. *Dose:* By mouth, 500 to 750 mg three times a day.

Nicorette is a chewing gum containing nicotine. It is used as an aid to stop smoking. It should not be used in pregnancy.

nicotinamide (niacinamide) has the effects of nicotinic acid. It is a member of the vitamin B group.

nicotinic acid (niacin) is a member of the vitamin B group. It is used to treat disorders of the circulation since it causes vasodilatation. It is also used to lower blood fat levels in arterial disease (atherosclerosis). *Adverse effects:* In doses used for this purpose it may cause flushing, dry skin, itching, skin rashes, nausea, vomiting, diarrhoea, headache, abdominal cramps, debility, loss of appetite, flare-up of peptic ulcers, jaundice, and increased blood sugar and uric acid levels. It may increase the effects of drugs used to treat raised blood pressure. *Dose:* The dose used to treat disorders of circulation is 50 to 250 mg daily in divided doses. Higher doses have been used to treat high blood fat levels.

nicotinic acid amide ◊ nicotinamide.

nicotinyl alcohol ◊ nicotinyl tartrate.

nicotinyl tartrate (Ronicol) is a vasodilator drug used to treat disorders of the circulation. It may produce flushing and faintness. Slight swelling of the face, nausea, vomiting and a fall in blood pressure may occur. It should be given with caution to patients with disorders of the arteries supplying the brain. *Dose:* By mouth, 25 to 50 mg four times daily.

nicoumalone (Sinthrome) is an anticoagulant drug with effects and uses similar to those described under phenindione. It may cause nausea, loss of appetite and dizziness. It is used to prevent blood from clotting. *Dose:* By mouth; 8 to 16 mg initially; maintenance, 4 to 12 mg daily according to blood tests.

Nidazol ◊ metronidazole.

nifedipine (Adalat, Adalat Retard) is used to treat angina and hypertension. It relaxes arterial muscles in the heart and peripheral circulation. *Adverse effects:* Headache, flushing and lethargy may occur. *Precautions:* It should be used with caution in patients with poor heart function or diabetes. It should not be used in women of childbearing age. *Dose:* By mouth, 10 to 20 mg two or three times daily.

Niferex tablets and **elixir** contain a polysaccharide-iron complex. *Dose:* By mouth, 2 tablets or 5 ml once or twice daily.

Night Nurse: Each 20 ml contains promethazine hydrochloride 20 mg, dextromethorphan hydrobromide 15 mg, paracetamol 500 mg, and alcohol 3·08 ml.

Nigroids pellets contain liquorice extract 68·6% and menthol 2·06%.

nikethamide stimulates the respiratory centre in the brain and also improves the circulation. It is used to treat clinical shock by intravenous injection of 0·5 to 2 g.

nilbite is used to prevent nail biting and thumbsucking. It contains capsicum oleoresin 0·25% and sucrose octoacetate 0·66%.

Nilstim ◊ methylcellulose.

nimodipine (Nimotop) is a calcium-channel blocker used to relieve spasm of brain arteries which may occur following bleeding between the membranes of the brain (subarachnoid haemorrhage). *Adverse effects:* Fall in blood pressure, flushing, headache, increased or decreased heart rate, transient abnormal tests of liver function. *Precautions:* Do not use in swelling of the brain (cerebral oedema), if the pressure inside the brain is increased, in patients with impaired kidney function, or in pregnancy. Check blood pressure at very regular intervals. Nimodipine is incompatible with PVC, avoid contact during treatment. *Dose:* 1 mg per hour by intravenous infusion for first two hours followed by 2 mg per hour for a minimum of five days, maximum of 14 days. Start with 0·5 mg per hour in patients who weigh 70 kg or less or who have an unstable blood pressure.

nimorazole (Naxogin-500) is used to treat trichomonal vaginitis. Sexual partners should also be treated even if they are free from symptoms. It is also effective against giardiasis, amoebiasis and acute ulcerative gingivitis. *Adverse effects:* Nausea and vomiting.

Intolerance to alcohol could possibly occur (see disulfiram) because it occurs with other nitroimidazoles. *Precautions:* It should not be given to breast-feeding mothers or to patients with disorders of their central nervous system. It should be used with utmost caution in pregnancy. It should not be used in patients with marked impairment of kidney function. *Dose:* By mouth for trichomoniasis, 2 g as a single dose with a main meal. For acute ulcerative gingivitis 500 mg twice daily for two days; for giardiasis or amoebiasis 500 mg twice daily for five days.

Nimotop intravenous infusion ◊ nimodipine.

nipastat is used as a preservative in cosmetics and medicines.

Nipride ◊ sodium nitroprusside.

niridazole is used to kill and remove guinea worms from tissues.

Nirolex Expectorant Linctus contains in each 5 ml guaiphenesin 50 mg, ephedrine hydrochloride 15 mg, menthol 1 mg, glycerol 1 ml, and sucrose 2·5 g.

Nitoman ◊ tetrabenazine.

Nitrados ◊ nitrazepam.

nitrazepam (Mogadon; Nitrados; Noctesed; Remnos; Somnite; Surem; Unisomnia) is a benzodiazepine used principally as a sleeping drug. *Adverse effects:* Nitrazepam may cause hangover and lightheadedness. In elderly patients it may cause confusion. *Precautions:* Nitrazepam may reduce ability to drive a motor vehicle or operate machinery. Alcohol and other depressants may increase the effects of nitrazepam. *Drug dependence:* Nitrazepam may cause dependence of the barbiturate/alcohol type. *Dose:* By mouth, 5 to 10 mg at night (half this dose in the elderly).

nitric acid is corrosive and has been used to 'burn' off warts. Its astringent actions have been used in the past to treat diarrhoea.

Nitrocine ◊ glyceryl trinitrate.

Nitrocontin Continus ◊ glyceryl trinitrate.

nitrofurantoin (Macrodantin; Urantoin; Furadantin) is an antibacterial drug. Its mode of action is unknown. It is excreted in high concentration in the urine and its principal use is in the treatment of infections of the urine which are prolonged and cannot be treated by other drugs. *Adverse effects:* Nausea, abdominal discomfort and drowsiness may occur on full dosage – these disappear on reduction of the dose. Skin rashes, nerve damage (peripheral neuritis) and an acute respiratory disorder (asthma) have been reported. These are more common in patients with impaired kidney function and patients on prolonged treatment with large doses. Blood disorders and liver damage may occur. *Precautions:* Nitrofurantoin should not be taken by patients with impaired kidney function or by patients with a genetic disease which causes a fault in glucose metabolism (deficiency of glucose-6-phosphate-dehydrogenase) since they may develop haemolytic anaemia. It should never be used in patients who have previously developed allergy or asthma whilst on nitrofurantoin. *Dose:* By mouth, 50 to 150 mg four times daily; preferably 5 to 8 mg per kg of body-weight for seven to fourteen days.

nitroglycerin ◊ glyceryl trinitrate.

Nitrolingual is an aerosol form of glyceryl trinitrate. *Dose:* 1 to 3 sprays under the tongue as required.

Nitronal injection contains glyceryl trinitrate ◊ glyceryl trinitrate.
nitrophenol is used to treat fungal skin infections.

nitrous ether spirit has the vasodilator effects of other nitrites. It has a slight diuretic action.

nitrous oxide is used for induction and maintenance of anaesthesia and, in sub-anaesthesia concentrations for pain relief in a variety of situations. It is also known as laughing gas.

Nivaquine ◊ chloroquine.

Nivea Creme is a water-in-oil emulsion prepared from solid alcohols of the cholesterol series and neutral hydrocarbons.

Nivemycin ◊ neomycin.

Nixoderm ointment is used to treat cuts and skin irritation. It contains benzoic acid 6%, salicylic acid 2·5% and precipitated sulphur 4·6%.

Nizatidine (Axid) is an H_2 receptor blocker used to heal and prevent stomach and duodenal ulcers. *Adverse effects:* Headache, weakness, chest pain, painful muscles, bad dreams, sleepiness, runny nose, sore throat, cough, itching, sweating, abnormal tests for liver function. *Warning:* Use with caution in patients with impaired kidney or liver function, in pregnancy or in breast-feeding mothers. *Dose:* By mouth, 300 mg in the evening for four to eight weeks or 150 mg morning and evening. Prevention of duodenal ulcers, 150 mg in the evening for up to twelve months.

Nizoral ◊ ketoconazole.

Nobrium ◊ medazepam.

Noctec ◊ chloral hydrate.

Noctesed ◊ nitrazepam.

Noltam tablets ◊ tamoxifen.

Noludar ◊ methyprylone.

Nolvadex ◊ tamoxifen.

Nolvadex Forte tablets contains tamoxifen 40 mg ◊ tamoxifen.

nonivamide is related to capsicum and is used as a rubefacient.

nonoxynol is a spermicide used in contraceptive preparations.

nonyl phenol ethylene oxide condensate is a surfactant.

Noradran syrup is used to treat bronchial asthma. Each 5 ml contains guaiphenesin 25 mg, diphenhydramine hydrochloride 5 mg, diprophylline 50 mg and ephedrine hydrochloride 7·5 mg. *Dose:* By mouth, 10 ml four hourly.

noradrenaline (Levophed; noradrenaline tartrate) is the chemical transmitter released by adrenergic nerves. It is used along with local anaesthetics to constrict blood vessels so that the anaesthetic works for a longer time; it is also used to treat clinical shock in order to try to keep the blood pressure up and the circulation diverted to the heart and brain. *Adverse effects* and *Precautions* ◊ adrenaline. *Dose:* 0·002 to 0·02 mg per minute by intravenous infusion according to the blood pressure of the patient.

Noratex cream contains cod-liver oil 2·15%, light kaolin 3·5%, talc 7·4%, wool fat 1·075% and zinc oxide 21·8%. Used to treat nappy rash, urinary rash and pressure sores.

Norcuron ◊ vecuronium bromide.

Nordox ◊ doxycycline.

norethisterone (Micronor; Noriday; Noristerat; Primolut N; S H 420; Utovlan, norethindrone; norethisterone acetate) is a progestogen. It is used to treat menstrual irregularities, to delay menstruation and to treat painful periods. It is included in several combined oral contraceptive pills and also in some progestogen-only oral contraceptive pills. *Adverse effects:* Norethisterone may cause headache, tension, depression, nausea, vomiting, breast fullness, fluid retention, weight gain, bleeding in between periods, deep voice, acne, hairiness, and masculinization of the unborn baby when doses of more than 15 mg a day are taken. Prolonged use may cause liver damage. *Precautions:* It should be taken with caution by patients with impaired liver function or a history of serious thrombosis. *Dose:* By mouth, 10 to 30 mg daily in divided doses.

Norflex ◊ orphenadrine.

Norgesic: Each tablet contains orphenadrine citrate 35 mg and paracetamol 450 mg. It is used as a pain reliever. *Dose:* 2 three times daily. Not recommended for children.

Norgeston tablets contain levonorgestrel 0·03 mg. It is a progestogen only oral contraceptive.

norgestrel is a progestogen.

Norgotin ear drops* contain ephedrine hydrochloride 1%, amethocaine hydrochloride 1%, chlorhexidine acetate 0·1% and propylene glycol 97·9%.

Noriday ◊ norethisterone.

Norimin tablets contain norethisterone 1 mg and ethinyloestradiol 0·035 mg. It is an oral contraceptive drug.

Norinyl-1: Each tablet contains norethisterone 1 mg and mestranol 0·05 mg. It is an oral contraceptive drug.

Norisen grass is used to treat allergy to pollens. It is prepared from 6 varieties of common grass pollen.

Noristerat injection ◊ norethisterone.

Norit capsules are used to treat diarrhoea. Each capsule contains activated charcoal 200 mg.

Normacol contains 62% sterculia. It is used to treat constipation. *Dose:* Gra-

nules by mouth, 1 to 2 heaped teaspoonfuls once or twice daily after meals or at bedtime.

Normasol Undine is a sterile solution of sodium chloride 0·9%.

Normax: Each capsule contains dioctyl sodium sulphosuccinate 60 mg and danthron 50 mg. It is used to treat constipation. *Dose:* 1 to 3 at night.

Normetic tablets contain amiloride hydrochloride 5 mg and hydrochlorothiazide 50 mg.

Normison ◊ temazepam.

nortriptyline (Allegron; Aventyl; nortriptyline hydrochloride) is a tricyclic antidepressant drug. It has effects and uses similar to those described under amitriptyline, but it produces less drowsiness. *Adverse effects* and *Precautions:* These are similar to those listed under amitriptyline. Nortriptyline should not be given to patients with glaucoma, patients who may develop retention of urine, patients with coronary artery disease or to patients with disordered heart rhythm. *Dose:* By mouth, 20 to 100 mg daily in divided doses.

Norval ◊ mianserin.

noscapine (narcotine, noscapine hydrochloride) is a cough suppressant. It is obtained from opium but it does not relieve pain or alter mood and it is unlikely to cause drug dependence. *Adverse effects:* Drowsiness, dizziness, headache, nausea and skin rash may occasionally occur. *Dose:* By mouth, 15 to 30 mg.

Nosor is used for nose sores due to colds. It contains eucalyptus oil 1%, pine oil 1%, dibromopropamidine isethionate 0·15%.

Nostroline contains eucalyptol 0·2%, menthol 0·3%, phenol 1·6%, and geranium oil 0·2%.

Nova-C chewable tablets contain vitamin A 1·5 mg and vitamin C 1 g.

Novantrone ◊ mitozantrone.

Novaprin ◊ ibuprofen.

Novasil Antacid Suspension contains in each 10 ml sodium bicarbonate 445 mg, light magnesium carbonate 333 mg, and peppermint oil 0·01 ml.

Novasil Antacid Tablets each contain sodium bicarbonate 15·6 mg, heavy kaolin 62·5 mg, calcium carbonate 220 mg, heavy magnesium carbonate 220 mg, and peppermint flavour 3·9 mg.

novobiocin (in Albamycin T; novobiocin calcium; novobiocin sodium) is an antibiotic. Bacterial resistance and adverse effects are common; its use should be restricted to certain infections by organisms resistant to other antibiotics and to infections of the gallbladder by organisms sensitive to novobiocin. *Adverse effects:* Nausea, vomiting, diarrhoea, abdominal colic, skin rashes and fever are fairly common. Novobiocin may produce blood disorders and impair liver function. *Precautions:* Novobiocin should not be given to children under six months of age and it should be given with caution during pregnancy.

Noxacorn Antiseptic Corn Remover contains benzocaine 2·2%, camphor 2·2%, salicylic acid 10·6%, iodine 0·11%, castor oil 2·6%, phenol 0·31%, and collodion to 100%.

Noxyflex solution (powder for reconstitution) contains noxythiolin 2·5 g and amethocaine hydrochloride 10 mg. It is used as a bladder irrigation to treat bladder infections.

Noxyflex S ◊ noxythiolin.

noxythiolin (Noxyflex-S) has antibacterial and antifungal actions and is used as a bladder washout in the treatment of bladder infections.

Noxzema Skin Cream contains camphor 0·37%, eucalyptus oil 0·12%, menthol 0·075%, clove oil 0·12%, and phenol 0·32%.

Nozinan ◊ methotrimeprazine.

Nubain injections (nalbuphine hydrochloride) ◊ nalbuphine.

Nucross Blackcurrant & Glycerine Pastilles are used to treat sore throats.

Nucross Bronchial Catarrh Pastilles are used to treat coughs and colds. Each pastille contains menthol 0·6%, peppermint oil 0·02%, aniseed oil 0·02%, creosote 0·15%, capsicin 0·001% and benzoin tincture 0·5%.

Nucross Children's Cough Syrup contains ipecacuanha tincture 6%, tolu syrup 18%, squill syrup 9%, anise oil 0·1%, squill vinegar 6%, chloroform spirit 3%, blackcurrant syrup 36% and glycerin 5%.

Nucross Glycerin, Lemon & Honey Linctus contains in each 5 ml squill syrup 0·5 ml, ipecacuanha liquid extract 0·02 ml, lemon oil 0·0013 ml, glycerin 0·25 ml, purified honey 0·5 g, citric acid 0·025 g and tolu syrup 0·5 ml.

Nucross Honey Glycerine & Lemon Pastilles are used to treat sore throats.

Nucross Menthol and Eucalyptus Pastilles are used to treat colds. Each pastille contains menthol 0·8% and eucalyptus oil 0·6%.

Nucross Pastilles of Gee's Linctus are used to treat coughs, each pastille contains opium tincture 1·25%, squill liquid extract 1·25%, benzoic acid 0·15%, cinnamic acid 0·01%, glacid acetic acid 0·83%, purified honey 9·68%, camphor 0·075% and aniseed oil 0·075%.

Nucross Toothache Tincture contains tannic acid 28·76%, creosote 1·25%, peppermint oil 12·5%, cassia oil 12·5% and clove oil 12·5%.

Nuelin ◊ theophylline.

Nuelin SA is a sustained-release form of theophylline.

Nulacin (each tablet contains milk, dextrins and maltose combined with magnesium trisilicate 230 mg, magnesium oxide 130 mg, calcium carbonate 130 mg, heavy magnesium carbonate 30 mg and peppermint oil). It is used to treat indigestion and peptic ulcers. *Dose:* 1 or more as required.

NU-K: Each tablet contains potassium chloride 600 mg in a sustained-release form.

Nuhome antiseptic liquid contains chlorophene 1·25%, dichloroxylenol 1·25%, and terpenes 4·5%.

Numotac ◊ isoetharine.

Nupercainal ◊ cinchocaine.

Nurofen ◊ ibuprofen.

Nurse Harvey's Gripe Mixture contains dill oil 0·069%, caraway oil 0·069%, weak ginger tincture 5·2%, sodium bicarbonate 1·33%, and syrup 15%.

Nurse Sykes Bronchial Balsam contains compound benzoin tincture 3·1%, capsicum tincture 0·26%, camphor 0·02%, acetic acid 1·5%, glycerol 6·25%, tolu syrup 25%, syrup 25%, alpha-glyceryl-guaiacol ether [guaiphenesin] 0·175%, and chloroform q.s.

Nurse Sykes Powders contain aspirin 41·33%, paracetamol 30%, caffeine 15%, and excipient to 100%.

Nu-Seals Aspirin: Each tablet contains aspirin 300 mg or 600 mg in an enteric coated form. *Dose:* By mouth, 300 to 900 mg twice or four times daily up to a maximum of 8 g daily.

nutmeg oil is used as an aromatic and carminative. It is also used as a rubefacient. Nutmeg appears to inhibit prostaglandin synthesis.

Nutraplus ◊ urea.

Nutrizym is a pancreatic preparation. Each tablet contains pancreatin 400 mg and ox bile 30 mg in the inner core and bromelains 50 mg in the outer layer. *Dose:* By mouth, 1 to 2 during meals.

nux vomica has the effects, uses and adverse effects of strychnine. It is present in some tonics.

Nybadex ointment contains hydrocortisone 1%, nystatin 100,000 units/g, dimethicone '350' 20%, and benzalkonium chloride 0·2%.

Nydrane ◊ beclamide.

Nylax Laxative Tablets each contain vitamin B_1 3 mg, phenolphthalein 60 mg, cascara dry extract 30 mg, aloin 2 mg, senna leaf 15 mg, and bisacodyl 2 mg.

Nyspes ◊ nystatin.

Nystaform cream and **ointment** contains nystatin 100,000 units/g and chlorhexidine 1%. **Nystaform HC** also contains hydrocortisone 0·5%.

Nystan ◊ nystatin.

nystatin (Nyspes, Nystan) is an antibiotic which is active against a wide range of fungi and yeasts. When given by mouth, little is absorbed. It is mainly used to treat *Candida* infections (e.g., thrush) of the skin, mouth, genitals and intestine. *Adverse effects:* It may rarely cause nausea, vomiting and diarrhoea. *Dose:* For intestinal infection, 1 to 2 million units per day in divided doses; vaginal moniliasis, pessaries containing 100,000 units, one or two at night for two weeks.

Nystavescent pessaries contain nystatin in a base that effervesces in contact with vaginal moisture. *Dose:* 1 or 2 inserted high into the vagina for 14 consecutive nights.

octaphonium (octaphonium chloride) is related to benzethonium. It is used as an antiseptic in skin applications.

Octapressin ◊ felypressin.

Octovit tablets contain vitamins and minerals.

octoxynol is an ether used in making water and oil emulsions and other drug preparations. It is also present in some spermicides.

octylphenoxypolyethoxyethanol ◊ octoxynol.

Ocusert Pilo 20 and **40** are devices used for applying pilocarpine to the eyes in patients suffering from glaucoma ◊ pilocarpine.

Ocusol eye drops contain sulphacetamide 5%, zinc sulphate 0·1% and cetrimide 0·01%.

Odd spot is used for acne. It contains allantoin 0·2%, hamamelis water 95% and chlorhexidine gluconate solution 0·25%.

oestradiol (Estraderm, Hormonin, Progynova, oestradiol benzoate; oestradiol monobenzoate, oestradiol valerate) is the most active of the naturally occurring oestrogens. It is used to treat menopausal symptoms and primary amenorrhoea. *Adverse effects* and *Precautions* ◊ ethinyloestradiol. *Dose:* By mouth, for the menopause 1 to 2 mg daily for 21 days with seven days free before the next course. By intramuscular injection for primary amenorrhoea, 1 to 5 mg at 1 to 14 day intervals. By implantation 25 to 50 mg every 36 weeks.

oestriol (Ovestin) is a naturally occurring oestrogen used to treat postmenopausal vaginal and vulval conditions. *Adverse effects* and *Precautions* ◊ ethinyloestradiol. *Dose:* By mouth, 0·25 to 0·50 mg daily.

oestrone (Harmogen; piperazine oestrone sulphate) is a naturally occurring oestrogen. It is used to treat menopausal symptoms. *Adverse effects* and *Precautions* ◊ ethinyloestradiol. *Note:* Piperazine oestrone sulphate 1·5 mg = oestrone 930 micrograms. *Dose:* By mouth, 1·5 to 4·5 mg daily for 21 days with seven days' break.

Oilatum cream contains arachis oil 21%; Oilatum emollient contains wool alcohol 5% and liquid paraffin 63·7%.

oil of bitter orange is used as a flavouring agent and carminative.

oil of cloves is obtained from dried flower buds, *Caryophyllus aromaticus*. It is used in mixtures to treat wind and indigestion, and in temporary dental fillings.

oil of pine needles has a pleasant aromatic odour and is used in rubefacients and in inhalants to treat coughs and colds.

oil of wintergreen ◊ methyl salicylate.

oily cream ◊ hydrous ointment.

Olbas Oil contains cajuput oil 18·5%, clove oil 0·1%, eucalyptus oil 35·45%, juniper berry oil 2·7%, menthol 4·1%, peppermint oil 35·45%, and wintergreen oil 3·7%.

Olbas Pastilles contain eucalyptus oil 1·16%, peppermint oil 1·12%, menthol 0·1%, juniper berry oil 0·067%, wintergreen oil 0·047%, and clove oil 0·0025%.

Olbetam capsules ◊ acipimox.

oleoresin capsicum ◊ capsicum.

olive oil is used as a nutrient, demulcent and mild purgative. It is used to soften ear wax and in skin applications.

Omega-H3: Each capsule contains aminobenzoic acid 50 mg, wheat-germ oil 100 mg, vegetable lecithin 20 mg, choline 100 mg, inositol 100 mg, rutin 10 mg, thiamine hydrochloride 15 mg, riboflavine 3 mg, pantothenic acid 3 mg, pyridoxine hydrochloride 1 mg, cyanocobalamin 20 micrograms, biotin 3 micrograms, folic acid 0·5 mg, ascorbic acid 60 mg, nicotinamide 15 mg, vitamin A 2,000 units, ergocalciferol 200 units, vitamin E 25 mg, ferrous sulphate 13·25 mg, ferrous fumarate 32 mg, calcium hydrogen phosphate 180 mg, magnesium sulphate 3·32 mg, zinc oxide 1·26 mg, copper sulphate 2·84 mg, and manganese sulphate 3·32 mg.

Omnopon ◊ papaveretum.

Omnopon-Scopolamine injections contain papaveretum 20 mg and hyoscine hydrobromide 400 micrograms in each ml. *Dose:* 1ml by subcutaneous or intramuscular injection pre-operatively.

On and Off Hair Removing Cream contains calcium thioglycollate.

Oncovin ◊ vincristine.

One-a-day Tablets each contain vitamin A palmitate 5,000 units, vitamin B_1 2 mg, vitamin B_2 2 mg, vitamin B_6 1 mg, vitamin B_{12} 2 micrograms, nicotinamide 20 mg, sodium ascorbate 50 mg, vitamin D 400 units, ferrous carbonate 15 mg, copper carbonate 0·75 micrograms.

One-Alpha capsules contain 0·25 or 1 microgram of alfacalcidol. It is used to treat patients suffering from renal bone disease, hypoparathyroidism and vitamin D resistant rickets. *Dose:* By mouth, 1 microgram daily (adults). **One-Alpha solution** contains 0·2 microgram/ml.

Opas Indigestion Powder contains sodium bicarbonate 20%, calcium carbonate 40%, and heavy magnesium carbonate 40%.

Opas Indigestion Tablets: Each contain sodium bicarbonate 68 mg, calcium carbonate 136 mg, and heavy magnesium carbonate 136 mg.

Opazimes: Each tablet contains dried aluminium hydroxide 160 mg, light kaolin 700 mg, morphine hydrochloride 250 micrograms, and belladonna dry extract 3 mg.

Operidine injection ◊ phenoperidine.

Ophthaine eyedrops contain proxymetacaine hydrochloride 0·5% ◊ proxymetacaine.

Ophthalmadine ◊ idoxuridine.

opiate squill linctus (Gee's Pastilles, Gee's Linctus) contains camphorated tincture of opium, and squill and tolu syrups. It contains about 0·8 mg of morphine in each 5 ml. It is used to treat coughs. *Dose:* 5 ml as required or as pastilles (each contains 2 ml of linctus) 1 to 2 to be sucked 3 to 4 times daily.

Opilon ◊ thymoxamine.

opium (raw opium; powdered opium) is discussed under the section on morphine and narcotic pain relievers. It has effects and uses similar to those described under morphine, which is its main constituent. It is more constipating than morphine alone.

Opobyl pills are a laxative, each containing aloes 20 mg, bile salts 50 mg, boldo extract 10 mg, euonymus 2 mg, desiccated liver 50 mg, and podophyllin 2 mg. *Dose:* 1 to 2 pills when required.

Optabs Eye Lotion Tablets contain phenylephrine hydrochloride 0·05%, adrenaline 0·6%, and acriflavine 0·005%.

Opticrom ◊ sodium cromoglycate.

Optimax tablets are used to treat depression. Each tablet contains tryptophan 500 mg, pyridoxine hydrochloride 5 mg and ascorbic acid 10 mg.

Optimax W V ◊ tryptophan.

Optimine ◊ azatadine.

Optrex Eye Drops contain hamamelis water 12·5%, allantoin 0·08%, and chlorbutol 0·06%.

Optrex Eye Lotion contains in 100 ml distilled witch hazel 12·95 g, allantoin 50 mg, salicylic acid 25 mg, chlorbutol 20 mg, zinc sulphate 4 mg and benzalkonium as a preservative.

Optrex Eye Ointment contains gramicidin 0·02% and aminacrine hydrochloride 0·02%.

Optrose Rose Hip Syrup contains ascorbic acid (vitamin C) not less than 110 mg per fl oz.

Opulets atropine single dose eyedrops contain atropine sulphate 1% ◊ atropine.

Opulets benoxinate single dose eyedrops contain oxybuprocaine hydrochloride 0·4% ◊ oxybuprocaine.

Opulets chloramphenicol single dose eyedrops contain chloramphenicol 0·5% ◊ chloramphenicol.

Opulets cyclopentolate single dose eyedrops contain cyclopentolate hydrochloride 1% ◊ cyclopentolate.

Opulets fluorescein single dose eyedrops contain fluorescein sodium 1%. It is used as a stain to diagnose damage to the cornea of the eye.

Opulets pilocarpine ◊ pilocarpine (eyedrops).

Opulets saline single dose eyedrops contain sodium chloride 0·9%. It is used for irrigation of the eye.

Orabase contains sodium carboxymethylcellulose, pectin and gelatin in equal parts. This ointment is used to protect lesions in the mouth.

Orabet ◊ metformin.

Oradexon ◊ dexamethasone.

Orahesive powder contains the same ingredients as Orabase and is used on moist body surfaces to protect them.

Orajel contains benzocaine 7·5%.

Oral-B gel is a local anaesthetic application. It contains lignocaine 0·6%, cetylpyridinium chloride 0·02%, cineole 0·1% and menthol 0·06%. *Dose:* Apply every 3 hours when required.

Oralcer is used to treat mouth ulcers. Each pellet contains clioquinol 35 mg and ascorbic acid 6 mg in sustained-release form. *Dose:* 6 to 8 pellets to be dissolved in the mouth near the ulcers on the first day, reducing to 4 to 6 daily from the second day. Treatment should not be continued over prolonged periods.

Oraldene mouth wash and gargle contains hexetidine 0·1%.

Oramorph solution for use by mouth ◊ morphine.

Orange & Halibut Vitamins: Each tablet contains vitamin A 2,500 units, vitamin D_2 200 units, and vitamin C 25 mg.

Orap ◊ pimozide.

Oratrol* ◊ dichlorphenamide.

Orbenin ◊ cloxacillin sodium.

orciprenaline (Alupent; orciprenaline sulphate) is used to treat asthma. Its effects are similar to those described under isoprenaline. *Adverse effects:* Rapid beating of the heart, headache, dizziness and nausea may occur. Difficulty in passing urine may also occur. *Precautions:* See warnings under isoprenaline, particularly the dangers of high doses. *Dose:* By mouth, 20 mg four times daily, or by a spray solution for inhalation or deep intramuscular injection.

Orimeten ◊ aminoglutethimide.

Orobronze: Each capsule contains canthaxanthin 30 mg.

Orovite contains B vitamins and vitamin C.

Orovite 7 is a multivitamin preparation. Each 5 g sachet of granules contains vitamin A 2,500 units (as palmitate), thiamine mononitrate 1·4 mg, riboflavine sodium phosphate 1·7 mg, nicotinamide 18 mg, pyridoxine hydrochloride 2 mg, ascorbic acid 60 mg, ergocalciferol 100 units.

orphenadrine (Biorphen; Disipal; Norflex; Norgesic; orphenadrine citrate; orphenadrine hydrochloride) is closely related to the antihistamine drug, diphenhydramine, but it has only weak antihistamine properties. It lifts the mood and relaxes spasm of skeletal muscles. It is used to treat Parkinsonism and muscle spasm due to injury (often combined with a pain reliever). *Adverse effects:* Insomnia, mental excitement, increased trembling (tremor), and nausea may occur.

These are usually dose-related. Anxiety, confusion and tremors have followed its combined use with dextropropoxyphene. *Precautions:* Orphenadrine should be used with caution in patients with glaucoma or urinary retention. *Dose:* Orphenadrine citrate: by mouth, 100 mg twice daily, or, by injection (intramuscular or intravenous), 60 mg once or twice a day. Orphenadrine hydrochloride: by mouth, 100 to 300 mg daily in divided doses, or, by intramuscular injection, 20 to 40 mg three times daily.

Ortho Dienoestrol Cream ◊ dienoestrol.

Ortho-Creme ◊ nonoxynol.

Ortho-forms pessaries contain nonoxynol '9' 5%.

Ortho-Gynest pessaries contain 500 micrograms of oestriol ◊ oestriol.

Ortho-Gynol jelly contains di-isobutyl phenoxypolyethoxyethanol 1%.

Ortho-Novin 1/50 is an oral contraceptive containing mestranol 0·05 mg and norethisterone 1 mg.

Ortracin Chewing Gum Pastilles contain tyrothricin 0·5 mg in each tablet.

Orudis ◊ ketoprofen.

Oruvail is a sustained-release form of ketoprofen 100 mg. *Dose:* 1 or 2 once daily with food.

Osmitrol ◊ mannitol.

Ospolot* ◊ sulthiame.

Ossopan ◊ hydroxyapatite.

Othoxicol syrup* is used to treat coughs. Each 5 ml contains codeine phosphate 10·95 mg, methoxyphenamine 16·9 mg and sodium citrate 325 mg.

Otosporin ear drops* contain neomycin sulphate 0·5%, polymyxin B 10,000 units, and hydrocortisone 1% in each 1 ml.

Ototrips ear drops* contain polymyxin B sulphate, bacitracin, and trypsin.

Otrivine nasal spray ◊ xylometazoline.

Otrivine-Antistin eye drops contain xylometazole 0·05% and antazoline sulphate 0·5%.

otto lavender ◊ lavender oil.

ouabain is a cardiac glycoside with actions similar to digoxin.

ouabain (strophanthin-G) ◊ digoxin.

Over-Nite contains in each 20 ml paracetamol 500 mg, diphenhydramine hydrochloride 10 mg, ephedrine hydrochloride 15 mg, and codeine phosphate 10 mg.

Ovestin ◊ oestriol.

Ovran tablets each contain levonorgestrel 0·25 mg and ethinyloestradiol 0·05 mg. It is an oral contraceptive drug.

Ovran 30 tablets each contain levonorgestrel 0·25 mg and ethinyloestradiol 0·03 mg. It is an oral contraceptive drug.

Ovranette tablets contain levonorgestrel 0·15 mg and ethinyloestradiol 0·03 mg. It is an oral contraceptive drug.

Ovysmen is an oral contraceptive containing ethinyloestradiol 0·035 mg and norethisterone 0·5 mg.

Owbridge's: Each 5 ml contains cetylpyridinium chloride 1·25 mg, anise oil 0·0025 ml, clove oil 0·0025 ml, acetic acid 0·06 ml, capsicum tincture 0·025 ml, strong ammonium acetate solution 0·16 ml.

Owbridge's Cold Control: Each liquid dose provides paracetamol 500 mg, phenylpropanolamine hydrochloride 25 mg, and ammonium chloride 300 mg.

oxamniquine (Mansil, Vansil) is used to treat infection caused by schistosoma mansoni. *Adverse effects:* These include abdominal and muscular pains, headache, dizziness, somnolence, nausea, diarrhoea, skin eruptions and insomnia. *Dose:* 7·5 mg to 30 mg per kg body-weight.

Oxanid ◊ oxazepam.

Oxatomide (Tinset) is an antihistamine which causes less drowsiness than the other antihistamines. *Adverse effects:* It may cause some drowsiness, weight gain and increase in appetite. *Precaution:* See antihistamines (pp. 125–30, 132–4). *Dose:* By mouth, 30 to 60 mg twice daily after food.

oxazepam (Oxanid) is a benzodiazepine anti-anxiety drug. Its effects and uses are similar to those described under chlordiazepoxide. *Adverse effects:* These are similar to those described under chlordiazepoxide. Oedema, nightmares, lethargy, slurred speech and blood disorders have also been reported. *Precautions* and *Drug dependence* ◊ chlordiazepoxide. *Dose:* By mouth, 10 to 30 mg daily in divided doses.

oxedrine (Sympatol; oxedrine tartrate) is used in the treatment of low blood pressure in shock. It is a sympathomimetic drug. *Adverse effects* and *Precautions* ◊ phenylephrine. *Dose:* By mouth, 20 to 30 drops three times daily; by injection, depends on the severity of the condition.

oxerutins (Paroven) are said to be useful in the treatment of cramps in the legs at night. *Dose:* 250 mg three times a day at mealtimes.

oxethazaine is a local anaesthetic. It is an ingredient of Mucaine, used to treat heartburn and hiatus hernia.

oxpentifylline (Trental) is a vasodilator drug which is claimed also to reduce the viscosity of the blood. It is used to treat disorders of the circulation. *Adverse effects:* These include nausea, dizziness and flushing. *Precautions:* It should be given with caution to patients with low blood pressure or severe coronary artery disease. It may affect the required dose of drugs used to treat diabetes or raised blood pressure. *Dose:* By mouth, 100 to 200 mg three times daily.

oxprenolol (Apsolox, Slow-ɼren; Trasicor, oxprenolol hydrochloride) is a beta-receptor blocking drug used to treat angina and disorders of heart rhythm and raised blood pressure. It has effects similar to those described under propranolol. *Dose:* By mouth; disorders of heart rhythm, 20 mg two or three times daily increasing until satisfactory results are obtained; in angina of effort, 40 to 160 mg three times daily. The dosage should be reduced or phased out if faintness associated with a slowing of the pulse and fall in blood pressure occur. (It is dangerous to stop it suddenly.) For raised blood pressure: 80 to 320 mg daily in divided doses if combined with a diuretic drug; or in the form of slow-release (Slow-Trasicor) tablets, 1 to 2 (160 mg each) once daily.

Oxy 5 lotion contains benzoyl peroxide 5%. **Oxy 10 lotion** contains benzoyl peroxide 10%. **Oxy Wash** contains benzoyl peroxide 10%.

oxybenzone is used as a sunscreen agent.

oxybuprocaine (Benoxinate) is a local anaesthetic used in eyedrops and is used for tonometry (the measurement of tension of the eyeball).

oxymel is a preparation of purified honey in acetic acid and water.

oxymetazoline (Afrazine; oxymetazoline hydrochloride) is used in 0·05% solution as a vasoconstrictor to relieve nasal congestion. *Adverse effects:* It may occasionally cause local stinging or burning, sneezing and dryness of the mouth and throat. Prolonged use may cause rebound congestion of the nose and a chronic blocked nose (drug-induced rhinitis).

oxymetholone (Anapolon) is an anabolic (body-building) steroid with effects, uses and adverse effects similar to those described under ethyloestrenol. It may impair liver function. *Dose:* By mouth, 5 to 30 mg daily.

Oxymycin ◊ oxytetracycline.

oxypertine (Integrin) is used to treat psychotic and related disorders. *Adverse effects:* It may cause drowsiness in high dosage and excitation in low dosage, and occasionally it causes nausea, vomiting, dizziness, dryness of the mouth, a fall in blood pressure and ataxia. It may also produce Parkinsonism effects and, rarely, disturbed liver function tests and blood disorders. Discomfort on looking at bright light (photophobia) and skin rashes have been reported. *Precautions:* It may interfere with ability to operate machinery and drive motor vehicles, and its effects are increased by alcohol, barbiturates, narcotics and other depressant drugs. It should not be given to patients taking M.A.O. inhibitor antidepressant drugs, or to patients who have received these drugs in the previous two weeks. *Dose:* By mouth; as a major tranquillizer, 80 to 120 mg daily in divided doses. Repeated liver function tests should be carried out and the drug should be stopped for one week out of four. It is also used to treat anxiety, but in a smaller dose of 30 to 40 mg daily in divided doses.

oxyphenisatin is a purgative.

oxyquinoline (hydroxyquinoline) is used in deodorants, and in cosmetics and toiletries. It has antibacterial and antifungal properties.

oxytetracycline (Berkmycen; Bisolvomycin; Chemocycline; Galenomycin; Imperacin; Oxymycin; Terramycin; Unimycin); oxytetracycline dihydrate and oxytetracycline hydrochloride (Berkmycen; Imperacin; Terramycin; Unimycin) is a tetracycline antibiotic. Its effects, uses and adverse effects are similar to those described under tetracycline. *Dose:* Oxytetracycline dihydrate: by mouth, 1 to 3 g daily in divided doses. Oxytetracycline hydrochloride: by mouth, 1 to 3 g daily in divided doses.

oxytocin (Syntocinon). Oxytocin injection contains an active principle from the posterior lobe of the pituitary glands. It may be prepared from animal glands or synthesized. It is used to stimulate the uterus to contract in order to start labour or during labour. Oxytocin may also be given by tablet to suck in the mouth or by nose spray. Its increasing use to start labour for non-medical reasons needs careful examination. *Adverse effects:* It may cause violent contractions of the uterus which can damage the tissues and cause the death of the baby from asphyxia. *Dose:* Varies according to use.

Pabrinex: High potency injections of vitamins B and C.

Pacitron ◊ tryptophan.

Paddington's Junior vitamins contain vitamin A_1 750 i.u., vitamin C 25 mg and vitamin D 125 i.u.

padimate is used as a sunscreen agent.

Paedialyte Rehydration Solution (RS) contains glucose 27·5 g, sodium chloride 3·8 g, sodium citrate 0·98 g, potassium citrate 2·16 g in 250 ml of sterile water. **Paedialyte Maintenance Solution (MS)** contains glucose 27·5 g, sodium chloride 2·05 g, sodium citrate 0·98 g and potassium citrate 2·16 g in 250 ml of sterile water. *Precautions:* Only for use by mouth. The treatment should not be given to a patient suffering from serious kidney disease or an intestinal obstruction. It should not be used to treat severe dehydration which requires intravenous fluids. *Dose:* Varies according to the condition of the patient. Paedialyte RS is used to treat dehydration and the MS is used as maintenance treatment following rehydration.

Paedo-Sed syrup* contains in each 5 ml dichloralphenazone 200 mg and paracetamol 100 mg. Used as sedative and pain reliever for young children. Check recommended dose carefully.

Palaprin Forte ◊ aloxiprin.

Paldesic ◊ paracetamol.

Palfium ◊ dextromoramide.

Paludrine ◊ proguanil.

palm kernel oil is used as a fatty basis for suppositories. It has also been used in chocolate.

Pameton tablets are used to relieve mild pain. Each tablet contains paracetamol 500 mg and dl-methionine 250 mg ◊ paracetamol ◊ methionine. *Dose:* 2 tablets every 6 hours; maximum dose 8 tablets daily.

Pan-A-Gel capsules contain royal jelly.

Pan-B-Gel capsules contain royal jelly.

Panacron spray is a nasal decongestant. It contains oxymetazoline hydrochloride 0·05%. **Panacron tablets** contain paracetamol 500 mg and phenylpropranolamine hydrochloride 12·5 mg.

Panadeine is a mild pain-reliever. Each tablet contains paracetamol 500 mg and codeine phosphate 8 mg in a sorbitol base. *Dose:* 2 four times daily.

Panadeine Forte tablets contain paracetamol 500 mg and codeine phosphate 15 mg ◊ paracetamol ◊ codeine.

Panadol ◊ paracetamol.

Panadol Junior sachets ◊ paracetamol.

Panaleve Elixir contains paracetamol 120 mg in each 5 ml.

Panasorb: Each tablet contains paracetamol 500 mg in a sorbitol base. *Dose:* 2 to 3 four times daily.

Pancrease capsules are used in conditions where there is a deficient production of pancreatic enzyme e.g., cystic fibrosis, chronic pancreatitis. Each capsule contains not less than 330 BP units of protease activity 2,900 BP units of amylase activity and 5,000 BP units of lipase activity. *Adverse effects:* Most frequently, gastrointestinal effects. Less frequently, allergic type reactions. *Precautions:* Food of pH over 5·5 can dissolve the protective shell. *Dose:* 1 or 2 capsules during each meal and one with snacks.

pancreatin is prepared from the pancreas of certain animals and contains enzymes which aid the digestion of fat, starch and protein. It is used in people who have pancreatic deficiency due to fibrocystic disease and pancreatitis. *Adverse effects:* It may cause soreness of the mouth. *Dose:* 1 to 6 g daily, with meals.

Pancreolauryl test is used to test exocrine pancreatic function.

Pancrex and **Pancrex V** preparations contain varying amounts of pancreatin and other pancreatic enzymes ◊ pancreatin.

pancuronium (Pavulon; pancuronium bromide) is a muscle-relaxant drug used along with general anaesthetics in surgical operations.

Panets: Each tablet contains paracetamol 500 mg.

Panets Baby Syrup: Each 5 ml contains paracetamol 120 mg in an orange-flavoured basis.

Panoxyl ◊ benzoyl peroxide.

pantothenic acid is considered to be a member of the vitamin B group. Although no deficiency disorder has ever been proved it is a common constituent of multivitamin preparations.

papain is a mixture of proteolytic enzymes from the juice of the unripe fruit

of *Carica papaya*. It is used as a meat tenderizer and in the clarification of beverages.

papaveretum (Omnopon) is an opium preparation. *Dose:* 10 to 20 mg by mouth or injection as required.

papaverine (papaverine hydrochloride) is an opium alkaloid and because it relaxes involuntary muscles it is used to treat colic of the gut or gall-bladder and bronchial asthma, and to dilate blood vessels in the limbs. *Adverse effects:* When given by mouth it can cause disorders of the heart rhythm. *Dose:* 60 to 300 mg by mouth; 30 to 100 mg by subcutaneous or intramuscular injection.

para-aminobenzoic acid ◊ aminobenzoic acid.

parabens is a preservative.

paracetamol (preparations include: Calpol, Paldesic, Panadol, Panasorb, Salzone; acetaminophen) is a mild pain reliever; it also reduces fever. Unlike aspirin it has no anti-inflammatory properties. It is a suitable alternative pain reliever for those patients who are sensitive to aspirin. *Adverse effects:* Skin rashes and blood disorders have been reported. Overdose may cause liver damage and therefore paracetamol is more dangerous, weight for weight, when taken in overdose than is aspirin. *Precautions:* Paracetamol should be taken with caution by patients with impaired kidney or liver function. It may increase the effects of certain anticoagulant drugs. *Dose:* By mouth, 500 to 1,000 mg. Maximum in 24 hours is 4,000 mg.

parachlorometaxylenol ◊ chloroxylenol.

Paracodol capsules contain paracetamol 500 mg and codeine phosphate 8 mg ◊ paracetamol and codeine.

Paracodol effervescent tablets contain paracetamol 500 mg and codeine phosphate 8 mg. It is a mild pain-reliever. *Dose:* 1 to 2 in water up to a maximum of 6 in twenty-four hours.

paradichlorobenzene is an insecticide.

Paradeine is a mild pain-reliever. Each tablet contains paracetamol 500 mg, codeine phosphate 10 mg, phenolphthalein 2·5 mg. *Dose:* 1 to 2 tablets 4 times daily.

paraffin (hard paraffin) is obtained from petroleum and is used to form a base for ointments.

paraffin (liquid paraffin), a mineral oil, is used as a laxative and as an emollient in the preparation of ointments, toiletries, hair creams and hand creams, etc.

paraffin, white soft and yellow soft, (Vaseline) are used in skin applications. They are obtained as emollients from petroleum.

parahydroxybenzoic acid esters are used as preservatives in medicines and foods. They are active against moulds, fungi and yeasts but less active against bacteria.

Parahypon is used as a mild pain-reliever. Each tablet contains paracetamol 500 mg, and caffeine 10 mg, codeine phosphate 5 mg. *Dose:* 1 to 2 four times daily.

Parake is used as a mild pain-reliever. Each tablet contains paracetamol 500 mg and codeine phosphate 8 mg. *Dose:* 2 tablets three or four times daily.

paraldehyde is a quick-acting sleeping drug and anti-convulsant. Because of its nasty smell, taste and part-excretion in the breath it is seldom used except in hospitals. *Adverse effects:* Because it irritates the stomach it is usually given by injection, which may be painful. Adverse effects are not common. Skin rashes may occur and rarely it may cause liver and kidney disorders. Nerve damage may occur if injected close to a main nerve. *Precautions:* If given by mouth or by rectum it should be well diluted. Intramuscular injections should not exceed more than 5 ml into any one site. It should not be given in plastic syringes and should be given with caution to patients with impaired liver function. It decomposes in light and heat to form acetic acid. Deaths from corrosive poisoning have occurred from using old paraldehyde; it should always be tested for acidity and discarded if acid. *Drug dependence:* Paraldehyde may produce dependence of the barbiturate/alcohol type. *Dose:* 5 to 10 ml by intramuscular injection or by mouth.

Paramax is used to treat acute attacks of migraine. Each tablet or sachet contains paracetamol 500 mg and metoclopramide 5 mg. See paracetamol and metoclopramide. *Dose:* By mouth, dissolve one tablet or the contents of one sachet in half a tumbler of water. 1 to 2 doses at onset of attack and 1 dose every four hours. Maximum of 6 sachets or 6 tablets in 24 hours.

Paramol is a mild to moderate pain-reliever. Each tablet contains paracetamol 500 mg and dihydrocodeine tartrate 10 mg. *Dose:* 1 to 2 every four hours as required during or after meals. Not for children under twelve years.

Paraplatin injection ◊ carboplatin.

Pardale is a mild pain-reliever. Each tablet contains paracetamol 400 mg, codeine phosphate 9 mg, and caffeine 10 mg. *Dose:* By mouth, 1 to 2 three or four times daily.

Parentrovite is a preparation of vitamins B and C in injectable form.

Parfenac cream ◊ bufexamac.

Parkinsons Glycerin, Lemon, Ipec Cough Mixture contains lemon juice 10%, glycerol 7%, ipecacuanha tincture 1%, dilute sulphuric acid 1·1%, ether 0·1%, chloroform 0·1%, camphor 0·03%, phosphoric acid 0·04%, benzoic acid 0·03%, and sucrose 50%.

Parkinsons Indian Brandee contains nitrous ether spirit 5%, capsicum tincture 2%, compound gentian tincture 0·04%, compound cardamom tincture 5%, glycerol 0·6%, sodium citrate 1·5%, and sucrose 35·6%.

Parkinsons Toothache Tincture contains camphor 18·8%, chloroform

0·4%, phenol 0·8%, clove oil 11·4%, benzalkonium chloride solution 0·2%, and industrial methylated spirit to 100%.

Parkinsons White Embrocation contains turpentine oil 15·5%, camphor 3·5%, industrial methylated spirit 9%, and acetic acid 7·5%.

Parlodel ◊ bromocriptine.

Parmid ◊ metoclopramide.

Parnate ◊ tranylcypromine.

Paroven ◊ oxerutins.

Parstelin: Each tablet contains tranylcypromine sulphate 10 mg and trifluoperazine hydrochloride 1 mg. It is an antidepressant drug. *Dose:* 1 morning and afternoon.

Parvolex ◊ acetylcysteine.

passion flower extract is said to have anti-spasmodic and sedative effects.

Pastilaid Indigestion Pastilles: Each contain aluminium hydroxidemagnesium carbonate co-dried gel 200 mg and magnesium trisilicate 200 mg.

Paton's Mouth Treatment contains wool fat 48·95%, yellow soft paraffin 48·95%, iodoform 0·05%, tannic acid 2%, and saccharin 0·05%.

Pavacol-D is used to treat coughs. Each 5 ml contains pholcodine 5 mg and aromatic and volatile oils. *Dose:* By mouth, 5 to 10 ml as required.

Pavulon ◊ pancuronium.

Paxadon (pyridixine hydrochloride) ◊ pyridoxine.

Paxalgesic tablets are a mild pain-reliever. Each tablet contains dextropropoxyphene hydrochloride 32·5 mg and paracetamol 325 mg. *Dose:* 2 three or four times daily, maximum dose of 8 daily.

Paxane ◊ flurazepam.

Paxidal tablets contain paracetamol 325 mg, meprobamate 135 mg and caffeine 65 mg ◊ paracetamol ◊ meprobamate. It is used to relieve mild pain. *Dose:* 2 tablets three times daily. *Warning:* It may cause drowsiness. If affected do not drive or operate machinery. It is better to avoid alcohol while taking the tablets.

Paxofen ◊ ibuprofen.

Paynocil is a mild pain-reliever. Each tablet contains aspirin 600 mg and glycine 300 mg.

P-chloro-m-cresol ◊ chlorocresol.

pectin is obtained from the rind of citrus fruits and apples. It is used to treat diarrhoea. It is also used in making cosmetics.

Ped-el is a replacement electrolyte therapy.

Pediclex Shampoo contains malathion 0·5%.

Pediclex Sprinkle 'n' Comb Lotion contains malathion 0·75%.

Pegina mixture is used to treat indigestion. It contains in each 5 ml aqueous extract of calumba 0·9 ml, alcohol extract of calamus root 0·03 ml, comfrey root 0·51 ml, dandelion root 0·03 ml, gentian root 0·071 ml and hydraslis 0·019 ml, capsicum tincture 0·008 ml, cascara liquid extract 0·172 ml, compound cardamom tincture 0·24 ml, liquorice liquid extract 0·012 ml, strong ginger tincture 0·01 ml, magnesium trisilicate 700 mg, magnesium sulphate 76·5 mg, papain 10 mg, pepsin 12 mg, and rhubarb 7 mg.

P.E.M. linctus is used to treat coughs and colds. Each 5 ml contains pholcodine 5 mg, ephedrine hydrochloride 10 mg, menthol 1·25 mg and guaiphenesin 12·5 mg.

pemoline (Volital) is said to produce effects between caffeine and amphetamine. It is used to treat over-active children. *Dose:* By mouth, children 6–12 years 10 to 20 mg twice daily. It may produce dizziness, sweating, headache, palpitations.

penamecillin (Havapen) has similar effects and adverse effects to benzylpenicillin. *Dose:* By mouth, 350 mg every 8 hours.

Penbritin ◊ ampicillin.

penbutolol (penbutolol sulphate) is a beta-receptor blocking drug used to treat raised blood pressure. *Adverse effects* and *Precautions:* ◊ propranolol. *Dose:* By mouth, 40 to 80 mg daily.

Pendramine ◊ penicillamine.

Penetrol Catarrh Lozenges: Each contain menthol 7·3 mg, ammonium chloride 26·25 mg, phenylephrine hydrochloride 5·5 mg, and creosote 1·8 mg.

Penetrol Inhalant contains menthol 17·5%, cajuput oil 2·5%, lavender oil 8%, eucalyptus oil 7·5%, otto lavender 4%, peppermint oil 0·2%, and industrial methylated spirit 60%.

penicillamine (Cuprimine; Distamine; Pendramine; penicillamine hydrochloride) is used to treat toxic metal poisoning (e.g., lead) and also to treat a disorder of copper metabolism found in Wilson's disease. It is also used to treat rheumatoid arthritis and related disorders. *Adverse effects:* It may produce headache, nausea, sore throat, fever, muscle and joint pains, skin rash, swollen glands and blood and kidney disorders. Rarely, severe allergic reactions occur, particularly with patients allergic to penicillin. Frequent blood and urine tests should be carried out during treatment. *Dose:* By mouth, 0·5 g to 0·75 g in divided doses, up to 2 g daily according to the disorder.

penicillin ◊ benzylpenicillin.

penicillin G ◊ benzylpenicillin.

penicillin G potassium ◊ benzylpenicillin.

penicillin G sodium ◊ benzylpenicillin.

penicillin V (phenoxymethylpenicillin potassium) ◊ phenoxymethylpenicillin.

penicillin V K ◊ phenoxymethylpenicillin.

penicillin V potassium ◊ phenoxymethylpenicillin.

Penidural ◊ benzathine penicillin.

Pennine Eye Drops contain zinc sulphate 0·05%, boric acid 1·6%, borax 0·16%, sodium potassium tartrate 0·2%, hamamelis water 5%, and phenylmercuric acetate 0·002%.

pentaerythritol (Mycardol; Cardiacap; pentaerythritol tetranitrate) is used to treat angina. Read section on drugs used to treat angina. Its effects and uses are similar to those described under glyceryl trinitrate. It is taken by mouth, takes about one hour to work and lasts about five hours. *Adverse effects* and *Precautions:* These are similar to those described under glyceryl trinitrate. *Dose:* By mouth, 20 to 30 mg four times daily, before meals.

pentazocine (Fortral) is a narcotic analgesic. *Adverse effects:* It may produce nausea, vomiting, dizziness, changes in mood and sweating. Headache, confusion and hallucinations may occur. These occur if the drug is taken by mouth or by injection; the latter may also cause constipation, pins and needles, breathlessness, a fall in blood pressure, retention of urine, allergic skin rashes and, rarely, depression of breathing. These adverse effects are more likely to occur if the patient is up and about rather than in bed. *Precautions:* Those which apply to morphine also apply to pentazocine. Its prolonged use may lead to drug dependence. *Dose:* By mouth, 25 to 100 mg every three to four hours up to a maximum of 600 mg in 24 hours. By subcutaneous or intramuscular injection, 20 to 60 mg every three to four hours.

pentobarbitone (pentobarbitone sodium; pentobarbital sodium; soluble pentobarbitone) is a barbiturate sleeping drug. *Dose:* By mouth, 100 to 200 mg at night.

Pentostam ◊ sodium stibogluconate.

Pepcid PM tablets ◊ famotidine.

Peplax are peppermint-flavoured tablets each containing phenolphthalein 130 mg.

peppermint oil is obtained from the dried leaves and flowering tops of *Mentha piperita*. There are two varieties, known as black peppermint and white peppermint. It is used as a carminative. Special capsules of peppermint oil (Colpermin; Mintec) are used to treat colic and distension of the abdomen, irritable bowel syndrome and spastic colon. *Adverse effects* of peppermint oil used in this way include heartburn, skin rashes, headache, slowing of the pulse rate, trembling and loss of control over voluntary movement (ataxia). *Precautions:* These preparations of peppermint oil should be used with caution in pregnancy. *Dose:* By mouth, one or two capsules of Colpermin or Mintec 3 times daily with water before meals.

pepsin is an enzyme secreted by the stomach that breaks down protein.

Peptard ◊ hyoscyamine.

Pepto-Bismol is an antacid. Each 5 ml contains bismuth salicylate 87.6 mg.

Dose: 30 ml every hour if necessary, maximum of 240 ml in a day.

Percutol ointment contains 2% glyceryl trinitrate.

Pergonal ◊ menotrophin.

perhexiline (perhexiline maleate) is used to prevent anginal attacks. *Adverse effects:* Postural hypotension, headache, dizziness, flushing, low blood sugar, weight loss and skin rash. Serious adverse effects may occur in patients who break the drug down slowly, these include severe nerve damage and liver damage. *Precautions:* It should not be used in patients with severe kidney or liver disorders. Regular checks on weight, blood sugar and liver function tests should be carried out during treatment as well as regular check-ups for nerve damage – e.g., pins and needles, headache, muscle weakness. *Dose:* By mouth, 50 to 100 mg twice daily. Its use is usually restricted to specialized units where other drug-treatments have failed.

Periactin ◊ cyproheptadine.

pericyazine (Neulactil) is a major tranquillizer. It has similar effects to chlorpromazine, but is more sedative. *Dose:* 10 to 75 mg daily.

Perifusin is an electrolyte therapy.

Permitabs contain 400 mg of potassium permanganate for making into a solution – one tablet dissolved in 4 litres of water makes a 0·1% solution ◊ potassium permanganate.

Pernivit: Each tablet contains acetomenapthone 7 mg and nicotinic acid 25 mg. This preparation is said to help in the treatment of chilblains. *Dose:* By mouth, 1 to 2 three times daily.

Pernomol paint is used to treat chilblains. It contains chlorbutol 2%, soap spirit 34%, phenol 0·95%, tannic acid 2·2% and camphor 10%. *Dose:* Apply to chilblains three or four times daily.

perphenazine (Fentazin) is a major tranquillizer. It may also be used in treating nausea and vomiting. *Adverse effects:* These are similar to those described under chlorpromazine but perphenazine produces less sedation. It may produce dryness of the mouth, blurred vision, restlessness, fatigue, headache and symptoms like those seen in Parkinsonism; at high doses these become more marked. *Precautions:* These are similar to those discussed under chlorpromazine. *Dose:* By mouth: for psychological disorders, 8 to 24 mg daily in divided doses; for nausea and vomiting, 4 mg three times daily.

Persantin ◊ dipyridamole.

Persomnia tablets: Each contains paracetamol 500 mg and codeine phosphate 8 mg.

Pertofran ◊ desipramine.

Peru balsam is a balsam exuded from the trunk of myroxylon balsamum. It has a mild antiseptic action by virtue of its content of cinnamic and benzoic acids. *Adverse effects:* May cause skin sensitization. It is used in ointments for the treatment of eczema and itching of the skin (pruritis) and in suppositories for the relief of haemorrhoids.

Per/Vac is Pertussis vaccine. It is a sterile suspension of killed Bordelella pertussis used for immunization against whooping-cough (Pertussis).

pethidine (pethidine hydrochloride; meperidine hydrochloride) is a synthetic narcotic pain-reliever. It has actions and uses similar to those described under morphine but it is not as powerful and its effects are less prolonged. It has little effect upon coughs. *Adverse effects:* It may cause a lift in mood, dizziness, sweating, dry mouth, nausea, vomiting, constipation and retention of urine. These are all much less frequent than with morphine. Injection into a vein may cause a fall in blood pressure. Its use during childbirth may depress the respiration of the baby at birth. *Precautions:* Pethidine should not be given to patients with severe liver disease or with gallbladder pains. Its effects are increased by M.A.O. inhibitor antidepressant drugs and possibly by some major tranquillizers (e.g., phenothiazines). *Drug dependence:* Pethidine may cause drug dependence of the morphine type. Tolerance is not always complete and addicts develop twitching, trembling, mental confusion and hallucinations. Sometimes convulsions and death may occur from pethidine dependence. Withdrawal symptoms come quicker than with morphine. *Dose:* By mouth, 50 to 100 mg; by subcutaneous or intramuscular injection, 25 to 100 mg; by intravenous injection, 25 to 50 mg.

Petrolagar emulsion (Blue label contains 7% liquid paraffin and 18% light liquid paraffin). It is used to treat constipation. *Dose:* 10 ml night and morning.

petrolatum ◊ paraffin yellow soft.

Petroleum ◊ paraffin, white soft and yellow soft.

petroleum jelly ◊ paraffin white soft and yellow soft.

Pevaryl ◊ econazole.

Phanodorm ◊ cyclobarbitone.

Pharmalgen is available as a treatment set. It contains bee or wasp venom (100 micrograms/ml). It is injected for the treatment of allergies to bee or wasp stings in graded doses to a maximum of 100 micrograms.

Pharmaton Capsules: Each containing dimethylaminoethanol bitartrate 26 mg, ginseng complex 200 mg, vitamin A 4,000 units, vitamin B_1 2 mg, vitamin B_2 2 mg, vitamin B_6 1 mg, vitamin B_{12} 1 microgram, vitamin C 60 mg, vitamin D 400 units, vitamin E 10 mg, nicotinamide 15 mg, calcium pantothenate 10 mg, rutin 20 mg, iron 10 mg, calcium 90·3 mg, phosphorus 70 mg, fluorine 200 micrograms, copper 1 mg, potassium 8 mg, manganese 1 mg, magnesium 10 mg, zinc 1 mg, with choline, inositol, linoleic acid and linolenic acid.

Pharmaton Ginseng Extract Capsules: Each contains 100 mg of standardized extract from Korean panax ginseng 500 mg.

Pharmidone is used to treat symptoms of the common cold. Each tablet contains codeine phosphate 10 mg, diphenhydramine hydrochloride 5 mg, paracetamol 400 mg, caffeine 50 mg.

Dose: 1 to 2 tablets every 4 hours, maximum 10 tablets daily.

Pharmorubicin injection is an anti-cancer drug containing epirubicin hydrochloride 10 mg or 50 mg ◊ epirubicin.

Phasal ◊ lithium.

Phazyme is a pancreatin preparation. Each tablet contains 60 mg activated dimethicone in two separate layers together with pancreatin and other pancreatic enzymes. *Dose:* By mouth, 1 to 2 tablets with meals or when required.

phenacetin is a mild pain-reliever and reduces fever. *Adverse effects:* Prolonged use may cause kidney damage, and large doses may damage the liver. *Warning:* Because of the link between kidney damage and pain relievers containing phenacetin it is suggested that phenacetin alone or in combination should no longer be used.

phenazocine (Narphen; phenazocine hydrobromide) is a synthetic pain reliever. It has effects and uses similar to those described under morphine. It is quicker in onset, lasts longer than morphine and is more effective. Tolerance develops more slowly. *Adverse effects* and *Precautions:* These are similar to those described under morphine. It may produce nausea, vomiting, dizziness and smallness of the pupils. It should not be used in patients who are unconscious, in convulsive disorders, in patients with impaired liver function, in alcoholism or in patients with underworking of their thyroid gland (myxoedema). *Drug dependence:* Phenazocine may produce drug dependence of the morphine type.

Dose: By mouth, 5 to 20 mg; by intramuscular injection, 1 to 3 mg; by intravenous injection, 0·5 to 1 mg.

phenazone by mouth has effects, uses and adverse effects similar to those described under phenacetin. It may cause skin rashes, large doses may cause nausea, drowsiness, coma and convulsions. Prolonged use may cause blood disorders. It is also used in ear drops.

phenazopyridine (phenazopyridine hydrochloride) was used to treat painful disorders of the bladder and urinary tract. *Adverse effects:* It may cause headache, vertigo and abdominal colic. *Precautions:* It may damage the red blood cells if given in high doses to patients with impaired kidney function. *Dose:* By mouth, 200 mg three times daily.

phenelzine (Nardil; phenelzine sulphate) is a monoamine oxidase inhibitor antidepressant drug. *Adverse effects:* Phenelzine causes a fall in blood pressure and giddiness. It may cause headache, trembling, restlessness, constipation, difficulty in passing water, dry mouth, blurred vision, skin rash, oedema, and impotence. Severe reactions may occur with certain foods and drugs and liver damage may occur. *Precautions:* Phenelzine should not be given to patients with impaired liver or heart function, to patients with disorders of the arteries supplying the brain (e.g., patients who have had a stroke), or to patients with epilepsy. If patients on phenelzine or other M.A.O. inhibitor drugs take certain drugs, a severe rise in blood pressure may occur, resulting in brain haemorrhage or heart failure. The following

drugs should therefore *not* be used: amphetamine, atropine, carbamazepine, chloroquine, dexamphetamine, ephedrine, ethamivan, fenfluramine, guanethidine, mephentermine, methoxamine, methylamphetamine, morphine, orciprenaline, pethidine, phenmetrazine, phenylephrine, phenylpropanolamine, pseudoephedrine, and reserpine. These drugs should not be given within two weeks of stopping M.A.O. inhibitor drugs. Certain foods contain chemicals that can produce dangerous reactions in patients who are taking M.A.O. inhibitors – these include cheese, pickled herrings, broad bean pods and protein extracts prepared from meat or yeast – e.g., Bovril, Marmite. Certain tricyclic antidepressant drugs should not be given at the same time or within two weeks of stopping M.A.O. inhibitor drugs and the effects of other drugs may be increased, e.g., antihistamines, barbiturates, some oral antidiabetic drugs and non-barbiturate hypnotics. Sensitivity to insulin may be increased and pethidine and other narcotic pain relievers have produced severe reactions. *Dose:* By mouth, 15 mg three times daily.

Phenergan ◊ promethazine.

Phenergan Compound Expectorant cough linctus contains promethazine hydrochloride 5 mg, ipecacuanha liquid extract 0·01 mg, potassium guaiacolsulphonate 45 mg and citric acid 65 mg in each 5 ml. *Dose:* 5 to 10 ml two to three times daily.

phenethicillin (Broxil; phenethicillin sodium) is a penicillin drug. It has effects, uses, and adverse effects similar to those described under phenoxy-

phenindamine

methylpenicillin. Although it gives rise to higher blood levels than phenoxymethylpenicillin it is less potent and therefore the effects of the two penicillins are similar. *Dose:* By mouth, 250 mg four times daily before meals.

phenindamine (Thephorin; phenindamine tartrate) is an antihistamine drug. Unlike other antihistamine drugs it does not produce drowsiness but it may cause stimulation. *Adverse effects:* It may cause nausea, dryness of the mouth, dizziness and stomach upsets. Insomnia and convulsions may occur. *Precautions:* As for antihistamine drugs. *Dose:* By mouth, 75 to 150 mg daily in divided doses.

phenindione (Dindevan; phenylindanedione) is used to stop the blood from clotting. Blood-clotting tests should be carried out at frequent intervals. *Adverse effects:* Early signs of overdose are bleeding gums or nose or elsewhere, and red blood cells in the urine. It may cause vomiting, diarrhoea, skin rashes and fever. Sore throat may be an early sign of allergy which may lead to blood disorders, liver damage, kidney damage and death. Phenindione may cause a brownish pigmentation of the finger nails, fingers and palms of the hands of person handling it. It sometimes colours the urine red. *Precautions:* It should be given with great caution to patients with impaired liver or kidney function. It should not be used in the later months of pregnancy or within three days of childbirth or surgery. Mothers who are taking phenindione should not breast feed their babies. Its effects may be increased by other drugs – methandienone, clofibrate, phenylbutazone (and similar anti-

rheumatic drugs). Its effects may be reduced by barbiturates, chloral hydrate, glutethimide and meprobamate. Aspirin and other salicylates may increase the danger of haemorrhage. *Dose:* By mouth; loading dose 200 mg on first day, 100 mg on second day, 50 to 150 mg daily maintenance dose.

pheniramine (Daneral-SA; pheniramine maleate) is an antihistamine drug. *Dose:* By mouth, 75 to 150 mg at night.

Phenistix is used to test for phenylpyruvate and salicylates in the urine.

phenmetrazine is used to suppress the appetite in the treatment of obesity. *Adverse effects:* These include dryness of the mouth, metallic taste, anorexia, nausea, constipation or diarrhoea, insomnia, headache, dizziness and tremor. *Dose:* 12·5 to 25 mg two or three times daily one hour before meals.

phenobarbitone (Luminal; Parabal; phenobarbitone sodium). Phenobarbitone is a barbiturate drug. It is used as a sedative and anti-convulsant. *Adverse effects:* Drowsiness may occur and elderly patients may become confused. Allergic reactions are rare and include skin rashes. *Precautions:* Phenobarbitone should be given with caution to the elderly, and those with impaired liver or kidney function. It should not be given to patients with acute intermittent porphyria. It may cause confusion in the presence of severe pain. Phenobarbitone may interfere with ability to drive motor vehicles and operate machinery. It increases the effects of alcohol and may make patients depressed. It affects enzymes in the liver, increasing the breakdown of certain drugs – folic acid, griseofulvin, phenylbutazone, phenytoin, and some anticoagulants. The effects of phenobarbitone and other barbiturates may be increased by other sedatives, diphenoxylate, mephenesin and possibly tricyclic antidepressant drugs. The blood level of the latter may be reduced by barbiturates. *Drug dependence:* Phenobarbitone may produce drug dependence of the barbiturate/alcohol type, which is characterized by a strong psychological dependence, intoxication resulting in sedation, sleep, coma, stupor, impaired judgement and unsteady gait, the development of tolerance and a dangerous physical dependence manifested by anxiety, insomnia, weakness, trembling, convulsions and delirium upon its withdrawal. Cross-tolerance with hypnosedative drugs may occur. *Dose:* By mouth, 30 to 125 mg daily in divided doses.

phenol is used as a disinfectant.

phenolphthalein is an irritant laxative. *Adverse effects* and *Precautions:* The adverse effects produced by laxatives are discussed in the section on drugs used to treat constipation. Phenolphthalein may cause abdominal cramps and, rarely, a skin rash, and may colour the urine red. It has occasionally caused protein to appear in the urine (albuminuria) and also free haemoglobin (the pigment in red blood cells) – this is called haemoglobinuria. *Dose:* By mouth, 50 to 300 mg.

phenoperidine (Operidine; phenoperidine hydrochloride) is a narcotic pain reliever used to produce analgesia during operations ◊ pethidine. *Dose:* Varies according to whether respiration is spontaneous or assisted.

phenoxybenzamine (Dibenyline) is an alpha-adrenoceptor blocking drug (see p. 000) and is used in the treatment of raised blood pressure and Raynaud's disease. *Adverse effects:* These include tachycardia (rapid heart beat), postural hypotension, dizziness, lassitude, nasal congestion, miosis, ejaculation. *Dose:* 10 mg twice daily.

phenoxyethanol is used as an antibacterial and antifungal agent.

phenoxymethylpenicillin (penicillin V) is a penicillin used by mouth to treat disorders such as tonsillitis and to prevent rheumatic fever. *Adverse effects* and *Precautions* ◊ entry under benzylpenicillin. *Dose:* By mouth, 250 to 500 mg every 6 hours at least 30 minutes before food.

Phensedyl linctus is a cough medicine. Each 5 ml contains codeine phosphate 9 mg, ephedrine hydrochloride 7·2 mg and promethazine hydrochloride 3·6 mg. *Warning:* It may cause drowsiness. If affected do not drive or operate machinery. Alcohol should be avoided.

Phensic tablets contain aspirin 325 mg and caffeine 50 mg ◊ aspirin ◊ caffeine.

phentermine (Duromine; Ionamin) is a sympathomimetic drug used as a slimming drug. Its adverse effects are similar to those described under amphetamines. It should be given with caution to patients with heart disease or overworking of their thyroid glands, and to those with psychological disturbances. *Dose:* 15 to 30 mg daily in one dose in the morning.

phentolamine (Rogitine; phentolamine hydrochloride; phentolamine mesylate) is a vasodilator drug used to treat disorders of the circulation. Phentolamine is used in a rare tumour of the adrenal glands called phaecochromocytoma in which the blood pressure increases. *Adverse effects:* It may cause rapid beating of the heart, anginal pain, flushing and occasionally vertigo. It should be used with caution in patients with coronary artery disease.

phenylbutazone (Butacote; Butazolidin; Butazone) is an anti-inflammatory drug used in hospital to treat rheumatic diseases such as ankylosing spondilitis. It has pain-relieving properties and reduces a high temperature. It is metabolized and excreted slowly and therefore its effects are prolonged. *Adverse effects:* Phenylbutazone causes salt retention, blocks iodine uptake by the thyroid gland and interferes with several enzyme processes in the body. Adverse effects are common and occur even when the dose does not exceed 400 mg daily. They include rashes, nausea, stomach upset, fluid retention (oedema), blurred vision, insomnia, and diarrhoea. Ulceration of the mouth, oesophagus (gullet), stomach or duodenum may occur leading to haemorrhage from these sites. Phenylbutazone may also cause damage to the liver, and blood disorders are not uncommon, occasionally resulting in death. Enlarged glands (including salivary glands) may occur and a generalized allergic reaction and

kidney failure have been reported. Adverse effects may occur within a few days of starting phenylbutazone and some patients may become sensitized so that a subsequent course of the drug may trigger off adverse effects. *Precautions:* Phenylbutazone should not be given to patients with a history of peptic ulcers. It should be used with caution by patients with impaired heart, liver or kidney function and by those with high blood pressure. Phenylbutazone increases the effects of acetohexamide, tolbutamide and certain anticoagulant drugs, and it may also increase the effects of phenytoin and some sulphonamides.

phenylephrine (phenylephrine hydrochloride) is a sympathomimetic drug included in numerous cold remedies and nasal drops and sprays. It constricts blood vessels and is used in anaesthesia, shock, and other states to combat a fall in blood pressure. It is also injected with local anaesthetics in order to prolong their effects. *Adverse effects:* It may cause pain and irritation at the site of injection. Overdose may cause headache, palpitation and vomiting. Nose drops may cause local irritation and eye drops may trigger off glaucoma. *Precautions:* Phenylephrine injections should not be given to patients with severe heart disease or blood pressure. Injections should be used with caution in patients with overworking thyroid glands and should not be given during, or within two weeks of stopping, treatment with M.A.O. inhibitor antidepressant drugs. *Dose:* 5 mg subcutaneously or intramuscularly, 0·5 mg intravenously.

phenylethyl alcohol is an antibacterial

agent used as a preservative in eye drops.

phenylindanedione ◊ phenindione.

phenylmercuric acetate has antibacterial and antifungal properties. It is used as a preservative in toiletries and cosmetics and also in chemical contraceptive creams.

phenylmercuric dinaphthylmethane ◊ hydrargaphen.

phenylmercuric nitrate is a mercury salt. It has antibacterial and antifungal properties. It is used as a preservative and in contraceptive creams.

phenylpropanolamine (phenylpropanolamine hydrochloride) has effects similar to those described under ephedrine but it is more active in constricting blood vessels and less active in dilating bronchi and as a stimulant. It is given by mouth in the treatment of snuffy noses, hay-fever and other allergic disorders. *Dose:* 25 to 50 mg by mouth in single doses only when required.

phenyl salicylate ◊ salol.

phenyltoloxamine is an antihistamine drug used in cough medicines, e.g., in Pholtex.

phenytoin and **phenytoin sodium** (Epanutin) are anti-convulsant drugs used to treat epilepsy. *Adverse effects:* Phenytoin may irritate the lining of the stomach and should be taken with plenty of water preferably after meals (although it is more effective if given before meals). Adverse effects are fairly frequent and are occasionally severe. These include dizziness, nausea and skin rashes which may be overcome by reducing the dose for a few days and then slowly increasing it. Tenderness and thickening of the gums may occur and hairiness (hirsutism). Other adverse effects include fever, ataxia, double vision, trembling, hallucinations and mental confusion. Severe blood disorders and skin rashes may occur. It may cause anaemia (megaloblastic anaemia) by interfering with folic acid metabolism. *Precautions:* It should be given with caution to patients on thyroid drugs and in pregnancy. *Dose:* By mouth, 50 to 200 mg three times daily.

Phillips Iron Tonic tablets: Each contain iron (as saccharated ferrous carbonate) 20 mg, dried yeast 170 mg, vitamin C 10 mg, vitamin B_1 160 micrograms, vitamin B_2 300 micrograms, and nicotinic acid 2 mg.

Phillips Tonic Yeast: Each tablet of brewers' yeast contains thiamine hydrochloride 110 micrograms, riboflavine 200 micrograms, nicotinic acid 1·4 mg, pyridoxine 9 micrograms, calcium pantothenate 12 micrograms, and other vitamins natural to brewers' yeast.

pHiso-Ac cream contains colloidal sulphur 6·4% and resorcinol 1·5%.

pHiso-Clear contains salicylic acid 0·5%, IMS 25·4%.

pHisoderm contains sodium octylphenoxyethoxyethyl ether sulphonate, lanolin derivatives, and petrolatum.

pHisohex contains chlorhexidine gluconate 1%.

pHiso-Med ◊ chlorhexidine.

pholcodine (Galphol) is used as a cough suppressant. It resembles codeine but does not cause constipation. *Dose:* By mouth, up to 60 mg daily in divided doses.

Pholcomed linctus: Each 5 ml contains pholcodine 5 mg and papaverine hydrochloride 1·25 mg. *Dose:* By mouth, 10 to 15 ml three or four times daily.

Pholcomed Diabetic linctus contains the same ingredients as Pholcomed, but is in a sugar-free form.

Pholcomed Expectorant is used to treat coughs. Each 5 ml contains guaiphenesin 62·5 mg and methylephedrine hydrochloride 0·625 mg. *Dose:* By mouth, 10 to 20 ml three times daily.

Pholtex is used to treat coughs. Each 5 ml contains pholcodine 15 mg and phenyltoloxamine 10 mg. *Dose:* 5 ml eight-hourly.

Pholtussa Mixture contains pholcodine 0·08%, ipecacuanha extract 1·5%, and blackcurrant syrup 50%.

Phortinea paint contains nitrophenol 2% in alcohol ◊ nitrophenol.

Phoserine Liquid contains cinchonidine sulphate 0·06% and quinine sulphate 0·47%.

Phosferine Tablets: Each contains cinchonidine sulphate 151 micrograms and quinine sulphate 703 micrograms.

Phosphate-Sandoz: Each effervescent tablet contains sodium acid phosphate 1·936 g, sodium bicarbonate 350 mg, and potassium bicarbonate 315 mg. This preparation is used to reduce excess levels of calcium in the blood. *Dose:* By mouth, up to 6 tablets dissolved in water daily.

phosphatides have no therapeutic effects. They occur in all animal and vegetable cells.

Phospholine-Iodide ◊ ecothiopate.

phosphoric acid: Dilute phosphoric acid has been given as a bitter to increase appetite.

phosphorus is an element essential for body function, and should be adequately provided in a normal diet.

phthalylsulphacetamide is a sulphonamide drug.

phthalyisulphathiazole has the antibacterial actions of the sulphonamides. It is slowly broken down in the gut, the bulk being excreted in the faeces. It was used to treat bowel infections. *Adverse effects:* Allergic reactions may occur in patients sensitized to sulphonamides, and skin disorders may occur. *Dose:* By mouth, 5 to 10 g daily in divided doses.

Phyldrox tablets are used to treat asthma. Each tablet contains ephedrine hydrochloride 11 mg, phenobarbitone 8 mg and theophylline 120 mg ◊ ephedrine ◊ phenobarbitone ◊ theophylline.

Phyllocontin tablets contain 225 mg aminophylline in a sustained-release form which reduces the incidence of gastric side-effects. *Dose:* 2 tablets morning and evening.

Phyllosan: Each tablet contains ferrous fumarate 35 mg, nicotinic acid 8·5 mg, thiamine hydrochloride 166 micrograms, riboflavine 333 micrograms, and ascorbic acid 5 mg.

Physeptone ◊ methadone.

physostigmine (eserine; physostigmine salicylate) acts upon the sympathetic division of the autonomic nervous system. It is used principally in eye drops to constrict the pupil and reduce the pressure inside the eyeball in the treatment of glaucoma.

Phytex is used to treat fungal infections of the skin and nails. It contains tannic acid, boric acid, salicylic acid, methyl salicylate and acetic acid. *Dose:* Apply morning, evening after bathing for at least 2 weeks after apparent cure.

Phytocil is used to treat tinea infections, e.g., athlete's foot. The cream contains phenoxypropanol, chlorophenoxyethanol, salicylic acid and menthol; the powder contains phenoxypropanol, chlorophenoxyethanol and zinc undecenoate. *Dose:* Apply 3 times daily.

phytolacca is the dried root of the poke plant. It has emetic, purgative and mildly narcotic properties.

phytomenadione (Konakion; vitamin K) occurs naturally and is involved in blood clotting. It is an antidote to overdosage with oral anticoagulant drugs and is used in bleeding disorders. Overdose may cause jaundice in newborn babies. If given into a vein it should be given very slowly because it may produce sweating, flushing, a sense of suffocation, and collapse. *Dose:* 10 to 20 mg daily by intramuscular or slow intravenous injection, or by mouth.

Pickles Chilbain Cream contains methyl nicotinate 1% and histamine acid phosphate 0·1%.

Pickles Corn Caps contain salicylic acid 40% and colophonium mass 60%.

Pickles Foot Ointment contains salicylic acid 50%.

Pickles Hard Skin Reducer contains salicylic acid 12·5%.

Pickles Mouth Treatment is used to treat mouth ulcers, it contains tannic acid 2% and iodoform 0·05%.

Pickles SCR contains salicylic acid 1·5%.

Pickles Smelling Salts contains strong ammonia solution 28·5%, pumilio pine oil 14·25%, and eucalyptus oil 14·25%.

Pickles Toothache Tincture contains lignocaine hydrochloride 0·7% and clove oil 10%.

Picolax oral powder contains sodium picosulphate 10 mg/sachet with magnesium citrate. It is used to evacuate the bowel before surgery, X-ray and endoscopy. *Dose:* One sachet in the morning and the second in the afternoon the day before the intervention. It acts within 3 hours.

Pilease contains ethyl aminobenzoate 6%, zinc oxide 5%, hexachlorophane 0·5%, starch 5%, wool fat 10%, and paraffin basis to 100%.

pilocarpine (pilocarpine hydrochloride; pilocarpine nitrate) has effects and uses similar to those described under physostigmine. It is used in eye drops to constrict the pupil and decrease the pressure inside the eyeball in patients with glaucoma. Its effect on the eye is less complete and of shorter duration than that produced by physostigmine and a slight increase in pressure in the eye may occur at first.

Pilogene Compound contains hamamelis 1·05%, almond oil 1·35%, and zinc oxide 0·9% in a saponaceous basis.

Pimafucin ◊ natamycin.

pimozide (Orap) is a major tranquillizer. *Adverse effects:* It may produce Parkinsonism, skin rashes, sugar in the urine, and liver disorders. *Precautions:* It should not be used in pregnancy. It should be used with caution in patients who are depressed and in those with epilepsy. *Dose:* 2 to 10 mg daily in a single dose.

pindolol (Visken) is a beta-receptor blocker used to treat angina and raised blood pressure. *Adverse effects:* Depression, diarrhoea, insomnia, headache, fatigue and dizziness due to

fall in blood pressure have been reported. *Precautions* ◊ propranolol. *Dose:* By mouth 2·5 to 15 mg daily for angina, 10 to 45 mg daily for raised blood pressure. Can be taken in single or divided doses.

pine oil is used in steam inhalations to treat coughs, and as a rubbing oil to treat sprains.

pipenzolate (Piptal; pipenzolate bromide) has similar effects to atropine. It is used in the treatment of colic of the gastrointestinal tract. *Dose:* 5 mg three times daily before meals and 5 mg at night.

piperacillin (Pipril; piperacillin sodium) is a penicillin antibiotic reserved for severe infections resistant to other penicillins. *Adverse effects* and *Precautions* ◊ benzylpenicillin. *Dose:* By injection, depends on the severity of the infection.

piperazine (Antepar, Ascalix; piperazine citrate, hydrate and phosphate). Piperazine is used to treat threadworms and roundworm infection. *Adverse effects:* These are very rare unless high and prolonged dosage is used, when the patient may develop dizziness, clumsiness, vomiting, pins and needles and blurred vision. *Precautions:* Do not use in patients who suffer from epilepsy, kidney failure or liver failure. Use with caution if breast feeding. *Dose:* By mouth, for adults, 2 g daily in divided doses for one week.

piperidolate (Dactil) is an atropine-like drug used to relieve intestinal colic and other disorders of the stomach and gut. *Adverse effects* and *Precautions* ◊ atropine. *Dose:* By mouth, 50 mg four times daily.

piperonyl butoxide is active against scabies and it has some insecticidal activities.

Piportil Depot is an oily depot injection of pipothiazine palmitate 50 mg/ml ◊ pipothiazine.

pipothiazine (Piportil Depot, pipothiazine palmitate) is a major tranquilizer. *Adverse effects* and *Precautions* ◊ chlorpromazine. *Dose:* By deep intramuscular injection – 25 mg test dose and then 25 to 50 mg after 28 days. Maintenance 50 to 100 mg every 4 weeks (max. 200 mg).

Pipril ◊ piperacillin.

Piptal ◊ pipenzolate.

Piptalin suspension is used to treat peptic ulcers. Each 10 ml contains pipenzolate 8 mg and activated dimethicone 80 mg. *Dose:* By mouth, 10 ml three or four times daily 15 minutes before eating.

pirbuterol (Exirel; pirbuterol hydrochloride) has similar actions to salbutamol and is used in the treatment of asthma. *Adverse effects* and *Precautions* ◊ salbutamol. *Dose:* By inhalation, up to 12 puffs daily, by mouth, 10 to 15 mg three to four times daily.

pirenzepine (Gastrozepin; pirenzepine hydrochloride) reduces secretion of acid in the stomach and has an ulcer healing effect. *Adverse effects:* These include dry mouth and blurred vision.

Dose: By mouth, 50 mg morning and night, for up to three months.

piretanide (Arelix) is a loop diuretic. For *Adverse effects* and *Precautions* ◊ frusemide. *Dose:* By mouth, 6 to 12 mg daily as a single dose in the morning.

Piriton ◊ chlorpheniramine.

piroxicam (Feldene) is an anti-rheumatic drug. *Adverse effects* and *Precautions* ◊ naproxen. It may produce oedema. *Dose:* By mouth, 20 to 40 mg daily in divided doses with meals.

Pitressin ◊ argipressin.

pivampicillin (Miraxid; Pondocillin) is a pro-drug ester of ampicillin. The pivampicillin is well absorbed from the gut and changed in the body to the active antibiotic ampicillin. *Uses, Adverse effects* and *Precautions* ◊ ampicillin. Repeated liver and kidney function tests should be carried out on patients receiving long-term treatment with pivampicillin. *Dose:* By mouth, 500 to 1,000 mg every 12 hours.

pivmecillinam (Miraxid; Selexid; pivmecillinam hydrochloride) is a pro-drug ester of mecillinam. The pivmecillinam is well absorbed from the gut and changed in the body to the active antibiotic mecillinam. It has similar actions and effects to the penicillins, and cephalosporins. *Adverse effects* and *Precautions* ◊ benzylpenicillin. They include gastro-intestinal upsets and rash. Dosage may need modification when kidney function is impaired. Routine liver and kidney function tests should be carried out in patients on long-term treatment. *Dose:* By mouth, 200 mg three to four times a day for urinary tract infections: for salmonellosis or carriers 1·2 to 2·4 g daily in divided doses. Take with water whilst standing up in order to avoid irritation of the gullet.

Piz Buin is a sunscreen preparation containing 2-ethylhexyl p-methoxycinnamate and oxybenzone.

pizotifen (Sanomigran; pizotifen malate) is chemically similar to amitriptyline. It has antihistamine properties and anticholinergic properties. It is used to prevent migraine attacks. *Adverse effects:* These include drowsiness, increase of appetite and gain in weight, nausea, dizziness, flushing of the face, muscle pains and mood changes. *Precautions:* It should not be given to patients in charge of moving machinery or where loss of attention could lead to an accident. It should not be given to patients with closed-angle glaucoma or to patients liable to retention of urine. *Dose:* By mouth, 0·5 mg three times daily. Up to maximum of 6 mg daily.

Placidex contains paracetamol 240 mg in each 10 ml.

Plancaps ◊ ferrous fumarate.

Plaquenil ◊ hydroxychloroquine.

Platinex ◊ cisplatin.

Platosin injection ◊ cisplatin.

Plesmet ◊ ferrous glycine sulphate.

Plex-Hormone* is used to treat hypogonadism. Each tablet contains methyltestosterone 5 mg, deoxycortone acetate 0·5 mg, ethinyloestradiol 2 micrograms and tocopheryl acetate 5 mg. *Dose:* 4 to 5 daily for 10 to 14 days.

Plex-Hormone injection* contains testosterone propionate 20 mg, deoxycortone acetate 0·5 mg, oestradiol benzoate 0·1 mg and tocopheryl acetate 20 mg/ml. *Dose:* By intramuscular injection 1 ml two to three times weekly for two weeks. Maintenance, 1 ml weekly.

plicamycin (mithracin) is an anticancer drug. *Adverse effects:* These include nausea, vomiting, diarrhoea, sore gums and mouth (stomatitis), headache and skin rashes. Blood levels of potassium, calcium and phosphorus may be reduced. It may cause damage to the bone marrow leading to blood disorders and bleeding, and reversible damage to the kidneys and liver. *Precautions:* It should not be used in pregnancy and should be given with caution to patients with impaired kidney, liver or bone-marrow function. *Dose:* Varies according to disorder being treated. It is also used to reduce raised blood calcium.

Plurivite M Tablets: Each contain vitamin A palmitate 5,000 units, thiamine hydrochloride 2 mg, riboflavine 2 mg, pyridoxine hydrochloride 1 mg, cyanocobalamin 2 micrograms, nicotinamide 20 mg, vitamin C (as sodium ascorbate) 50 mg, calciferol solution 400 units, iron (as ferrous carbonate) 15 mg, and copper (as copper carbonate) 0·75 mg.

Plurivite Tablets: Each contain vitamin A palmitate 4,000 units, thiamine hydrochloride 2 mg, riboflavine 2 mg, pyridoxine hydrochloride 1 mg, cyanocobalamin 2 micrograms, nicotinamide 20 mg, ascorbic acid 50 mg, calciferol solution 400 units, vitamin E 5 mg, and calcium pantothenate 5 mg.

P.M.T. Tablets: Each contain pyridoxine hydrochloride 20 mg.

Pneumovax is a polyvalent pneumonia vaccine for the immunization of persons for whom the risks of contracting pneumococcal pneumonia is unusually high.

podophyllum is an irritant when applied to the skin and mucous membranes. It is used in skin paints and ointments to treat warts.

Point-Two ◊ fluoride.

Pol/vac (Poliomyelitis vaccine inactivated and oral). The oral vaccine is a suspension of live attenuated strains of poliomyelitis virus. The inactivated vaccine is used for active immunization when the oral vaccine cannot be used, e.g., in pregnancy.

poldine (Nacton; poldine methylsulphate) is an atropine-like drug. It reduces gastric secretion, is long acting and is used to treat peptic ulcers and conditions associated with an increased production of acid in the stomach. *Adverse effects* and *Precautions:* These are similar to those described under atropine. *Dose:* By mouth, 4 mg every six hours.

Pollen-B tablets: Each contain bee-collected pollen 150 mg.

Pollinex is used to treat allergy to pollens. It is prepared from 10 varieties of common grass pollen.

poloxamer is a surface-active agent used to treat constipation.

Polyalk suspension is used to treat indigestion and peptic ulcers. Each 5 ml contains dimethicone 125 mg, aluminium hydroxide 440 mg, and magnesium oxide 70 mg. *Dose:* By mouth, 5 to 10 ml between meals and at bedtime. **Tablets** contain 500 mg of dried aluminium hydroxide and 250 mg of activated dimethicone – dose 1 to 2 tablets chewed or sucked when required.

Polybactrin soluble powder for reconstitution for bladder irrigation contains polymyxin B sulphate 75,000 units, neomycin sulphate 20,000 units and bacitracin 1,000 units.

Polycal contains carbohydrate (as maltodextrin syrup) 94·5%. Maltodextrin is prepared from corn starch and provides a source of glucose.

Polycrol: Each tablet contains activated dimethicone 25 mg, aluminium hydroxide gel 275 mg and magnesium hydroxide 100 mg. It is used to treat indigestion and peptic ulcers. *Dose:* 1 to 2 tablets three or four times daily between meals and at bedtime. It is also available as a gel.

Polycrol Forte preparations contain the same ingredients as Polycrol but the amount of dimethicone is increased.

polydimethylsiloxane ◊ activated dimethicone.

Polydine ◊ povidone-iodine.

polyethylene glycol ◊ macrogol.

Polyfax antibiotic ophthalmic ointment and skin ointment contains polymyxin B sulphate 10,000 units and bacitracin zinc 500 units/g.

polyhydroxyaluminium sodium carbonate is an antacid.

Polygeline ◊ gelatin.

polymethylsiloxane is activated dimethicone – a silicone used in antacids used as a dispersant.

polymyxin B (Aerosporin; polymyxin B sulphate) is an antibiotic. It is used in ointments, sprays, drops and powders and is taken by mouth to treat infections of the gut. It may also be given by injection. *Adverse effects:* When given by injection it may cause dizziness and sensory sensations, particularly over the face, hands and feet (this suggests that it is toxic to nerves); rarely, it may damage the kidneys and produce nerve damage leading to paralysis of respiration. These adverse effects do not occur when the drug is taken by mouth; but adverse effects may occur when it is applied to large raw areas, especially burns. Fever and pain at the site of injection may occur. *Precautions:* It should be given with caution to patients with impaired kidney function. *Dose:* By mouth, 1 to 2 million units daily in divided doses; by intravenous injection, dose varies according to disorder being treated.

polynoxylin (Anaflex, Ponoxylan) has antibacterial and antifungal actions and is used in creams, powders and lozenges for the treatment of infections.

polyoestradiol (Estradurin, polyoestradiol phosphate) is broken down in the body to oestradiol ◊ oestradiol. It is used in the treatment of cancer of the prostate. *Dose:* By deep intramuscular injection, 40 to 160 mg every four weeks.

polyoxyethylene derivative of wool fat ◊ wool fat.

polysorbate 60 is an emulsifier.

Polytar preparations contain cade oil and extracts of tar.

polythiazide (Nephril) is a diuretic with effects, uses and adverse effects similar to those described under chlorothiazide. *Dose:* By mouth, 1 to 4 mg daily.

Polytrim eye drops and **ointment** contain trimethoprim 1 mg and polymyxin B sulphate 10,000 units in each 1 ml.

Polyvinyl alcohol is used in aerosol sprays which dry rapidly when applied to the skin and form a soluble plastic protective film.

polyvinylpyrrolidone ◊ povidone.

Polyvite capsules are a multivitamin preparation.

Ponderax ◊ fenfluramine.

Ponderax P A capsules contain fenfluramine hydrochloride 60 mg in slow-release form. ◊ fenfluramine.

Pondocillin ◊ pivampicillin.

Pondocillin Plus tablets contain pivampicillin 250 mg and pivmecillinam 200 mg ◊ pivampicillin and pivmecillinam.

Ponoxylan ◊ polynoxylin.

Ponstan ◊ mefenamic acid.

Ponstan Forte: Each capsule contains mefenamic acid 500 mg.

Portia athletic rub is a rub containing capsicum ointment 4·5%, methyl salicylate 0·75% and menthol 0·9%.

Posalfilin ointment is used to treat plantar warts (verrucae). It contains salicylic acid 25% and podophyllum resin 20%.

posterior pituitary extract (Di-Sipidin) is used in the treatment of diabetes insipidus. *Dose:* By insufflation into the nose, the contents of 2 or 3 capsules daily.

Potaba: Each capsule or tablet contains potassium p-aminobenzoate 500 mg.

Potaba +6 tablets contain pyridoxine hydrochloride 1 mg in addition to potassium p-aminobenzoate ◊ pyridoxine.

potassium: Many diuretic drugs which are used to reduce fluid retention (oedema), caused by heart, liver or kidney disorders, may result in a loss of potassium salts. This loss is usually corrected by giving potassium salts by mouth. *Adverse effects:* Potassium salts are irritant when taken by mouth;

they may cause ulceration of the stomach or intestine with bleeding and obstruction. When given with a thiazide diuretic they may cause similar effects. *Precautions:* Potassium salts should be taken well diluted and given with caution to patients with impaired kidney function or adrenal insufficiency. *Dose:* This depends upon the salt used and the patient's requirements.

potassium acetate is used in the prevention and treatment of potassium deficiency. It is also used as a food preservative.

potassium acid tartrate is used as a saline purgative. It also has a mild diuretic effect and has been used in dusting powder for surgical rubber gloves.

potassium p-aminobenzoate (Potaba) is considered to belong to the B-group of vitamins. It has been used in the treatment of various fibrotic disorders such as sclerodema, that involve excessive hardening of tissues. *Dose:* 12 g daily in divided doses.

potassium bicarbonate is used in the prevention and treatment of potassium deficiency.

potassium bitartrate ◊ cream of tartar.

potassium bromide was widely used as a sedative. *Adverse effects:* During prolonged use bromide accumulates in the body; this may give rise to symptoms of bromide intoxication (bromism) which include skin rashes, nausea, vomiting, mental dullness, poor memory, apathy, loss of appetite, constipation and drowsiness. These symptoms disappear if the drug is stopped but get worse if the drug is continued, leading to insomnia, restlessness, disorientation, hallucinations, delirium, stupor and coma.

potassium chloride (Slow-K) is used in the prevention and treatment of potassium deficiency. It is also used as a table salt substitute.

potassium citrate makes the urine less acid and is used to treat inflammation of the bladder and urethra. It may also be used as a potassium supplement.

potassium clorazepate (Tranxene) is a benzodiazepine anti-anxiety drug. *Adverse effects* and *Precautions* ◊ chlordiazepoxide. *Dose:* By mouth, 15 mg at night.

potassium guaiacolsulphonate is used as an expectorant to treat coughs. It is of doubtful value.

potassium hydroxyquinoline (potassium hydroxyquinoline sulphate) is used in skin applications as an antibacterial, antifungal, deodorant, and keratolytic. It is used in an anti-acne preparation (Quinoderm).

potassium hypophosphite ◊ glycerophosphates and hypophosphites.

potassium iodide is used in cough medicines as an expectorant, to treat underworking of the thyroid gland due to iodine deficiency, and in skin applications as an antiseptic. *Adverse effects* ◊ iodine.

potassium metabisulphate is an antioxidant used as a preservative in medicines and food.

potassium molybdate ◊ molybdendum.

potassium monopersulphate and sodium chloride yield sodium hypochlorite (a disinfectant) in aqueous solution – Milton crystals, Napisan.

potassium nitrate acts as a diuretic. It is used as a preservative in foods.

potassium permanganate has disinfectant, deodorizing and astringent properties. It is used as a cleansing agent and as a gargle or mouthwash when diluted with water. It is also used for certain skin conditions, e.g., athlete's foot. *Adverse effect:* It may cause corrosive burns.

potassium sulphate has been used as a saline laxative.

potassium tartrate ◊ potassium acid tartrate.

Potter's Asthma Cigarettes contain the active principles of stramonium leaves equivalent to 0·15% of alkaloids calculated as hyoscyamine.

Potter's Asthma Remedy contains the active principles of stramonium leaves equivalent to 0·12% of alkaloids calculated as hyoscyamine.

Potter's Catarrh Pastilles contain sylvestris pine oil 0·41%, pumilio pine oil 0·41%, eucalyptus oil 0·02%, creosote 0·2%, menthol 0·83%, thymol 0·02%, and aqueous extractive from althaea 0·5%.

Potter's Children's Cough Pastilles contain honey 90 mg, glycerol 22 mg, menthol 430 micrograms, and creosote 120 micrograms.

Potter's **Dermacreme Ointment** contains menthol 0·015%, methyl salicylate 3%, liquefied phenol 1%, starch 8%, zinc oxide 8%, hard paraffin 5%, wool fat 3·25%, and yellow soft paraffin to 100%.

Potter's **Gee's Linctus Pastilles** contain concentrated camphorated opium tincture 0·075 ml, squill liquid extract 0·03 ml, benzoic acid 0·6 mg, cinnamic acid 0·25 mg, glacial acetic acid 0·02 ml and purified honey 0·2 ml.

Potter's **Glycerin and Blackcurrant Pastilles** are used to treat throat irritation.

Potter's **Glycerin, Lemon and Honey Pastilles** are used to treat coughs and colds.

Potter's **Glycerin of Thymol Pastilles** contain thymol 0·04%, menthol 0·003%, cineole 0·06%, pine oil 0·02%, glycerol 3·0% and methyl salicylate 0·004%.

Potter's **Menthol and Eucalyptus Pastilles** contain menthol 0·8% and eucalyptus oil 0·6%.

Potter's **Psoriasis Ointment** contains starch 5%, sublimed sulphur 7%, zinc oxide 7%, phytolacca 0·5%, butamyrate citrate 0·18%, hydrous wool fat 28%, and yellow soft paraffin to 100%.

Potter's **Skin Clear Ointment** contains phenol 0·33%, starch 17%, sulphur sublimed 5%, zinc oxide 23%, and yellow soft paraffin to 100%.

Potter's **Varicose Vein Ointment** contains boric acid 3·7%, cade oil 2·3%, emulsifying wax 2·4%, hamamelis liquid extract 7·4%, hard paraffin 1·85%, wool alcohol 1·48%, zinc oxide 3·57%, and yellow soft paraffin to 100%.

Potter's **Walk Easy Ointment** contains salicylic acid 12·5%.

povidone (polyvinylpyrrolidone) is used in the preparation of tablets and as a carrier of drugs such as penicillin, insulin and iodine to prolong their action. It is also used in lubricant eye drops and in solutions to make the wearing of contact lenses more comfortable.

povidone-iodine (Disadine DP) is used in skin and mouth applications as an antiseptic. ◊ iodine.

Powerin tablets: Each contain paracetamol 200 mg, caffeine 45 mg, and aspirin 300 mg.

PP Tablets each contain gentian extract 6 mg, valerian liquid extract 12 mg, passion flower extract (1 in 1) 6 mg, theobromine 15 mg, paracetamol 150 mg, caffeine 7·5 mg, and kola liquid extract 12 mg.

PR Spray is a refrigerant skin spray, contains dichlorodifluoromethane 15% and trichlorofluoromethane 85%. It evaporates readily from the skin to produce a cooling, pain-relieving effect. *Precautions:* Not to be used on inflamed or broken skin. *Dose:* Spray for 3 to 5 seconds, repeating if necessary up to a maximum of 9 sprays daily.

Practolol* (Eraldin) is a beta-receptor blocking drug. It was used to treat irregularities of heart rate and rhythm and in the treatment of angina and raised blood pressure. It had effects and uses similar to those described under propranolol but it had less effect upon respiration. *Adverse effects:* Practolol damaged the eyes, produced diminished tear production, conjunctivitis, corneal damage and occasionally impairment or loss of vision. These effects were noted in patients who received practolol for periods ranging from a few weeks to several years. There were also reports of skin rashes like psoriasis. Mild eye changes and the skin rashes usually recovered when the drug was stopped but not the corneal damage. There were reports of deafness, a scarring (sclerosis) peritonitis, and a general disease called systemic lupus erythematosus. This is an inflammatory disease that can affect skin, joints, lungs, heart, spleen, lymph nodes, and kidneys. *Dose:* By injection 2 mg/ml. It is only used in hospitals.

Pragmatar ointment contains tar distillate 4%, sulphur 3% and salicylic acid 3%.

Praminil ◊ imipramine.

pramoxine (pramoxine hydrochloride) is a local anaesthetic used on the skin.

Praxilene ◊ naftidrofuryl.

prazepam is a benzodiazepine anti-anxiety drug with similar effects to diazepam. *Dose:* 5 to 60 mg daily.

praziquantel (Biltricide) is used to kill schitosomes (worms that live in the genito-urinary veins). *Dose:* 40 mg/kg body-weight as a single oral dose.

prazosin (Hypovase; prazosin hydrochloride) is used to treat raised blood pressure. *Adverse effects:* These include dizziness, headache, drowsiness, lack of energy, nausea, dry mouth, weakness, blurred vision, frequency of passing urine, congestion of the nose, nervousness, depressed mood, constipation, skin rashes, diarrhoea, fainting and itching. These are usually related to dose and may disappear on continuation of treatment or on reducing the dose. There are a few reported cases of unconsciousness after the first dose. *Dose:* By mouth, 0·5 mg the first evening, 0·5 mg three times a day for seven days, 1 mg three times a day for seven days, then gradually increasing to a maximum daily dose of 20 mg. Also used to treat benign enlargement of the prostate gland. Maximum dose 2 mg twice daily.

Precortisyl ◊ prednisolone.

Predenema ◊ prednisolone.

Predfoam rectal foam contains prednisolone metasulphobenzoate sodium ◊ prednisolone. *Precautions:* Protect the can from sunlight and do not expose to temperatures above 50°C. Do not pierce or burn the can.

Prednesol ◊ prednisolone.

prednisolone (preparations include: Codelsol; Delta-Phoricol; Deltacortril Enteric; Deltalone; Deltastab; Precortisyl; Predenema; Predfoam; Prednesol; Predsol; Sintisone; prednisolone acetate; prednisolone sodium metasulphobenzoate; prednisolone sodium phosphate; prednisolone steaglate) is a corticosteroid. It has effects and uses similar to those described under cortisone but it is effective in a much smaller dose and has weaker salt retention effects. Because of this it is preferred to cortisone as an anti-inflammatory drug in the treatment of such disorders as rheumatoid arthritis, rheumatic fever and asthma. Read section on corticosteroids. *Adverse effects* and *Precautions:* These are similar to those described under cortisone. *Dose:* By mouth, 10 to 100 mg daily in divided doses.

prednisone (Decortisyl, Econosone) is converted in the liver to prednisolone and there is no significant difference between the effects of the two substances.

Predsol (prednisolone sodium phosphate) is used in eye and ear drops, retention enemas and suppositories. ◊ prednisolone.

Prefil is a slimming drug. It contains sterculia 55% and guar gum 5%. *Dose:* By mouth, two 5 ml spoonfuls of granules swallowed with water, 30 minutes before each meal.

Pregaday tablets contain ferrous fumarate 304 mg and folic acid 0·35 mg. *Dose:* 1 daily.

Pregnavite Forte F is a compound iron preparation. Each tablet contains ferrous sulphate 84 mg (25·2 mg iron), folic acid 120 micrograms, vitamin A 1,333 units, thiamine hydrochloride 500 micrograms, riboflavine 500 micrograms, nicotinamide 5 mg, pyridoxine hydrochloride 330 micrograms, ascorbic acid 13·3 mg, vitamin D 133 units, calcium phosphate 160 mg.

Premarin contains conjugated oestrogens. It is used to treat menopausal symptoms. Tablets of 0·625 mg, 1·25 mg and 2·5 mg are available and also a vaginal cream.

Premiums: Each tablet contains magnesium trisilicate 0·04 g, dried aluminium hydroxide gel 0·125 g, light magnesium carbonate 0·15 g, chalk 0·25 g and peppermint oil 0·0042 g.

Prempak 0·625 is used to treat menopausal symptoms. It comprises a calendar pack containing 21 maroon tablets of conjugated oestrogens 625 micrograms and 7 white tablets of norgestrel 500 micrograms. *Dose:* 1 maroon tablet daily for 14 days starting on 5th day of cycle or at any time if cycles have ceased or are infrequent, then 1 white and 1 maroon tablet daily for 7 days, followed by a 7 day interval.

Prempak 1·25 is used to treat menopausal symptoms. It comprises a calendar pack containing 21 yellow tablets of conjugated oestrogens 1·25 mg and 7 white tablets of norgestrel 500 micrograms. *Dose:* As Prempak 0·625 but starting with 1 yellow tablet daily.

Prempak-C 0·625 is used to treat menopausal symptoms. It comprises a calendar pack containing 28 maroon tablets of conjugated oestrogens 625 micrograms and 12 light brown tablets of norgestrel 150 micrograms. *Dose:* 1 maroon tablet daily, starting on 1st day of cycle or at any time if cycles have ceased or are infrequent then 1 maroon and 1 brown tablet daily for 12 days. Subsequent courses should be repeated without intervals.

Prempak-C 1·25 is used to treat meno-pausal symptoms. It comprises a calendar pack containing 28 yellow tablets of conjugated oestrogens 1·25 mg and 12 light brown tablets of norgestrel 150 micrograms. *Dose:* As Prempak-C 0·625 but starting with 1 yellow tablet daily.

Prenatol cream helps prevent stretch marks during pregnancy. It contains hydroxyproline 2·45%.

prenylamine (Synadrin; prenylamine lactate) is used to treat angina. *Adverse effects:* It may cause nausea, vomiting and diarrhoea. Skin rashes, flushing and drowsiness may occur. *Precautions:* It should not be used in patients with impaired liver function or with heart failure. *Dose:* By mouth, 60 mg three times daily.

Preparation H Ointment contains the alcohol-soluble extract of 2 g of live yeast cells per g (Bio-Dyne), shark-liver oil 3%, and phenylmercuric nitrate 0·01% and **Suppositories** each containing the alcohol-soluble extract of 72 mg of live yeast cells, shark-liver oil 72 mg, and phenylmercuric nitrate 0·24%.

Pressimmune ◊ antilymphocyte immunoglobulin.

Prestim is used to treat raised blood pressure. Each tablet contains timolol 10 mg and bendrofluazide 2·5 mg.

Prestim forte is used to treat raised blood pressure. Each tablet contains timolol maleate 20 mg and bendro-fluazide 5 mg.

Priadel ◊ lithium.

prilocaine (Citanest; prilocaine hydro-chloride) is a local anaesthetic with similar effects and uses to lignocaine but it produces fewer adverse effects. Overdose may cause chemical change inside the red blood cells (methaemo-globinaemia) and it should therefore not be used in patients with anaemia; similarly it should not be used in pregnancy because of this risk.

Primalan ◊ mequitazine.

primaquine (primaquine phosphate) is an antimalarial drug. *Adverse effects:* Common adverse effects of high dosage are nausea, abdominal pain and blood disorders. Adverse effects on the blood occur more frequently in patients with a genetic fault which leads to an abnormality of glucose metabolism. *Dose:* By mouth, prevention, 30 to 60 mg once a week along with 300 mg of chloroquine; treatment, 15 mg daily for fourteen days.

Primes Premiums: Each tablet contains magnesium trisilicate 40 mg, dried aluminium hydroxide 125 mg, magnesium carbonate 150 mg, calcium carbonate 250 mg, and peppermint oil.

primidone (Mysoline) is an anti-convulsant used to treat epilepsy. *Adverse effects:* It may cause drowsiness, ataxia, nausea, vomiting, vertigo, irritability, headache, visual disturbances, fatigue and general de-bility, and occasionally skin rashes. These are usually mild and disappear with reduction of dosage. Other adverse effects include thirst, passing a lot of water, oedema, and impaired sexual function. Anaemia may occur (megaloblastic anaemia) which responds to folic acid treatment. *Dose:* By mouth, 750 to 1,000 mg daily in divided doses.

Primolut N ◊ norethisterone.

Primoteston Depot contains testosterone for injection.

Primperan ◊ metoclopramide.

Prioderm ◊ malathion.

Pripsen (each 10 g sachet contains piperazine phosphate 4 g and sennosides A and B 14 mg) ◊ piperazine and sennosides. Used to treat threadworms. *Dose:* 1 sachet is a single dose.

Pro-Actidil ◊ triprolidine.

Pro-Banthine ◊ propantheline.

probenecid (Benemid) is used to treat gout. It increases the excretion of urates by the kidneys. This results in a reduction of the raised blood uric acid level (which occurs in gout) and slowly causes removal of urate deposits (tophi) from the tissues. It is of no use in treating an acute attack of gout and is only used to prevent the frequency of acute attacks. Treatment must usually be continued for life. Probenecid also reduces the excretion of penicillins and of the antibiotics cephalexin and cephalothin. It therefore increases the plasma level of these drugs, which is directly related to their effectiveness. *Adverse effects:* These are rare with doses up to 1 g daily. Above this dose nausea, vomiting, skin rashes and fever may occur. These are more likely to occur in patients with impaired kidney function. *Precautions:* Acute

attacks of gout may be precipitated in the first few weeks or months of treatment with probenecid, particularly with high doses. Daily dosage should not be interrupted because this allows the blood uric acid level to rise. Aspirin, citrates and salicylates should not be given with probenecid because they antagonize its effects. *Dose:* By mouth, 500 mg twice daily.

probucol (Lurselle) is used to reduce high blood fat levels. *Adverse effects:* Nausea, vomiting, diarrhoea, abdominal pain and flatulence, hypersensitivity reactions and angioneurotic oedema. *Precautions:* It should not be used in breast-feeding mothers. Avoid pregnancy during and for six months after stopping treatment. *Dose:* By mouth, 500 mg twice daily with food.

procainamide (Procainamide Durules; Pronestyl; procainamide hydrochloride) has effects upon the heart rate and rhythm. *Adverse effects:* In high dosage it may cause loss of appetite, nausea, vomiting, and diarrhoea. Rapid injections into a vein may cause a sudden fall in blood pressure and disorders of heart rhythm. Prolonged administration may produce joint pains, skin rashes, chest pains and a blood disorder (these signs and symptoms are known as lupus erythematosus). It may also cause abdominal pain, enlargement of the liver, confusion, itching, and allergic reactions – fever and skin rashes. *Precautions:* Procainamide should not be given to patients with bronchial asthma, allergy to the drug, impaired kidney function, disorders of the heart affecting the conduction of nervous impulses, and during treatment with sulphonamide drugs. It should be used with caution in patients with digoxin intoxication. *Dose:* By mouth, 250 mg six hourly; by slow intravenous injection, up to 1 g in a 2·5 per cent solution under E.C.G. control.

Procainamide Durules ◊ procainamide.

procaine (procaine hydrochloride) is a short-acting local anaesthetic.

procaine penicillin (Depocillin; procaine benzylpenicillin; procaine penicillin G) is a salt of benzylpenicillin ◊ benzylpenicillin. It is given by intramuscular injection and creates a depot from which the benzylpenicillin is slowly released into the blood-stream. It can therefore be given only once daily. Large doses given more than once daily may cause adverse effects due to release of procaine and leave painful lumps at the site of injection. *Dose:* 300 to 900 mg daily by deep intramuscular injection.

procarbazine (Natulan) is an anticancer drug. *Adverse effects:* These include loss of appetite, nausea, vomiting, sore mouth and gums (stomatitis), diarrhoea, pain, fever and infections. Skin rashes, bleeding, disorders of the heart and circulation, loss of hair (alopecia), impaired liver function and general itching have been recorded. Mood changes and nerve damage may occasionally occur and in children trembling, convulsions and unconsciousness have been reported. *Precautions:* It should not be used in pregnancy. It should be used with caution in patients with impaired kidney and liver function and it should not be

used if there is evidence of impaired bone-marrow function. It is a monoamine oxidase inhibitor drug and therefore special precautions about food and other drugs should be taken (◊ phenelzine). It may increase the depressant effects upon the brain of antihistamines, narcotic pain relievers and phenothiazine major tranquillizers. It can produce a disulfiram-like effect with alcohol. *Dose:* Varies according to the disorder being treated.

prochlorperazine (Buccastem; Stemetil; Vertigon; prochlorperazine maleate) is a major tranquillizer. It has effects and uses similar to those described under chlorpromazine but it is less sedating and is more effective in treating nausea and vomiting. It is also effective in treating vertigo and Ménière's disease. *Adverse effects:* These are similar to those described under chlorpromazine. Adverse effects occur less frequently than with chlorpromazine but Parkinsonism is more common. Dryness of the mouth, dizziness, fall in blood pressure, and rapid beating of the heart may occur occasionally. Drowsiness is frequent and jaundice and blood disorders have been reported. Severe Parkinsonism may occur in ill children and can be very alarming. *Precautions:* It should be given with great caution to children; other precautions are similar to those described under chlorpromazine. *Dose:* For nausea, vomiting or vertigo: 10 to 30 mg daily in divided doses by mouth, or by suppository or intramuscular injection (12·5 mg). For psychological disorders: by mouth, 15 to 100 mg daily in divided doses.

Procol are sustained-action capsules each containing isopropamide iodide 3·4 mg and phenylpropanolamine hydrochloride 50 mg.

Proctofibe contains fibrous grain extract 375 mg and fibrous citrus extract 94 mg and it is used as a bulk laxative. *Dose:* By mouth, 4 to 12 tablets daily with water, in divided dose.

Proctofoam H C foam aerosol is used to treat proctitis etc. It contains hydrocortisone acetate 1% and pramoxine hydrochloride 1%. *Dose:* 1 applicatorful rectally two to three times daily.

Proctors' Pinelyptus Pastilles contain menthol 0·548%, eucalyptus oil 0·842%, abietis oil 0·12%, and sylvestris pine oil 0·12%.

Proctosedyl: Each 1 g of ointment and suppository contains hydrocortisone 5 mg, cinchocaine hydrochloride 5 mg and framycetin sulphate 10 mg. It is used to treat haemorrhoids, and pruritus ani.

procyclidine (Arpicolin; Kemadrin; procyclidine hydrochloride) is used to treat Parkinsonism. It decreases rigidity and tremor, and improves muscle coordination and mobility of the patient. It has little effect upon salivation. It is an atropine-like drug. *Adverse effects* and *Precautions:* These are similar to those described under atropine. Drowsiness, ataxia, giddiness, blurred vision, confusion, nausea and vomiting may occur. These usually disappear when the dose is reduced. *Dose:* By mouth, 7·5 to 30 mg daily in divided doses.

Prodexin is used to treat indigestion and peptic ulcers. Each tablet contains aluminium glycinate 900 mg and magnesium carbonate 100 mg. *Dose:* By mouth, 1 to 2 when required.

Profasi ◊ chorionic gonadotrophin.

proflavine (proflavine hemisulphate) is used as an antiseptic and disinfectant in skin applications and eye drops.

Proflex ◊ ibuprofen.

Progesic ◊ fenoprofen.

progesterone (Cyclogest) is a naturally occurring female sex hormone. Read section on female sex hormones. It is used to treat heavy and irregular periods, habitual abortion and premenstrual syndrome. *Adverse effects:* Acne, urticaria (nettle-rash), weight gain, breast discomfort, stomach upsets, changes in libido, changes in menstrual cycle and occasionally jaundice. Injection may be painful. *Precautions:* It should not be used in undiagnosed vaginal bleeding, breast cancer, or missed abortion. It should be used with caution in breast-feeding mothers and in patients suffering from diabetes, raised blood pressure or kidney, liver or heart disease. *Dose:* By vagina or rectum 200 to 400 mg twice daily from 14th to 28th day of menstrual cycle. By intramuscular injection for habitual abortion, 5 to 10 mg daily or up 20 mg 2 to 3 times weekly. For menstrual disorders 5 to 10 mg daily for 5 to 10 days before periods.

proguanil (Paludrine; proguanil hydrochloride) is used to prevent and treat malaria. *Adverse effects:* These rarely occur except with large doses which may cause vomiting and abdominal pain. *Precautions:* It should always be given after meals. *Dose:* By mouth; suppressive dose, 100 to 200 mg daily.

Progynova ◊ oestradiol.

Pro-Hyd 50 capsules: Each contains procaine hydrochloride 50 mg and haematoporphyrin hydrochloride 200 micrograms.

prolintane is a weak central nervous stimulant, having a similar effect to caffeine ◊ caffeine. It is found in the multivitamin preparation Villescon.

Proluton Depot ◊ hydroxyprogesterone.

promazine (Sparine; promazine hydrochloride) is a major tranquillizer with effects and uses similar to those described under chlorpromazine. *Adverse effects* and *Precautions:* These are similar to those described under chlorpromazine. Dizziness and drowsiness occur frequently but a fall in blood pressure and Parkinsonism are not as frequent as with chlorpromazine. *Dose:* By mouth, 25 to 100 mg three or four times daily. By intramuscular or intravenous injection, 50 mg every eight hours.

promethazine (Phenergan; Sominex; promethazine hydrochloride; Avomine; promethazine theoclate) is an antihistamine drug. The hydrochloride is used as an antihistamine and the theoclate as an anti-vomiting drug. *Adverse effects:* These are discussed under the section on antihistamine drugs. Adverse effects include dryness of the mouth, throat and nose, ab-

dominal pain with vomiting and diarrhoea. The most common adverse effect is drowsiness, which can interfere with the ability to drive a motor vehicle or operate machinery. Other adverse effects include inability to concentrate, lassitude, dizziness, muscle weakness, incoordination, headache, blurred vision, irritability, loss of appetite and noises in the ears (tinnitus). Stimulation may occur, particularly in children and infants, causing excitability and nightmares after even one dose. Blood disorders and jaundice have been reported and skin sensitivity to sunlight may occur. *Precautions:* Promethazine may increase the sedative effects of alcohol, sleeping drugs, sedatives, and tranquillizers. The effects of antidepressant drugs and atropine-like drugs may also be increased. It should be used with caution in patients with impaired liver function. Patients should be warned about the dangers of driving motor vehicles and operating machinery and of the dangers of taking alcohol whilst on promethazine. *Dose:* By mouth, 25 to 50 mg daily (usually at night); by deep intramuscular injection, up to 50 mg.

Prominal ◊ methylphenobarbitone.

Prondol ◊ iprindole.

Pronel capsules are used to treat brittle and flaking finger nails. Each capsule contains gelatin 320 mg.

Pronestyl ◊ procainamide.

Propaderm-A ointment contains beclomethasone dipropionate 0·025%, chlortetracycline hydrochloride 3% in soft paraffin.

Propain is a mild pain-reliever which also contains an antihistamine drug. Each tablet contains codeine phosphate 10 mg, diphenhydramine hydrochloride 5 mg, paracetamol 400 mg and caffeine 50 mg. *Dose:* By mouth, 1 to 2 four-hourly, to a maximum of 10 tablets in 24 hours.

propamidine isethionate ◊ dibromopropamidine isethionate.

propanidid (Epontol) is used as an anaesthetic for short operations.

propantheline (Pro-Banthine; propantheline bromide) is an atropine-like drug. It is used to treat peptic ulcers because it reduces gastric secretions and spasm. It may also be used to treat intestinal colic, spasms of the gall-bladder ducts and spasms of the ureters, and to control excessive salivation. *Adverse effects:* These are similar to those described under atropine. *Precautions:* These are similar to those described under atropine. It should be used with caution in patients with glaucoma and in those with enlarged prostates. *Dose:* By mouth, 15 mg three times daily.

Propine ◊ dipivefrin.

propionic acid is an antifungal drug used as preservative.

Pro-Plus Tablets: Each contains caffeine 50 mg.

propoxyphene ◊ dextropropoxyphene.

propranolol (Angilol; Apsolol; Bedranol; Berkolol; Half-Inderal LA; Inderal; Sloprolol; propranolol hydrochloride) is a beta-receptor blocking drug. It is used to treat disorders of heart rhythm and angina, and also raised blood pressure. *Adverse effects:* Nausea, vomiting, diarrhoea, insomnia, lassitude and ataxia may occur. Sensory sensations in the hands, blood disorders, skin rashes and visual hallucinations may occur less frequently. Heart failure and wheezing (bronchospasm) may also occur. *Precautions:* Propranolol should not be given to patients with bronchial asthma, bronchospasm or partial heart block. It should be given to patients with congestive heart failure only when they have been treated with digoxin. It should be given with caution to patients on anti-diabetic drugs. It should not be withdrawn suddenly. *Dose:* Disordered heart rhythm, 10 to 30 mg three or four times daily; angina, 60 to 240 mg daily in divided doses; raised blood pressure, 40 to 120 mg daily initially, increasing to 120 to 360 mg daily in divided doses as maintenance treatment; anxiety disorders, start with 40 mg three times daily and increase weekly according to desired effects. Inderal-LA contains 160 mg propranolol in sustained-release form.

propylene glycol is used as a vehicle for drugs and as a vehicle for flavouring agents in foods.

propylene phenoxetol ◊ phenoxyethanol.

propyl hydroxybenzoate is used as a preservative in drug preparation.

propylthiouracil is a drug used to treat overworking of the thyroid gland. It has effects, uses and adverse effects similar to those described under carbimazole. *Dose:* By mouth; initially, 200 to 600 mg daily in divided doses, reducing to a maintenance dose of about 50 to 200 mg daily.

Prostigmin ◊ neostigmine.

Prostin E2 ◊ dinoprostone.

Prostin F2 alpha ◊ dinoprost.

Prostin VR ◊ alprostadil.

protamine (protamine sulphate) neutralizes the anti-blood clotting effects of heparin. *Dose:* 50 mg intravenously.

Prothiaden ◊ dothiepin.

prothionamide (Trevintix) is a drug used to treat tuberculosis. It should be given with at least one and preferably two other anti-tuberculous drugs in order to prevent the risk of development of resistant strains of bacteria. Read section on drugs used to treat tuberculosis. *Adverse effects* and *Precautions:* These are similar to those described under ethionamide. It should not be used in pregnancy and it may cause liver damage. *Dose:* By mouth, 0·5 to 1 g daily in divided doses or as a single dose.

protirelin (TRH) is used as an agent to diagnose overworking of the thyroid gland.

protriptyline (Concordin; protriptyline hydrochloride) is a tricyclic antidepressant drug. Its effects and uses are similar to those described under imipramine. *Adverse effects:* These are similar to those discussed under imipramine. Rashes may develop due to

sunlight sensitivity of the skin. *Precautions:* These are similar to those described under imipramine. Exposure to strong sunlight should be avoided. *Dose:* By mouth, 15 to 60 mg daily in divided doses.

Pro-Ven Gel contains benzoyl peroxide 2·5%.

Pro-Vent sustained-release capsules ◊ theophylline.

Provera ◊ medroxyprogesterone.

Pro-Viron ◊ mesterolone.

proxymetacaine (Ophthaine) is a local anaesthetic used in eye drops and because it causes less initial stinging than other local anaesthetics, it is useful for children.

prune (aqueous extract) has purgative and demulcent properties.

Pru-Sen contains senna leaf 5%, figs 10%, prunes 1·67%, raisins 3·33%, and dates 80%.

Pruven gel contains benzoyl peroxide 2·5%.

pseudoephedrine (Galpseud; pseudoephedrine hydrochloride) has effects and uses similar to those described under ephedrine. It is used to relieve nasal and bronchial congestion, particularly in bronchial asthma. *Adverse effects* and *Precautions* ◊ ephedrine. *Dose:* 60 to 180 mg daily in divided doses by mouth.

Psoradrate cream contains dithranol and urea and is used to treat psoriasis.

Psoriderm is a preparation of tar available as a Bath Emulsion, Cream and Scalp lotion for treating psoriasis.

Psorigel contains tar solution 7·5%. It is used to treat psoriasis.

Psorin is used for treating psoriasis and contains dithranol 0·16%, crude coal tar 1%, salicylic acid 1·6%.

psyllium (flea seed) absorbs and retains water and is therefore used as a bulk laxative. *Dose:* 5 to 15 g.

pteroylglutamic acid ◊ folic acid.

Pulmadil inhaler and **Pulmadil auto:** These are aerosols containing rimiterol which are used in treating bronchial asthma.

Pulmicort ◊ budesonide.

Pulmo Bailly: Each 5 ml contains guaiacol 75 mg, codeine 7 mg, and phosphoric acid 75 mg.

pumilio pine oil has a pleasant aromatic odour and is used in inhalations and rubefacients.

Pump-Hep infusion ◊ heparin.

Puri-Nethol ◊ mercaptopurine.

Puritabs are used to purify water. Each tablet contains sodium dichloroisocyanurate 17 mg.

Pylatum Regulators contain senna leaf 5%, cascara dry extract 56%, aloin 16%, colocynth 6%, ginger oleoresin 4%, peppermint oil 4%, and hard soap 1·5%.

Pyopen ◊ carbenicillin.

Pyralvex oral paint contains anthraquinone glycosides 5% and salicylic acid 1%.

pyrantel (Combantrin; pyrantel embonate) is used to treat threadworm, roundworm, hookworm, whipworm and trichostrongyliasis. It may cause nausea and vomiting. It should be given with caution to patients with impaired liver function. *Dose:* Adults and children over six months of age, 10 mg per kg of body-weight as a single dose by mouth. Maximum dose 1 g, repeated in 24 to 48 hours if necessary.

pyrazinamide (in Rifater; Zinamide) is a drug used to treat tuberculosis. *Adverse effects:* Liver damage with fever, anorexia, enlargement of the liver, jaundice, severe liver failure, vomiting, painful joints, skin rash, (urticaria) and sideroblastic anaemia. *Precautions:* It should be given with caution to patients with impaired kidney function, diabetes and gout. It should *not* be given to patients with liver damage. *Dose:* By mouth, 20 to 30 mg per kg daily, max. 3 g hourly.

pyribenzamine ◊ tripelennamine.

pyridostigmine (pyridostigmine bromide) acts on the parasympathetic division of the autonomic nervous system. It is used in the treatment of myasthenia gravis, and has a similar but longer action than neostigmine. *Adverse effects:* These include salivation, abdominal cramps and diarrhoea. Increased muscular weakness is a symptom of overdosage. *Precautions:* Contra-indicated in intestinal or urinary obstruction and should be used with caution in patients with asthma or Parkinson's disease. *Dose:* By mouth, 0·3 to 1·2 g daily in divided doses. An injection is also available.

pyridoxine (Benadon; pyridoxine hydrochloride) is vitamin B_6.

pyrimethamine (Daraprim) is used to prevent malaria. Prolonged use may damage the production of red blood cells by interfering with folic acid use. Skin rashes may occur occasionally. *Dose:* Suppression of malaria, 25 to 50 mg weekly.

pyrithione zinc has antibacterial and antifungal properties. Its use is similar to selenium sulphide in the treatment of seborrhoeic dermatitis and dandruff. It is an ingredient of some proprietary shampoos.

Pyrogastrone is used to treat indigestion and peptic ulcers. Each tablet contains carbenoxolone sodium 20 mg, magnesium trisilicate 60 mg, aluminium hydroxide 240 mg, and a base containing sodium bicarbonate and alginic acid. *Dose:* By mouth, 1 chewed three times daily after meals and 2 at night.

Q-Guard first aid cream contains cetrimide 0·35% and benzalkonium chloride solution 0·3%.

Q-Panol Elixir contains in each 5 ml paracetamol 120 mg.

quassia is from the dried stem of Jamaica quassia. It is a bitter which has been used to treat threadworms, in a lotion to treat body lice and as a flavouring agent.

Quatoral Lozenges: Each contains tyrothricin 1 mg, benzocaine 5 mg, and cetylpyridinium chloride 1·5 mg.

Quellada lotion ◊ gamma benzene hexachloride.

Quench cream is used to treat burns. It contains aminacrine hydrochloride 0·1%.

Questran ◊ cholestyramine.

Quick Action Cough Cure: Each dose provides dextromethorphan hydrobromide 3·75 mg and guaiphenesin 25 mg.

Quick Kwells tablets each contain hyoscine hydrobromide 300 micrograms.

Quicksol: Read section on insulins.

quinalbarbitone sodium (Seconal Sodium, secobarbital sodium) is a barbiturate sleeping drug. *Dose:* By mouth, 100 to 200 mg at night.

quinestradol is an oestrogen used to treat post-menopausal vulva and vaginal disorders. *Adverse effects* and *Precautions* ◊ ethinyloestradiol. *Dose:* By mouth, 0·5 mg twice daily for two to three weeks depending on the disorder being treated.

Quinicardine ◊ quinidine.

quinidine (Kiditard; Kinidin Durules; Quinicardine; quinidine sulphate) prolongs the resting period of the heart and reduces its rate. It is used to treat disorders of heart rhythm. *Adverse effects:* Patients may be allergic to quinidine and develop noises in the ears, vertigo, visual disturbances, headache, confusion, skin rash, loss of appetite, nausea, vomiting, diarrhoea, pain in the chest, abdominal cramps and fever. Fall in blood pressure, difficulty in breathing, blueness (cyanosis) and collapse may also occur. *Precautions:* It should not be given to allergic patients – this should be tested for by giving a small dose initially. Quinidine should not be used in severe heart disorders or to treat irregular heart rhythms due to overworking of the thyroid gland. It may increase the effects of some anticoagulants and some muscle-relaxant drugs. *Dose:* By mouth, 200 to 400 mg 3 or 4 times daily.

quinine (quinine bisulphate; quinine acid sulphate; quinine hydrochloride) was previously used to treat malaria but has largely been replaced by less toxic and more effective drugs. It is now only used in malarial infections resistant to other drugs. It is also used to treat night cramps. *Adverse effects:* Deafness, noises in the ears, visual disturbances, giddiness and trembling may occur. *Dose:* By mouth 300 to 600 mg at night for cramps.

Quinocort cream contains potassium hydroxyquinoline sulphate 0·5% and hydrocortisone 1%.

Quinoderm (**cream** and **lotio-gel**) is used to treat acne. It contains benzoyl peroxide 10%, potassium hydroxyquinoline sulphate 0·5% in an astringent base.

Quinoderm with Hydrocortisone cream is the same as Quinoderm with added hydrocortisone 1%.

Quinoped cream contains benzoyl peroxide 5% and potassium hydroxyquinoline sulphate 0·5%.

Rab/Vac is Rabies Vaccine. It is an inactivated suspension of suitable strains of rabies virus.

Rabro is used to treat indigestion and peptic ulcers. Each tablet contains deglycyrrhinized liquorice 400 mg, magnesium oxide 100 mg, calcium carbonate 500 mg and frangula 25 mg. *Dose:* By mouth, 1 to 2 chewed three times daily after meals.

Radian-B Spirit Liniment contains menthol 1·4%, aspirin 1·2%, camphor 0·6%, and methyl salicylate 0·6%, in alcohol. **Radian-B Spray** is prepared from the same ingredients but contains no alcohol.

Radian Massage Cream contains menthol 2·54%, camphor 1·43%, methyl salicylate 0·42%, and water-soluble capsicin 0·042%.

Radian Warm-up Sports Rub contains capsicin and methyl salicylate in a lotion basis.

Radox bath salts contain extracts of herbs with witch hazel, horsechestnut, rosemary, hops, and camomile; sea salt with salts of calcium, magnesium, and sodium; a mixture of sodium carbonate and sodium bicarbonate; and soapless cleansing agents.

Ralgex Balm contains methyl nicotinate 1%, histamine dihydrochloride 0·05%, and capsicin 0·12%.

Ralgex Embrocation contains turpentine oil 22%, dilute acetic acid 30%, and dilute ammonia solution 14%.

Ralgex Embrocation Stick contains glycol salicylate 3·01%, ethyl salicylate 3·01%, methyl salicylate 0·6%, capsicin 1·67%, and menthol 6·19%.

Ralgex Spray contains glycol salicylate 4·8%, ethyl salicylate 4·8%, methyl salicylate 0·96%, and methyl nicotinate 1·6%.

Ramodar tablets ◊ etodolac.

ranitidine (Zantac) is an H_2 antihistamine which blocks acid production in the stomach and is used to treat peptic ulcers. *Adverse effects:* Headache and rashes. *Precautions:* It should be used with caution (lower doses) in patients suffering from impaired kidney function, and like any other drug in pregnant and breast-feeding women. *Dose:* By mouth 150 mg twice daily for 4 weeks, maintenance dose 150 mg at bedtime. By slow intravenous injection, 50 mg every 6 to 8 hours; or intravenous infusion, 25 mg/hour for 2 hours repeated if necessary, after 6 to 8 hours.

Rapifen injection ◊ alfentanil.

raspberry leaf contains a drug which relaxes the smooth muscle of the uterus and gut in *some animals*. It is a traditional remedy for painful and heavy periods and for use before and during childbirth. It has also been used as an astringent gargle.

Rastinon ◊ tolbutamide.

rauwolfia are the plants from which reserpine is obtained.

Rayglo BKB: Each tablet contains buchu extract 10 mg and methylene blue 4 mg.

Rayglo Chest Rub contains camphor 6·1%, menthol 2·03%, cedar wood oil 0·5%, eucalyptus oil 2%, nutmeg oil 0·1%, thyme oil 0·1%, gauiacol 0·0011%, turpentine oil 6·1%, pine oil 3%, Peru balsam 0·05%, and white soft paraffin to 100%.

Rayglo Laxative Tablets: Each contains phenolphthalein 125 mg.

Rayglo Toothache Tincture contains camphor 10%, sandarac substitute 10%, and clove 5%.

razoxane (Razoxin) is an anti-cancer drug. *Adverse effects:* Nausea, vomiting, diarrhoea, skin rashes, alopecia, blood disorders, oesophagitis and pneumonitis may occur in patients receiving radiotherapy to the chest. *Precautions:* It should not be used in pregnancy or for breast-feeding mothers. The white cell count should be monitored regularly. *Dose:* By mouth, 125 mg tablets in a dose which varies according to the disorder being treated.

Razoxin ◊ razoxane.

R.B.C. antihistamine cream contains antazoline hydrochloride 1·8%, calamine 8%, camphor 0·1% and cetrimide 0·5%.

rectified spirits (dilute alcohols) ◊ alcohol.

Redelan Effervescent tablets each contains vitamin A 5,500 units, thiamine mononitrate 1·2 mg, riboflavine sodium phosphate 1·8 mg, pyridoxine hydrochloride 1·6 mg, cyanocobalamin 1·4 micrograms, nicotinamide 15 mg, calcium pantothenate 13 mg, ascorbic acid 75 mg, ergocalciferol 400 units, and DL-alpha-tocopheryl acetate 10 mg.

Redeptin ◊ fluspirilene.

Red Kooga are a range of preparations containing Korean panax ginseng.

Redoxon tablets each contain ascorbic acid 25, 50, 200, or 500 mg. **Redoxon Effervescent** tablets each contain ascorbic acid 1 g; in standard, blackcurrant, lemon, or orange flavours.

red-poppy syrup is used as colouring and sweetening agent.

Refolinon tablets and injection ◊ folinic acid.

Regaine liquid contains minoxidil, 20 mg per ml. It is used to treat male-type baldness in men only. Minoxidil has been used since 1980 to treat raised blood pressure during which time it was noted to cause an increase growth of hair. After several trials it is now marketed as a liquid to apply locally on the scalp in male-type baldness. This type of baldness is characterized by recession of the frontal hair line and thinning of the hair on the crown. Regaine produces a moderate regrowth of hair in about 39% of males if it is applied to bald areas daily for 12 months. Very little regrowth takes place in the first four months and if none is seen after 12 months it is unlikely that regrowth will occur. Best results occur in men who have been bald for 2 to 10 years and have a bald patch on their crown of less than 10 cm diameter. Once treatment is stopped the baldness recurs within about 2 to 3 months and will be as extensive as if treatment had never been used. *Adverse effects:* Dermatitis, overgrowth of hair outside area of application, swelling of ankles (oedema), chest pain, changes in blood pressure and pulse rate, shortness of breath, dizziness, headache. *Precautions:* Do not use on broken skin. Monitor blood pressure at regular intervals. Its safety is not established for use in men under 18 years of age and over 65 years of age. *Dose:* 1 ml applied to bald area twice daily. Maximum daily dose 2 ml. Wash hands thoroughly after use.

Regulan ◊ ispaghula.

Reguletts tablets each contain phenolphthalein 120 mg in a chocolate basis.

Rehibin ◊ cyclofenil.

Rehidrat: Each sachet contains sodium chloride 440 mg, potassium chloride 380 mg, sodium bicarbonate 420 mg, citric acid 440 mg, glucose 4·09 g, sucrose 8·07 g, and laevulose 70 mg. It is used to treat fluid and salt loss in diarrhoea. Each sachet should be added to 250 ml of water.

Relaxit Micro-enema contains sodium citrate 450 mg, sodium lauryl sulphate 75 mg, sorbic acid 5 mg in a viscous solution in each 5 ml single-dose disposable pack with nozzle.

Relcofen ◊ ibuprofen.

Relcol Tablets contain paracetamol 240 mg, quinine bisulphite 1 mg, ephedrine 7·5 mg.

Relefact LH–RH ◊ gonadorelin.

Relefact LH–RH/TRH ◊ gonadorelin.

Relifex ◊ nabumetone.

Remnos ◊ nitrazepam.

Rendells spermicidal contraceptive pessaries contain monoxynols '10' and '11' 5% in a base containing palm kernel oil.

Rennie Tablets: Each contains chalk 680 mg and light magnesium carbonate 80 mg.

reproterol (Bronchodil; reproterol hydrochloride). It has similar effects to, and the same adverse effects as salbutamol, and is used to treat bronchial asthma. *Dose:* By aerosol spray, 1 to 2 inhalations repeated after 3 to 6 hours as necessary.

Rescufolin powder in vials contains folinic acid (as calcium folinate) is used to treat patients after large doses of methotrexate.

reserpine (Serpasil) is obtained from the roots of rauwolfia. It depresses the brain, produces sedation, lowers the blood pressure and slows the heart rate. It is used to treat patients with high blood pressure. It takes about three to six days to work, accumulates in the body and its effects continue for some time after it is stopped. It should not be used as a tranquillizer to treat patients with anxiety and psychoses. *Adverse effects:* Common adverse effects include lethargy, stuffiness of the nose, drowsiness, dreams, stomach upsets, diarrhoea and vertigo. Breathlessness, increase in weight and skin rashes may occur. High doses may cause flushing, insomnia, redness of the eyes, slowing of the pulse and occasionally Parkinsonism and severe depression which may lead to suicide. Salt retention with swelling (oedema), blurred vision, disturbances of ejaculation, peptic ulcers and nose bleeds have been reported. On the whole adverse effects are mild and pass off on reduction of dosage or if the drug is stopped. *Precautions:* It should be used with caution in patients with psychological symptoms, particularly if they are depressed. It should also be used with caution in patients with peptic ulcers, ulcerative colitis, heart disorders and asthma or bronchitis. It may cause a fall in blood pressure in patients under anaesthetic. *Dose:* By mouth, to treat high blood pressure: 0·1 to 0·5 mg daily.

Resolve granules is a mild pain-reliever and antacid formulation designed to counter the effects of overindulgence in food and alcohol. Each sachet contains paracetamol 500 mg, anhydrous citric acid 1185 mg, sodium bicarbonate 808 mg, potassium bicarbonate 715 mg, sodium carbonate 153 mg and vitamin C 200 mg, in a base containing glucose.

Resonium-A is used to treat high blood potassium levels (hyperkalaemia), it consists of sodium polystyrene sulphonate powder.

resorcin ◊ resorcinol.

resorcinol (resorcinol monoacetate) stops itching and is used in skin ointments because it causes skinning. Prolonged use of large amounts on the skin can cause underworking of the thyroid gland because it may be absorbed and interfere with the production of thyroid hormones.

Ress-Q Pastilles, each contain benzalkonium chloride 600 micrograms, tinct. benzoin co. 10 mg, and menthol 2 mg.

Restandol ◊ testosterone undecanoate.

Retcin ◊ erythromycin.

Retin-A ◊ tretinoin.

retinol is vitamin A.

Retrovir ◊ zidovudine.

Revlon ZP11 Formula Medicated Hair Dressing contains zinc pyrithione 0·5% and **Medicated Shampoo** contains zinc pyrithione 1%.

Rheomacrodex ◊ dextran.

Rheumaban Cream contains histamine acid phosphate 0·1%, eucalyptus oil 3%, methyl nicotinate 1·5%, camphor oil 2%, glycol salicylate 7·5%, and pumilio pine oil 3%.

Rheumacin LA is a sustained-release capsule of indomethacin 75 mg ◊ indomethacin.

Rheumox ◊ azapropazone.

Rhinocort metered dose nasal aerosol ◊ budesonide.

Rhuaka herbal syrup is used to treat indigestion, flatulence and constipa-tion. Each 5 ml contains cascara liquid extract 0.05 ml, rhubarb concentrated infusion 0·05 ml, senna concentrated infusion 0·15 ml, compound cardamom tincture 0·018 ml and liquorice liquid extract 0·075 ml.

rhubarb is obtained from *Rheum palmatum* grown in China and Tibet. It is used as an irritant laxative. In very small doses it is astringent and is included in some preparations to treat diarrhoea.

ribavirin (Virazid) is an antiviral drug with a broad spectrum of activity against certain viruses which cause chest diseases in children and infants. *Adverse effects:* Worsening of chest disorder, bacterial pneumonia, pneumothorax, increase in reticulocytes in the blood. *Precautions:* Monitor patient and equipment because drug may precipitate and block tubing. *Dose:* By aerosol or nebulization, 20 mg per ml of solution for 12 to 18 hours a day for a minimum of 3 days and a maximum of 7 days.

riboflavine sodium phosphate ◊ riboflavine (vitamin B_2).

riboflavine (vitamin B_2) is a member of the vitamin B group.

ribonucleic acid is obtained from living cells. It has been tried as a tonic.

Ridaura tablets ◊ see auranofin.

Rifadin ◊ rifampicin.

rifampicin (Rifadin; in Rifater; Rimactane) is used to treat tuberculosis. *Adverse effects:* These include nausea, jaundice and blood disorders.

Alterations of liver function tests may occur and allergic reactions have been reported. It may colour the urine, sputum and tears red. *Precautions:* It should not be used during the first three months of pregnancy and in patients with obstructive disorders of their gall-bladder system. It should be given with caution to alcoholics and to patients who have had previous drug allergies. *Dose:* By mouth, 450 to 600 mg daily before breakfast.

Rifater tablets are used in the treatment of pulmonary tuberculosis. Each tablet contains isoniazid 50 mg, pyrazinamide 300 mg and rifampicin 120 mg ◊ isoniazid ◊ pyrazinamide ◊ rifampicin. *Dose:* Depends on weight of patient, 3 tablets daily (under 40 kg), 4 tablets daily (40–49 kg), 5 tablets daily (50–64 kg), 6 tablets daily (over 65 kg).

Rifinah is used to treat tuberculosis. Each '150' tablet contains rifampicin 150 mg and isoniazid 100 mg; each '300' tablet contains rifampicin 300 mg and isoniazid 150 mg. *Dose:* Taken as a single dose before breakfast: '150' tablets (patients under 50 kg), 3 tablets daily, '300' tablets (patients over 50 kg), 2 tablets daily.

Rikospray Balsam is an aerosol containing benzoin 12·5% and prepared storax 2·5%. It is used to treat bed sores, cracked nipples and skin fissures.

Rikospray Silicone is an aerosol containing aluminium dihydroxyallantoinate 0·5%, cetylpyridinium chloride 0·02% in a silicone base. It is used to treat bed sores and nappy rash.

Rimactane ◊ rifampicin.

Rimactazid is used to treat tuberculosis. Each '150' tablet contains rifampicin 150 mg and isoniazid 100 mg; each '300' tablet contains rifampicin 300 mg and isoniazid 150 mg. *Dose:* Taken as a single dose before breakfast: '150' tablets (patients under 50 kg), 3 tablets daily, '300' tablets (patients over 50 kg), 2 tablets daily.

Rimevax is a brand of measles vaccine.

Rimifon ◊ isoniazid.

rimiterol (Pulmadil; rimiterol hydrobromide) has effects and uses similar to those described under salbutamol. It is a selective $beta_2$-adrenoreceptor stimulant used to treat asthma and bronchospasm. It does not cause the rapid beating of the heart produced by isoprenaline and similar drugs. *Adverse effects:* It may produce a fall in blood pressure causing dizziness and fainting. Anxiety, tremor and rapid beating of the heart may occur. *Precautions:* It should be used with caution in patients with high blood pressure and overworking of their thyroid gland. *Dose:* 1 to 3 puffs. Not to be repeated for at least half an hour and no more than 24 puffs in 24 hours, i.e. eight treatments.

Rimso-50 is used to relieve the symptoms of cystitis. It contains dimethyl sulphoxide 50%.

Rinstead Gel contains benzocaine 2%, sodium ricinoleate 0·1%, chloroxylenol 0·1%, clove oil 0·1%, myrrh 0·1%, glycerol 10%, CMC 2%, and SVR 30%.

Rinstead Pastilles each contain menthol 0·37 mg, myrrh 1·25 mg, sodium ricinoleate 0·62 mg, chloroxylenol 0·75 mg, phenolphthalein 0·75 mg, and tartaric acid 3·25 mg.

ritodrine (Yutopar; ritodrine hydrochloride) is a sympathomimetic drug which is used to relax the womb in premature labour. *Adverse effects:* These include vomiting, flushing, sweating, low blood pressure and rapid heart beat. *Precautions:* It should not be given to women taking antidepressants, beta-blocking drugs or drugs used to treat raised blood pressure.

Rivotril ◊ clonazepam.

Roaccutane ◊ isotretinoin.

Ro-A-Vit injection contains vitamin A (retinol) 300,000 units (as palmitate)/ml. *Dose:* By deep intramuscular injection, 150,000 to 300,000 units monthly, increased to weekly in acute deficiency states.

Ro-A-Vit tablets contain vitamin A (retinol) 50,000 units (as acetate).

Robaxin ◊ methocarbamol.

Robinul ◊ glycopyrronium.

Robinul Neostigmine injection contains the anticholinergic drug, glycopyrronium 0·5 mg and the anticholinesterase drug neostigmine 2·5 mg in each ml. Used as a premedication before a general anaesthetic to dry up secretions ◊ glycopyrronium and neostigmine.

Robitussin cough liquid contains guaiphenesin 100 mg/5 ml. *Dose:* 5 to 10 ml every 2 to 3 hours.

Robitussin cough soother, Junior cough soother are both used in the treatment of dry coughs, they each contain dextromethorphan hydrobromide ◊ dextromethorphan.

Robitussin Plus is used to treat coughs and nasal congestion. Each 5 ml contains guaiphenesin 100 mg and pseudoephedrine 30 mg.

Roc Total Sunblock 15A + Broc is a sunscreen preparation containing a cinnamic ester and zinc oxide. SPF 15.

Rocaltrol ◊ calcitriol.

Roccal ◊ benzalkonium.

Rochelle salt is sodium potassium tartrate and is used as a laxative.

Roferon-A (interferon alfa-2a(rbe)) is a human protein produced by recombinant DNA techniques. It is used to treat AIDS-related Kaposi's sarcoma and hairy cell leukaemia. *Adverse effects:* Flu-like symptoms, fever, chills, headaches, malaise, painful joints and muscles, lethargy, weakness, fatigue, drowsiness, nervousness, sleepiness, convulsion, pins and needles and numbness in the arms and legs, tremor, changes in blood pressure, disorders of heart rhythm and rate, heart failure, strokes, loss of appetite, nausea, diarrhoea, vomiting, raised liver function tests, blood disorders. *Precautions:* Do not use in patients who are allergic to it or related drugs, or in patients with severe heart, kidney or liver disease or convulsions. Patients on treatment should practise contraception. *Dose:* By intramuscular or subcutaneous injection. Dose varies according to disorder being treated.

Rogitine ◊ phentolamine.

Rohypnol ◊ flunitrazepam.

Ronicol ◊ nicotinyl tartrate.

Ronicol Timespan tablets contain nicotinyl tartrate 150 mg in sustained-release form. *Dose:* By mouth 1 to 2 night and morning.

Ronson antiseptic disinfectant contains chloroxylenol.

rose geranium oil ◊ geranium oil.

rose-hip syrup is a source of vitamin C.

rosemary oil is a carminative and is mildly irritant. It is principally used as rosemary spirit in hair lotions, soap and liniments.

rosewater ointment (cold cream) contains rosewater 20 ml, white beeswax 18 g, borax 1 g, almond oil 61 g and rose oil 0·1 ml.

rosin ◊ colophony.

Rosoxacin ◊ acrosoxacin.

Roter: Each tablet contains bismuth subnitrate 300 mg, magnesium carbonate 400 mg, sodium bicarbonate 200 mg and frangula 25 mg. It is used to treat indigestion and peptic ulcers. *Dose:* 2 three times daily.

Rotersept is a spray application of chlorhexidine gluconate 0·2% ◊ chlorhexidine.

Rowachol: Each capsule contains borneol 5 mg, camphene 5 mg, cineole 2 mg, menthol 32 mg, menthone 6 mg, pinene 17 mg in olive oil. It raises biliary cholesterol solubility and is used to help dissolve cholesterol gallstones.

Rowatinex solution contains anethole 400 mg, borneol 1 g, camphene 1·5 g, cineole 300 mg, fenchone 400 mg, pinene 3·1 g and olive oil to 10g.

royal jelly (Queen Bee Jelly) is a milky-white viscid secretion from the salivary glands of the worker hive bee. It is essential for the development of queen bees. It is a complex mixture of proteins, amino acids, lipids, carbohydrates, fatty acids and vitamins (particularly pantothenic acid). One constituent is 10-hydroxydec-2-enoic acid which has antibacterial properties. It is used as a tonic to ward off the effects of ageing without any substantiated evidence of its effects. It is also incorporated in some cosmetics.

Rub/Vac is a Rubella vaccine (live). It is used for active immunization against rubella (German measles).

Ruban contains glycol salicylate 2%, methyl nicotinate 0·75%, capsicum oleoresin 0·2%, in a non-greasy basis.

Ruthmol ◊ potassium chloride.

rutin is obtained from buckwheat. It is claimed to be used in disorders producing capillary bleeding and fragility but evidence of its value is inconclusive.

Rutivite Tablets each contain dried buckwheat (leaf and flower) equivalent to 30 mg of rutin.

Rybarvin inhaler is used to treat bronchial asthma. It contains atropine methonitrate 0·1%, adrenaline 0·4%, papaverine hydrochloride 0·08% and benzocaine 0·08%. *Dose:* Using Rybarvin inhaler, inhale deeply for 1 to 2 minutes three times daily.

Rynacrom nasal insufflator or spray ◊ disodium cromoglycate. Used for allergic runny nose.

Rynacrom Compound nasal spray is used to treat nasal allergy. It contains sodium cromoglycate 2% (2·5 mg/metered spray) and xylometazoline hydrochloride 0·025%.

Rythmodan ◊ disopyramide.

Rythmodan Retard tablets contain disopyramide 250 mg in a sustained-release form. *Dose:* By mouth 1 to 1½ twice daily.

saccharin (saccharin sodium) is an artificial sweetening drug. Rarely it may produce sensitivity of the skin to sunlight.

safrol ◊ sassafras oil.

Sainsbury's Cold Powders each contain paracetamol 1 g, phenylephrine hydrochloride 10 mg, and vitamin C 60 mg.

St James' Balm is used to treat eczema. It contains zinc oxide 20%, ichthammol 2·8%, urea 0·1%, and salicylic acid 0·1%.

Salactol paint contains salicylic acid 16·7% and lactic acid 16·7%. It is used to treat warts.

Salazopyrin ◊ sulphasalazine.

Salazopyrin enema (3 g in 100 ml) ◊ sulphasalazine.

salbutamol (Aerolin; Asmaven; Cobutolin; Ventodisks; Ventolin; Volmax; salbutamol sulphate) has effects and uses similar to those described under isoprenaline. Its main effects, however, are on the bronchi rather than the heart. It is therefore used to treat asthma and bronchospasm. It does not cause the rapid beating of the heart produced by isoprenaline and similar drugs. *Adverse effects:* These are similar but less marked than those produced by isoprenaline. Muscle trembling may occur after using salbutamol by mouth. *Precautions:* It should not be used by patients with high blood pressure, heart disorders and overworking of the thyroid gland. *Dose:* By aerosol spray, 0·1 mg (in one discharge); 1 to 2 inhalations at no less than four-hourly intervals. Salbutamol sulphate; by mouth as tablets or elixir, 6 to 16 mg daily in divided doses.

Salcatonin (Calsynar) is closely related to calcitonin and is used in the treatment of Paget's Disease. *Adverse effects* and *Precautions* ◊ calcitonin. *Dose:* 50 to 100 units three times weekly.

salicylamide has effects and uses similar to those described under aspirin but it is less effective. *Dose:* By mouth, 300 to 1,000 mg three times daily.

salicylic acid (Anthranol) is used in skin applications because it kills bacteria and fungi and causes skinning. It is also used in rheumatic liniments. It can cause dermatitis and prolonged extensive use may cause toxic effects.

Salivix is used to treat the symptom of dry mouth. It contains buffered malic acid.

salol (phenyl salicylate) is a sunscreen agent.

Salonair is a spray used for muscular and rheumatic pain. It contains methyl salicylate 1·15%, glycol salicylate 1·75%, menthol 3·2%, camphor 3%, squalane 0·5% and benzyl nicotinate 0·04%.

salsalate (Disalcid) is used to treat rheumatic disorders. It is broken down slowly in the body to salicylic acid. *Adverse effects* and *Precautions* ◊ aspirin. *Dose:* 500 mg to 1 g three or four times daily.

Saltair Lotion contains magnesium trisilicate 2·05%, bismuth carbonate 0·25%, aldioxa 0·5%, hexachlorophane 0·1%, starch 11%, kaolin, light 0·7%, zinc oxide 27·5%, and silicon dioxide 0·35%.

Saluric ◊ chlorothiazide.

Salzone ◊ paracetamol.

Samaritan Anti-midge Cream contains dimethyl phthalate 1% and diethyltoluamide 15%.

Samaritan Chilblain Cream contains methyl nicotinate 1·5%, phenol 0·5%, camphor 1·5%, and benzocaine 4%.

Samaritan Menthol and Wintergreen Cream contains methyl salicylate 12·5% and menthol 1% in a water-miscible basis.

Sanatogen contains casein 94·5%, sodium glycerophosphate 5%, and glyceryl mono-oleate 0·5%.

Sanatogen High C Tablets each contain ascorbic acid 1·020 g and riboflavine 300 micrograms, with tartaric acid and adipic acid.

Sanatogen Junior Vitamins Tablets each contain vitamin A acetate 2,500 units, vitamin C 50 mg, and vitamin D_2 200 units.

Sanatogen Multivitamins Tablets each contain vitamin A 4,000 units, vitamin B_1 1·2 mg, vitamin B_2 1·8 mg, vitamin C 30 mg, vitamin D_2 400 units, vitamin E 2 mg, nicotinamide 12 mg, potassium iodide 130 micrograms.

Sanatogen Multivitamins Plus Iron contain vitamin A acetate 4,000 units, vitamin B_1 1·2 mg, vitamin B_2 1·8 mg, nicotinamide 12 mg, coated ascorbic acid 30 mg, vitamin D_2 400 units, vitamin E 0·5 mg, potassium iodide 130 micrograms, and ferrous fumarate 45·6 mg.

Sanatogen Vitamin C Tablets each contain ascorbic acid 75 mg.

Sanatogen Vitamin E Tablets each contain vitamin E 100 mg.

sandarac substitute is a substitute for sandaraca resin (gum juniper) used as a temporary filling for carious teeth.

Sanderson's Cough Linctus contains in each 5 ml compound cardamom tincture 0·2 ml and citric acid 1·4 mg.

Sanderson's Throat Specific Mixture contains in each 5 ml squill extract 0·025 ml, capsicum liquid extract 0·025 ml, quassia extract 0·008 ml, and acetic acid 0·113 ml. **Pastilles** each contain honey 145 mg, squill vinegar 96 mg, capsicum· oleoresin 19 micrograms, tolu tincture 3 mg, menthol 1·5 mg, benzoic acid 0·966 mg, eucalyptus oil 0·376 mg, and cinnamic acid 37·5 micrograms.

Sandimmun ◊ cyclosporin.

Sando-K are effervescent tablets which contain potassium bicarbonate and potassium chloride equivalent to 470 mg of potassium and 285 mg of chloride. Used to treat deficiency of potassium. *Dose:* By mouth, 2 to 4 daily according to need.

Sandocal effervescent tablets contain calcium, sodium, potassium and vitamin C; are used for deficiency disorders of calcium. *Dose:* 1 to 5 tablets daily.

Sandoglobulin injection ◊ immunoglobulin.

Sanoid medicated plaster for boils. It consists of 2 plasters containing hexachlorophene 0·75% and 1 healing plaster containing aminacrine hydrochloride 0·1%.

Sanomigran ◊ pizotifen.

sanguis dracunis is a constituent of Fennings' Original Mixture.

sarsaparilla decoction is used as a flavouring agent in medicines. It is obtained from sarsaparilla roots.

sassafras oil is obtained from dried sassafras bark or roots. It should not be taken internally since it can damage the liver. It has rubefacient properties and it kills body lice. There are many more suitable alternatives.

Saventrine ◊ isoprenaline.

Savloclens solution contains chlorhexidine 0·05% and cetrimide 0·5%.

Savlodil solution contains chlorhexidine 0·015% and cetrimide 0·15%.

Savlon antiseptic lozenges contain chlorhexidine hydrochloride 5 mg.

Savlon Antiseptic Cream contains cetrimide 0·5% and chlorhexidine gluconate 0·1%.

Savlon Antiseptic Liquid contains chlorhexidine gluconate 0·3% and cetrimide 3%.

Savlon Babycare Cream contains cetrimide 0·5%.

Savlon Dry First Aid Spray aerosol contains povidone-iodine 0·5%.

Saxin ◊ saccharin.

Schering PC₄ is a post-coital (morning-after) oral contraceptive. Each tablet contains levonorgestrel 0·25 mg and ethinyloestradiol 0·05 mg. *Dose:* 2 tablets as soon as possible after coitus (up to 72 hours) then 2 tablets 12 hours later.

Scheriproct ointment and suppositories contain prednisolone, cinchocaine, hexachlorophane and clemizole. Used to treat haemorrhoids, and pruritus ani.

Scholl Antiseptic Foot Balm contains halquinol 0·4%, menthol 0·5%, methyl salicylate 0·1%, and basis to 100%.

Scholl Athlete's Foot Gel and **Powder** contains chlorphenesin 1%, zinc oxide 20%, and talc 79%.

Scholl Athlete's Foot Treatment (S1) contains borotannic complex 9·9% and methyl salicylate 0·76%.

Scholl Corn and Callous Salve contains salicylic acid 39%, eucalyptus oil 1%, and anhydrous lanolin to 100%.

Scholl Corn Removing Liquid contains salicylic acid 11·25% and camphor 2·8%.

Scholl Fixo Corn Plasters: The spread material contains salicylic acid 40%.

Scholl Foot Powder contains salicylic acid 3% and aluminium chlorhydroxide 10%.

Scholl Ingrown Toenail Treatment contains potassium acetate 3%, triethanolamine 10%, and urea 10%.

Scholl Zino Corn, Callous, and Bunion Pads are plasters with medicated discs impregnated with salicylic acid 40%.

scoline ◊ suxamethonium.

scopolamine ◊ hyoscine.

Scott's Cod Liver Oil Capsules each contain vitamin A 625 units and vitamin D 62·5 units in 315 mg of codliver oil.

Scott's Emulsion: Each 5 ml contains cod-liver oil 1·68 g, calcium hypophosphite 48 mg, sodium hypophosphite 24 mg.

S.C.R. is used for cradle cap, it contains salicylic acid 1·5%, empiwax 10% and white petroleum jelly 20%.

SDV is a preparation used to treat allergies in individuals. It is especially formulated and prepared from a range of over 200 specific allergens to which a patient may be sensitive. There is a maximum of 8 allergens in any one vaccine.

Sea-Cal is a calcium and vitamin D supplement, it contains calcium 500 mg and vitamin D 125 i.u.

Sea-legs Tablets: Each contains meclozine hydrochloride 12·5 mg.

Seal-a-bite is a flexible collodian containing chlorhexidine acetate 0·05%.

Seba Med Soap-free Liquid Cleanser contains amino acids, nicotinic acid, nicotinamide, lactic acid, vitamin B_6, vitamin H, and vitamin F. **Soap-free Cleansing Bar** contains amino acids, cholesterol, lecithin, phosphatides, glycerides, and vitamins.

Sebbix Shampoo contains purified coal fraction 0·25% stated to be therapeutically equivalent to crude coal tar 2%, with sodium sulphosuccinated undecylenic monoalkylolamide 1%.

Secaderm Salve contains phenol 2·4%, terebene 5·25%, melaleuca oil 5·6%, rectified oil of turpentine 6%, and resin 26%.

Secadrex is used to treat raised blood pressure. Each tablet contains acebutolol 200 mg and hydrochlorothiazide 12·5 mg. *Dose:* By mouth, 1 to 2 daily.

Seclodin ◊ ibuprofen.

Seconal Sodium ◊ quinalbarbitone sodium.

Secron: Each 5 ml contains phenylpropanolamine hydrochloride 7·5 mg and guaiphenesin 30 mg.

Sectral ◊ acebutolol.

Securon ◊ verapamil.

Securon MID ◊ verapamil.

Securon SR is a sustained-release preparation of verapamil ◊ verapamil.

Securopen ◊ azlocillin.

Sek Ointment contains sodium propionate 12·1%, propionic acid 1·5%, sodium octoate 9·8%, zinc octoate 4·9%, and docusate sodium 0·15%.

selegiline (Eldepryl; selegiline; hydrochloride) is a monoamine oxidase-B inhibitor. Unlike other monoamine oxidase inhibitors it does not cause episodes of hypertension. It is used together with levodopa in the treatment of Parkinsonism. *Adverse effects:* These include low blood pressure, confusion, agitation and nausea. *Precautions:* The adverse effects of levodopa may be increased, and the dosage

may need to be reduced. *Dose:* 5 to 10 mg in the morning.

Selenium is a trace element required in the diet.

Selenium-ACE: each tablet contains vitamin C 100 mg, selenium yeast 80 mg (50 micrograms Se), vitamin A 500 units, and vitamin E (natural) 50 units.

selenium sulphide (Lenium; Selsun; selenium sulphide) is used as a shampoo. When taken by mouth it is very dangerous. Repeated use as a shampoo may result in loss of hair. It should not be used on inflamed skin or on broken skin and it should not enter the eyes.

selenium yeast ◊ dried yeast ◊ selenium.

Selexid ◊ pivmecillinam.

Selexid suspension (100 mg in a single-dose sachet) ◊ pivmecillinam.

Selexidin ◊ mecillinam.

Selora is a table salt substitute containing potassium chloride.

Selsun ◊ selenium.

Semi-Daonil tablets contain 2·5 mg glibenclamide.

Senade tablets and **elixir laxative** contain sennosides A and B 13·5 mg (as the calcium salt) in each tablet or 5 ml of elixir. *Dose:* 1 to 3 tablets or 10 ml elixir at bedtime.

senega (Seneca snakeroot) contains two glycosidal saponins which irritate the stomach lining and give rise to reflex stimulation of bronchial secretion. It is used as a cough expectorant.

senna is an irritant laxative.

sennosides A and **B** are the principal active ingredients of senna fruit; used as a laxative.

Senokot contains sennosides A and B in granules or syrup. ◊ sennosides A and B.

Sensodyne Toothpaste contains strontium chloride 10%.

Sential cream contains hydrocortisone 0·5%, urea 4%, and sodium chloride 4% in a water-miscible base ◊ hydrocortisone and urea.

Seominal is an old treatment for raised blood pressure. Each tablet contains phenobarbitone 10 mg, theobromine 325 mg and reserpine 0·2 mg. *Dose:* By mouth, 1 daily.

Septex No. 2 cream contains sulphathiazole 4·44% and zinc oxide 7·4%.

Septrin ◊ co-trimoxazole.

Serc ◊ betahistine.

Sereen tablets: Each contains hyoscine hydrobromide 300 micrograms.

Serenace ◊ haloperidol.

Serophene ◊ clomiphene.

Serpasil ◊ reserpine.

Serpasil-Esidrex is used to treat raised blood pressure. Each tablet contains reserpine 0·15 mg and hydrochlorothiazide 10 mg. *Dose:* By mouth, 2 to 3 daily.

Serum gonadotrophin* ◊ gonadotraphin.

serum gonadotrophin is a pituitary hormone occasionally used to stimulate the ovaries in the treatment of female infertility.

Setlers tablets: Each contain calcium carbonate 534 mg and light magnesium carbonate 72 mg. Used to treat indigestion and peptic ulcers.

Seven Rubbing Oils contains rectified camphor oil 0·9%, clove oil 0·18%, cajuput oil 0·18%, sweet birch oil 0·18%, amber oil 0·36%, eucalyptus oil 0·36%, expressed mustard oil 16·2%, methyl salicylate 0·9%, and camphor 1·08%.

Seven Seas consists of cod-liver oil.

Seven Seas Capsules each contain 0·3 ml of cod-liver oil, providing vitamin A 600 units, vitamin D 60 units, and vitamin E 0·3 units.

Seven Seas Cherry Flavour consists of cod-liver oil with cherry flavouring.

Seven Seas Orange Syrup contains per 10 ml: cod-liver oil 2·8 g, vitamin A 4,000 units, vitamin B_6 0·7 mg, vitamin C 35 mg, vitamin D 400 units, and vitamin E 3 mg, with concentrated orange juice and polyunsaturates.

S H 420 ◊ norethisterone.

shark liver oil is obtained from the livers of various sharks. It has a high content of vitamin A.

Siberian fir oil has a pleasant odour and is used as a flavouring agent. It is included in preparations which relieve nasal congestion.

Si-Ko Toothpaste contains silica-hydro-glycero-gel 67·8%, emulsifying agent 1·2%, essential oils 0·5%, sodium fluoride 0·2%, cream of tartar 29·8%, and buffers 0·5%.

silica-hydro-glycero-gel is used in medicines and toiletries as a suspending, disintegrating and anti-caking agent. In granular form it is used as a desiccant.

silicone ◊ dimethicone.

silicon dioxide is used as a suspending agent, thickener and filler in medicines. It is also used as anti-caking agent. It is used in homoeopathic medicines.

Siloxyl is used to treat indigestion and peptic ulcer. Each tablet contains aluminium hydroxide 500 mg and dimethicone 250 mg. *Dose:* By mouth, 1 to 2 tablets chewed or sucked between meals and at bedtime.

silver acetate has similar uses to silver nitrate in creams, eye lotions and eye drops. It has been used in anti-smoking preparations.

silver nitrate is used as a caustic, astringent and antiseptic in skin applications. It has also been used in eye applications. Continued application to surfaces leads to a blue-black discoloration (argyria) due to deposition of silver granules in the tissues.

silver sulphadiazine cream (Flamazine) is a sulphonamide antibacterial drug used to treat infection in burns, leg ulcers and pressure sores. *Adverse effects:* Allergic reactions may occur. *Precautions:* It should be used with caution in patients suffering from impaired kidney and liver function. *Dose:* Apply daily to burns, to leg ulcers apply at least 3 times a week.

simethicone (◊ dimethicone) is used as a water repellent in barrier creams and skin applications.

Simpkins Antiseptic Throat Lozenges contain weak iodine solution 1·13%, menthol 0·04%, and phenol 0·02%.

Simpkins Bronchial Catarrh Lozenges contain cinnamon oil 0·02%, menthol 0·12%, and compound benzoin tincture 1·1%.

Simpkins Children's Cough Lozenges contain ipecacuanha extract 0·0026 ml, squill extract 0·0026 ml, menthol 1·3 mg, chloroform spirit 0·0013 ml, glycerol 0·021 ml, anise oil 0·0026 ml, and tolu extract.

Simpkins Menthol & Eucalyptus Drops contain menthol 0·25% and eucalyptus oil 0·215%.

Simpkins Menthol & Eucalyptus Mini-Tabs contain eucalyptus oil 0·95% and menthol 0·52%.

Simpkins Teddy Cough Lozenges contain anise oil 0·0013 ml, peppermint oil 0·0013 ml, coltsfoot extract 0·00054 ml, menthol 0·48 mg, ipecacuanha extract 0·00036 ml, squill extract 0·00036 ml and chloroform spirit 0·00048 micrograms.

Simplene eye drops contain adrenaline 0·5% or 1%.

Simpson's foot ointment is used to treat athlete's foot. It contains potassium iodine 0·25%, sublimed sulphur 3%, salicylic acid 0·187%, camphor 2%, zinc oxide 0·25%, zinc stearate 1·67% and menthol 0·2%.

Sinemet Plus contains levodopa 100 mg and carbidopa 25 mg. *Dose:* 1 to 8 tablets daily.

Sinemet 275 contains 25 mg of carbidopa and 250 mg levodopa. It is used to treat Parkinsonism. It is also available with 10 mg of carbidopa and 100 mg of levodopa in each tablet (**Sinemet 110**). *Dose:* By mouth, initially according to the patient's needs and previous treatment. Maintenance dose is 3 to 6 tablets daily.

Sine-Off: Each tablet contains aspirin 325 mg, phenylpropanolamine hydrochloride 18·75 mg, and chlorpheniramine maleate 2 mg.

Sinequan ◊ doxepin.

Sinitol ◊ ibuprofen.

Sinthrome ◊ nicoumalone.

Sintisone ◊ prednisolone.

Sinutab contains paracetamol 500 mg and phenylpropanolamine hydrochloride 12·5 mg.

Siopel cream contains silicone 10% and cetrimide 0·3%. ◊ It is used as a protective skin application.

Sketofax ◊ dimethylphthalate.

Skintex Medicinal Cream contains chloroxylenol 0·25%, glycerol 18%, castor oil 10%, and camphor 0·5%.

Slim-Line chewing gum contains benzocaine 6 mg in each tablet.

Slim-Nite capsules contain three amino acids.

slippery elm was used as a demulcent and in poultices. Its use as a flavouring agent in food is prohibited.

Sloan's Liniment contains methyl salicylate 2·65%, camphor 0·63%, pine oil 6·77%, turpentine oil 48·9%, and capsicum oleoresin 0·72%.

Slo-indo ◊ indomethacin.

Slo-Phyllin is used to treat bronchial asthma. Each capsule contains either 60 mg, 125 mg or 250 mg of theophylline in a sustained-release form. *Dose:* By mouth, 250 to 500 mg twice daily.

Sloprolol is a slow-release capsule containing propranolol hydrochloride 160 mg ◊ propranolol.

Slow-Fe are slow-release tablets of dried ferrous sulphate 160 mg. *Dose:* 1 to 2 once daily.

Slow-Fe Folic: Each tablet contains ferrous sulphate 160 mg and folic acid 0·04 mg in a slow-release form. *Dose:* By mouth, 1 to 2 daily.

Slow-K ◊ potassium chloride.

Slow-Pren (oxprenolol) slow-release capsules ◊ oxprenolol.

Slow-Trasicor ◊ oxprenolol, slow-release.

Smokers Supplement: Each tablet contains ascorbic acid 500 mg, cysteine 10 mg, pyridoxine hydrochloride 5 mg, and thiamine hydrochloride 20 mg.

Snef Nasal Drops contain phenylephrine hydrochloride 0·25% in an iso-osmotic basis.

Sno Phenicol ◊ chloramphenicol.

Sno Pilo ◊ pilocarpine.

Sno Tears ◊ polyvinyl alcohol.

Snowfire Healing Tablets contain benzoin 0·02%, citronella oil 0·06%, thyme oil 0·01%, clove oil 0·04%, cade oil 0·04%, lemon oil 0·01%, in a soft paraffin basis.

Snufflebabe contains camphor 3·5%, menthol 1·5%, pine oil 0·5%, cedar oil 0·25%, thyme oil 0·5%, and cajuput oil 1%.

soap liniment is a rheumatic rub. It contains oleic acid 4g, potassium hydroxide solution 14 ml, alcohol (90%) 70 ml, camphor 4 g, rosemary oil 1·5 ml and water to 100 ml. It is used in the treatment of sprains and bruises.

sodium acid phosphate is given by mouth to render the urine more acid. It is also given with sodium phosphate in the treatment of high blood calcium levels. It is poorly absorbed from the gut and retains water in the lumen. It is administered rectally as an enema to clear the bowel before operations and it is used as a saline laxative by mouth.

sodium alginate ◊ alginic acid.

sodium alkyl sulphates have detergent properties and are used in medicated shampoos and as skin cleansers.

Sodium Amytal ◊ amylobarbitone sodium.

sodium ascorbate ◊ ascorbic acid.

sodium aurothiomalate ◊ gold.

sodium benzoate is used as an antibacterial and antifungal drug in mouth washes and in surgical instrument sterilization fluids and preservatives.

sodium bicarbonate is used as an antacid.

sodium bisulphate is used in drug preparations as a preservative.

sodium borate ◊ borax.

sodium calciumedetate (Ledclair) is used to treat poisoning by heavy metals, especially lead.

sodium carbonate is used in some skin lotions as a water softener and to relieve skin irritation.

sodium carboxymethylcellulose ◊ carboxymethylcellulose.

sodium cellulose phosphate (Calcisorb) is used in patients with high blood calcium levels. It reduces calcium absorption from food. It may cause diarrhoea and it should not be used in patients with congestive heart failure, or impared kidney function. *Dose:* By mouth, 5 g; 3 times daily with food.

sodium chloride is common salt.

sodium citrate (Cymalon) is used to make the urine less acid; as a very mild diuretic, in some laxatives and enemas; to prevent milk from forming large curds when feeding infants; to stop blood from clotting in laboratory instruments; and to wash out the bladder after an operation.

sodium cromoglycate (Intal) is used to prevent attacks of asthma due to allergy, and as Lomusol and Rynacrom for allergic runny nose (allergic rhinitis). It appears to block certain processes in the allergic reaction. It is taken by inhalation into the lungs or up the nose. It may be taken alone or with isoprenaline to prevent bronchospasm due to inhalation of the powder. *Adverse effects:* It may cause irritation of the throat and bronchi, especially during infective illnesses. Sudden withdrawal may trigger off an attack of asthma, particularly in those patients where it has permitted a reduction in corticosteroid dose. *Dose:* Intal, by inhalation, 20 mg every three to twelve hours; Rynacrom (10 mg), 1 capsule insufflated up each nostril four times daily. Also available as a nose spray (Lomusol, Rynacrom) and eye drops (Opticrom). Also ◊ Nalcrom.

sodium ferric citrate ◊ iron.

sodium fluoride ◊ fluoride.

sodium fusidate (Fucidin) is an antibacterial drug. It is effective against bacteria which have developed a resistance to penicillin. *Adverse effects:* Mild abdominal upsets may occur. Skin rashes and jaundice have been reported. *Precautions:* Abdominal upsets are reduced if the drug is given with food. *Dose:* By mouth, 1 to 2 g daily in divided doses.

sodium glycerophosphate and other glycerophosphates were used in the belief that they would help to build up tissues after illness. They form a source of phosphorus in the diet but this has never been shown to be of any value. Tonics containing sodium glycerophosphate and other glycerophosphates are still widely used.

sodium hypochlorite (Chlorasol) solutions release chlorine and are used as disinfectants and antiseptics. They should be protected from the light and not stored for more than three or four months.

sodium hypophosphite ◊ glycerophosphates and hypophosphites.

sodium lauryl ether sulphate has detergent properties and is used in medicated shampoos and as a skin cleanser.

sodium lauryl sulphate is used as a detergent skin cleanser and in shampoos.

sodium magnesium aluminium citrate is used in tablet making.

sodium monofluorophosphate ◊ fluoride.

sodium nitrite has effects and uses similar to but less marked than those described under glyceryl trinitrate. It is used to treat angina. It is also used to treat cyanide poisoning. *Adverse effects* and *Precautions:* These are similar to those described under glyceryl trinitrate. *Dose:* By mouth, 30 to 120 mg.

sodium nitroprusside (Nipride) is a vasodilator drug used to treat heart-failure, severe hypertension, and to maintain a low blood pressure during surgery. *Adverse effects:* Nausea, vomiting, headache, dizziness, palpitations and chest pain (reduce the infusion rate). *Precautions:* It should be used with caution in patients suffering from hypothyroidism, or severe impairment of their kidney function. It should not be used in patients with liver failure, vitamin B_{12} deficiency (e.g., pernicious anaemia). *Dose:* Hypertensive crisis, by intravenous infusion 0·5 to 1·5 micrograms/kg/minute. Heart failure, by intravenous infusion 10 to 15 micrograms/minute, range 10 to 200 with a maximum of 400 micrograms/minute. As it is converted into cyanide in the body it is important that blood level monitoring should be carried out.

sodium octoate has some antifungal properties.

sodium octylphenoxyethoxyethyl ether sulphonate has detergent properties.

sodium oleate has detergent properties.

sodium o-phenylphenate tetrahydrate is used as a preservative and disinfectant.

sodium perborate monohydrate dissolves in water, releasing oxygen and hydrogen peroxide. It has mild anti-septic and deodorant properties and is used to prepare a mouth wash used to treat mouth and gum conditions.

sodium phosphate when taken by mouth acts as a saline laxative and produces a watery evacuation of the bowels. It can be used as an enema. It may be given by mouth or intravenously in the treatment of calcium and phosphorus disorders.

sodium picosulphate (Laxoberal) is broken down in the intestinal tract to form an irritant compound that acts as a laxative. *Dose:* 5 to 15 mg (5 to 15 ml) at night.

sodium polymetaphosphate is included in dusting powders in the treatment of excessive sweating and as a protection against athlete's foot.

sodium polystyrene sulphonate (Resonium-A) is a resin used to reduce potassium absorption from the food in patients suffering from high blood levels of potassium. *Dose:* 15 g four times daily, by mouth or as a rectal suspension.

sodium potassium tartrate is used as a saline laxative which produces a watery evacuation of the bowels. It is used as a stabilizer in cheese and meat products in some countries.

sodium propionate is an antifungal drug. It is used in skin applications.

sodium propyl-p-hydroxybenzoate is used as a preservative in food and medicines.

sodium ricinoleate is a powder made up of a mixture of the sodium salts of the fatty acids from castor oil.

sodium salicylate is a mild pain-reliever and it brings down high temperature. It is rapidly excreted and frequent doses are required. It irritates the stomach and therefore sodium bicarbonate was often given with it to prevent this. However, this merely increased its rate of excretion and reduced its effectiveness. It is seldom used now except in acute rheumatic fever. *Adverse effects* and *Precautions:* These are similar to those described under aspirin.

sodium salts of alkyl ether sulphate and sulphosuccinates have detergent properties and are used in medicated shampoos and as skin cleaners.

sodium stibogluconate (Pentostam) is used to treat Leishmaniasis. *Adverse effects:* Anorexia, vomiting, coughing, substernal pain. *Precautions:* IV injections should be given slowly and stopped if coughing or substernal pain occurs. It should not be given to patients suffering from pneumonia, myocarditis, nephritis, hepatitis. *Dose:* 600 mg daily by intravenous or intramuscular injections.

sodium sulphate (Glauber's salts) is used as a saline laxative. It may also be used to replace body sodium and in lotions for dressing wounds.

sodium sulphosuccinated undecylenic monoalkylolamide has antifungal properties ◊ undecenoic acid.

sodium tartrate is used as a purgative and in some countries as a stabilizer in meat products.

sodium tauroglycocholate has been given by mouth to assist the emulsification and absorption of fats, and fat-soluble vitamins in patients who have a deficiency of bile secretion.

sodium tetraborate ◊ borax.

sodium valproate (Epilim) is used to treat epilepsy. *Adverse effects:* Nausea, stomach upsets, transient loss of hair, oedema, blood disorders. It may damage the liver and rarely cause death. It may also produce pancreatitis. *Precautions:* Careful and regular tests of liver function and tests of blood function (e.g., platelets) should be carried out. It may give false positive tests for ketones in diabetes. *Dose:* By mouth, 600 to 2,600 mg daily in divided doses after food according to response. Blood levels of the drug should be regularly monitored.

Sofradex eye and **ear drops** contain framycetin 0·5%, dexamethasone 0·05%, and gramicidin 0·005%.

Soframycin ◊ framycetin.

Solarcaine Cream contains benzocaine 1% and triclosan 0·2%. **Solarcaine Lotion**, benzocaine 0·5% and triclosan 30·2%. **Solarcaine Spray**, benzocaine 5% and triclosan 0·1%.

Solardryl is a sunscreen cream containing benzyl salicylate, benzyl cinnamate, and methyl and propyl hydroxybenzoates.

Solasil contains hamamelis liquid extract 1·5%, almond oil 1·35%, zinc oxide 0·9%, camphor 0·1%, and menthol 0·1%.

Soleze contains dibromopropamidine isethionate 0·15% in an emollient basis.

Solis ◊ diazepam.

Solivito N vitamin injections contain thiamine 3·0 mg, riboflavine 3·6 mg, pyridoxine 4 mg, cyanocobalamin 5 micrograms, nicotinamide 40 mg, folic acid 0·4 mg, biotin 60 micrograms, pantothenic acid 15 mg, ascorbic acid 100 mg in each vial.

Solivito is a supplementary vitamin injection containing a range of vitamins.

Soliwax capsules for removing wax from the ears contain dioctyl sodium sulphosuccinate 5%.

Solmin tablets contain aspirin 300 mg and glycine 133 mg.

Solpadeine is a mild pain-reliever. Each effervescent tablet contains paracetamol 500 mg, codeine phosphate 8 mg and caffeine 30 mg in a sorbitol base. *Dose:* By mouth, 2 tablets dissolved in water three or four times daily.

Solprin (neutral soluble aspirin) ◊ aspirin.

Solu-Cortef (soluble hydrocortisone for injection) ◊ hydrocortisone.

Solu-Medrone powder for injection ◊ methylprednisolone.

Solution 41 contains salicylic acid 0·07% and triclosan 0·05%.

Solvazinc effervescent tablets contain zinc sulphate 200 mg (equivalent to 45 mg of zinc) ◊ zinc sulphate.

Somatonorm injection is used in the treatment of short stature caused by decreased or absent secretion of pituitary growth hormone. It contains

somatrem (methionyl human somatotrophin) corresponding to 4 i.u. human somatotrophin (growth hormone).

Sominex ◊ promethazine.

Somnite ◊ nitrazepam.

Soneryl ◊ butobarbitone.

Soni-Slo capsules contain either 20 or 40 mg isosorbide dinitrate in sustained-release form. *Dose:* By mouth, 40 to 120 mg daily in two or three divided doses.

Soothadent contains lignocaine hydrochloride 2%.

Soothake contains benzyl alcohol 5%, clove oil 5%, benzocaine 7·5%, wool fat 12·5%, and basis to 100%.

sorbic acid has antibacterial and antifungal properties and is used as a preservative in cosmetics, medicines and foods.

Sorbichew (chewable tablets) ◊ isosorbide dinitrate.

Sorbid SA: Each capsule contains isosorbide dinitrate 40 mg in sustained-release form.

sorbide nitrate ◊ isosorbide dinitrate.

sorbitan monostearate is an emulsifier.

sorbitol is used as a sugar substitute in diabetic food. It is used as a sweetening agent in drug preparations and is present in some creams and toothpastes. Excessive amounts in the diet may cause wind, abdominal distension and diarrhoea.

Sorbitrate ◊ isosorbide dinitrate.

Sotacor ◊ sotalol.

sotalol (Beta-Cardone; Sotacor; Tolerzide; sotalol hydrochloride) is a beta-receptor blocker used to treat angina, raised blood pressure and disorders of heart rhythm. *Adverse effects* and *Precautions* ◊ propranolol. *Dose:* By mouth, angina, 240 to 480 mg daily in divided doses; raised blood pressure, 240 to 640 mg daily in divided doses; disorders of heart rhythm, 120 to 240 mg daily in divided doses.

Sotazide is used to treat raised blood pressure. Each tablet contains sotalol 160 mg and hydrochlorothiazide 25 mg.

Sotol effervescent mouthwash tablets contain sodium bicarbonate, tartaric acid, sodium benzoate, saccharin, menthol and thymol.

Sovol Liquid: Each 5 ml contains aluminium hydroxide 200 mg, magnesium hydroxide 200 mg, and dimethylpolysiloxane 25 mg.

Sovol Tablet: Each contains aluminium hydroxide-magnesium carbonate co-dried gel 300 mg, magnesium hydroxide 100 mg, and dimethylpolysiloxane 25 mg

soya lecithin ◊ lecithin.

soya oil is prepared from soya beans, it has a high content of unsaturated fatty acids. It is given intravenously to patients who are unable to take any nutrients orally. It is also used as a base in bath oils.

Sparine ◊ promazine.

Spasmonal ◊ alverine citrate.

spearmint oil is obtained from the dried leaves and flowering tops of spearmint (mint). It is used as a flavouring agent and as a carminative.

spectinomycin (Trobicin) is an antibiotic used to treat gonorrhoea. *Adverse effects:* It may produce dizziness, nausea, chills, nettle-rash (urticaria) and pain at the infection site. *Dose:* By deep intramuscular injection, males 2 g and females 4 g.

Spectraban Sunscreen ◊ dimethylaminobenzoate.

Spectralgen is used to treat allergy to pollens. It is available either as a single species from any one of seven varieties of common grasses or trees, or as a four-grass mix, or as a three-tree mix.

spermaceti is a solid wax from the mixed oils from the head, blubber and carcase of the sperm whale.

Spiretic ◊ spironolactone.

Spiroctan ◊ spironolactone.

Spiroctan-M ◊ canrenoate potassium.

Spirolone ◊ spironolactone.

spironolactone (Aldactone; Diatensec; Laractone; Spiretic; Spiroctan; Spirolone) inhibits the effects of a corticosteroid called aldosterone, which is produced by the adrenal glands. Since aldosterone produces retention of sodium and loss of potassium from the urine spironolactone does the reverse, and thus increases sodium loss and potassium retention. It is therefore used as a diuretic to treat patients with fluid retention caused by certain heart and other disorders which are associated with an increased production of aldosterone by the adrenal glands. *Adverse effects:* It may cause headache and when taken in large doses, drowsiness. Skin rashes may also occur; these clear when the drug is stopped. Ataxia, mental confusion, hairiness (hirsutism), irregular periods and swelling of the breasts have been reported. *Precautions:* It should be given with caution to patients with impaired kidney function. *Dose:* By mouth, 50 to 200 mg daily.

Spotoway Antiseptic Cream contains extrapone No. 4 Special 0·5% and chlorhexidine gluconate solution 1%.

Spotoway Lotion contains chlorhexidine gluconate solution 0·5%, cetrimide 0·04%, and industrial methylated spirit 10%.

Sprilon spray contains dimethicone 2·0% and zinc oxide 20% in a propellent with several skin protective bases.

Squalane is used in ointment bases to increase permeability through the skin.

squill (*Scilla*) has an effect upon the heart like digitalis but it is poorly absorbed and irritates the stomach, producing nausea and vomiting. In small doses it is a common constituent of cough mixtures.

squill oxymel ◊ squill.

squill vinegar ◊ squill.

Stabillin V-K ◊ phenoxymethylpenicillin.

Stafoxil ◊ flucloxacillin.

stannic oxide (tin oxide) has been used to treat boils, acne and tapeworms.

stanozolol (Stromba) is an anabolic (body-building) steroid used to treat debility. *Adverse effects* and *Precautions* ◊ ethyloestrenol. *Dose:* By mouth, 5 mg daily. By deep intramuscular injections 50 mg every 2 to 3 weeks. It has been used as a fibrinolytic to treat Raynaud's disease.

Staphcil ◊ flucloxacillin.

starch is used in protective skin applications. It is used in the manufacture of some tablets and is included in some enemas as a base.

Staycept ◊ nonoxynol.

stearic acid is used as a lubricant in the manufacture of tablets.

Steedman's Teething Jelly contains cetylpyridinium chloride 0·02% and ethyl nicotinate 0·0025%.

Steiner Treatment Shampoo contains zinc omadine 1%.

Stelazine ◊ trifluoperazine.

Stemetil ◊ prochlorperazine.

sterculia is a gum used as a laxative.

Steribath concentrate solution contains iodine-nonoxynol complex (4·5% available iodine) per sachet.

Sterogyl-15 ◊ calciferol.

Steriwipe contains chlorhexidine 0·015% and cetrimide 0·15%.

Sterotabs Tablets: Each contains halazone 4 mg.

Ster-Zac Bath Conc contains 2% triclosan.

Ster-Zac DC Skin Cleanser cream contains hexachlorophane 3%.

Ster-Zac Powder contains hexachlorophane 0·33%, zinc oxide 3%, talc 88·67% and starch 8%.

Stesolid is an injection of diazepam 5 mg/ml.

Stiedex ◊ desoxymethasone.

stilboestrol is the most widely used synthetic oestrogen. Read section on female sex hormones. For uses ◊ ethinyloestradiol. Stilboestrol is also used to treat breast cancer and prostatic cancer. *Adverse effects:* These include nausea, vomiting and fluid retention and in males loss of libido and gynaecomastia. For other *Adverse effects* and *Precautions* ◊ ethinyloestradiol. *Dose:* Varies according to the disorder being treated.

Stingo aerosol contains trichlorofluoromethane 85% and dichlorodifluoromethane 15%.

Stings Cream contains diphenhydramine hydrochloride 2% and menthol 1%.

Stomosol Liquid Concentrate contains chlorhexidine gluconate solution 5%, benzalkonium chloride solution (50%) 20%, and cetomacrogol '1000' 10%.

Stop 'n' Grow contains denatonium benzoate 0·14%, sucrose octa-acetate 7·69%.

storax has actions similar to Peru balsam. It is used as an ointment in the treatment of scabies and other parasitic disorders. It is an ingredient of benzoin inhalation.

stramonium (thornapple leaf; stramonium leaf) has effects similar to belladonna. It is an ingredient of powders which are burned and the fumes inhaled to relieve asthma. This procedure often makes bronchitis worse and there are much more effective drugs available.

Strepsils lozenges each contain amylmetacresol 600 micrograms and dichlorobenzyl alcohol 1·2 mg. **Strepsils Honey and Lemon** contain the same active ingredients in a flavoured basis.

Streptase ◊ streptokinase.

streptodornase is an enzyme used in combination with streptokinase to remove tissue exudates and coagulated blood from body cavities.

streptokinase (Kabikinase, Streptase) is an enzyme used to dissolve thromboses. *Adverse effects:* Bleeding, rashes, fever and allergic reactions. *Precautions:* It should be used with caution in patients suffering from atrial fibrillation or recovering from streptococcal infections. It should not be used during periods, pregnancy, in patients with bleeding disorders, in severe hypertension or in patients who have had surgery in the preceding 72 hours or have a streptococcal infection. *Dose:* By intravenous infusion, 250,000 to 600,000 units over 30 minutes then 100,000 units every hour for up to one week.

streptomycin (streptomycin sulphate) is an antibiotic. It is effective against a wide range of bacteria but it is used particularly to treat tuberculosis. *Adverse effects:* After intramuscular injections the patient may develop pain at the site of injection and peculiar sensations around the mouth, vertigo, headache, and lassitude. Allergic reactions are common and patients may develop skin rashes, swollen glands and fever. More severe adverse effects may result from streptomycin's effects upon the nerves supplying the ear and organs of balance. These may come on suddenly and disappear when the drug is withdrawn, but permanent deafness and damage to the organ of balance may develop slowly and even come on after the drug has been stopped. In high doses kidney damage, blood disorders and liver damage may develop. *Precautions:* Great caution is needed when giving streptomycin to patients with impaired kidney or liver function, to the elderly, and to premature infants. It should not be used in pregnancy because the baby could be born deaf. It should not be used in patients with ear disorders or disorders of their organ of balance or in patients who are allergic to it. To prevent the development of resistant bacteria it should be used with other antituberculous drugs in the treatment of tuberculosis. *Dose:* By intramuscular injection, 0·5 to 1 g daily.

Stress B supplement is a vitamin supplement.

Stromba ◊ stanozolol.

strontium chloride is used as a 10% toothpaste for the relief of dental hypersensitivity.

strophanthin-G (ouabain) ◊ digitalis.

strychnine stimulates all parts of the nervous system and has been used in tonics, bitters and laxatives. *Adverse effects:* May cause convulsions and it should not be used.

Stubit lozenges are used as an aid to stop smoking; they contain essential oils and purified tobacco extract.

Stugeron ◊ cinnarizine.

Stugeron Forte ◊ cinnarizine.

Sublamin liquid contains benzoic acid 4·85%, salicylic acid 3%, benzalkonium chloride solution 0·1%, and cetylpyridinium chloride 0·05%.

Sublimaze injection ◊ fentanyl.

succinylcholine ◊ suxamethonium.

succinylsulphathiazole (Sulfasuxidine) has effects, uses and adverse effects similar to those described under phthalylsulphathiazole. It is an antibacterial drug used to treat infections of the gut. *Dose:* By mouth, 10 to 20 g daily in divided doses.

sucralfate (Antepsin) is used to treat peptic ulcers. It may interfere with the absorption of drugs such as tetracycline. *Adverse effects:* Constipation.

Precautions: It should be used with caution in patients with impaired kidney function. *Dose:* By mouth, 1 to 2 g four times a day.

Sucrets are throat lozenges each containing hexylresorcinol 2·4 mg.

sucrose is refined sugar.

Sucrose octa-acetate is used as an alcohol denaturant.

Sudafed is used to treat symptoms of the common cold. Each tablet and 10 ml elixir contains 60 mg pseudoephedrine. **Sudafed expectorant** also contains 200 mg guaiphenesin per 10 ml; **Sudafen-Co** tablets also contain paracetamol 500 mg.

Sudocrem cream is used to treat urinary rash and pressure sores. It contains benzyl alcohol 0·39%, benzyl benzoate 1·01%, benzyl cinnamate 0·15%, wool fat 4% and zinc oxide 15·25%.

Suleo shampoo ◊ carbaryl.

Suleo-C lotion ◊ carbaryl.

Suleo-M lotion ◊ malathion.

sulfadoxine is a sulphonamide drug. It has a long duration of action and is used to treat leprosy. It is given with pirimethamine in the treatment and prophylaxis of falciparum malaria resistant to other therapies. *Adverse effects* and *Precautions* ◊ Section on sulphonamides. *Dose:* By mouth, intramuscular or intravenous injections – varies according to the disorder being treated.

sulfametopyrazine (Kelfizine W) is a long-acting sulphonamide drug. Read section on sulphonamides. *Dose:* By mouth, 2 g once weekly.

Sulfomyl ◊ mafenide.

Sulfamylon* ◊ mafenide.

Sulfamylon cream is used to treat skin infections. It contains mafenide 8·5% ◊ mafenide.

Sulfasuxidine ◊ succinylsulphathiazole.

sulindac (Clinoril) is an anti-rheumatic drug with uses and effects similar to those described under indomethacin. *Dose:* By mouth, 100 to 200 mg twice daily with food.

sulphacetamide (Albucid; sulphacetamide sodium) is a sulphonamide drug. It is used chiefly as eye drops to treat infections of the eye (conjunctivitis). Read section on sulphonamides.

sulphadiazine is a sulphonamide. Read section on sulphonamides. *Dose:* By mouth, 3 g initially and then up to 4 g daily in divided doses.

sulphadimethoxine (Madribon) is a long-acting sulphonamide. Read section on sulphonamides. *Dose:* By mouth, 2 g daily initially and then 1 g daily.

sulphadimidine (Sulphamezathine) is a sulphonamide. Read section on sulphonamides. *Dose:* By mouth for infections, 3 to 6 g daily in divided doses; for urinary infections, 2 to 4 g daily in divided doses.

sulphafurazole is a sulphonamide; it is long acting and reaches a high concentration in the urine, and was used to treat infections of the bladder and kidneys. Read section on sulphonamides. *Dose:* By mouth, 2 to 6 g daily in divided doses.

sulphaguanidine is a sulphonamide. It is not readily absorbed and is used to treat infections of the gut such as bacillary dysentery. Because of its effects on the bacteria in the gut it may cause fungal infections (e.g., thrush) and deficiency of vitamin B. Read section on sulphonamides. *Dose:* By mouth, 6 to 20 g daily in divided doses.

sulphamethoxazole is a sulphonamide. It is now frequently combined with trimethoprim as co-trimoxazole (Bactrim, Septrin).

Sulphamezathine ◊ sulphadimidine.

sulphamoxole is a sulphonamide.

sulphanilamide is a sulphonamide used topically in the treatment of ear and nose infections.

sulphapyridine (M & B 693) is a sulphonamide which is now rarely used except in a serious skin disorder called dermatitis herpetiformis. Read section on sulphonamides.

sulphasalazine (Salazopyrin) is used to treat ulcerative colitis and Crohn's disease. *Adverse effects:* Nausea, vomiting, epigastric discomfort, headache, vertigo, tinnitus, rashes, fever, minor haematological abnormalities such as Heinz-body anaemia, reversible neutropenia, folate malabsorption; rarely frank haemolytic anaemias, pancreati-

tis, agranulocytosis, Stevens–Johnson syndrome, neurotoxicity, photosensitization, polyarteritis nodosa, allergic myocarditis, pulmonary fibrosis, reversible azoospermia. Urine may be coloured orange. *Precautions:* It should not be given to patients with a known allergy to salicylates and sulphonamides. It should be used with caution in pregnancy, in patients with impaired kidney and liver function. Adequate fluid intake must be maintained to prevent crystals developing in the kidneys and repeated blood and urine tests should be carried out. *Dose:* By mouth, acute attack 1 g 4 times daily, maintenance 500 mg 4 times daily. By rectum 0·5 to 1 g night and morning. Bed-time enema 3 g to be retained for at least one hour.

Sulphatriad: Each tablet contains sulphathiazole 185 mg, sulphadiazine 185 mg and sulphamerazine 130 mg. Read section on sulphonamides. *Dose:* By mouth, 2 tablets four to six hourly.

sulphaurea has the properties of a sulphonamide drug and is used to treat urinary tract infection. Read section on sulphonamides. *Dose:* By mouth, 1 g three times daily.

sulphinpyrazone (Anturan) reduces the blood uric acid level and is used as long-term treatment for gout. It increases uric acid excretion by the kidneys. It is no use for treating acute attacks of gout. *Adverse effects:* It may cause nausea, vomiting and abdominal pain and aggravate peptic ulcers. At the beginning of treatment it may trigger off acute attacks of gout. Blood disorders may occasionally occur with prolonged treatment. *Precautions:* It should be given with caution to patients with impaired kidney function or to those who have had peptic ulcers in the past. It should not be given to patients with active peptic ulcers. It may increase the effects of certain anti-blood clotting drugs, insulin and other anti-diabetic drugs, and its effects are decreased by aspirin and other salicylates. *Dose:* By mouth, 100 to 800 mg daily in divided doses for gout. As an anti-thrombosis drug, e.g. after recent myocardial infarction. By mouth, 200 mg four times daily with meals, starting one month after heart attack.

sulphur has been widely used as a mild antiseptic in skin applications.

sulphuric acid has been used in dilute forms as an astringent to treat diarrhoea and occasionally as a bitter to stimulate the appetite.

sulpiride (Dolmatil; Sulpitil) is an antipsychotic drug used to treat schizophrenia. *Adverse effects* and *Precautions* are similar to those described under chlorpromazine. It should not be used in patients suffering from severe kidney, liver or blood disease, nor should it be used in patients suffering from a phaeochromocytoma. Reduced dosage is necessary in elderly people and patients with impaired kidney function. *Dose:* By mouth, 400 to 1,800 mg daily in divided doses twice daily. Maximum daily dose of 2,400 mg.

Sulpitil ◊ sulpiride.

sulthiame (Ospolot*) is an anticonvulsant used to treat certain forms of epilepsy. *Adverse effects:* The most usual are loss of appetite, loss of energy, and ataxia. These usually go in a few days. Children may develop breathlessness. Other adverse effects include sensory sensations on the face, hands and feet; dizziness, nausea, loss of weight and mental changes. Abdominal pains, drooling, insomnia, blood disorders and increased fits have been reported. *Precautions:* It should be used with caution in patients with impaired kidney function. It is not recommended for the treatment of petit mal epilepsy. *Dose:* By mouth, up to 200 mg three times daily.

Sultrin pessaries and **vaginal cream** contain a mixture of sulphonamides. *Dose:* 1 pessary or 1 applicatorful vaginally twice daily for 10 days.

Sunnimax tablets each contain vitamin A 4,500 units, vitamin D 450 units, and vitamin C 40 mg.

Sunscreen lotion contains menthyl salicylate, glycerin and borax.

Sunspot Healing Paint contains camphor 8%, benzoin 2%, ethylene glycol 0·02%, benzalkonium chloride 0·1%, allantoin 0·4%, isopropyl alcohol (90%) to 100%.

Super Plenamins tablets: Each contain vitamin A 5,000 units, vitamin B_1 2·25 mg, vitamin B_2 2·25 mg, vitamin B_3 500 micrograms, vitamin B_6 100 micrograms, vitamin B_{12} 2 micrograms, vitamin C 40 mg, vitamin D 300 units, vitamin E 2 mg, nicotinamide 20 mg, dried ferrous sulphate 51 mg, calcium 75 mg, phosphorus 58 mg, magnesium 10 mg, iodine 150 micrograms, copper 750 micrograms, manganese 1·25 mg, potassium 3 mg, and zinc 1 mg.

Super Zinc-C is a zinc and vitamin C supplement.

Superfact ◊ buserelin.

Supren ◊ ibuprofen.

Surama Medicated Cigarettes contain cascarilla bark 1·5%, cubeb fruit 1·5%, benzoin 1·5%, stramonium leaf 92·5%, eucalyptus oil 1·5%, menthol 0·5%, and pumilio pine oil 1%.

Surbex T is a multivitamin preparation. Each tablet contains thiamine mononitrate 15 mg, riboflavine 10 mg, nicotinamide 100 mg, pyridoxine hydrochloride 5 mg, ascorbic acid 500 mg.

Sure Shield Adult Travel Tablets: Each contains chlorbutol 150 mg.

Sure Shield Antibactic Throat Lozenges each contain tyrothricin 1 mg and cetylpyridinium chloride 1·5 mg.

Sure Shield Bronchial Mixture: Each 5 ml contains ammonium bicarbonate 50 mg, squill liquid extract 0·021 ml, ipecacuanha liquid extract 0·0085 ml, senega liquid extract 0·0145 ml, liquorice extract 0·425 ml, glycerol 310 mg, tolu syrup 0·245 ml, capsicin 0·000125 ml, and treacle 1·75 g.

Sure Shield Catarrh Pastilles contain creosote 0·2%, pumillo pine oil 0·52%, sylvestris pine oil 0·39%, eucalyptus oil 0·2%, menthol 0·83% and thymol 0·2%.

Sure Shield Children's Cough Pastilles contain anise oil 0·4%, lemon oil 0·05%, ipecacuanha liquid extract 0·11%, benzoic acid 0·11%, squill liquid extract 0·22%, tolu solution 0·33% and tartaric acid 0·44%.

Sure Shield Children's Travel Tablets: Each contains chlorbutol 75 mg.

Sure Shield Diarrhoea Mixture: Each 5 ml contains sodium bicarbonate 125 mg, light kaolin 470 mg, compound rhubarb tincture 0·0625 ml, catechu tincture 0·125 ml, chalk 32 mg, and aromatic ammonia solution 0·195 ml.

Sure Shield Doctors' Catarrh Pastilles contain menthol 0·36%, creosote 0·18% and sylvestris pine oil 0·36%.

Sure Shield Dyspepsia Tablets: Each contain bismuth carbonate 11·25 mg, heavy magnesium carbonate 62·5 mg, sodium bicarbonate 43·75 mg, calcium carbonate 400 mg, pepsin 870 micrograms, pancreatin 625 micrograms, capsicin 50 micrograms.

Sure Shield Extra Strong Bronchial Cough Mixture: Each 5 ml contains ammonium bicarbonate 50 mg, squill liquid extract 0·021 ml, ipecacuanha liquid extract 0·0085 ml, capsicin 0·0001 ml, treacle 1·75 g, tolu syrup 0·245 ml, glycerin 310 mg, liquorice extract 0·0425 ml and senega liquid extract 0·0145 ml.

Sure Shield Footballer's Linctus: Each 5 ml contains menthol 12·5 mg, anise oil 0·0125 ml, tolu syrup 0·5 ml, capsicum tincture 0·167 ml, euphorbia liquid extract 0·05 ml, coltsfoot liquid extract 0·05 ml, and treacle 2·75 g.

Sure Shield Glycerin, Lemon and Honey contains glycerin 0·25 g, purified honey 0·5 g, citric acid 42 mg and lemon oil 0·008 ml.

Sure Shield Glycerin, Lemon and Honey with Ipecacuanha liquid contains in each 5 ml glycerin 0·25 g, purified honey 0·5 g, lemon oil 0·004 ml, ipecacuanha liquid extract 0·01 ml, squill vinegar 0·125 ml, tolu solution 0·025 ml and citric acid 42 mg.

Sure Shield Indian brandee is used to treat colic pains. Each 5 ml contains compound rhubarb tincture 0·095 ml, nitrous ether spirit 0·25 ml, solvent ether 0·1 ml and strong ginger tincture 0·04 ml.

Sure Shield Iodised Throat Tablets contain iodine (free and combined) 0·0478%, methyl salicylate 0·0617%, phenol (free and combined) 0·379%, menthol 0·228%, citric acid 0·446%, and cetylpyridinium chloride 0·044%.

Sure Shield Mouth Ulcer Tablets: Each contain amylmetacresol 500 micrograms, ascorbic acid 25 mg, and cetylpyridinium chloride 1·5 mg.

Sure Shield Sure-Lax Tablets: Each contain phenolphthalein 90 mg and natural raspberry juice.

Sure Shield Rum Cough Elixir contains in each 5 ml cocillana liquid extract 0·02 ml, squill liquid extract 0·01 ml, senega liquid extract 0·01 ml, cascara liquid extract 0·125 ml, ipecacuanha tincture 0·125 ml, menthol 460 micrograms, and Jamaica rum 2·5 ml.

Surem ◊ nitrazepam.

Surgam ◊ tiaprofenic acid.

Surgolene Liquid contains liquefied phenol 0·63%, hydrochloric acid 0·4%, salicylic acid 0·045%, and iodine 0·11%.

Surmontil ◊ trimipramine.

Suscard Buccal ◊ glyceryl trinitrate.

Sustac (slow-release glyceryl trinitrate) ◊ glyceryl trinitrate.

Sustamycin capsules contain tetracycline hydrochloride 250 mg in a sustained-release form. *Dose:* By mouth, 1 twice daily.

Sustanon injections contain three testosterone compounds formulated so that blood levels are maintained for a long period after injection.

suxamethonium (Anectine, Brevidil M, Scoline; succinylcholine chloride; suxamethonium chloride, suxamethonium bromide) is a depolarizing voluntary muscle relaxant used in surgery. *Adverse effects* and *Precautions:* It may cause slowing of the heart rate, irregularities of heart rhythm and arrest of the heart. Fever and allergic reactions may occur and patients up and about soon after surgery may develop pains in their chest, abdomen, trunk, shoulders and neck. Prolonged absence of breathing (apnoea) may occur in some patients due to a low level of the enzyme (cholinesterase) which breaks down the chemical transmitter called acetylcholine. This low level may occur in patients with impaired liver function and severe anaemia. The drug should not be used in such patients and it should not be used for eye surgery.

suxethonium (Brevidil E, suxethonium bromide) has similar actions and effects to those described under suxamethonium. *Dose:* Intravenous injection 1 to 1·25 ml per kg.

S.V.C. is an acetarsol vaginal preparation ◊ acetarsol.

SVR is 90% alcohol (ethanol).

Swarm cream contains dibromopropamidine isethionate 0·15%, mepyramine maleate 1·5%, and calamine 10%.

sweet birch oil is used as a rubefacient ◊ wintergreen oil.

Sweetex pellets ◊ saccharin.

Syl is a barrier cream containing dimethicone and benzalkonium chloride in a base.

Sylphen Tablets contain paracetamol 300 mg, ephedrine hydrochloride 5 mg, and caffeine 30 mg.

sylvestris pine oil is present in so-called pine disinfectants to give them a nice smell.

Symmetrel ◊ amantadine.

Sympatol ◊ oxedrine.

Synacthen ◊ tetracosactrin.

Synadrin ◊ prenylamine.

Synalar cream and **ointment** ◊ fluocinolone.

Synalar C cream and **ointment** contains fluocinolone acetonide 0·025% and clioquinol 3%.

Synalar N cream and **ointment** contains fluocinolone acetonide 0·025% and neomycin sulphate 0·5%.

Syndol is a mild pain-reliever. Each tablet contains paracetamol 450 mg, codeine phosphate 10 mg, doxylamine succinate 5 mg and caffeine 30 mg. *Dose:* 1 to 2 tablets, every 4 to 6 hours, maximum 8 tablets daily.

Synflex ◊ naproxen.

Synkavit (menadiol sodium diphosphate, soluble vitamin K) is used to treat patients with malabsorption syndrome and to antagonize the effects of oral anticoagulants (see Part Two).

Synogist ◊ sodium sulphosuccinated undecylenic monoalkylolamide.

Synphase is an oral contraceptive having 12 white tablets and 9 yellow tablets. Each white tablet contains norethisterone 0·5 mg and ethinyloestradiol 0·035 mg. Each yellow tablet contains norethisterone 1 mg and ethinyloestradiol 0·035 mg.

Syntaris ◊ flunisolide.

Syntocinon ◊ oxytocin.

Syntometrine: Each 1 ml ampoule contains ergometrine maleate 0·5 mg and oxytocin 5 units. Used during labour to contract the uterus. *Dose:* 1 ml by intramuscular injection as necessary.

Syntopressin ◊ lypressin.

Synuretic is a diuretic containing amiloride hydrochloride 5 mg and hydrochlorothiazide 50 mg.

Syraprim ◊ trimethoprim.

Sytron elixir contains the iron salt sodium iron edetate. *Dose:* By mouth, 5 to 10 ml three times daily.

Tabassan tablets each contain ephedrine hydrochloride 15 mg, theobromine 30 mg, and salicylamide 60 mg.

Tabmint chewing gum contains silver acetate 6 mg, ammonium acetate 14·5 mg, sodium chloride 11 mg, and cocarboxylase 25 micrograms in each tablet.

Tachyrol (dihydrotachysterol) ◊ vitamin D.

Tagamet ◊ cimetidine.

talampicillin (Talpen; talampicillin hydrochloride) in the body turns into ampicillin ◊ ampicillin. *Dose:* By mouth, 250 to 500 mg three times daily.

talc is used in dusting powders. Prolonged and intense use may cause scarring of the lungs through inhalation.

Talpen ◊ talampicillin.

Tambocor (flecainide acetate) ◊ flecainide.

Tamofen ◊ tamoxifen.

tamoxifen (Noltam; Nolvadex; Tamofen) has anti-oestrogenic properties, probably because it competes with oestrogen at sites of action. It is used to treat cancer of the breast and also to treat infertility where it has been demonstrated that the patient is suffering from anovulatory menstrual cycles. *Adverse effects:* Hot flushes, vaginal bleeding, and pruritus vulvae, gastro-intestinal discomfort, lightheadedness and fluid retention. It may reduce the platelet count in the blood. *Precautions:* It should not be given in pregnancy. High blood calcium levels have been observed in patients with secondary bone tumours treated with tamoxifen. *Dose:* By mouth, 10 mg twice daily.

Tampovagan: Each pessary contains stilboestrol 0·5 mg and lactic acid 5%.

Tancolin paediatric cough linctus contains ascorbic acid 12·35 mg, citric acid 45·85 mg, dextromethorphan hydrobromide 2·62 mg, glycerol 655 mg, sodium citrate 99·56 mg, and theophylline 15 mg in each 5 ml. *Dose:* 2·5 to 15 ml, 3 times daily according to the age of the child.

Tanderil Chloramphenicol ointment contains chloramphenicol 1% and oxyphenbutazone 10%.

tannic acid has been used as an astringent in throat lozenges, gargles and skin preparations, and to treat diarrhoea and cases of poisoning. Deaths from liver damage have been reported following its use on burns and when it has been mixed with enemas for X-ray examinations.

tannin ◊ tannic acid.

tar is used as an anti-itching drug in skin applications. It is used to treat eczema and psoriasis.

Taractan ◊ chlorprothixene.

taraxacum (Dandelion root) has been used as a bitter tonic and also as a mild laxative.

Tarcortin cream contains hydrocortisone 0·5% and tar extract 5%.

tarta~ic acid is used to make fizzy drinks and tablets.

Taumasthman* is used to treat bronchial asthma. Each tablet contains theophylline 100 mg, phenazone 100 mg, caffeine 50 mg, ephedrine hydrochloride 10 mg, atropine sulphate 0·3 mg. *Dose:* By mouth, 1 to 3 tablets daily, after meals.

Tavegil ◊ clemastine.

TCP First Aid Gel contains TCP Liquid Antiseptic 80% in a gel basis.

TCP Liquid Antiseptic is an aqueous solution containing halogenated phenols and salicylic acid made from chlorine 0·4%, iodine 0·005%, phenol 0·63%, and sodium salicylate 0·052%, with the partial elimination of ionizable halides.

TCP Ointment contains TCP liquid antiseptic 6·4%, iodine 0·2%, methyl salicylate 1·3%, precip. sulphur 1·5%, kaolin 8·5%, with camphor 1·3%, tannic acid 0·4%, salicylic acid 0·4%, and glycerol 2·4%.

TCP Throat Pastilles: Active ingredients are TCP Liquid Antiseptic 10% (1·74 mg); available in blackcurrant and lemon flavours.

Tears Naturale contain dextran 0·1% and hypromellose 0·3%.

Tedral SA is a sustained-release form of Tedral. *Dose:* By mouth, 1 tablet night and morning.

Teejel applications contain choline salicylate 8·7% and cetalkonium chloride 0·1%.

Tegretol ◊ carbamazepine.

Tellodont gargle and mouthwash tablets each contain sodium benzoate 5%, peppermint oil 0·9%, thymol 0·3%, menthol 1·2%, cinnamon oil 0·3%, methyl salicylate 0·3%, and saccharin 0·1%, in an effervescent basis.

Tellora Powder for preparing mouthwash contains menthol, thymol, sodium benzoate, cetrimide, clove oil, aniseed oil, saccharin, sodium bicarbonate, tartaric acid, and empicol.

temazepam (Normison) is a benzodiazepine drug used as a hypnotic. It produces similar actions and effects to diazepam. *Adverse effects:* Include drowsiness, dizziness on waking and morning headaches. Skin rashes and gastro-intestinal symptoms have been reported. *Precautions:* Small doses should be used in the elderly. Temazepam interferes with ability to drive motor vehicles and operate moving machinery. Its effects may be increased by alcohol. *Dose:* By mouth, 10 to 60 mg at night.

Temetex ◊ diflucortolone.

Temgesic ◊ buprenorphine.

Tempulin: Read section on insulins.

10 Hour Capsules: Each contains paracetamol 150 mg, noscapine 10 mg, terpin hydrate 30 mg and phenylephrine hydrochloride 5 mg.

Tenavoid for P.M.T. Each tablet contains bendrofluazide 3 mg and meprobamate 200 mg. *Dose:* By mouth, 1 tablet three times daily for 5 to 8 days before expected onset of period.

Tenoret 50 is used to treat raised blood pressure. Each tablet contains atenolol 50 mg, and chlorthalidone 12·5 mg. *Dose:* By mouth, 1 daily.

Tenoretic is used to treat raised blood pressure. Each tablet contains atenolol 100 mg and chlorthalidone 25 mg. *Dose:* By mouth, 1 daily.

Tenormin ◊ atenolol.

Tensilon ◊ edrophonium.

Tensium ◊ diazepam.

Tenuate Dospan is a slow-release preparation of diethylpropion.

Teoptic eyedrops contain carteolol hydrochloride 1% or 2%. Carteolol is a beta-blocker used to treat glaucoma. *Adverse effects* and *Precautions:* Carteolol may be absorbed into the blood stream and interact with other drugs, e.g., verapamil, to produce adverse effects. It should not be used in patients who suffer from asthma or a slow pulse rate ◊ propranolol. *Dose:* Apply eyedrops twice daily.

terazosin (Hytrin) is used to treat raised blood pressure. It is a selective alpha-receptor blocker. *Adverse effects* include dizziness, lassitude, ankle swelling and a fall in blood pressure upon standing from a sitting or lying position (orthostatic or postural hypotension). *Precautions:* It should be used with caution in patients with impaired liver function and in patients with a history of fainting. *Dose:* By mouth, at night, 2 to 10 mg daily.

terbutaline (Bricanyl; Monovent; terbutaline sulphate) is a bronchodilator drug used to treat bronchial asthma. *Precautions:* It should not be used in patients with heart failure, high blood pressure or overworking of their thyroid glands. *Dose:* By inhaler, 0·25 mg per puff, 1 to 2 puffs when required, to a maximum of 8 in twenty-four hours. Bricanyl is available as tablets, syrup, inhaler, nebuhaler, spacer inhaler, respiratory solution and as sustained-release tablets (Bricanyl SA).

Tercoda cough elixir. Each 5 ml contains codeine phosphate 8 mg, terpin hydrate 8 mg, menthol 4 mg, peppermint oil 0·01 ml and other volatile oils. *Dose:* By mouth, 5 to 10 ml three times a day.

terebine closely resembles turpentine oil. It is an aromatic ingredient in some throat pastilles.

terfenadine (Triludan) is an antihistamine with similar effects to promethazine. The incidence of drowsiness and impaired driving ability is lower with this drug. *Dose:* By mouth, 60 mg twice daily.

terlipressin is a derivative of vasopressin which is used in the treatment of bleeding oesophageal varices ◊ vasopressin.

terodiline (Terolin) is an atropine-like drug used to treat frequency and incontinence of urine. *Adverse effects and Precautions* ◊ atropine. It should not be used if there is an obstruction to the flow of urine (e.g., an enlarged prostate gland) or in severe liver or gall-bladder disease. *Dose:* By mouth, 12·5 to 25 mg twice daily. Elderly people, 12·5 mg twice daily.

Terolin ◊ terodiline.

Teronac ◊ mazindol.

Terperoin Elixir: Each 5 ml contains codeine phosphate 10·4 mg, menthol 5 mg, terpin hydrate 20 mg, in a flavoured syrup basis.

Terperoin Pastilles contain pine oil 0·05%, cineole 0·028%, ipecacuanha liquid extract 0·014%, terpin hydrate 0·64%, codeine phosphate 0·097%, and menthol 0·14%.

terpineol is used as a disinfectant, flavouring agent and a solvent.

terpin hydrate is used as a cough expectorant. It may produce stomach pains and should be taken after meals.

Terpoin cough elixir: Each 5 ml contains codeine phosphate 15 mg, guaiphenesin 50 mg, terpin hydrate 9·15 mg, cineole 4·15 mg, and menthol 18·3 mg. *Dose:* By mouth, 5 to 10 ml three hourly.

Terra-Cortril ear drops contain oxytetracycline hydrochloride 0·5%, hydrocortisone acetate 1·5% and polymyxin B sulphate 10,000 units; **topical ointment** contains oxytetracyline hydrochloride 3% and hydrocortisone 1%; **aerosol spray:** oxytetracycline 0·5%, hydrocortisone 0·17%.

Terra-Corril Nystatin cream contains hydrocortisone 1%, nystatin 100,000 units/g and oxytetracycline 3% (as calcium salt).

Terramycin ◊ oxytetracycline.

Tertroxin ◊ liothyronine.

testosterone (Restandol; Sustanon; testosterone phenylpropionate; testosterone propionate; testosterone undecenoate) is a male sex hormone. *Adverse effects:* Testosterone may cause increase in skeletal weight, salt and water retention, oedema, increased number of small blood vessels in the skin, raised blood calcium, and increased bone growth. Prolonged use of high doses (300 mg monthly) in women produces masculinization – hairiness (hirsutism), deep voice, decrease in breast size, enlargement of the clitoris, increased libido and acne. *Precautions:* It should be used with extreme caution in pregnancy, in patients with cancer of the prostate and in patients with disorders of the circulation, kidneys or any other condition where an increased retention of fluids would cause trouble. Phenobarbitone may reduce its effects by increasing its breakdown in the liver. *Dose:* By implant under the skin, 100 to 600 mg. Other preparations of testosterone may be taken by mouth or injection.

Test Sixty are packs of 8 tablets each containing lobeline hydrochloride 2 mg, and 30 lozenges each containing methylcellulose 187 mg, oil of bitter orange 2 mg, peppermint oil 6 mg, and bergamot oil 2 mg.

TET/Vac/ads is tetanus vaccine (adsorbed).

Tetmosol ◊ monosulfiram.

tetrabenazine (Nitoman) is used to treat movement disorders due to Huntington's chorea, senile chorea, and related disorders. *Adverse effects:* Drowsiness, stomach upsets, depression, and Parkinsonism-like effects. *Dose:* By mouth, 75 to 200 mg daily according to age and response, in divided doses.

Tetrabid ◊ tetracycline.

Tetrachel ◊ tetracycline.

tetrachloroethylene is used to treat hookworm infections. *Adverse effects:* Occasionally nausea and headache or drowsiness may be experienced.

tetracosactrin (Synacthen, Synacthen Depot) is a synthetic polypeptide with corticotrophic activity. ◊ corticotrophin. It is structurally similar to natural corticotrophin, which is usually obtained from pigs and may produce allergic reactions. The most antigenic portion has been excluded in tetracosactrin. *Adverse effects* ◊ corticotrophin. It may produce allergic reactions such as itching and flushing. It may be used in patients allergic to pig corticotrophin. *Dose:* By intravenous infusion 250 micrograms in 500 ml over 6 hours or intramuscular injection 250 micrograms every 3 to 4 hours. By depot injection (Synacthen Depot) 0·5 to 1 mg twice weekly but varies according to response.

tetracycline (Achromycin; Economycin; Tetrabid; Tetrachel; Tetrex; tet-racycline hydrochloride) is a tetracyclinc antibiotic. *Adverse effects:* These are common to all tetracyclines. They include nausea, wind, vomiting and diarrhoea. Overgrowth of resistant bacteria and fungi may cause thrush, sore tongue, sore lips, irritation around the anus and the vagina. Alteration of the bacterial content of the bowel may cause diarrhoea and vitamin B deficiency. Serious adverse effects may be produced in patients with impaired kidney function. These include loss of appetite, nausea, vomiting and weakness. Large doses given intravenously have produced death in pregnant women due to liver damage. Tetracycline is deposited in bone, teeth and nails causing discoloration. When given in late pregnancy or to young infants it may interfere with the growth of the child's bones and teeth. Allergic reactions may occur, producing fever and skin rashes. *Precautions:* Tetracycline should not be given to pregnant women or infants, and preferably not to children under twelve years of age, because of its effects on bone and teeth. It decomposes on storage and may cause nausea and alterations in the chemistry of the blood and urine. *Dose:* By mouth, 250 mg four times daily.

tetrahydrozoline is a sympathomimetic drug used as a nasal decongestant (tetrahydrozoline hydrochloride) in drops and sprays to treat the common cold. *Adverse effects:* It may produce irritation at the site of use and overdose may produce unconsciousness and a drop in body temperature, particularly in infants. *Precautions:* It should be used with caution in patients with raised blood pressure, overworking of their thyroid glands, and glaucoma. It should not be used in children under two years of age.

Tetralysal ◊ lymecycline.

Tetrex ◊ tetracycline. It is a tetracycline phosphate complex.

T/Gel shampoo contains coal tar extract 2%.

Thalamonal is a severe pain-reliever. Each 1 ml of injection contains droperidol 2·5 mg and fentanyl 0·05 mg. *Dose:* 1 to 2 ml by intramuscular injection.

thebaine is in opium.

thenyldiamine is an antihistamine with similar properties to promethazine, but is less potent and has a shorter duration of action.

thenylpyramine ◊ methapyrilene.

theobromine has a weak diuretic effect on the kidneys. It is present in tea, coffee, cocoa and cola. It has practically no stimulating effect upon the brain. It dilates coronary and other arteries and was widely used in the past to treat angina. It was also used to treat high blood pressure, usually combined with phenobarbitone. *Adverse effects:* It may produce nausea and loss of appetite in high doses. *Dose:* By mouth, 300 to 600 mg.

Theodrox: Each tablet contains aminophylline 195 mg and dried aluminium hydroxide gel 260 mg. It is used to treat bronchial asthma. *Dose:* 1 three times daily and 1 at night.

Theo-Dur tablets contain theophylline 200 or 300 mg in a sustained-release form. *Dose:* By mouth, 200 to 300 mg 12 hourly.

theophylline (Biophylline; Labophylline; Lasma; Nuelin; Nuelin S A; Pro-Vent; Sibidal SR; Slophyllin; Theo-Dur; Uniphyllin Continus) is used to treat bronchial asthma and also heart failure. *Adverse effects:* Depend on the blood levels and include palpitations, nausea, vomiting, anorexia and stomach upsets. With very high blood levels severe adverse effects may occur – cramps, convulsions and disorders of heart rhythm. *Precautions:* The dose should be reduced in liver disease, epilepsy, heart disease, breast feeding, elderly patients and in fever. *Dose:* By mouth, 60 to 250 mg 3 to 4 times daily after food. By rectum as suppositories, 300 to 600 mg daily. Smoking can affect response.

theophylline sodium glycinate is used for the same purposes as theophylline.

Thephorin ◊ phenindamine.

Theraderm 5 and **10 gel** ◊ benzoyl peroxide.

thiabendazole (Mintezol) is used to treat infestation with threadworm and other intestinal worms. *Adverse effects:* Vomiting, vertigo and gastric discomfort may occur 3 to 4 hours after a dose. *Dose:* 25 mg per kg bodyweight morning and evening on 1 or 2 occasions.

thiamine (Benerva; thiamine hydrochloride; thiamine mononitrate; aneurine hydrochloride; vitamin B) is vitamin B_1.

Thiaver: Each tablet contains veratrum alkaloids 4 mg and epithiazide 4 mg. It is used to treat raised blood pressure.

thiethylperazine (Torecan; thiethylperazine maleate) has effects similar to chlorpromazine and is used to treat nausea and vomiting. *Adverse effects* and *Precautions:* It may produce Parkinsonism and should not be used in children under fifteen years. *Dose:* 10 mg two to three times daily.

thioguanine (Lanvis) is an anti-cancer drug with adverse effects and precautions similar to those described under mercaptopurine. *Dose:* Initially by mouth, 2 mg per kg of body-weight daily; maintenance dose according to patient's needs.

thiomersal (Merthiolate) is a mercury drug used as an antibacterial and antifungal agent for cleaning the skin.

thiopentone sodium is a fast-acting barbiturate which is used by intravenous injection as a general anaesthetic.

thioridazine (Melleril; thioridazine hydrochloride) is a major tranquillizer. It has effects and uses similar to those described under chlorpromazine but it has little effect in stopping nausea and vomiting or in reducing body temperature. It produces fewer Parkinsonism symptoms than chlorpromazine. *Adverse effects:* Thioridazine may cause drowsiness, dizziness, dryness of the mouth, skin rashes, production of milk (galactorrhoea), fall in blood pressure, disorders of heart rhythm, fluid retention, weight gain, blood disorders, irritation of the stomach and nasal stuffiness. Large doses may damage vision by causing pigmentation of the retina (this may be produced within four to eight weeks of treatment with a dose of 1 g or more daily). It may cause changes in the electric tracings of the heart and it may produce sunlight sensitivity of the skin. *Precautions* ◊ chlorpromazine. *Dose:* By mouth, 30 to 600 mg daily in divided doses.

thiotepa is an anti-cancer drug. *Adverse effects:* These include nausea, vomiting, headache, fever, allergic reactions, loss of hair (alopecia), loss of periods (amenorrhoea) and reduced sperm production. It is very damaging to bone marrow, producing severe blood disorders. *Precautions:* It should not be used in pregnancy, in the presence of infections, or in patients with severe blood disorders. It should be used with utmost caution if impaired bone-marrow function is suspected. *Dose:* Varies according to the disorder and patient being treated.

thonzylamine (thonzylamine hydrochloride) is an antihistamine similar to promethazine, but it is less potent and shorter acting.

Thornton & Ross Diarrhoea Mixture contains in each 5 ml aromatic chalk powder 250 mg and catechu 40 mg.

Thornton & Ross Indian Brandee contains in each 5 ml potassium nitrate 25 mg, ether 0·05 ml, compound rhubarb tincture 0·75 ml, capsicum tincture 0·125 ml, and compound cardamom tincture 0·05 ml.

Thornton & Ross Indigestion Mixture: Each 5 ml contains aluminium oxide

150 mg, light magnesium oxide 118 mg, aromatic cardamom tincture 0·05 ml; and peppermint oil 0·0004 ml.

Thornton & Ross Vapour Rub contains menthol 2·5%, camphor 2·5%, methyl salicylate 2·75%, eucalyptus oil 2·5%, turpentine oil 5%, pine oil 1%, thyme oil 0·2%, and creosote 0·025%.

Thovaline aerosol and ointment contains talc, kaolin, zinc oxide, cod-liver oil and wool fat. It is used as protective skin applications.

Three Flasks Bronchial Emulsion contains liquid paraffin 25%, anise oil 0·2%, pumilio pine oil 0·05%, cinnamon oil 0·05%, calcium hypophosphite 1·2%, sodium hypophosphite 1·2%, glycerol 5%, and compound benzoin tincture 1%.

Three Flasks Cold Sore Lotion contains camphor 1·1%, menthol 1·1%, diethyl phthalate 0·825%, and benzoin tincture (meth.) 84·475%.

Three Flasks Corn & Wart Solvent contains pyroxylin 1·27%, Canada balsam 4·7%, zinc chloride 1·7%, salicylic acid 12%, castor oil 2·85%, and colophony 2·4%.

Three Flasks Juniper Pills each contain bearberry extract (aqueous 5–2) 16·2 mg, buchu extract (aqueous 8–3) 16·2 mg, capsicum 16·2 mg, squill 16·2 mg, potassium nitrate 65 mg, aloin 9·7 mg, juniper oil 4 mg, and methylene blue 4 mg.

Three Flasks Nail Bite Lotion contains soap spirit 50%, capsicum oleoresin 0·1%, and quassia extract 0·2%.

Three Flasks Proflavine Cream contains proflavine hemisulphate 0·1%.

Three Flasks Tooth-Ache Solution contains menthol 2%, phenol 0·9%, clove oil 6%, camphor 4%, chloroform 0·95%, colour q.s., and IMS to 100%.

Three Noughts Cough Syrup contains anise oil 0·04%, clove oil 0·01%, cassia oil 0·02%, spearmint oil 0·01%, ether 0·1%, chloroform 0·65%, chloroform spirit 0·66%, alcoholic (90%) tincture of capsicum (1–5) 0·08%, ipecacuanha liquid extract 0·19%, cetylpyridinium chloride 0·018%, acetic acid 0·9%, and benzoic acid 0·05%.

threonine is an amino-acid which is an essential constituent of the diet to form body protein.

Throat Chest and Lung Drops are lozenges each containing clove oil 0·0014 ml, eucalyptus oil 0·0021 ml, anise oil 0·0028 ml, peppermint oil 0·0028 ml, ginger extract 0·0014 ml, menthol 0·14 mg, with citric acid, benzoic acid, and chloroform spirit.

Throaties Original Flavour contain benzoin tincture 0·5%, menthol 0·45%, aniseed oil 0·1%, peppermint oil 0·025%, and capsicin 0·001%. **Throaties Catarrh Pastilles:** Active ingredients are menthol 0·6%, abietis pine oil 0·3%, sylvestris pine oil 0·3%, and creosote 0·2%.

Throaties, Lemon Honey & Menthol: Active ingredients are honey 2·4%, lemon oil 0·3%, and menthol 0·09%.

thurfyl salicylate is a rubefacient used in Transvasin cream.

thyme oil is used as a carminative, antispasmodic and anti-microbial. It is also used as a rubefacient and counter-irritant.

thymol is an antiseptic used in mouth washes, gargles and skin applications. It is irritant.

thymoxamine (Opilon; thymoxamine hydrochloride) is a vasodilator drug, used to treat disorders of the circulation. *Adverse effects:* It may produce nausea, headache, diarrhoea, flushing and dizziness. *Precautions:* It should be given with caution to patients with coronary artery disorders and disorders of blood pressure. It should not be given to children. *Dose:* By mouth, 40 mg four times daily.

thyroid (dry thyroid, thyroid extract; thyroid gland) is an extract of thyroid glands; it has effects and uses similar to those described under thyroxine. *Dose:* By mouth, 30 to 250 mg daily.

thyrotrophin-releasing hormone ◊ protirelin.

Thytropar injection is thyrotrophin (thyroid stimulating hormone).

thyroxine (Eltroxin; thyroxine sodium; levothyroxine sodium) is a thyroid hormone used to treat under-working of the thyroid gland. *Adverse effects:* Too large a dose may produce sweating, rapid beating of the heart, diarrhoea, restlessness, excitability, irregularities of heart rhythm and angina. It may also produce pain in the arms or legs and make worse the symptoms of osteoarthritis. *Precautions:* It has a delayed and cumulative effect and may take up to two weeks to be effective; the dose must therefore be controlled carefully. It should be used with caution in patients with heart disorders. It may increase the effects of drugs used to prevent blood clotting and its effects may be increased by phenytoin and aspirin. *Dose:* By mouth, 0·05 to 0·3 mg daily.

tiaprofenic acid (Surgam) is an anti-rheumatic drug. *Adverse effects* and *Precautions* ◊ ibuprofen. *Dose:* 600 mg daily, in divided doses after food.

Ticar ◊ ticarcillin.

ticarcillin (Ticar; ticarcillin disodium) is a broad-spectrum penicillin antibiotic. ◊ penicillins. *Dose:* By slow intravenous injection over 3 to 4 minutes or by intravenous infusion over 30 to 40 minutes. 15 to 20 g daily in divided doses. For urinary tract infections by intramuscular or slow intravenous injection 3 to 4 g daily in divided doses.

Tiempe ◊ trimethoprim.

Tigason ◊ etretinate.

Tiger Balm contains menthol, camphor, clove oil, and cajuput oil.

Tilade aerosol ◊ nedocromil.

Tildiem tablets contain diltiazem hydrochloride 60 mg ◊ diltiazem.

Tilloderm White Tar Ointment contains lanolin 39·3%, soft paraffin 46·7%, zinc oxide 10%, resorcin 4%, cresol 0·002%.

Timentin injections contain clavulanic acid with ticarcillin. Timentin 3·2 g contains 200 mg of clavulanic acid with 3 g of ticarcillin. Timentin 1·6 g contains 100 mg with 1·5 g, and Timentin 800 mg contains 50 mg with 750 mg ◊ clavulanic acid and ticarcillin. *Precautions:* It should not be used in patients allergic to penicillin.

Timocort cream contains 1% hydrocortisone ◊ hydrocortisone.

Timodine cream contains nystatin 100,000 units, hydrocortisone 0·5%, benzalkonium chloride 0·2% and dimethicone 350 10% in each 10 g.

timolol (Betim, Blocadren) is a beta-receptor blocking drug used to treat hypertension and angina. *Adverse effects* and *Precautions* ◊ propranolol. *Dose:* By mouth for raised blood pressure. 15 to 45 mg daily; for angina 15 to 45 mg daily.

Timoped cream contains tolnaftate 1% and triclosan 0·25% ◊ tolnaftate ◊ triclosan.

Timoptol eye drops are used to treat glaucoma ◊ timolol.

tin powder: There is no evidence to suggest that it has any therapeutic value.

Tinaderm preparation ◊ tolnaftate.

Tinaderm M cream contains nystatin in addition to tolnaftate.

tincture of myrrh ◊ myrrh.

Tineafax ointment and **dusting powder** ◊ zinc undecenoate.

tinidazole (Fasigyn) is an antibacterial drug similar to metronidazole. It is used to treat anaerobic bacterial infections. *Adverse effects* and *Precautions* ◊ metronidazole. *Dose:* By mouth, 500 mg twice daily. By intravenous infusion 800 mg daily.

Tinoxid Tablets contain tin powder 110 mg and stannic oxide 19·5 mg.

Tinset ◊ oxatomide.

tioconazole (Trosyl) is a broad spectrum antifungal drug used to treat fungal infections of the nails. *Adverse effects:* Rarely local irritation, local allergic reactions. *Precautions:* Do not use in patients allergic to the drug or to other related drugs (imidazoles). Do not use in pregnancy. *Dose:* Apply solution to affected areas every twelve hours.

titanium (titanium dioxide) is used as a skin protective and also as a sunscreen agent. It is included in some face powders and cosmetics.

Titralac is used to treat indigestion and peptic ulcers. Each tablet contains calcium carbonate 420 mg and glycine 180 mg. *Dose:* By mouth, 1 to 2 tablets when required.

Tixylix cough linctus contains promethazine hydrochloride 1·5 mg and pholcodine 1·5 mg in each 5 ml. *Dose:* By mouth, 10 to 20 ml three times daily.

Tobralex ◊ tobramycin.

tobramycin (Nebcin, Tobralex) has effects similar to gentamicin. *Adverse effects* and *Precautions* ◊ gentamicin. *Dose:* 3 to 5 mg per kg of body-weight daily in divided doses by intramuscular injection or intravenous infusion.

tocainide (Tonocard; tocainide hydrochloride) is used to treat disorders of heart rhythm. It produces similar effects to lignocaine. *Dose:* By mouth or injection, depending on severity of condition.

tocopheryl (Ephynal, Vita-E; tocopherol, tocopheryl acetate, tocopheryl acid succinate, vitamin E) is a vitamin. The minimum daily requirements are not clear, a deficiency has only been found in premature babies. It is said to delay ageing of the skin, but this has not been proved.

tocopheryl acid succinate ◊ tocopheryl.

Today sponge is a vaginal contraceptive containing nonoxynol-9. The sponge should be positioned directly over the cervix.

tofenacin (tofenacin hydrochloride) is used to treat depression in elderly patients. It is a metabolite of orphenadrine. *Precautions:* It should not be used in patients with glaucoma or prostate problems. *Dose:* Up to 240 mg daily in divided doses.

Tofranil ◊ imipramine.

Tolanase ◊ tolazamide.

tolazamide (Tolanase) is an oral antidiabetic drug. *Adverse effects:* It may cause nausea, vomiting, diarrhoea, loss of appetite, dizziness, weakness, nervousness and skin rashes. *Dose:* By mouth, 100 to 1,000 mg daily.

tolbutamide (Glyconon; Rastinon) is a drug used to treat diabetes. It is taken by mouth and has effects and uses similar to those described under chlorpropamide but it works for a shorter time. *Adverse effects:* These are similar to those described under chlorpropamide. Skin rashes and intolerance to alcohol may occur and, rarely, blood disorders and jaundice. *Precautions* ◊ chlorpropamide. Sulphonamides and phenylbutazone may increase its blood sugar lowering effects. *Dose:* By mouth, 500 mg to 2,000 mg daily in divided doses.

Tolectin DS ◊ tolmetin.

Tolerzide is used to treat raised blood pressure. Each tablet contains sotalol 80 mg and hydrochlorothiazide 12·5 mg. *Dose:* By mouth 1 daily.

tolmetin (Tolectin) is an antirheumatic drug. *Adverse effects* and *Precautions* ◊ naproxen. *Dose:* By mouth, 0·6 to 1·8 g daily in divided doses after meals.

tolnaftate (Timoped; Tinaderm) is an antifungal drug. It is used in creams or powders to treat ringworm and other fungal infections of the skin. It is not active against thrush or bacteria. In treating tinea infections of the nails or scalp it should be used along with general treatments such as griseofulvin.

tolu (tolu balsam) has very mild antiseptic properties and is used in cough mixtures as a flavouring agent.

Tonivitan A and D syrup contains ferric ammonium citrate 150 mg, vitamin A 700 units, ergocalciferol 70 units, calcium glycerophosphate 25 mg, copper sulphate 400 micrograms and manganese glycerophosphate 400 micrograms 15 ml.

Tonivitan B is a vitamin B complex preparation. Each 5 ml of syrup contains thiamine hydrochloride 500 micrograms, riboflavine 400 micrograms, nicotinamide 2·5 mg, pyridoxine hydrochloride 16·5 micrograms, calcium glycerophosphate 20 mg, manganese glycerophosphate 5 mg.

Tonocard ◊ tocainide.

Topal is an antacid. Each tablet contains dried aluminium hydroxide 30 mg, light magnesium carbonate 40 mg and alginic acid 200 mg. *Dose:* 1 to 3 tablets to be chewed between meals and at bed-time.

Topex lotion contains benzoyl peroxide 5%.

Topex Acne Cream contains benzoyl peroxide 5%.

Topiclens is a solution of sodium chloride 0·9% which is used for irrigating eyes and wounds.

Topicycline solution is used in the topical treatment of acne, it contains 2·2 mg/ml of tetracycline hydrochloride.

Topilar cream and ointment ◊ fluclorolone.

Toracsol solution is used to treat acne. It contains cetrimide 2·8%, benzalkonium bromide 0·2% and hexachlorophane 3%.

Torbetol contains cetrimide 0·7%, benzalkonium bromide 0·05%, and hexachlorophane 0·75%.

Torbetol Shampoo contains cetrimide 17·5% and benzalkonium bromide 2·5%.

Torecan ◊ thiethylperazine.

Totavit Capsules each contain vitamin A 5,00 units, ergocalciferol 400 units, thiamine hydrochloride 1·5 mg, riboflavine 1·2 mg, pyridoxine hydrochloride 0·5 mg, nicotinamide 10 mg, ascorbic acid 30 mg, tocopheryl acetate 1 unit, copper (as copper sulphate) 0·1 mg, iron (as ferrous sulphate) 15 mg, calcium 24 mg, phosphorus 18·5 mg, and DL-methionine 30 mg.

Touch and Go Toothache Tincture contains camphor 10%, menthol 1·25%, chloroform 7·5%, ether 7·5%, cajuput oil 2·5%, clove oil 3·12%, and tolu balsam 1·25%.

Trace elements essential for life include: chromium, cobalt, copper, manganese, molybdenum, nickel, selenium, tin, vanadium and zinc. Fluorine, iodine, iron and silicon are also considered essential.

Tracrium (atracurium besylate) ◊ atracurium.

tragacanth is a gum used as a laxative and suspending agent.

tramazoline is a nasal decongestant related to naphazoline.

Tramil 500 capsules contain paracetamol 500 mg and caffeine 32 mg ◊ paracetamol ◊ caffeine.

Trancopal ◊ chlormezanone.

Trancoprin is a mild pain-reliever. Each tablet contains aspirin 300 mg and chlormezanone 100 mg. *Dose:* By mouth, 1 to 2 tablets three times daily.

Trandate ◊ labetalol.

tranexamic acid (Cyklokapron) is a fibrin stabilizer and is used to treat haemophilia and severe haemorrhage associated with surgery and in patients suffering from the bleeding disease haemophilia. *Adverse effects* and *Precautions* ◊ aminocaproic acid. *Dose:* Depends on the severity of the condition.

Transiderm-Nitro 5 and 10 patches contain glyceryl trinitrate in a form that is absorbed slowly through the skin. *Dose:* Apply 1 patch to the chest wall, and remove after 24 hours, replacing with a new patch at a new site.

Transvasin cream contains ethyl nicotinate 2%, hexyl nicotinate 2%, thurfyl salicylate 14% and benzocaine 2% in a base. It is a rubefacient containing a local anaesthetic cream used to treat muscle aches and pains.

Tranxene ◊ potassium clorazepate.

tranylcypromine (Parnate; tranylcypromine sulphate) is an M.A.O. inhibitor antidepressant drug. Unlike other drugs of this group its effects persist for only about two to three days after withdrawal. *Adverse effects:* These are similar to those discussed under phenelzine. *Precautions:* These are important and are discussed under phenelzine. *Dose:* By mouth, 20 to 60 mg daily in divided doses, reducing to a maintenance dose of about 20 mg daily.

Trasicor ◊ oxprenolol.

Trasidrex is used to treat raised blood pressure. Each tablet contains oxpre-nolol 160 mg in slow-release form and cyclopenthiazide 0·25 mg.

Trasylol ◊ aprotinin.

Travasept 100 antiseptic solution contains chlorhexidine and cetrimide; use undiluted for the treatment of wounds.

Traveltabs ◊ chlorbutol.

Travogyn ◊ isoconazole.

trazodone (Molipaxin; trazodone hydrochloride) is an antidepressant drug. *Adverse effects:* Nausea, vomiting, constipation, diarrhoea, loss of weight, dry mouth, changes in the heart rate, fall in blood pressure, headaches, drowsiness, blurred vision, dizziness, insomnia and confusion. *Precautions:* It should be used with utmost caution in patients who drive motor vehicles or operate moving machinery. It should not be used in patients with impaired function of their kidneys or liver. It should not be used during the first three months of pregnancy. *Dose:* By mouth, 100 to 150 mg daily in divided doses. Maximum daily dose is 600 mg.

Tremonil ◊ methixene.

Trental ◊ oxpentifylline.

treosulfan (Treosulfan) is an anti-cancer drug. *Adverse effects:* Treosulfan has a depressing effect upon bone-marrow producing blood disorders. It produces gastro-intestinal pain, nausea and vomiting, skin rashes and alopecia. Stomatitis may occur if patients chew the capsule. *Precautions:* It should not be used in pregnancy or in breast-feeding mothers.

Blood tests should be carried out at frequent intervals. *Dose:* By mouth, 1 g daily in four divided doses for one month; then repeated for one month after a month's interval without the drug.

tretinoin (Retin-A) is a derivative of vitamin A which causes the top layer of skin to peel off more quickly. It is used to treat acne. *Precautions:* It may cause increased sensitivity to sunlight. *Dose:* Apply the lotion or gel twice daily.

Trevintix ◊ prothionamide.

TRH ◊ thyrotrophin-releasing hormone.

Tri-ac lotion is used to treat acne, it contains ethyl lactate 10% and zinc sulphate 0·3%.

Tri-Adcortyl ointment and **cream** contains in each 1 g triamcinolone acetonide 1 mg, neomycin 2·5 mg, gramicidin 0·25 mg and nystatin 100,000 units.

Tri-Adcortyl Otic ear ointment contains gramicidine 0·025%, neomycin 0·25%, nystatin 3·33% and triamcinolone acetonide 0·1%.

Triadol ◊ benorylate.

triamcinolone (Adcortyl, Kenalog, Ledercort, Lederspan) has the effects, uses and adverse effects of cortisone. Read corticosteroids in Part Two. *Adverse effects:* It is less likely to cause an increase in appetite than the other members of the group and it does not cause salt and water retention. It may cause dizziness, loss of appetite, muscle weakness, sleepiness and flushing after meals. *Dose:* By mouth, 4 to 48 mg daily in divided doses. Triamcinolone acetonide (Adcortyl) is used in creams, lotions, ointments and injections. Triamcinolone hexacetonide (Kenalog, Lederspan) is used in injections.

Triamco: Each diuretic tablet contains triamterene 50 mg and hydrochlorothiazide 25 mg ◊ triamterene and hydrochlorothiazide.

triamterene (Dytac; Frusene) is a diuretic drug. It is weaker than the thiazide diuretics but it causes potassium retention rather than loss. It does not trigger off underlying diabetes. *Adverse effects:* It may cause nausea, vomiting, diarrhoea, headache, fall in blood pressure, dry mouth, skin rashes and dizziness. Loss of calcium in the urine as well as other disturbances of salts and water balance may occur. *Precautions:* Triamterene should be used with caution by patients with impaired kidney or liver function or with diabetes. Periodic checks should be made on the blood salts. *Dose:* By mouth, 150 to 250 mg daily in divided doses.

triazolam (Halcion) is a benzodiazepine drug used as a hypnotic. ◊ benzodiazepines in Part Two. *Dose:* By mouth, 0·25 mg before retiring (0·125 mg for elderly patients).

Tribiotic spray application contains neomycin sulphate 500,000 units, bacitracin zinc 10,000 units and polymyxin B sulphate 150,000 units per aerosol unit.

trichloroacetic acid is used as a caustic and keratolytic to treat warts. It is also used in dilute solution (1%) as an astringent for sweaty feet.

trichlorofluoromethane is a propellant in aerosol sprays. It has a cooling effect on the skin.

trichloromonofluoromethane ◊ trichlorofluoromethane.

triclocarban (Cutisan) has antiseptic properties and is used in preparations to treat infected skin conditions.

triclofos is used as a sedative and sleeping drug. It has effects similar to those described under dichloralphenazone. *Adverse effects, Precautions* and *Drug dependence:* These are similar to those described under dichloralphenazone. Headache and skin rashes may occur and triclofos may increase the effects of alcohol. *Dose:* By mouth, 1 to 2 g at night.

triclosan (Aquasept, Timoped) has antibacterial properties and is used in surgical scrubs, soaps, deodorants and to prevent bacterial growth in the treatment of athlete's foot with tolnaftate.

trichloroethylene (Trilene) is a weak anaesthetic agent and poor muscle relaxant, but a potent pain-reliever. It can be used to supplement nitrous-oxide anaesthesia in major surgery.

Tridesilon cream and **ointment** ◊ desonide.

Tridil ◊ glyceryl trinitrate.

triethanolamine is combined with fatty acids as an emulsifying agent in soap manufacturing.

trifluoperazine (Stelazine; trifluoperazine hydrochloride) is a major tranquillizer. It has effects and uses similar to those described under chlorpromazine, but it is effective in smaller doses. It may stimulate rather than sedate. *Adverse effects:* These are similar to those discussed under chlorpromazine. Mild adverse effects include drowsiness, dizziness, agitation, insomnia, stuffy nose and sweating. High doses may produce Parkinsonism symptoms and peculiar stiffness and trembling of muscles (dystonias and akathisia) particularly of the face, eyes, neck, tongue and throat (especially in children). These symptoms are not always reversible on stopping the drug. It may, rarely, cause blood disorders, jaundice and discharge of milk from the breasts (galactorrhoea). *Precautions* ◊ chlorpromazine. *Dose:* By mouth, 2 to 30 mg daily in divided doses; to prevent nausea or vomiting, 1 to 6 mg daily in divided doses.

trifluperidol (Triperidol) is a major tranquillizer similar to haloperidol. *Dose:* 0·5 mg daily initially, increasing as required by 0·5 mg at three to four day intervals.

trihexyphenidyl ◊ benzhexol.

tri-iodothyronine ◊ liothyronine.

Trilene ◊ trichloroethylene.

Trilisate: Each tablet contains 500 mg of the choline magnesium salt of aspirin ◊ aspirin. *Dose:* 2 to 3 tablets twice daily.

Trilostane (Modrenal) stops the synthesis of both mineralocorticoids and glucocorticoids by the adrenal glands. It is used to treat overworking of the adrenal glands (e.g., Cushing's syndrome and primary hyperaldosteronism). *Adverse effects:* Rarely flushing, nausea and runny nose. *Precautions:* In patients with impaired kidney and liver functions the blood levels of corticosteroids and electrolytes should be carefully monitored. A hormonal contraceptive should not be used in women undergoing this treatment. *Dose:* 60 mg 4 times daily for at least 3 days and then adjusted – usual dose range 120 to 480 mg daily in divided doses.

Triludan ◊ terfenadine.

trimeprazine (Vallergan; trimeprazine tartrate) produces antihistamine effects and also major tranquillizer effects like those described under chlorpromazine. However, its main effect and use is to prevent itching. It is slow to work and its effects last a long time. *Adverse effects:* It frequently produces drowsiness and occasionally dizziness, dryness of the mouth, skin rashes, blood disorders and Parkinsonism. *Precautions:* These are similar to those described under chlorpromazine. It should be given with caution to patients with impaired liver function. *Dose:* By mouth to prevent itching, 10 to 40 mg daily.

trimetaphan (Arfonad; trimetaphan camsylate) has effects and uses similar to those described under pempidine. It is used to treat raised blood pressure. *Dose:* Slowly by intravenous infusion in a dose according to the condition being treated.

trimethoprim (Ipral; Monotrim; Syraprim; Tiempe; Trimogal; Trimopan; Unitrim) is an antibacterial drug. It is active against the same range of bacteria as the sulphonamides, with which it produces a synergistic effect. It is often given combined with the sulphonamide, sulphamethoxazole. This combination is known as co-trimoxazole (Bactrim or Septrin). Read section on sulphonamides. *Adverse effects:* Nausea, vomiting and diarrhoea, itching and rashes. When used over a prolonged period it may produce anaemia because it interferes with the body's use of folic acid, which is essential for the manufacture of blood. *Precautions:* It should be given with caution to patients with impaired kidney function. It should not be given during pregnancy and when it is used over a prolonged period blood tests should be carried out at appropriate intervals of time. *Dose:* By mouth 100 to 300 mg every 12 hours. By slow intravenous injection or infusion 150 to 250 mg every 12 hours.

trimipramine (Surmontil; trimipramine maleate) is a tricyclic antidepressant drug. It has effects and uses similar to those described under imipramine but it is more sedating. *Adverse effects* and *Precautions:* These are similar to those described under imipramine. Drowsiness is common and so is rapid beating of the heart, dryness of the mouth and blurred vision. Trembling and stiffness of muscles (Parkinsonism) may rarely occur. *Dose:* By mouth, 25 to 125 mg daily in divided doses.

Trimogal ◊ trimethoprim.

Trimopan ◊ trimethoprim.

Trimovate cream and **ointment** contains clobetasone butyrate 0·05%, nystatin 100,000 units/g and tetracycline 3%.

trinitrin ◊ glyceryl trinitrate.

Trinity Ointment contains eucalyptus oil 8·33%, zinc ointment 25%, hydrous wool fat 25%, soft paraffin to 100%.

Trinordiol is a triphasic oral contraceptive. Read section on oral contraceptive drugs.

Tri-Novum is a triphasic oral contraceptive. Seven white tablets containing ethinyloestradiol 35 micrograms, norethisterone 0·5 mg; seven light peach-coloured tablets containing ethinyloestradiol 35 micrograms, norethisterone 0·75 mg; seven peach-coloured tablets containing ethinyloestradiol 35 micrograms, norethisterone 1 mg.

Triogesic*: Each tablet contains phenylpropanolamine hydrochloride 12·5 mg and paracetamol 500 mg. Each 5 ml of elixir contains 3 mg of phenylpropanolamine and 125 mg of paracetamol. Used to relieve the symptoms of the common cold. *Dose:* 1 to 2 tablets three- to four-hourly.

Triolinctus is a cough medicine. Each 5 ml contains pholcodine 5 mg, pseudoephedrine hydrochloride 20 mg, chlorpheniramine maleate 2 mg, syrup 5·25 g and glycerol 600 mg.

Triominic*: Each tablet contains phenylpropanolamine hydrochloride 50 mg, mepyramine maleate 25 mg and

pheniramine maleate 25 mg; each 5 ml of syrup contains 12·5 mg, 6·25 mg and 6·25 mg respectively. Used to relieve the symptoms of the common cold. *Dose:* 1 six- to eight-hourly, 10 ml syrup four-hourly; maximum, 3 tablets or 4 doses of syrup in 24 hours.

tripelennamine is an antihistamine drug.

Triperidol ◊ trifluperidol.

Triplopen: Each single-dose vial contains penicillin sodium 500,000 units, procaine penicillin 250,000 units and benethamine penicillin 500,000 units. Read section on antibiotics. *Dose:* By deep intramuscular injection, 1 vial every two to three days.

tripotassium di-citrate bisthumate ◊ DeNol.

triprolidine (Actidil; Pro-Actidil; triprolidine hydrochloride) is an antihistamine drug. *Adverse effects* and *Precautions:* These are similar to those described under promethazine. *Dose:* By mouth, 5 to 7·5 mg daily.

Triptafen preparations contain a mixture of amitriptyline and perphenazine in various doses. Used as an antidepressant drug.

Trisequens is used to treat menopausal symptoms. It comprises a calendar pack of 12 blue tablets containing oestradiol 2 mg and oestriol 1 mg; 10 white tablets containing oestradiol 2 mg, oestriol 1 mg and norethisterone acetate 1 mg and 6 red tablets containing oestradiol 1 mg and oestriol 500 micrograms. *Dose:* 1 blue tablet, starting on 5th day of menstrual cycle or at any time if cycles have stopped or are infrequent then one tablet daily in sequence (without interruption).

trisodium edetate (Limclair) is used to treat high blood calcium levels and also to remove lime burns in the eye. *Adverse effects:* Nausea, diarrhoea, cramps, overdose may produce kidney damage. *Precautions:* It should be used with caution in patients suffering from tuberculosis. Repeated blood calcium levels should be carried out. It should *not* be used in patients with impaired kidney function. *Dose:* By slow intravenous infusion up to 70 mg per kg daily over 2 to 3 hours. *For use in the eye* dilute 1 ml to 50 ml with sterile purified water.

Trisonovin cream contains resorcinol 2% and sulphur 8%.

Trivax is a brand name of diphtheria, tetanus and pertussis (whooping cough) vaccine.

Trivax-AD is a vaccine used for primary vaccination of children. Diphtheria, tetanus, and pertussis vaccine, absorbed.

Trobicin ◊ spectinomycin.

tropicamide eye drops (Mydriacyl) have effects and uses similar to those described under atropine.

Tropium ◊ chlordiazepoxide.

Trosyl nail solution ◊ tioconazolē.

trypsin is an enzyme that breaks down protein. It is used to help clear up ulcers, · abscesses and similar inflammatory conditions. It has no effect on healthy tissue.

Tryptizol ◊ amitriptyline.

tryptophan (Optimax WV; Pacitron) is an amino-acid which is an essential constituent of the diet. It is used to treat depression. *Adverse effects:* These include nausea, loss of appetite and drowsiness. *Precautions:* When used along with a monoamine oxidase inhibitor drug it may produce a drunken state. *Dose:* By mouth, 500 mg tablets, 2 to 12 daily.

TSH ◊ thyrotrophin.

TUB/VAC/BCG is Bacillus Calmette-Guérin vaccine. It is used for active immunization against tuberculosis.

Tubarine ◊ tubocurarine.

Tuberculin PPD is used to test for tuberculosis.

tubocurarine (Jexin; Tubarine; tubocurarine chloride) is a muscle relaxant which is used along with general anaesthetics in surgical operations. Its effects are increased by ether. *Adverse effects* and *Precautions:* It increases the fall in blood pressure produced by the general anaesthetic halothane and its effects in depressing respiration may be increased by quinidine and some antibiotics. Patients with impaired liver function may be resistant to tubocurarine.

Tuinal: Each capsule contains equal quantities of quinalbarbitone and amylobarbitone in 100 mg and 200 mg strengths. It is used as a sleeping drug and sedative. *Dose:* 100 to 200 mg at bedtime.

Tums: Each tablet contains calcium carbonate 500 mg and peppermint oil 1·1 mg.

Tunes, Cherry Menthol contain tolu balsam 0·036%, menthol 0·162%, thyme oil 0·0025%, and camphor 0·0086%.

Tunes, Honey Menthol contain menthol 0·135%, anethole 0·114%, cinnamon oil 0·018%, peppermint oil 0·015%, eucalyptol 0·015%, with sugar, glucose syrup, and honey.

turpentine oil is used in some indigestion mixtures, enemas, and irritant skin applications as a rubefacient.

Tusana Cough Linctus contains in each 5 ml dextromethorphan hydrobromide 5 mg, ipecacuanha liquid extract 0·025 ml, and tolu syrup 3·71 ml.

Tussils Cough Lozenges each contain dextromethorphan hydrobromide 2·5 mg and phenylephrine hydrochloride 500 micrograms.

Tussobron Cough Suppressant Syrup contains in each 5 ml dextromethorphan hydrobromide 5 mg, ephedrine hydrochloride 10 mg, and ammonium chloride 37·5 mg.

tyloxapol is a surface-active agent used in inhalants to dissolve sputum (e.g., Alevaire).

Tymasil ◊ natamycin.

Typhoid/vac is typhoid vaccine. It is a suspension of killed salmonella typhi and it is used for active immunization against typhoid.

Tyrocane Paediatric lozenges each contain cetylpyridinium chloride 2·5 mg.

Tyrocane Throat Lozenges contain tyrothricin 500 micrograms, cetylpyridinium chloride 2·5 mg, and benzocaine 5 mg.

Tyroco Throat Lozenges each contain tyrothricin 1 mg, benzocaine 5 mg, cetylpyridinium chloride 4 mg.

Tyromycin Lozenges contain tyrothricin 1 mg, benzocaine 5 mg, cetylpyridinium chloride 1 mg.

tyrothricin has antibacterial properties and is used in skin applications and throat lozenges.

Tyrozets throat lozenges contain tyrothricin 1 mg and benzocaine 5 mg.

T-Zone Decongestant Tablets each contain salicylamide 324 mg, caffeine 16·2 mg, ephedrine sulphate 4 mg, atropine sulphate 120 micrograms, magnesium hydroxide 65 mg, sodium citrate 16·2 mg, and dried aluminium hydroxide 16·2 mg.

Ubretid ◊ distigmine.

Ukidan ◊ urokinase.

Ulcaid Tablets contain benzocaine 5 mg, cetylpyridinium chloride 2·5 mg, and tyrothricin 0·5 mg.

Ulcanon ◊ tannic acid.

Ultra Cleancut Spray solution contains benzalkonium chloride solution (50%) 2%, lignocaine hydrochloride 0·5%.

Ultra Plastron Spray Dressing contains benzocaine 1%, cetrimide 0·1%, polyvinylpyrrolidone co-polymer 3%.

Ultra Steriflow Eye Wash contains sodium acid phosphate 0·52%, sodium phosphate 1·19%, sodium chloride 0·48%.

Ultra Throat Lozenges contain benzalkonium chloride solution (50%) 0·0006 ml.

Ultracach Analgesic Capsules contain paracetamol 300 mg, caffeine 30 mg.

Ultradal Antacid Stomach Tablets contain light magnesium carbonate 60 mg, magnesium trisilicate 150 mg, dried aluminium hydroxide gel 90 mg, calcium carbonate 105 mg.

Ultradil cream and **ointment** ◊ fluocortolone.

Ultrakool Aerosol Spray contains trichlorofluoromethane 85%, dichlorodifluoromethane 15%.

Ultralanum Plain cream contains fluocortolone hexanoate 0·25% and fluocortolone pivalate 0·25%.

Ultralanum Plain ointment contains fluocortolone 0·25% and fluocortolone hexanoate 0·25%.

Ultralief Tablets contain salicylamide 200 mg, paracetamol 200 mg, caffeine 25 mg.

Ultraproct ointment contains cinchocaine hydrochloride 0·5%, clemizole undecenoate 1%, fluocortolone hexanoate 0·095% and fluocortolone pivalate 0·092%.

Ultraproct suppositories contain cinchocaine hydrochloride 1 mg, clemizole undecenoate 5 mg, fluocortolone hexanoate 630 micrograms, fluocortolone pivalate 610 micrograms.

undecenoic acid (Mycota; undecylenic acid) is an antifungal drug.

undecylenic acid ◊ undecenoic acid.

Unguentum Merck is an emollient cream.

Unichem Throat & Catarrh Pastilles contain menthol 0·62%, sylvestris pine oil 0·31%, peppermint oil 0·31%, and thymol 0·073%.

Uniflu Plus Gregovite C comprises a composite pack of pairs of tablets: Uniflu mauve tablets containing caffeine 30 mg, codeine phosphate 10 mg, diphenhydramine hydrochloride 15 mg, paracetamol 500 mg and phenylephrine hydrochloride 10 mg; Gregovite C yellow tablets containing ascorbic acid 300 mg. *Dose:* 1 of each tablet every 4 hours.

Unigesic is a mild pain-reliever, each tablet contains paracetamol 500 mg and caffeine 30 mg. *Dose:* By mouth, 1 to 2 four-hourly as required.

Unigest is used to treat indigestion and peptic ulcer. Each tablet contains aluminium hydroxide gel 450 mg and dimethicone 400 mg. *Dose:* 1 or 2 sucked or chewed after meals and at bedtime.

Unihep ◊ heparin.

Unimycin ◊ oxytetracycline.

Uniparin ◊ heparin.

Uniparin Calcium injections contain 25,000 units/ml of heparin calcium for injection under the skin ◊ heparin.

Uniphyllin Continus tablets contain theophylline 200 mg in a sustained-release form. *Dose:* By mouth, 400 to 800 mg once daily.

Uniprofen ◊ ibuprofen.

Uniroid ointment contains cinchocaine hydrochloride 0·5%, hydrocortisone 0·5%, neomycin sulphate 0·5%, polymixin B sulphate 6,250 units/g.

Uniroid suppositories contain cinchocaine hydrochloride 5 mg, hydrocortisone 5 mg, neomycin sulphate 10 mg and polymyxin B sulphate 12,500 units.

Unisomnia ◊ nitrazepam.

Unitrim ◊ trimethoprim.

Univer capsules ◊ verapamil.

Uracil Mustard ◊ uramustine.

uramustine (Uracil Mustard) is an anti-cancer drug. *Adverse effects:* It may produce nausea, vomiting, diarrhoea, changes in mood, skin rashes and loss of hair (alopecia). It damages bone marrow, producing blood disorders. *Precautions:* It should not be used in pregnancy, in patients with an infection, or in patients with severe blood disorders. It should be given with utmost caution to patients with impaired bone-marrow function. *Dose:* Varies according to disorder being treated.

Urantoin ◊ nitrofurantoin.

urea (Aquadrate; Calmurid; carbamide) has been used as an osmotic diuretic. It may cause nausea and vomiting by mouth. Injection into a vein may produce headache, nausea, vomiting, a fall in blood pressure and inflammation at the site of injection. It should not be used in patients with impaired kidney function. It is also used in skin creams to counteract dryness.

Ureaphil ◊ urea.

Uriben ◊ nalidixic acid.

Urisal sachets are used for the relief of cystitis. Each sachet contains the equivalent of 4 g sodium citrate. *Precautions:* It should not be used in pregnancy, heart disease, hypertension or renal disorders.

Urispas ◊ flavoxate.

Urizide ◊ bendrofluazide.

urokinase (Ukidan) is an enzyme used to dissolve blood clots in the body. *Dose:* By injection, varies depending on the condition being treated.

Uromide is used to treat urinary tract infections. Each tablet contains sulphaurea 500 mg and phenazopyridine hydrochloride 50 mg.

Uromitexan ◊ mesna.

Uro-tainer sachets are for preparing solutions to maintain indwelling urinary catheters. They contain sodium chloride 0·9% or chlorhexidine acetate 0·02% or mandelic acid 1% or citric acid 3·23%, light magnesium oxide 0·38%, sodium bicarbonate 0·7%, disodium edetate 0·01% or citric acid 6%, gluconolactone 0·6%, light magnesium carbonate 2·8%, disodium ederate 0·01% in sterile solution.

ursodeoxycholic acid (Destolit) is used to dissolve gallstones. *Adverse effects* and *Precautions* ◊ chenodeoxycholic acid. Diarrhoea occurs less frequently than with chenodeoxycholic acid and liver damage has not been reported. *Dose:* By mouth, 8 to 10 mg per kg body-weight at bedtime or daily in divided doses for up to 2 years.

Ursofalk capsules ◊ ursodeoxycholic acid.

Uticillin ◊ carfecillin.

Utovlan ◊ norethisterone.

uva ursi ◊ bearberry.

Uvicool contains para-aminobenzoic acid.

Uvistat sunscreen ◊ mexenone.

Vadarex Nasal Inhaler contains menthol 225 mg, rectified camphor oil 0·01 ml, cedar wood oil 0·05 ml, pine oil 0·05 ml, camphor 25 mg, creosote 0·02 ml, and methyl salicylate 0·02 ml.

Vadarex Wintergreen Ointment contains sweet birch oil 0·12%, cajuput oil 0·12%, eucalyptus oil 1%, menthol 0·5%, and methyl salicylate 9%.

Vaginyl ◊ metronidazole.

Valda pastilles are used to treat sore throats, coughs and colds. Each pastille contains menthol 3·28 mg, eucalyptol 0·451 mg, thymol 0·016 mg,

terpineol 0·016 mg and guaicacol 0·016 mg.

Valderma Antiseptic Cream contains di-8-hydroxyquinoline *p*-aminosalicylate 0·3% in a water-miscible basis.

Valderma cream is used to treat acne. It contains potassium hydroxyquinoline sulphate 0·2% and chlorocresol 0·2%.

valerian (liquid extract) has been used to treat nervous disorders and as a carminative.

Valium ◊ diazepam.

Vallergan ◊ trimeprazine.

Vallex cough linctus: Each 5 ml contains trimeprazine 2·5 mg, menthol 1·2 mg, phenylpropanolamine 10 mg, guaiphenesin 25 mg, citric acid 65 mg, sodium citrate 200 mg, and ipecacuanha extract 0·015 ml. *Dose:* By mouth, 5 to 10 ml two or three times daily.

Valoid ◊ cyclizine.

Valomel Hand Lotion contains hydrogen peroxide solution 2·5%, chlorocresol 0·25%, benzoin tincture 1%, and glycerol 14%.

Valpeda Foot Balm contains halquinol 0·3%.

Vanamil tablets each contain dried aluminium hydroxide 200 mg, magnesium hydroxide 200 mg, and activated dimethicone 20 mg.

Vancocin ◊ vancomycin.

vancomycin (Vancocin; vancomycin

hydrochloride) is an antibiotic. It is given by intravenous injection to treat serious infections caused by bacteria resistant to other antibiotics and orally for antibiotic-induced colitis. *Adverse effects:* Leakage into the surrounding tissues at the site of injection causes pain and tissue damage. The drug may cause nausea, fever and skin rashes and large doses or prolonged treatment may cause irreversible deafness, particularly in patients with impaired kidney function. *Precautions:* It should not be given to patients with impaired kidney function. *Dose:* By slow, diluted intravenous injection, 500 mg slowly every 6 hours; By mouth, 125 mg every 6 hours.

vanillylnonamide (nonivamide) is used as a rubefacient.

Vanispot cream contains resorcinol 2%, precipitated sulphur 8%, hexachlorophane 0·25%, and titanium dioxide 3%.

Vansil ◊ oxamniquine.

Vapex Inhalant contains menthol 17·5, linalyl acetate 0·468%, eucalyptus oil 4·687%, lavender oil 4·687%, bornyl acetate 0·416%, essential oil of camphor 1·5%, and alcohol (IMS) 70·742%.

Var/vac is a smallpox vaccine.

Varemoid: Each tablet contains hydroxyethylrutosides 100 mg.

Variclene gel contains brilliant green 0·5% and lactic acid 0·5%.

Vascardin ◊ isosorbide dinitrate.

Vaseline: Brands of white and yellow petroleum jelly.

Vaseline Intensive care Anti-dandruff Shampoo contains pyrithione zinc 1% w/w.

Vaseline Medicated Shampoo contains triclosan 0·2%.

Vasocon-A eye drops contain antazoline 0·5% and naphazoline 0·05%.

Vasogen silicone cream contains dimethicone 20%, zinc oxide 7·5% and calamine 1·5%. It is a protective cream.

Vasolastine injection is used to treat disorders of the circulation. It contains enzymes of lipid metabolism 8000 units, tyrosinase 4000 units and amineoxidase 4000 units.

vasopressin (Pitressin) is used to treat and diagnose a disorder known as diabetes insipidus in which the patient cannot concentrate his urine and drinks and passes water excessively. It acts directly on the kidney, producing an anti-diuretic effect.

Vasoxine ◊ methoxamine.

Vaydar Vapour-Rub contains menthol 2·7%, camphor 5·7%, turpentine oil 5%, eucalyptus oil 2·5%, cedar wood oil 0·5%, pine oil 1%, and chloroxylenol 0·1%.

V-Cil-K ◊ phenoxymethylpenicillin.

vecuronium bromide (Norcuron) is a non-depolarizing muscle relaxant used during surgical operations. It has a short to medium duration of action.

See discussion on muscle relaxants in Part Two. *Dose:* By intravenous injection initially 80 to 100 micrograms per kg, then 30 to 50 micrograms per kg according to patient's response.

Vedax-slim is a slimming preparation.

veegum ◊ aluminium magnesium silicate.

VeetO Cream and **Lotion** contain calcium and potassium thioglycollates, in an oil-in-water basis.

Veganin is a mild pain-reliever. Each tablet contains aspirin 250 mg, paracetamol 250 mg and codeine phosphate 9·58 mg. *Dose:* 1 to 2 when required. Maximum 8 in 24 hours.

vegetable lecithin ◊ lecithin.

Velbe ◊ vinblastine.

Velosef ◊ cephradine.

Veno's Adult Formula Cough Mixture: Each 5 ml contains noscapine hydrochloride 8·5 mg and liquid glucose 4·25 g.

Veno's Honey and Lemon Cough Mixture contains in each 5 ml, lemon juice 1 ml, honey 250 mg, ammonium chloride 30 mg, and ipecacuanha liquid extract 0·003 ml.

Veno's Night Time sugar-free syrup contains, in each 5 ml, chlorpheniramine maleate 2 mg and dextromethorphan hydrobromide 3·75 mg ◊ chlorpheniramine and dextromethorphan.

Veno's Original Cough Mixture contains camphor 0·02%, aniseed oil 0·03%, capsicum tincture 0·12%, liquid glucose 63·5%, and molasses 34%.

Ventide metered aerosols contain salbutamol 100 micrograms, and beclomethasone dipropionate 50 micrograms in each dose. **Ventide Rotacaps** contain 400 micrograms and 200 micrograms respectively.

Ventodisks ◊ salbutamol. The disk device has eight blisters on a circular disk. Each blister contains 200 or 400 micrograms of salbutamol powder mixed with powdered lactose. The particle size of the salbutamol is small enough to be breathed into the lungs whereas the powdered lactose is deposited in the mouth and throat. To use the device the patient raises the lid which punctures the blister with a needle and the patient inhales the powdered contents of the blister.

Ventolin ◊ salbutamol.

Vepesid ◊ etoposide.

Veractil ◊ methotrimeprazine.

Veracur gel contains formaldehyde solution 1·5%.

verapamil (Berkatens; Cordilox; Securon; Univer; verapamil hydrochloride) is used to prevent attacks of angina and disorders of heart rhythm. *Adverse effects:* These include nausea, vomiting and allergic reactions. After intravenous injection it may cause blushing and transient heart block if injected rapidly. *Precautions:* It may reduce the blood pressure in patients being treated with antihypertensive drugs, and so a reduction in the dose of antihypertensive drug may be required. It should not be used in acute heart disorders and it should be used with caution in patients with low blood pressure, slow heart rate or partial heart block. *Dose:* By mouth, 40 to 80 mg three times daily. By slow intravenous injection, in doses of 5 mg up to three times daily.

veratrum alkaloids (alkavervir) are a group of drugs obtained from the veratrum plant, that were used to lower raised blood pressure. They should no longer be used for this purpose.

Verdiviton is a multivitamin preparation. Each 5 ml of syrup contains thiamine mononitrate 667 micrograms, riboflavine 334 micrograms, nicotinamide 5 mg, pyridoxine hydrochloride 167 micrograms, cyanocobalamin 5 micrograms, calcium glycerophosphate 36·7 mg, dexpanthenol 334 micrograms, manganese glycerophosphate 3·34 mg, potassium glycerophosphate 6·7 mg, sodium glycerophosphate 26·7 mg.

Vericaps are used for the removal of verrucae on the feet (plantar warts). Each cap contains podophyllin 20% and linseed oil 20%.

Veripaque enema powder for reconstitution contains oxyphenisatin 50 mg in 3 g.

Vermox ◊ mebendazole.

Verrugon contains salicylic acid 50% and glycerol 7%.

Vertactil ◊ methotrimeprazine.

Vertigon capsules contain prochlorperazine 10 mg or 15 mg in sustained-release form. *Dose:* By mouth, 10 to 30 mg daily.

Verucasep gel is used to treat warts. It contains glutaraldehyde 10%.

Vesagex ◊ cetrimide.

Vibramycin ◊ doxycycline.

Vibrocil nasal drops, nasal gel and nasal spray contain dimethindene maleate 0·025%, phenylephrine 0·25%, and neomycin 0·35%.

Vicks Coldcare capsules contain paracetamol 325 mg, dextromethorphan hydrobromide 10 mg and phenylpropanolamine hydrochloride 12·5 mg.

Vicks Cough Calmers lozenges each contain dextromethorphan 4·05 mg and benzocaine 2·4 mg.

Vicks Double-Action Medicated Lozenges each contain menthol 7·04 mg, camphor 0·24 mg, and eucalyptus oil 2·35 mg.

Vicks Expectorant Cough Syrup: Each 5 ml contains guaiphenesin 50 mg, sodium citrate 200 mg, and cetylpyridinium chloride 1·25 mg.

Vicks Inhaler contains menthol 125 mg, camphor 50 mg, methyl salicylate 5 mg, and oil of pine needles 10 mg.

Vicks Lozenges each contain menthol 1·74 mg and vitamin C 3·9 mg; available in menthol, lemon, blackcurrant, and wild cherry flavours.

Vicks Lozenges, Lemon Plus each contain menthol 2·75 mg and vitamin C 100 mg.

Vicks Medinite: Each 30-ml dose contains ephedrine sulphate 8 mg, doxylamine succinate 7·5 mg, paracetamol 600 mg, dextromethorphan hydrobromide 15 mg, and alcohol 19%.

Vicks Sinex Nasal Spray contains oxymetazoline hydrochloride 0·05%, menthol 0·025%, camphor 0·015%, and eucalyptol 0·0075% in a buffered aqueous solution. **Sinex Nose Drops** contain the same active ingredients.

Vicks Vapo-lem is used in the relief of cold and flu symptoms. Each sachet contains paracetamol 500 mg, guaiphenesin 100 mg, phenylephrine 10 mg, vitamin C 50 mg.

Vicks VapoRub contains menthol 2·82%, camphor 5·25%, turpentine oil 4·77%, eucalyptus oil 1·35%, nutmeg oil 0·48%, cedar wood oil 0·45%, thymol 0·1%.

Victory-V lozenges contain gum arabic, liquorice extract, glucose syrup, ether, linseed oil and sugar.

vidarabine is an antiviral drug similar to idoxuridine. It is used to treat herpes zoster. Vira-A is a preparation for use in the eyes.

Vi-Daylin is a multivitamin preparation. Each 5 ml of syrup contains vitamin A 3,000 units (as palmitate), thiamine hydrochloride 1·5 mg, riboflavine 1·2 mg, nicotinamide 10 mg, pyridoxine hydrochloride 1 mg, ascorbic acid 50 mg, ergocalciferol 400 units.

Videne preparations contain povidone-iodine.

Videne dusting-powder ◊ povidone-iodine.

Vidopen ◊ ampicillin.

Vigranon B is a vitamin B complex preparation. Each 5 ml of elixir contains thiamine hydrochloride 5 mg, riboflavine 2 mg, nicotinamide 20 mg, pyridoxine hydrochloride 2 mg, panthenol 3 mg.

Villescon is a tonic containing various B vitamins and a stimulant drug called prolintane. *Dose:* 1 tablet or 10 ml after breakfast and before 4 p.m.

viloxazine (Vivalan; viloxazine hydrochloride) is used as an antidepressant drug. *Adverse effects:* It may produce nausea and loss of appetite. *Precautions:* It may increase the effects of phenytoin and certain drugs used to treat raised blood pressure, e.g. debrisoquine, guanethidine and bethanidine. *Dose:* By mouth, 150 to 300 mg daily in divided doses.

vinblastine (Velbe; vinblastine sulphate) is used as an anti-cancer drug. *Adverse effects:* These include nausea, vomiting, diarrhoea, mood changes, loss of hair (alopecia), nerve damage and convulsions. It damages bone marrow producing blood disorders, and can affect the nerves supplying the bladder (producing retention of urine) and the gut (producing paralysis). Injections may be painful and can produce irritation and phlebitis at the site. *Precautions:* It should not be used in pregnancy or in patients with an infection. It should be given with utmost caution to patients with impaired bone-marrow function. *Dose:* Up to 10 mg weekly by intravenous injection.

vincristine (Oncovin; vincristine sulphate) is used as an anti-cancer drug. *Adverse effects:* These include nausea, vomiting, constipation, mood changes, loss of hair (alopecia), nerve damage and convulsions. It damages bone marrow, producing blood disorders, and can affect the nerves supplying the bladder (producing retention of urine) and the gut (producing paralysis). Injections may be painful and can produce irritation and phlebitis at the site. *Precautions:* It should not be used in pregnancy or in patients with an infection. It should be given with utmost caution to patients with impaired bone-marrow function. It may cause severe constipation and therefore enemas or laxative may be needed. *Dose:* Varies according to disorder being treated.

vindesine (Eldisine) is an anti-cancer drug. *Adverse effects:* Dysphagia, anorexia, nausea, vomiting, constipation, skin rashes, alopecia, blood disorders, malaise, fever, rigors, and nerve damage. *Precautions:* Careful monitoring of the white blood cells and red blood cells is necessary. Careful monitoring of the patient for nerve damage is important and abdominal pain should be treated with great caution since vindesine may produce paralysis of the gut. *Dose:* By intravenous infusion in a dose which varies according to the disorder being treated.

Vine's Anti-Scurf Hair Dressing contains *p*-chloro-*m*-cresol 0·25% sodium alkyl sulphates 0·25%, alkyl aliphatic

esters 8·7%, aliphatic alcohols 4·9%, cholesterol 0·37%, lanosterol 0·3%, sulphur 1·97%, and carbamide 0·98%.

Vioform ◊ clioquinol.

Vioform-Hydrocortisone cream, lotion and **ointment** contain clioquinol 3% and hydrocortisone 1%.

Vira-A ◊ vidarabine.

Virazid powder to make up into an aerosol or nebulizer solution ◊ ribaviran.

Virormone injection ◊ methyltestosterone.

Virormone-Oral ◊ methyltestosterone.

Visclair ◊ methylcysteine.

Vi-Siblin ◊ ispaghula.

Visine Eye Drops contain tetrahydrozoline hydrochloride 0·05% and benzalkonium chloride solution (50%) 0·02%.

Viskaldix is used to treat raised blood pressure. Each tablet contains pindolol 10 mg and dopamide 5 mg.

Visken ◊ pindolol.

Vista-Methasone N nasal drops contain betamethasone sodium phosphate 0·1% and neomycin sulphate 0·5%.

Vita-E ◊ tocopheryl acetate.

Vita-Glucose Tablets contain dextrose with not less than 40 mg ascorbic acid in each 28 g.

Vitamin E suspension ◊ alpha tocopheryl acetate.

Vitaplus Multivitamins tablets: Each contains vitamin A 2,500 units, B_1 1·1 mg, B_2 1·5 mg, B_6 1·0 mg, B_{12} 4·0 micrograms, nicotinamide 17 mg, folic acid 25 micrograms, vitamin C 30 mg, vitamin D 100 units, vitamin E 5 mg.

Vitaplus Multivitamins with Iron tablets: Each contain vitamin A 2,500 units, B_1 1·1 mg, B_2 1·5 mg, B_6 1·0 mg, B_{12} 4·0 micrograms, nicotinamide 17 mg, folic acid 25 micrograms, vitamin C 30 mg, vitamin D 100 units, vitamin E 5 mg, iron, as ferrous fumarate, 15 mg.

Vitathone Chilblain Cream contains methyl nicotinate 1·25%, azulene 0·05%, and dimethicone 3%.

Vitathone Chilblain Tablets: Each contain acetomenaphthone 7 mg and nicotinic acid 25 mg.

Vitavel syrup contains vitamins A, B, C and D, and glucose.

Vitocee Tablets: Each contain vitamin A 750 micrograms, vitamin C 25 mg, and cholecalciferol 5 micrograms.

Vitrite Multi-Vitamin Syrup: Each 5 ml contains vitamin A 2,000 units, cholecalciferol 200 units, vitamin E 1·5 mg, nicotinamide 9 mg, thiamine hydrochloride 0·7 mg, riboflavine 0·85 mg, pyridoxine hydrochloride 0·35 mg, and ascorbic acid 17·5 mg.

Vivalan ◊ viloxazine.

Vocalzone Pastilles contain menthol 1%, peppermint oil 0·5%, myrrh 0·25%, and liquorice extract 1·1%.

Volital ◊ pemoline.

Volmax controlled release tablets of salbutamol ◊ salbutamol.

Voltarol ◊ diclofenac.

Voltarol Retard: Each tablet contains diclofenac sodium 100 mg in a sustained-release form.

Vosene contains thymol 0·1%, resorcinol 0·03%, coal tar solution 3·3%, rosemary oil 0·1%, and biomin (sulphosuccinated undecylenic monoalkylolamide) 2·5%.

Vykmin E: Each capsule contains retinol 2,000 units, cholecalciferol 200 units, vitamin E 100 mg, vitamin B_1 1·2 mg, vitamin B_2 1·8 mg, vitamin B_6 100 micrograms, vitamin B_{12} 1 microgram, vitamin C 40 mg, nicotinamide 12 mg, calcium pantothenate 1 mg, manganese 500 micrograms, potassium 3 mg, zinc 1 mg, iodine 150 micrograms, molybdenum 100 micrograms, iron 15 mg, and calcium phosphate 92·34 mg.

Vykmin Fortified capsules each contains retinol 5,000 units, ergocalciferol 350 units, vitamin B_1 1·2 mg, riboflavine 1·8 mg, vitamin B_6 100 micrograms, vitamin B_{12} 1 microgram, vitamin C 40 mg, vitamin E 2 mg, nicotinamide 12 mg, calcium pantothenate 1 mg, dried ferrous sulphate 51 mg, potassium molybdate 340 micrograms, manganese sulphate 2·2 mg, potassium sulphate 6·68 mg, potassium iodide 200 micrograms, zinc sulphate 4·4 mg, and calcium phosphate 92·34 mg.

warfarin (Marevan; warfarin sodium) is an anticoagulant drug. It is used to stop the blood from clotting and has effects and uses similar to those described under phenindione. *Adverse effects:* Loss of hair (alopecia) and nettle-rash (urticaria) may occur. Early signs of overdosage are bleeding from the gums or elsewhere and red blood cells in the urine. *Precautions:* It should be given with caution to patients with impaired liver or kidney function. It should not be used in the last few months of pregnancy or within three days of childbirth. It should not be used by mothers who are breast feeding their babies or within three days of a surgical operation. Its effects may be increased by aspirin, other salicylates, clofibrate, dextrothyroxine, disulfiram, oxyphenbutazone, phenylbutazone, and possibly by anabolic steroids, antibiotics and quinidine. Its effects are reduced by barbiturates, glutethimide, griseofulvin, and possibly by corticosteroids. *Dose:* By mouth, 30 to 50 mg daily initially reducing to a maintenance dose of 3 to 10 mg daily.

Wartex Ointment contains salicylic acid 50% and glycerol 7%.

Wasp-Eze is an aerosol for insect-bite relief containing mepyramine maleate 0·5% and benzocaine 1%.

Waxaid ear drops contain paradichlorobenzene 2%, chlorbutol 5%, turpentine oil 10%, arachis oil to 100%.

Waxsol ear drops contain dioctyl sodium sulphosuccinate 5%.

Waxwane ear drops contain turpentine oil 15%, terpineol 5%, and chloroxylenol 0·2%, in arachis oil.

Welldorm ◊ dichloralphenazone.

Wellferon (interferon alfa-N_1 (1ns)) is a highly purified blend of natural human alfa-interferons obtained from human lymphoblastoid cells. It is used to treat hairy cell leukaemia. *Adverse effects:* Fever, chills, headache, malaise, painful muscles (flu-like symptoms), loss of appetite, loss of weight, lethargy, weakness, depression, confusion, apathy and coma, seizures, changes in blood pressure, disorders of heart rhythm, blood disorders, nausea, vomiting, diarrhoea, alopecia, raised liver function tests, kidney and liver damage and changes in the chemistry of the blood, skin rashes, pins and needles and numbness in the arms and legs and painful joints. *Precautions:* Use with caution in patients with kidney, heart, liver or nervous disease or mental disturbances. Use with caution in patients with asthma. Do not drive or operate moving machinery. No information available on its safety in breast-feeding and pregnancy. *Dose:* By intramuscular injection, dose varies according to severity of disorder.

wheat-germ oil is a source of vitamin E.

white liniment is a rub containing turpentine oil 25%, ammonium chloride 1·25%, dilute ammonia solution 4·5%, oleic acid 8·5% and water 62·5%.

Whitfield's ointment (benzoic acid compound mixture) ◊ benzoic acid.

Wigglesworth Acne Cream contains resorcinol 0·5%, precipitated sulphur 1%, cetylpyridinium chloride 0·5%, and isopropyl myristate 2%.

Wigglesworth Adults' Bronchial Balsam contains potassium citrate 9·06%, potassium iodide 0·47%, ipecacuanha liquid extract 0·3%, camphorated opium tincture 4·05%, liquorice liquid extract 2·5%, and cetylpyridinium chloride 0·03%.

Wigglesworth Calamine and Mepyramine Lotion is used to treat skin rashes, insect bites and stings. It contains calamine 15%, mepyramine maleate 1% and glycerol 10%.

Wigglesworth Chilblain Ointment contains phenol 1%, camphor 6%, and Peru balsam 2%.

Wigglesworth Children's Cherry Cough Linctus contains in each 5 ml squill liquid extract 0·02 ml, ipecacuanha liquid extract 0·003 ml, wild cherry syrup 0·08 ml, camphor 2 mg, glycerol 0·12 ml, and honey 350 mg.

Wigglesworth Children's Cough Balsam contains potassium citrate 3%, ipecacuanha liquid extract 0·1%, and liquorice liquid extract 2·5%.

Wigglesworth Glycerin Lemon & Honey with Ipecacuanha contains glycerol 12·5%, purified honey 30%, ipecacuanha liquid extract 0·42%, and lemon oil 0·04%.

Wigglesworth Golden Ear Drops contain rectified camphor oil 15%, cineole 7·5%, nutmeg oil 0·4%, terpineol 2%, and arachis oil to 100%.

Wigglesworth Infants' Nasal Drops

contain ephedrine hydrochloride 0·5%.

Wigglesworth Junior Expectorant contains in each 5 ml dextromethorphan hydrobromide 3·75 mg, ephedrine hydrochloride 2·5 mg, phenylephrine hydrochloride 2·5 mg, ipecacuanha liquid extract 0·0037 ml, and sucrose 4·25 g.

Wigglesworth Mentholated Balsam contains purified honey 5·17%, glacial acetic acid 0·86%, liquorice liquid extract 1·29%, formaldehyde solution 0·02%, menthol 0·005%, and syrup 25·86%.

Wigglesworth Rapid Energy Release Tablets each contain caffeine 50 mg, nicotinic acid 5 mg, riboflavine 1 mg, and thiamine hydrochloride 1 mg.

Wigglesworth Syrup of Honey, Glycerin & Blackcurrant with Ipecacuanha contains purified honey 14%, glycerol 5%, blackcurrant syrup 5%, ipecacuanha liquid extract 0·2%, tolu syrup 7·6%, citric acid 0·75%, glacial acetic acid 0·25%, and sucrose 50%.

Wigglesworth Vitamin ACD Tablets each contain vitamin A 4,000 units, vitamin D 550 units, vitamin C 25 mg.

Windcheaters capsules contain activated dimethicone 100 mg for the treatment of wind ◊ dimethicone.

Wintergreen oil (sweet birch oil) has the same effects as methyl salicylate. It is used in liniments and ointments for the relief of pain in rheumatic disorders.

Wintogeno contains capsicin 0·3%,

thymol 0·11%, eucalyptol 0·11%, menthol 2·6%, methyl salicylate 12·2%.

Witch Doctor Gel contains witch hazel liquid extract 81·5%, propylene glycol 7%, and alkoyl diethanolamide 0·75%.

witch hazel (hamamelis water) is used on sprains and bruises as a cooling agent.

Witch Stik is a witch hazel extract containing not less than 65% alcohol.

Woodward's baby cream contains benzalkonium chloride solution 0·02 ml and cetrimide 100 mg.

Woodward's Gripe Water contains dill water, concentrated 3·6%, sodium bicarbonate 1%, ginger tincture 1·25%, rectified spirit 3·67%, and syrup 15%.

Woodward's teething balm: Each 100 ml contains lignocaine base 300 mg, benzyl alcohol 300 mg, myrrh tincture 0·8 ml and menthol 60 mg.

wool alcohols are used as emulsifiers in the preparation of ointments.

wool fat (anhydrous lanolin) is a fatlike substance removed from the wool of sheep. It may produce skin sensitization.

X.89 Geriomar capsules: Each contain parā-aminobenzoic acid 25 mg, haematoporphyrin hydrochloride 250 micrograms, 2-dimethylaminoethanol hydrogen tartrate 15 mg, with traces of minerals and excipients.

Xanax ◊ alprazolam.

xipamide (Diurexan) is a diuretic. *Adverse effects* and *Precautions* ◊ bendrofluazide. *Dose:* By mouth, 20 to 40 mg daily as a single dose in the mornings.

X-Prep mixture is used to evacuate the bowel before radiological examination. It contains sennosides A 142 mg ◊ sennoside A.

Xylocaine ◊ lignocaine.

Xylocard ◊ lignocaine.

Xylodase cream contains lignocaine 50 mg and hyaluronidase 150 micrograms (50 units)/g.

xylometazoline (Otrivine) is used as a nasal decongestant. It is used to treat the common cold. It may rarely cause stinging, dry nose, headache, palpitations and drowsiness and insomnia.

Xyloproct ointment contains aluminium acetate 3·5%, hydrocortisone acetate 0·275%, lignocaine 5%, and zinc oxide 18%. *Dose:* Apply several times daily.

Xyloproct suppositories contain aluminium acetate 50 mg, hydrocortisone acetate 5 mg, lignocaine 60 mg, zinc oxide 400 mg. *Dose:* 1 suppository at night and after defecation.

Xylose-BMS powder is a diagnostic agent used to test absorption from the gut, it contains d-xylose.

Xylotox ◊ lignocaine.

yeast is used as a source of vitamin B. Large doses may cause diarrhoea.

Yeast Pac Medicated contains coal tar solution 0·6%, bentonite 2·3%, precipitated sulphur 3%, zinc oxide 13%, kaolin 36·2%, and dried yeast 1·9%.

Yeast-Vite: Each tablet contains salicylamide 162 mg, caffeine 50 mg, thiamine hydrochloride 167 micrograms, riboflavine 167 micrograms, and nicotinamide 1·5 mg.

Yel/Vac is yellow fever vaccine.

yellow soft paraffin is an emollient and protective agent. It is also known as petroleum jelly. It is a purified semisolid mixture of hydrocarbons obtained from petroleum.

Yestamin tablets are a tonic.

Yomesan ◊ niclosamide.

Yutopar ◊ ritodrine.

Zaditen ◊ ketotifen.

Zadstat ◊ metronidazole.

Zagreb is an antivenom for snake bite. It is used for adder bites, the only indigenous venomous snake in the United Kingdom.

Zam-Buk contains eucalyptus oil 5%, camphor 1·8%, thyme oil 0·5%, colophony 2·5%, and sassafras oil 0·65%.

Zantac ◊ ranitidine.

Zanthine Tablets each contain caffeine 30 mg and dextrose 150 mg.

Zarontin ◊ ethosuximide.

ZeaSORB is a dusting powder containing aldioxa 0·2%, chloroxylenol 0·5%, pulverized maize core 45%.

Zefringe Sachets: Each contains paracetamol 800 mg and caffeine 60 mg in an effervescent basis.

Zenoxene cream contains 1% hydrocortisone ◊ hydrocortisone.

zidovudine (Retrovir) is an antiviral drug used in the treatment of AIDS. *Adverse effects* include damage to the blood-forming tissues in the bone marrow, affecting red blood cell production causing anaemia, and affecting the production of white blood cells. It also causes nausea, vomiting and loss of appetite, headache, abdominal pain, skin rash, fever, painful muscles, pins and needles, and insomnia. *Precautions:* Blood tests should be carried out before and every 2 weeks during the first 3 months of treatment, and then every month after that. It should not be used in patients who are allergic to it, or in patients with very low numbers of white blood cells or with severe anaemia. *Dose:* By mouth, 3·5 mg per kilogram of body weight every 4 hours.

Zinacef ◊ cefuroxime.

zinamide ◊ pyrazinamide.

zinc is an essential element in nutrition and it is a constituent of many enzyme systems. Zinc salts are used topically as mild astringents and may help skin ulcer healing.

zinc acetate is used as an astringent in eye drops.

Zinc amino acid chelate ◊ zinc.

zinc and salicylic acid paste (Lassar's paste) contains zinc oxide 24%, salicylic acid 2%, starch 24% and white soft paraffin 50%. It is used to remove excess skin.

zinc bacitracin ◊ bacitracin.

zinc chloride is used as a caustic and astringent. It is also used as a deodorant and mouth wash.

zinc octoate has similar uses to zinc stearate.

zinc oleostearate ◊ zinc stearate.

zinc omadine ◊ pyrithione zinc.

zinc oxide is used in bandages and skin applications.

zinc pyrithione ◊ pyrithione zinc.

zinc stearate is used as a protective and soothing application alone or in the form of a cream. *Warning:* It should *not* be applied to infants.

zinc sulphate is used as an astringent in skin applications, mouth washes and eye lotions. It has been given by mouth in the treatment of pressure sores. It irritates mucous membranes and may produce inflammation, ulceration and perforation of the stomach.

zinc sulphate lotion contains zinc sulphate 1% and is used for skin ulcers.

zinc undecenoate (zinc undecylenate) is an antifungal drug.

zinc undecylenate ◊ zinc undecenoate.

Zincast Baby Cream contains zinc oxide 7·5%, wool fat 4%, and castor oil 4·5%.

Zincfrin eye drops contain zinc sulphate 0·25% and phenylephrine hydrochloride 0·12%.

Zincold 23 contains zinc gluconate 23 mg and vitamin C 50 mg.

Zincomed capsules contain zinc sulphate 220 mg.

Zincosol ◊ zinc sulphate.

Zinnatt capsules ◊ cefuroxime.

Zoladex depot injection (biodegradable) ◊ goserelin.

Zonulysin: Each injection contains alphachymotrypsin 300 USP unit ◊ chymotrypsin.

Zovirax ◊ acyclovir.

Z Span spansules are sustained-release capsules of zinc sulphate monohydrate 61·8% (equivalent to 22·5 mg of zinc) ◊ zinc sulphate.

Zubes Lemon and Honey Cough Lozenges contain menthol 0·1%, lemon oil 0·22%, citric acid 1·5%, and honey 5%. **Zubes Original** contain anise oil 0·2%, peppermint oil 0·13%, clove oil 0·02%, menthol 0·3%, camphor 0·01%, tolu balsam 0·07%, benzoin 0·07%, capsicum tincture 0·02%, gingerin 0·02%, aqueous extract of horehound (1 in 15), quassia (1 in 48), and coltsfoot leaf (1 in 60) 0·015%, with sucrose and liquid glucose.

Zyloric ◊ allopurinol.

Zymafluor ◊ fluoride.

Drug Interactions

These are some examples of drug interactions. Always check with your pharmacist whether any drugs you are taking may react with others and do not forget that alcohol, tobacco and caffeine (in tea or coffee) are drugs.

Drug affected	Drug interacting	Effect
Adrenaline	Beta-adrenoreceptor blocking drugs	Potentiation of hypertensive effect (increases blood pressure raising effects)
Aldosterone antagonists	Captopril, potassium supplements, trilostane	Hyperkalaemia (raised blood potassium)
Amiloride	Captopril, potassium supplements, trilostane	Hyperkalaemia (raised blood potassium)
Aminoglycosides	Ethacrynic acid, frusemide	Increased ototoxicity (ear damage)
Anaesthetics	Antihypertensive drugs, beta-adrenoreceptor blocking drugs, chlorpromazine	Potentiation of hypotensive effect (increases blood pressure lowering effects)
	Adrenaline, isoprenaline, levodopa	Arrhythmias (disordered heart rhythms) with halothane, cyclopropane, trichloroethylene
Anti-arrhythmic drugs	Any combinations of two or more	Increased myocardial depression (damps down the function of the heart muscle)
Anticholinergic drugs	Amantadine, antidepressants, antihistamines, disopyramide, phenothiazine derivatives	Increased side-effects, dry mouth, urine retention, confusional states, etc.

Drug affected	Drug interacting	Effect
Anti-diabetic drugs (oral and insulin)	Alcohol, beta-adrenoreceptor blocking drugs, monoamine-oxidase inhibitors	Potentiation (increases the blood sugar lowering effects)
	Corticosteroids, corticotrophin, diazoxide, diuretics, bumetanide, frusemide, thiazides, oral contraceptives	Antagonism (works against the blood sugar lowering effects)
Anti-epileptics	Antidepressants, phenothiazine derivatives	Antagonism (works against the anti-convulsant effects)
Antihypertensive drugs (drugs used to treat raised blood pressure)	Anti-inflammatory analgesics, such as indomethacin, phenylbutazone; carbenoxolone, corticosteroids, corticotrophin, oestrogens, oral contraceptives	Reduced blood pressure lowering effects
	Alcohol, antidepressants, hypnotics, sedatives, tranquillizers, fenfluramine, levodopa, vasodilators such as nitrates, nifedipine, verapamil	Potentiation (increases blood pressure lowering effects)
Aspirin	Metoclopramide	Potentiation (increases effects)
Azathioprine	Allopurinol	Potentiation-increased toxicity (increased effects leading to increased adverse effects)
Beta-adrenoreceptor blocking drugs	Ergotamine	Peripheral vasoconstriction (produces closing down of blood vessels in hands and feet – cold extremities)
	Indomethacin	Antagonism of antihypertensive effect (works against blood pressure lowering effects)

Drug affected	Drug interacting	Effect
	Nifedipine	Severe hypotension (drop in blood pressure) and heart failure occasionally
	Prenylamine	Increased myocardial depression (damps down the function of the heart muscle)
	Sympathomimetic amines such as adrenaline, amphetamines, phenylephrine	Severe hypertension (raised blood pressure) reported
Betahistine	Antihistamines	Antagonism (works against the desired effects)
Bethanidine	Sympathomimetic amines (including some common cold remedies); mazindol, pizotifen, tricyclic antidepressants	Antagonism (works against the desired effects)
Bumetanide	Acetazolamide, carbenoxolone, corticosteroids, corticotrophin	Hypokalaemia (low blood potassium)
Captopril	Potassium supplements, potassium sparing diuretics	Hyperkalaemia (raised blood potassium)
Carbamazepine	Cimetidine, dextropropoxyphene, isoniazid	Potentiation (increased effects)
Carbenoxolone	Amiloride, spironolactone	Inhibition of ulcer healing
Cephaloridine	Ethacrynic acid, frusemide, gentamicin	Increased nephrotoxicity (kidney damage)
Cephalosporins	Ethacrynic acid, frusemide, gentamicin	Increased nephrotoxicity (kidney damage)
Cephalothin	Ethacrynic acid, frusemide, gentamicin	Increased nephrotoxicity (kidney damage)
Cephamandole	Alcohol	'Antabuse' reaction (see antabuse)

Drug affected	Drug interacting	Effect
Chloramphenicol	Phenobarbitone	Reduced plasma concentrations (reduced blood levels, therefore less effective)
Chlordiazepoxide	Cimetidine, disulfiram	Potentiation because of decreased hepatic metabolism (increased effects because of decreased breakdown by the liver)
Chlormethiazole	Cimetidine	Potentiation (increased effect)
Chlorpromazine	Antacids	Reduced absorption from the gut, therefore less effective in normal doses
Chlorpropamide	Bezafibrate, chloramphenicol, clofibrate, co-trimoxazole, oxyphenbutazone, phenylbutazone, sulphinpyrazone	Potentiation (increased effects)
	Alcohol	Flushing in susceptible patients
	Rifampicin	Reduced effect
Cimetidine	Antacids	Reduced absorption from the gut, therefore less effective in normal doses
Clonidine	Beta-adrenoreceptor blocking drugs	Increased risk of clonidine withdrawal hypertension
	Tricyclic antidepressants	Antagonism (works against the desired effects)
Corticosteroids	Carbenoxolone, diuretics, bumetanide, ethacrynic acid, frusemide, thiazides	Increased potassium loss (in the urine)

Drug affected	Drug interacting	Effect
Corticotrophin	Carbenoxolone, diuretics, bumetanide, ethacrynic acid, frusemide, thiazides	Increased potassium loss (in the urine)
Cortisone	Barbiturates, carbamazepine, phenytoin, primidone, rifampicin	Reduced effect
Cyclosporin	Ketoconazole	Increased plasma (blood levels) concentrations of cyclosporin, therefore increased risk of adverse effects
Dapsone	Probenecid	Reduced excretion (via the kidneys), increased adverse effects
Debrisoquine	Sympathomimetic amines (including some common cold remedies), mazindol, pizotifen, tricyclic antidepressants	Antagonism (works against the desired effects)
Dexamethasone	Barbiturates, carbamazepine, phenytoin, primidone, rifampicin	Reduced effect
	Aminoglutethimide	Reduced effect
Diazepam	Cimetidine, disulfiram	Potentiation because of decreased hepatic metabolism (increased effects because of reduced breakdown in the liver)
Diflunisal	Antacids	Reduced absorption from the gut, therefore less effective in normal doses
Digoxin	Amiodarone, quinidine	Potentiation (increased effects). Halve maintenance dose of digoxin

Drug affected	Drug interacting	Effect
	Nifedipine, verapamil	Potentiation may occur (increased effects)
Digoxin and other cardiac glycosides	Carbenoxolone, diuretics, bumetanide, ethacrynic acid, frusemide, thiazides	Increased toxicity
	Cholestyramine, colestipol	Reduced absorption from the gut, therefore less effective in normal doses
	Phenobarbitone, rifampicin	Inhibition (digitoxin only), blocks its actions
Disopyramide	Diuretics, bumetanide, ethacrynic acid, frusemide, thiazides	Toxicity increased by hypokalaemia (low blood potassium)
	Amiodarone	Increased risk of ventricular arrhythmias (serious disorders of heart rhythm)
Diuretics	Anti-inflammatory analgesics, such as indomethacin; carbenoxolone, corticosteroids, corticotrophin, oestrogens	Antagonism (works against the desired effects)
Doxycycline	Barbiturates, carbamazepine, phenytoin	Reduced plasma concentrations (blood levels) leading to reduced effectiveness
Drugs for Parkinsonism	Haloperidol, phenothiazine derivatives, methyldopa, metirosine, metoclopramide, reserpine, tetrabenazine	These have extra-pyramidal side-effects (Parkinsonism-like)
Ethosuximide	Carbamazepine	Reduced plasma concentrations (blood levels) leading to reduced effectiveness of ethosuximide, therefore less effective.

Drug affected	Drug interacting	Effect
	Phenytoin, sodium valproate	Increased plasma concentrations of ethosuximide, therefore more risk of adverse effects
Frusemide	Acetazolamide, carbenoxolone, corticosteroids, corticotrophin	Hypokalaemia (low blood potassium)
Gentamicin	Ethacrynic acid, frusemide	Increased ototoxicity (ear damage)
Griseofulvin	Phenobarbitone	Antagonism (works against the desired effects)
Guanethidine	Sympathomimetic amines (including some cold remedies), mazindol, pizotifen, tricyclic antidepressants	Antagonism (works against the desired effects)
Haloperidol	Metoclopramide	Increased risk of extra-pyramidal effects (Parkinsonism-like)
Heparin	Aspirin, dipyridamole	Potentiation (increases the effects)
Hydrocortisone	Barbiturates, carbamazepine, phenytoin, primidone, rifampicin	Reduced effect
Hypnotics and sedatives	Alcohol, antidepressants, antihistamines, narcotic analgesics	Potentiation (increases the effects)
Indapamide	Carbenoxolone, diuretics, bumetanide, frusemide, thiazides, xipamide	Hypokalaemia (low blood potassium)
Indomethacin	Probenecid	Increased plasma (blood levels) concentrations, therefore more risk of adverse effects
Ketoconazole	Antacids, anticholinergic drugs, cimetidine	Decreased absorption, therefore less effective in normal doses

Drug affected	Drug interacting	Effect
Ketoprofen	Probenecid	Increased plasma concentrations (blood levels) therefore more risk of adverse effects
Labetalol	Cimetidine	Potentiation possible because of reduced metabolism (increased effects because of reduced breakdown)
Latamoxef	Alcohol	'Antabuse' reaction (see antabuse)
Levodopa	Chlordiazepoxide, diazepam	Antagonism, occasionally (works against the desired effects)
	Metoclopramide	Increased plasma (blood levels), concentrations of levodopa, therefore more risk of adverse effects
	Pyridoxine	Antagonism (works against the desired effects). Does not occur if dopa decarboxylase inhibitor also given
Lignocaine	Diuretics, bumetanide, ethacrynic acid, frusemide, thiazides	Antagonized by hypokalaemia (effects reduced by low blood potassium)
	Propranolol	Increased risk of lignocaine toxicity
Lincomycin	Kaolin mixtures	Reduced absorption from the gut, therefore less effective in normal doses
Lithium	Diuretics, sodium depletion; diclofenac, indomethacin, phenylbutazone	Potentiation (increases the effects)

Drug affected	Drug interacting	Effect
	Acetazolamide, aminophylline, sodium bicarbonate	Increased lithium excretion by the kidneys, therefore reduced effects
	Haloperidol	Increased risk of extra-pyramidal effects (Parkinsonism-like)
Mercaptopurine	Allopurinol	Potentiation- increased toxicity (increased effects leading to increase in adverse effects)
Metformin	Alcohol	Increased risk of lactic acidosis
Methotrexate	Aspirin, phenylbutazone, probenecid	Delayed excretion by the kidneys (increased risk of adverse effects)
	Anti-epileptics, co-trimoxazole, pyrimethamine	Increased anti-folate effect leading to anaemia
Metirosine	Haloperidol, metoclopramide, phenothiazine derivatives	Increased risk of extra-pyramidal effects (Parkinsonism-like)
Metoclopramide	Anticholinergic drugs such as atropine, benzhexol, propantheline; narcotic analgesics	Antagonism – they have opposing effects on gastro-intestinal activity – they work against each other on the stomach nerves
Metronidazole	Alcohol	'Antabuse' reaction (see antabuse)
Mexiletine	Diuretics, bumetanide, ethacrynic acid, frusemide, thiazides	Antagonized by hypokalaemia (made worse by low blood potassium)
	Atropine, narcotic analgesics	Delayed absorption from the gut, therefore less effective in normal doses

Drug affected	Drug interacting	Effect
	Acetazolamide, antacids	Reduced excretion (by kidneys) in alkaline urine may increase plasma concentrations (blood levels) (leading to increased risk of adverse effects)
Monoamine oxidase inhibitors	Sympathomimetic amines such as amphetamines, common cold remedies, ephedrine, fencamfamin, fenfluramine, levodopa, oxypertine, pemoline	Hypertensive crisis (a sudden and severe rise in blood pressure). NB. can occur up to two weeks after stopping M.A.O.I.
	Narcotic analgesics, reserpine, tetrabenazine, tricyclic antidepressants, zimeldine	CNS excitation, hypertension (the brain is stimulated and the blood pressure rises)
	Tryptophan	CNS excitation (the brain is stimulated). Reduce dose of tryptophan
Monosulfiram	Alcohol	'Antabuse' reaction (see antabuse)
Muscle relaxants	Colistin, polymyxin B, lithium, propranolol, quinidine	Potentiation (increased effects)
Nalidixic acid	Probenecid	Reduced excretion by kidneys, increased adverse effects
Naproxen	Probenecid	Increased plasma (blood levels) concentrations leading to risk of increased adverse effects
Nitrofurantoin	Probenecid	Reduced excretion (by the kidneys), increased adverse effects

Drug affected	Drug interacting	Effect
Noradrenaline	Beta-adrenoreceptor blocking drugs	Potentiation of hypertensive effect, (increase of blood pressure raising effects)
Oral anticoagulants. Coumarins such as warfarin	Aminoglutethimide, barbiturates, carbamazepine, dichloralphenazone, glutethimide, griseofulvin, oral contraceptives, primidone, rifampicin, vitamin K	Inhibition (blocks the desired effects)
	Alcohol, amiodarone, anabolic steroids, aspirin, azapropazone, bezafibrate, cephamandole, chloral hydrate, chloramphenicol, cimetidine, clofibrate, co-trimoxazole, danazol, dextrothyroxine, dipyridamole, latamoxef, metronidazole, miconazole, neomycin, oxyphenbutazone, phenylbutazone, sulphinpyrazone, sulphonamides, thyroxine	Potentiation (increases the effects)
	Allopurinol, diflunisal, feprazone, flurbiprofen, mefenamic acid, piroxicam, sulindac and possibly other anti-inflammatory analgesics, cholestyramine, dextropropoxyphene, indomethacin, nalidixic acid, paracetamol (regular treatment or high doses), phenytoin, tetracyclines	Potentiation may occur (increases the effects)
Oral contraceptives	Barbiturates, carbamazepine, dichloralphenazone, phenytoin, primidone, rifampicin	Reduced effect
	Oral antibiotics, such as ampicillin, tetracycline	Reduced effect, risk probably small

Drug affected	Drug interacting	Effect
Oral iron	Magnesium trisilicate; tetracyclines	Reduced absorption from the gut, therefore less effective in normal doses
Paracetamol	Cholestyramine	Reduced absorption from the gut, therefore less effective in normal doses
	Metoclopramide	Potentiation (increased effects)
Penicillamine	Oral iron, zinc sulphate	Reduced absorption from the gut, therefore less effective in normal doses
Phenindione	Oral contraceptives, vitamin K	Inhibition (blocks the desired effects)
	Anabolic steroids, aspirin, bezafibrate, cholestyramine, clofibrate, dipyridamole, neomycin, thyroxine	Potentiation (increases the effects)
Phenobarbitone	Phenytoin, sodium valproate	Increased sedation (drowsiness)
Phenothiazine derivatives	Metoclopramide	Increased risk of extra-pyramidal effects (Parkinsonism-like)
Phenoxymethyl penicillin	Neomycin	Reduced absorption from the gut, therefore less effective in normal doses
Phenylbutazone	Cholestyramine	Reduced absorption from the gut, therefore less effective in normal doses
Phenytoin	Azapropazone, chloramphenicol, cimetidine, co-trimoxazole, diazepam,	Potentiation (increased effects)

Drug affected	Drug interacting	Effect
	disulfiram, isoniazid, phenylbutazone, sulphinpyrazone, sulthiame, viloxazine	
	Aspirin, sodium valproate	Transient potentiation (increased effects)
Pivampicillin	Antacids	Reduced absorption from the gut, therefore less effective in normal doses
Prednisolone	Barbiturates, carbamazepine, phenytoin, primidone, rifampicin	Reduced effect
Prednisone	Barbiturates, carbamazepine, phenytoin, primidone, rifampicin	Reduced effect
Primidone	Phenytoin, sodium valproate	Increased sedation (drowsiness)
Probenecid	Aspirin	Inhibition (blocks the desired effects)
Procarbazine	Alcohol	'Antabuse' reaction (see antabuse)
Propranolol	Cimetidine	Potentiation because of decreased hepatic metabolism (increases effects because of reduced breakdown in the liver)
Quinidine	Diuretics, bumetamide, ethacrynic acid, frusemide, thiazides	Toxicity increased by hypokalaemia (low blood potassium)
	Amiodarone	Increased risk of ventricular arrhythmias (serious disorders of the heart rhythm)
Sodium valproate	Carbamazepine, phenobarbitone, phenytoin, primidone	Reduced plasma (blood levels) concentrations of valproate, therefore less effective

Drug affected	Drug interacting	Effect
Sulphinpyrazone	Aspirin	Inhibition (blocks the desired effects)
	Pyrazinamide	Antagonism (works against the desired effects)
Sulphonylureas	Bezafibrate, chloramphenicol, clofibrate, co-trimoxazole, oxyphenbutazone, phenylbutazone, sulphinpyrazone	Potentiation (increased effects)
Suxamethonium	Cyclophosphamide, ecothiopate eye drops, neostigmine, propanolol, thiotepa	Potentiation (increased effects)
	Digoxin	Arrhythmias (disorders of heart rhythm)
Tetrabenazine	Metoclopramide	Increased risk of extra-pyramidal effects (Parkinsonism-like)
Tetracyclines	Antacids, dairy products, oral iron, sucralfate, zinc sulphate	Reduced absorption from the gut, therefore less effective in normal doses
Theophylline	Cimetidine, erythromycin, influenza vaccine, oral contraceptives	Potentiation (increased effects)
Thiazides	Acetazolamide, carbenoxolone, corticosteroids, corticotrophin	Hypokalaemia (low blood potassium)
Thiopentone	Sulphonamides	Potentiation (increased effects)
Thyroxine	Cholestyramine	Reduced absorption from the gut, therefore reduced effects in normal doses
	Fenclofenac, phenylbutazone, phenytoin	False low total plasma-thyroxine

Drug affected	Drug interacting	Effect
		concentration, may lead doctors to increase dose
Tocainide	Diuretics, bumetanide, ethacrynic acid, frusemide, thiazides	Antagonized by hypokalaemia (effects worked against by low blood potassium)
Tolbutamide	Bezafibrate, chloramphenicol, clofibrate, co-trimoxazole, oxyphenbutazone, phenylbutazone, sulphinpyrazone	Potentiation (increased effects)
	Rifampicin	Reduced effect
Triamterene	Captopril, potassium supplements, trilostane	Hyperkalaemia (high blood potassium)
	Indomethacin	Decreased kidney function reported
Tricyclic antidepressants	Alcohol	Potentiation (increased effects) of sedative effect
	Oral contraceptives	Reduced effect
	Phenothiazines	Increased adverse effects
Tubocurarine	Aminoglycosides, clindamycin, lincomycin, magnesium salts	Potentiation (increased effects)
Vancomycin	Cholestyramine	Antagonism (works against the antibacterial effects)
Vasoconstrictors	Tricyclic antidepressants	Potentiation (increased effects)
Verapamil	Beta-adrenoreceptor blocking drugs	Asystole (heart stops beating) hypotension (low blood pressure)

Index

FOR THE BEST IN PAPERBACKS, LOOK FOR THE

In every corner of the world, on every subject under the sun, Penguin represents quality and variety – the very best in publishing today.

For complete information about books available from Penguin – including Pelicans, Puffins, Peregrines and Penguin Classics – and how to order them, write to us at the appropriate address below. Please note that for copyright reasons the selection of books varies from country to country.

In the United Kingdom: Please write to *Dept E.P., Penguin Books Ltd, Harmondsworth, Middlesex, UB7 0DA*

In the United States: Please write to *Dept BA, Penguin, 299 Murray Hill Parkway, East Rutherford, New Jersey 07073*

In Canada: Please write to *Penguin Books Canada Ltd, 2801 John Street, Markham, Ontario L3R 1B4*

In Australia: Please write to the *Marketing Department, Penguin Books Australia Ltd, P.O. Box 257, Ringwood, Victoria 3134*

In New Zealand: Please write to the *Marketing Department, Penguin Books (NZ) Ltd, Private Bag, Takapuna, Auckland 9*

In India: Please write to *Penguin Overseas Ltd, 706 Eros Apartments, 56 Nehru Place, New Delhi, 110019*

In Holland: Please write to *Penguin Books Nederland B.V., Postbus 195, NL–1380AD Weesp, Netherlands*

In Germany: Please write to *Penguin Books Ltd, Friedrichstrasse 10–12, D–6000 Frankfurt Main 1, Federal Republic of Germany*

In Spain: Please write to *Longman Penguin España, Calle San Nicolas 15, E–28013 Madrid, Spain*

In France: Please write to *Penguin Books Ltd, 39 Rue de Montmorency, F–75003, Paris, France*

In Japan: Please write to *Longman Penguin Japan Co Ltd, Yamaguchi Building, 2–12–9 Kanda Jimbocho, Chiyoda-Ku, Tokyo 101, Japan*

The Beginner's Cookery Book Betty Falk

Revised and updated, this book is for aspiring cooks of all ages who want to make appetizing and interesting meals without too much fuss. With an emphasis on healthy eating, this is the ideal starting point for would-be cooks.

The Pleasure of Vegetables Elisabeth Ayrton

'Every dish in this beautifully written book seems possible to make and gorgeous to eat' – *Good Housekeeping*

French Provincial Cooking Elizabeth David

'One could cook for a lifetime on this book alone' – *Observer*

Jane Grigson's Fruit Book

Fruit is colourful, refreshing and life-enhancing; this book shows how it can also be absolutely delicious in meringues or compotes, soups or pies.

A Taste of American Food Clare Walker

Far from being just a junk food culture, American cuisine is the most diverse in the world. Swedish, Jewish, Creole and countless other kinds of food have been adapted to the new environment; this book gives some of the most delicious recipes.

Leaves from Our Tuscan Kitchen Janet Ross and Michael Waterfield

A revised and updated version of a great cookery classic, this splendid book contains some of the most unusual and tasty vegetable recipes in the world.

FOR THE BEST IN PAPERBACKS, LOOK FOR THE 🐧

COOKERY IN PENGUINS

Simple French Food   Richard Olney

'There is no other book about food that is anything like it . . . essential and exciting reading for cooks, of course, but it is also a book for eaters . . . its pages brim over with invention' – Paul Levy in the *Observer*

The Vegetarian Epicure   Anna Thomas

Mouthwatering recipes for soups, breads, vegetable dishes, salads and desserts that any meat-eater or vegetarian will find hard to resist.

A Book of Latin American Cooking   Elisabeth Lambert Ortiz

Anyone who thinks Latin American food offers nothing but *tacos* and *tortillas* will enjoy the subtle marriages of texture and flavour celebrated in this marvellous guide to one of the world's most colourful *cuisines*.

Quick Cook   Beryl Downing

For victims of the twentieth century, this book provides some astonishing gourmet meals – all cooked in under thirty minutes.

Josceline Dimbleby's Book of Puddings, Desserts and Savouries

'Full of the most delicious and novel ideas for every type of pudding' – *Lady*

Chinese Food   Kenneth Lo

A popular step-by-step guide to the whole range of delights offered by Chinese cookery and the fascinating philosophy behind it.

FOR THE BEST IN PAPERBACKS, LOOK FOR THE

COOKERY IN PENGUINS

Fast Food for Vegetarians   Janette Marshall

Packed with ideas for healthy, delicious dishes from Caribbean vegetables to rose-water baklava, this stimulating book proves that fast food does not have to mean junk food.

More Easy Cooking for One or Two   Louise Davies

This charming book, full of ideas and easy recipes, offers even the novice cook good wholesome food with the minimum of effort.

The Cuisine of the Rose   Mireille Johnston

Classic French cooking from Burgundy and Lyonnais, including the most succulent dishes of meat and fish bathed in pungent sauces of wine and herbs.

Good Food from Your Freezer   Helge Rubinstein and Sheila Bush

Using a freezer saves endless time and trouble and cuts your food bills dramatically; this book will enable you to cook just as well – perhaps even better – with a freezer as without.

Roy Ackerman's Recipe Collection

Here is a treasure-trove of recipes that have been created by some of the top chefs in the very best restaurants in the British Isles. Handwritten and beautifully illustrated, it is a stunning selection of their favourite dishes, gathered together to recreate memories of a special experience.

Budget Gourmet   Geraldene Holt

Plan carefully, shop wisely and cook well to produce first-rate food at minimal expense. It's as easy as pie!

FOR THE BEST IN PAPERBACKS, LOOK FOR THE

THE PENGUIN COOKERY LIBRARY – A SELECTION

The Foods and Wines of Spain   Penelope Casas

'I have not come across a book before that captures so well the unlikely medieval mix of Eastern and Northern, earthy and fine, rare and deeply familiar ingredients that make up the Spanish kitchen' – *Harpers and Queen*. 'The definitive book on Spanish cooking . . . a jewel in the crown of culinary literature' – Craig Claiborne

An Omelette and a Glass of Wine   Elizabeth David

'She has the intelligence, subtlety, sensuality, courage and creative force of the true artist' – *Wine and Food* 'Her pieces are so entertaining, so original, often witty, critical yet lavish with their praise, that they succeed in enthusing even the most jaded palate' – Arabella Boxer in *Vogue*

English Food   Jane Grigson

'Jane Grigson is perhaps the most serious and discriminating of her generation of cookery writers, and *English Food* is an anthology all who follow her recipes will want to buy for themselves as well as for friends who may wish to know about *real* English food . . . enticing from page to page' – Pamela Vandyke Price in the *Spectator*

Mediterranean Seafood   Alan Davidson

'Mr Davidson has a gift for conveying memorable information in a way so effortless that his book makes lively reading for its own sake' – Elizabeth David. 'The best book ever written on this, or possibly any other subject' – Auberon Waugh

Classic Cheese Cookery   Peter Graham

Delicious, mouthwatering soups, starters, main meals and desserts using cheeses from throughout Europe make this tempting cookery book a must for everyone with an interest in the subject. Clear, informative and comprehensive, it is a book to return to again and again.

PENGUIN HEALTH

Acupuncture for Everyone   Dr Ruth Lever

An examination of one of the world's oldest known therapies used by the Chinese for over two thousand years.

Aromatherapy for Everyone   Robert Tisserand

The use of aromatic oils in massage can relieve many ailments and alleviate stress and related symptoms.

Chiropractic for Everyone   Anthea Courtenay

Back pain is both extremely common and notoriously difficult to treat. Chiropractic offers a holistic solution to many of the causes through manipulation of the spine.

Herbal Medicine for Everyone   Michael McIntyre

An account of the way in which the modern herbalist works and a discussion of the wide-ranging uses of herbal medicine.

Homoeopathy for Everyone   Drs Sheila and Robin Gibson

The authors discuss the ways in which this system of administering drugs – by exciting similar symptoms in the patient – can help a range of disorders from allergies to rheumatism.

Hypnotherapy for Everyone   Dr Ruth Lever

This book demonstrates that hypnotherapy is a real alternative to conventional healing methods in many ailments.

Osteopathy for Everyone   Paul Masters

By helping to restore structural integrity and function, the osteopath gives the whole body an opportunity to achieve health and harmony and eliminate ailments from migraines to stomach troubles.

Spiritual and Lay Healing   Philippa Pullar

An invaluable new survey of the history of healing that sets out to separate the myths from the realities.

FOR THE BEST IN PAPERBACKS, LOOK FOR THE 🐧

PENGUIN HEALTH

Audrey Eyton's F-Plus   Audrey Eyton

'Your short cut to the most sensational diet of the century' – *Daily Express*

Baby and Child   Penelope Leach

A beautifully illustrated and comprehensive handbook on the first five years of life. 'It stands head and shoulders above anything else available at the moment' – Mary Kenny in the *Spectator*

Woman's Experience of Sex   Sheila Kitzinger

Fully illustrated with photographs and line drawings, this book explores the riches of women's sexuality at every stage of life. 'A book which any mother could confidently pass on to her daughter – and her partner too' – *Sunday Times*

Food Additives   Erik Millstone

Eat, drink and be worried? Erik Millstone's hard-hitting book contains powerful evidence about the massive risks being taken with the health of the consumer. It takes the lid off the food we have and the food industry.

Living with Allergies   Dr John McKenzie

At least 20% of the population suffer from an allergic disorder at some point in their lives and this invaluable book provides accurate and up-to-date information about the condition, where to go for help, diagnosis and cure – and what we can do to help ourselves.

Living with Stress   Cary L. Cooper, Rachel D. Cooper and Lynn H. Eaker

Stress leads to more stress, and the authors of this helpful book show why low levels of stress are desirable and how best we can achieve them in today's world. Looking at those most vulnerable, they demonstrate ways of breaking the vicious circle that can ruin lives.

FOR THE BEST IN PAPERBACKS, LOOK FOR THE

PENGUIN HEALTH

The Prime of Your Life   Dr Miriam Stoppard

The first comprehensive, fully illustrated guide to healthy living for people aged fifty and beyond, by top medical writer and media personality, Dr Miriam Stoppard.

A Good Start   Louise Graham

Factual and practical, full of tips on providing a healthy and balanced diet for young children, *A Good Start* is essential reading for all parents.

How to Get Off Drugs   Ira Mothner and Alan Weitz

This book is a vital contribution towards combating drug addiction in Britain in the eighties. For drug abusers, their families and their friends.

Naturebirth   Danaë Brook

A pioneering work which includes suggestions on diet and health, exercises and many tips on the 'natural' way to prepare for giving birth in a joyful relaxed way.

Pregnancy   Dr Jonathan Scher and Carol Dix

Containing the most up-to-date information on pregnancy – the effects of stress, sexual intercourse, drugs, diet, late maternity and genetic disorders – this book is an invaluable and reassuring guide for prospective parents.

Care of the Dying   Richard Lamerton

It is never true that 'nothing more can be done' for the dying. This book shows us how to face death without pain, with humanity, with dignity and in peace.